PEDIATRIC NEUROPSYCHOLOGY

THE SCIENCE AND PRACTICE OF NEUROPSYCHOLOGY
A Guilford Series

Robert A. Bornstein, *Series Editor*

Pediatric Neuropsychology: Research, Theory, and Practice
Keith Owen Yeates, M. Douglas Ris, and H. Gerry Taylor, Editors

The Human Frontal Lobes: Functions and Disorders
Bruce L. Miller and Jeffrey L. Cummings, Editors

PEDIATRIC NEUROPSYCHOLOGY

Research, Theory, and Practice

Edited by

Keith Owen Yeates
M. Douglas Ris
H. Gerry Taylor

Foreword by Arthur Benton

THE GUILFORD PRESS
New York   London

© 2000 The Guilford Press
A Division of Guilford Publications, Inc.
72 Spring Street, New York, NY 10012
www.guilford.com

Printed in the United States of America

This book is printed on acid-free paper.

Last digit is print number: 9 8 7 6 5 4 3 2

Library of Congress Cataloging-in-Publication Data

Pediatric neuropsychology : research, theory, and practice / edited by
Keith Owen Yeates, M. Douglas Ris, H. Gerry Taylor ; foreword by
Arthur Benton.
       p.   cm. (The science and practice of neuropsychology)
    Includes bibliographical references and index.
    ISBN 1-57230-507-X
    1. Pediatric neuropsychology.   I. Yeates, Keith Owen.   II. Ris, M. Douglas.
III. Taylor, H. Gerry.   IV. Series.
    [DNLM: 1. Nervous System Diseases—Adolescence. 2. Nervous System
Diseases—Child. 3. Nervous System Diseases—Infant. 4. Neuropsychology—
Adolescence. 5. Neuropsychology—Child. 6. Neuropsychology—Infant.
WS 340 P37137 1999]
RJ486.5 .P435   1999
618.92′8—dc21
                                                    99-049880

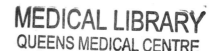

To my wife, Nan, and my daughters, Kiernan and Taylor—
you make it all worthwhile.

—K. O. Y.

To my sons, Geoff, Greg, and Andrew—lenses that focus my life
and provide clarity of purpose.

—M. D. R.

To Kay, Nat, and Jake—my home base.

—H. G. T.

ABOUT THE EDITORS

Keith Owen Yeates, PhD, ABPP-CN, is an associate professor in the Department of Pediatrics at The Ohio State University College of Medicine and Public Health. He also directs the Pediatric Neuropsychology Program and the Postdoctoral Program in Pediatric Neuropsychology at Columbus Children's Hospital. Dr. Yeates currently serves as Vice President of the Association of Postdoctoral Programs in Clinical Neuropsychology. He sits on several editorial boards and is actively involved in grant-funded research on the neurobehavioral outcomes associated with closed-head injury and with spina bifida and hydrocephalus. He is especially interested in the effects of these childhood brain disorders on memory functioning.

M. Douglas Ris, PhD, ABPP-CN, is an associate professor in the Department of Pediatrics at the University of Cincinnati College of Medicine, and holds a joint appointment in the Psychology Department at the University of Cincinnati. Dr. Ris established and directs both the Neuropsychology Program and the Pediatric Neuropsychology Postdoctoral Program at Cincinnati Children's Hospital Medical Center. He has served as Vice President of the Association of Postdoctoral Programs in Clinical Neuropsychology, and currently serves on the Board of Directors of the American Board of Clinical Neuropsychology. He maintains active research programs on the neurobehavioral effects of pediatric brain tumors, sickle cell disease, and environmental lead.

H. Gerry Taylor, PhD, ABPP-CN, is a professor in the Department of Pediatrics at Case Western Reserve University School of Medicine. He holds joint appointments in the Departments of Psychology and Psychiatry. He is also a neuropsychologist in the Division of Behavioral Pediatrics and Psychology at Rainbow Babies and Children's Hospital in Cleveland, Ohio. Dr. Taylor currently serves as Secretary of the American Academy of Clinical Neuropsychology. He has been active on several editorial boards, and has served as a grant reviewer for federal funding agencies. He has received research grants to study the consequences of high-risk conditions arising in infancy and early childhood, including meningitis, leukemia, closed-head injury, and low birthweight. His research interests also encompass methods of assessment and early identification of learning disabilities.

CONTRIBUTORS

Vicki A. Anderson, PhD, Department of Psychology, University of Melbourne, Parkville, Victoria, Australia

Elizabeth H. Aylward, PhD, Department of Radiology, University of Washington, Seattle, Washington

Michael Balthazor, PhD, Department of Psychology, Child Development Center, The Hospital for Sick Children, Toronto, Ontario, Canada

Ida Sue Baron, PhD, ABPP-CN, Independent Practice, Potomac, Maryland

Bruce G. Bender, PhD, Department of Pediatrics, National Jewish Medical and Research Center, Denver, Colorado

Daniel B. Berch, PhD, Office of Educational Research and Improvement, U.S. Department of Education, Washington, DC

Jane Holmes Bernstein, PhD, Department of Psychiatry, Harvard Medical School, Boston, Massachusetts; Neuropsychology Program, Department of Psychiatry, Children's Hospital, Boston, Massachusetts

Naomi Breslau, MD, Department of Psychiatry, Henry Ford Hospital, Detroit, Michigan

Jerel E. Del Dotto, PhD, ABPP-CN, Department of Neuropsychology, Foote Memorial Hospital, Jackson, Michigan

Martha B. Denckla, MD, Developmental Cognitive Neurology, Kennedy Krieger Institute, Baltimore, Maryland; Departments of Pediatrics and Psychiatry, Johns Hopkins University School of Medicine, Baltimore, Maryland

Maureen Dennis, PhD, Department of Surgery, Faculty of Medicine, University of Toronto, Toronto, Ontario, Canada; Department of Psychology and Research Institute, The Hospital for Sick Children, Toronto, Ontario, Canada

Kim N. Dietrich, PhD, Department of Environmental Health, Division of Biostatistics and Epidemiology, University of Cincinnati College of Medicine, Cincinnati, Ohio

Eileen B. Fennell, PhD, ABPP-CN, Department of Clinical and Health Psychology, University of Florida, Gainesville, Florida

Jack M. Fletcher, PhD, ABPP-CN, Departments of Pediatrics and Neurosurgery, University of Texas–Houston Medical School, Houston, Texas

Royal Grueneich, PhD, Department of Psychology, St. Louis Children's Hospital, St. Louis, Missouri; Department of Clinical Neurology, Washington University School of Medicine, St. Louis, Missouri

Sue M. Ingram, MS, Department of Psychology, Georgia State University, Atlanta, Georgia

Nicholas S. Krawiecki, MD, Department of Pediatrics, Emory University School of Medicine, Atlanta, Georgia

Kris A. Kullgren, PhD, Department of Psychology, Georgia State University, Atlanta, Georgia

Betty Kurczynski, MD, Department of Pediatrics, Robert C. Byrd Health Sciences Center, West Virginia University Medical School, Charleston, West Virginia

Bartlett D. Moore, III, PhD, Division of Pediatrics and Department of Neuro Oncology, University of Texas M. D. Anderson Cancer Center, Houston, Texas

Robin D. Morris, PhD, Department of Psychology, Georgia State University, Atlanta, Georgia

Phyllis J. Mullenix, PhD, Department of Radiation Oncology, Harvard Medical School, Boston, Massachusetts; Department of Psychiatry, Children's Hospital, Boston, Massachusetts

Hope Northrup, MD, Department of Pediatrics, University of Texas—Houston Medical School, Houston, Texas

Bruce Pennington, PhD, Department of Psychology, University of Denver, Denver, Colorado

Erin M. Picard, PhD, Bloorview MacMillan Center, Toronto, Ontario, Canada

Margaret B. Pulsifer, PhD, Department of Psychiatry and Behavioral Sciences, Johns Hopkins University School of Medicine, Baltimore, MD

M. Douglas Ris, PhD, ABPP-CN, Department of Pediatrics, University of Cincinnati College of Medicine, Cincinnati, Ohio; Division of Psychology, Children's Hospital Medical Center, Cincinnati, Ohio

Byron P. Rourke, PhD, FRSC, ABPP-CN, Department of Psychology, University of Windsor, Windsor, Ontario, Canada; Child Study Center, Yale University, New Haven, Connecticut

Joanne F. Rovet, PhD, Departments of Pediatrics and Psychology, Faculty of Medicine, University of Toronto, Toronto, Ontario, Canada; Department of Psychology, The Hospital for Sick Children, Toronto, Ontario, Canada

Elsa Shapiro, PhD, Departments of Pediatrics and Neurology, University of Minnesota, Minneapolis, Minnesota

Gregory B. Sharp, MD, Departments of Pediatrics and Neurology, University of Arkansas for Medical Sciences, Little Rock, Arkansas

H. Gerry Taylor, PhD, ABPP-CN, Department of Pediatrics, Case Western Reserve University, Cleveland, Ohio; Department of Psychology, Rainbow Babies and Children's Hospital, Cleveland, Ohio

Deborah P. Waber, PhD, Department of Psychiatry, Harvard Medical School, Boston, Massachusetts; Department of Psychiatry, Children's Hospital, Boston, Massachusetts

Marilyn Welsh, PhD, Department of Psychology, University of Northern Colorado, Greeley, Colorado

Jane Williams, PhD, Department of Pediatrics, University of Arkansas for Medical Sciences, Little Rock, Arkansas

Keith Owen Yeates, PhD, ABPP-CN, Department of Pediatrics, The Ohio State University, Columbus, Ohio; Department of Psychology, Columbus Children's Hospital, Columbus, Ohio

SERIES EDITOR NOTE

Pediatric Neuropsychology: Research, Theory, and Practice, edited by Keith Yeates, Douglas Ris, and Gerry Taylor, is the second volume in The Science and Practice of Neuropsychology series. The volume reflects the vital integration between theory, research, and practice, which is fundamental to all disciplines working in the field of neuropsychology, and presents a broad coverage of the disorders affecting neuropsychological development.

In this series, neuropsychology is defined broadly as the study of brain–behavior relationships, incorporating the perspectives of a range of related disciplines. Although some of the volumes will undoubtedly be of greater interest to specific subsets of readers, it is intended that the series be of interest to scientists and practitioners in all the disciplines that address brain–behavior relationships. A wide range of topics will be covered and will include reviews of emerging technologies and their potential impact on the science and clinical understanding of neuropsychology.

This volume is a timely reflection of the increasing interest in neurobehavioral disorders in children. Studies of maturing nervous systems provide a unique opportunity for fundamental insights into the organization and development of cognitive systems, and offer clues to the basis of deficit and recovery in mature nervous systems. Furthermore, the neuropsychological impacts of some disorders, such as neurogenetic and metabolic disorders, are best studied in children. Future developments in gene therapies will likely have their most profound effects in the treatment of children. This volume provides a contemporary and future-oriented view of the issues and concepts in neuropsychological development that will be the focus of scientific investigation and clinical application in the coming decades.

ROBERT A. BORNSTEIN, PhD

FOREWORD

The evolution of clinical neuropsychology into a major area of research and practice during the second half of the 20th century is a rather striking phenomenon. Before 1950 detailed study of the behavioral consequences of cerebral dysfunction, and of the factors responsible for that dysfunction, was pursued by only a few neurologists, psychologists, and psychiatrists—the names of Kurt Goldstein and Walther Poppelreuter in Germany, and Shepherd Ivory Franz in the United States, come to mind. But as a legacy of the carnage of World War II, coupled with advances in physiological and behavioral analysis, the field rapidly expanded in the 1950s when Ward Halstead, Henry Hécaen, Hans-Lukas Teuber, Oliver Zangwill, and other investigators established clinical neuropsychology as a distinctive discipline.

Attention was initially focused on brain–behavior relationships in adult patients. Although there was always some interest in the behavioral sequelae of cerebral dysfunction in children (reflected, for example, in the studies of Randolph Byers, Elizabeth Lord, Alfred Strauss, and their coworkers), expansion of the field of pediatric neuropsychology occurred somewhat later. It was in the 1960s that the clinical picture of the "clumsy child" (renamed *developmental dysgnosia and dyspraxia*) was described, specific reading disability (renamed *developmental dyslexia*) was investigated from a neuropsychological standpoint, and the concept of *minimal brain dysfunction* was formulated to account for these and a myriad of other behavioral disabilities in children. Since that time pediatric neuropsychology has become a flourishing area of inquiry and practice, generating new knowledge and deeper understanding, with the result that today the evaluation and management of children with documented or suspected brain dysfunction by the well-informed neuropsychologist are incomparably more insightful and effective than was the case 20 years ago.

This book is an admirable example of the fruits of that remarkable progress. Gone are the rather simple generalizations that were so often characteristic of state-of-the-art reviews not many years ago. The complexity and variability of the neurological bases of these disorders, which recent neuropathological and physiological study has brought to light, no longer permit such generalizations. The chapters of the book cover in detail and with uncommon acumen the behavioral sequelae of neurological and non-neurological diseases of children with which neuropsychologists are frequently called upon to deal. Presenting new findings and correcting mistaken assumptions, they reflect a new and higher level of understanding and judgment; this is bound to have a salutary influence on clinical practice.

The authors of these splendid chapters are to be congratulated. Thanks to their contributions and those of others of their generation, pediatric neuropsychology has come of age.

ARTHUR BENTON, PHD

PREFACE

The origins of this book can be traced to a series of discussions among the three of us during which we bemoaned the dearth of books available in the field of pediatric neuropsychology. In particular, we felt a need for a book that would provide an overview of neurological and medical conditions frequently seen in the practice of pediatric neuropsychology. At that time, there were various books available on the neuropsychology of learning disabilities, attention-deficit/hyperactivity disorder, and other developmental syndromes, but few that focused on the neuropsychology of pediatric neurological and medical conditions. We thought that a book that described the conditions, reviewed the neuropsychological outcomes with which they were associated, critiqued the existing research, suggested avenues for future exploration, and discussed the clinical implications of the existing knowledge base would make a valuable contribution to the field. Although some books devoted to pediatric neuropsychology have been published since our initial discussions (e.g., Baron, Fennell, & Voeller, 1995), there still remains a need for a volume of the sort we envisioned. We believe that the current text meets that need.

Our plan for the book was to combine reviews of the research on specific disorders with discussions of theoretical issues and clinical applications. We explicitly excluded learning disabilities, attention-deficit/hyperactivity disorder, and other developmental disorders, focusing instead on neurological and medical conditions that affect children and adolescents and that often result in referrals to pediatric neuropsychologists (Yeates, Ris, & Taylor, 1995). Most of the conditions we selected for inclusion are common in clinical practice, although we have included some that are less common or even unusual. All of the disorders have been topics of research that address critical issues regarding the neurobehavioral outcomes associated with childhood medical illnesses. Thus, while certainly not exhaustive, the book encompasses a broad range of disorders, all of which have been the subject of neuropsychologists' attention.

The book begins with a chapter by Maureen Dennis that provides an elegant conceptual discussion of the biological, environmental, and developmental variables affecting neurobehavioral outcomes in childhood medical disorders. It also highlights the need for future research that is prospective, longitudinal, and multivariate in nature. Dennis describes an outcome algorithm that may eventually be applied to children with specific disorders to predict their long-term cognitive and behavioral functioning. Her perspective offers an overarching framework for the book as a whole.

Following the introductory chapter are 16 chapters devoted to specific neurological or medical conditions. They are divided into two sections of 8 chapters each. The first section concerns primary disorders of the central nervous system: early hydrocephalus, epilepsy, brain tumors, closed-head injuries, meningitis, neurofibromatosis, metabolic and neuro-degenerative disorders, and exposure to neurotoxicants. The second section concerns central nervous system dysfunction associated with other medical disorders: prematurity and low birthweight, Turner syndrome, phenylketonuria, acute lymphoblastic leukemia, sickle cell disease, diabetes, renal disease, and human immunodeficiency virus (HIV).

In a desire to ensure that the chapters on specific disorders (those in Parts II and III of the book) provided similar types of information, we asked the authors to follow a common format. Most of these chapters begin with a section describing the condition's epidemiology, as well as its associated pathophysiology and neuropathology. The next sections include a description of the neurobehavioral outcomes associated with the disorder, as well as a critique of the existing research from both conceptual and methodological perspectives. The chapters generally conclude with a discussion of future directions for research on the disorder in question.

The book continues with two chapters that focus on the clinical implications of the knowledge base described in the preceding chapters. Although the book is not intended as a "how-to" guide to neuropsychological assessment and evaluation, we believe that it should include some consideration of how research on the neuropsychological consequences of medical conditions is brought to bear on clinical practice. We therefore have asked two well-known pediatric neuropsychologists to share their clinical insights. Jane Holmes Bernstein describes a broad conceptual framework for neuropsychological assessment; she enumerates a set of principles that mesh well with the approach to research advocated by Dennis in her introductory chapter. Ida Sue Baron describes how the results of neuropsychological assessment can be used to guide intervention, and provides illustrative examples of the link between assessment and intervention derived from her own practice.

The book concludes with a commentary by Byron Rourke, who was asked to discuss each of the chapters pertaining to a specific disorder (Chapters 2–17), as well as the book as a whole. His comments are insightful and thought-provoking. He was not asked to comment on the chapters pertaining to clinical practice; any perceived omission in that regard is by design. We are indebted to Rourke for sharing his thoughts in his inimitable style.

We believe that this volume provides a unique contribution to the field of pediatric neuropsychology. It spans a wide range of medical and neurological conditions, and it provides current, in-depth reviews of empirical research on those conditions. The chapters have been written by recognized experts in the field of pediatric neuropsychology who have been actively involved in research on their chapter topics. Finally, and perhaps most importantly, the book explores the boundaries of current research, theory, and practice by highlighting lacunae in the existing knowledge base. Thus the book not only demonstrates how the knowledge base in pediatric neuropsychology has grown in recent decades, but also foreshadows the scientific and professional journey to come. In so doing, it helps to ensure that we do not reach beyond our scientific boundaries when working clinically with children. Indeed, the book presents principles of assessment and intervention precisely to encourage a closer examination of these practices in light of our existing knowledge.

We hope that the book appeals to a wide audience of scientists and practitioners, including neuropsychologists, pediatric and child clinical psychologists, school psychologists, pediatric neurologists, child psychiatrists, behavioral–developmental pediatricians, and speech pathologists. We also intend it to be useful to graduate students, predoctoral psychology interns, and postdoctoral residents in neuropsychology.

The book could not have been completed without the help of many individuals, all of whom deserve our gratitude. We would like to thank the authors for their contributions.

We appreciate the time and energy that they devoted to writing their chapters, and their willingness to respond to our editorial suggestions for revisions. We also would like to thank our former and current students, interns, and residents for the inspiration that they provided to undertake editing the book in the first place. Our editors at The Guilford Press, Sharon Panulla and Rochelle Serwator, who have shepherded the book toward completion with just the right blend of encouragement and exhortation, deserve our thanks as well. We should also thank Robert Bornstein for inviting us to include the book in The Science and Practice of Neuropsychology series. Finally, we want to thank our families for their ongoing support and understanding. Without them, our work would be empty of purpose and meaning.

KEITH OWEN YEATES
M. DOUGLAS RIS
H. GERRY TAYLOR

REFERENCES

Baron, I. S., Fennell, E. B., & Voeller, K. K. S. (1995). *Pediatric neuropsychology in the medical setting.* New York: Oxford University Press.

Yeates, K. O., Ris, M. D., & Taylor, H. G. (1995). Hospital referral patterns in pediatric neuropsychology. *Child Neuropsychology, 1,* 56–62.

CONTENTS

PEDIATRIC NEUROPSYCHOLOGY

PART I

Introduction

1

CHILDHOOD MEDICAL DISORDERS AND COGNITIVE IMPAIRMENT: BIOLOGICAL RISK, TIME, DEVELOPMENT, AND RESERVE

MAUREEN DENNIS

The last few years have seen a burgeoning interest in the neurobehavioral outcomes of medical conditions that affect the developing central nervous system (CNS). The effect of medical condition on outcome is neither transparent nor direct. Neurobehavioral outcome is the result, not only of the biological risk associated with a medical condition, but also of development, time and reserve. Current research derived from studies of diseases, lesions, or symptoms suggests that neurobehavioral outcome or cognitive phenotype may be thought of as an outcome algorithm that expresses the *biological risk* associated with the medical condition, moderated by the child's *development*; by the *time since onset* of the condition; and by the *reserve* available within the child, family, school, and community (Figure 1.1).

This chapter considers four questions related to childhood medical disorders that affect the CNS:

- What is a cognitive phenotype?
- Which factors set biological risk?
- How do development, time since onset, and reserve moderate biological risk?
- What is the general form of an outcome algorithm?

These questions have practical implications for diagnosis and management, as well as theoretical relevance to the search for a developmental perspective on these disorders.

COGNITIVE PHENOTYPE

A *cognitive phenotype* is the appearance of mental and behavioral skills. It is neither a table of test scores nor a description of test performance, although derivation of scores

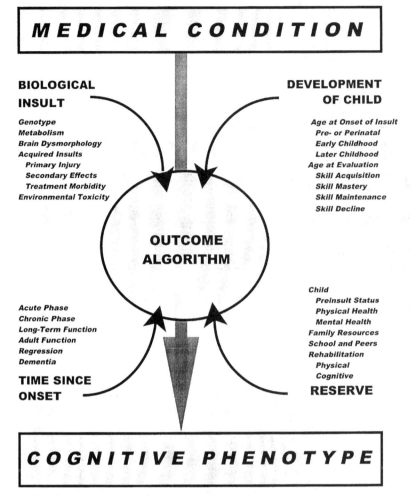

FIGURE 1.1. The relation between medical disorder and outcome, set by biological risk and moderated by development, time, and reserve.

and understanding of how they were derived both contribute to establishing a phenotype. Cognitive phenotype involves five concepts: modal profile; variability; core deficits; challenge level; and phenocopy.

Modal Profile

The *modal profile* of a medical disorder is the most typical set of cognitive strengths and weaknesses associated with it. For some well-studied conditions, robust modal profiles have been identified. For example, individuals with Turner syndrome have difficulty with spatial analysis; children with hydrocephalus have difficulty in graphomotor skills, spatial attention, mathematics, and reading comprehension. As more childhood medical disorders are studied in relation to functional cognitive models (see Welsh & Pennington, Chapter 12, this volume), a broader delineation of modal profiles is likely to emerge.

Variability

Part of what is measured in a neuropsychological assessment is *variability* in cognitive phenotype, which should not routinely be dismissed as error variance. Variability in performance over time is part of what defines some cognitive functions.

Variability around a modal cognitive profile is typical of most medical conditions, just as is medical variability. Variability may itself be the outcome measure; for instance, variable performance over time on attention tasks could be a marker of a deficit in attention for a particular condition. Variability is sometimes more closely associated with the markers of brain disorder (e.g., positive neuroimaging findings in sickle cell disease; Ris & Grueneich, Chapter 14, this volume) than is level of performance.

Within a group with a childhood medical disorder, variations in medical status are common. These variations may be principally related to cognitive outcome. For early-onset hydrocephalus, variability in cognitive phenotype is related to physical symptoms (e.g., eye movement disorders), to medical severity (e.g., level of spinal cord lesion), and to specific brain dysmorphologies (e.g., in the cerebellum, midbrain, corpus callosum, and posterior cortex) (Fletcher, Dennis, & Northrup, Chapter 2, this volume).

For many medical conditions, variability around a modal profile may reflect the precision with which modal problems have been identified. More precise identification of modal weaknesses and strengths may yield smaller variations across individuals and studies than often occurs with measurement tools that are psychometrically derived rather than model-driven.

Variability in phenotype merits study not as error variance, but as a clue to mechanism of disease action. This is most obvious in conditions in which dose–response issues are in the foreground (e.g., toxic exposure), but it also applies more broadly to all medical conditions that affect children's cognitive functioning.

Core Deficits

Core deficits are an important part of the cognitive phenotype. Going beyond a modal or typical profile, a *core deficit* is a cognitive impairment defined in terms of underlying processes that is robust across various levels of disorder severity and mental ability.

In approaching childhood medical conditions, one strategy has been to study individuals with severe forms of mental retardation to search for islands of preserved functioning. An alternative strategy is to study conditions across a range of IQ levels, the rationale being that cognitive deficits varying with IQ are likely to share more general cognitive processing resources, whereas cognitive deficits that persist in higher-IQ groups are more likely to be core deficits.

Cognition in children with early hydrocephalus has been investigated with respect to core deficits (Barnes & Dennis, 1992, 1996, 1998; Dennis & Barnes, 1993; Dennis, Hendrick, Hoffman, & Humphreys, 1987; Dennis, Jacennik, & Barnes, 1994). These children attend to objects but not locations, remember and learn facts but not procedures, and process reference but not inference (Dennis, Barnes, & Hetherington, 1999).

The identification of core language deficits in hydrocephalus is of particular interest. Some language tasks vary with IQ in this disorder, while others do not. Children with hydrocephalus are relatively proficient at language tasks in which meaning is not context-dependent. These tasks, which vary with a child's IQ, include word recognition, phonological analysis skills, single-word comprehension, and understanding idiomatic expressions.

Children with hydrocephalus have difficulty with language tasks in which meaning must be contextually computed. These tasks, which are relatively invariant across IQ level, include making inferences, understanding written or oral texts, and processing nonidiomatic figurative language (e.g., novel metaphors or similes).

Difficulty in computing meaning from context may be considered to be a core deficit in hydrocephalus. First, it is relatively independent of intelligence; that is, it is demonstrable even in individuals with average or above-average IQ. Second, it is a deficit specific to discourse contexts; that is, it cannot be accounted for by limitations in other language skills, such as vocabulary. Finally, it is specific to derivation of a particular form of meaning; that is, it is apparent when meaning must be constructed from a discourse context, but is not associated with context-independent meaning.

Challenge Level

Challenge level also contributes to defining the cognitive phenotype. Children with medical conditions may manage routine neuropsychological tasks, but may fail as the challenge level is increased and the skill must be instantiated under demand conditions involving multitasking and/or distraction.

Inability to retain functionality under challenge can be a sensitive sign of neuropsychological morbidity. Adult survivors of medulloblastoma and age-matched controls both perform poorly on gait tasks under conditions of physical or cognitive challenge; however, the challenges reduce the performance of the medulloblastoma (but not control) group to the level of clinical impairment (Dennis, Hetherington, Spiegler, & Barnes, 1999).

Clinically, impairment in individuals with severe medical disorders is readily demonstrated on low-challenge tasks. Failure on high-challenge tasks is one definition of subclinical impairment in individuals who may superficially appear cognitively intact. The presence of subclinical impairment is relevant to understanding the ability to function under everyday demands of multitasking and distraction. To evaluate the ecological validity of the test instruments, it is also useful to compare individual performances on low- and high-challenge tasks.

Measurement of cognitive skill under conditions of challenge may reveal impairments not observable on tasks that measure routine skill performance. It is perhaps the deficits revealed under challenge that are the truer measure of the impact of the medical condition on the CNS.

Cognitive Phenocopies

Cognitive phenocopies are phenotypes that are superficially alike but that are found on inspection to arise from fundamentally different cognitive processes. A comparison of reading comprehension deficits in head injury and congenital hydrocephalus illustrates this concept. Both conditions involve some perturbation of white matter—in hydrocephalus because of dysmorphologies and secondary effects of raised intracranial pressure, but in head injury because of diffuse axonal injury. Reading comprehension, which is poor in both conditions, is related to a processing speed bottleneck in one condition and to an inability to compute contextually derived meaning in the other. Children with head injury decode words slowly, and decoding speed is related to reading comprehension in this condition (Barnes, Dennis, & Wilkinson, 1999). Children with hydrocephalus, on the other hand, decode words as rapidly as peers; their reading comprehension is related to semantic integration, not to reading speed (Barnes, Faulkner, & Dennis, 1999).

It is important to pursue the study of cognitive profiles across conditions, in order to establish whether similar profiles are phenocopies or the results of similar biological mechanisms. Children with Turner syndrome and children with congenital hydrocephalus have deficits in spatial function, as well as impairments related to compromise of the posterior cortex (Reiss et al., 1993; Fletcher et al., 1996). Although the functional and structural abnormalities associated with these conditions appear to be related, there are no detailed comparisons spatial processing in the two groups. Similarly, children with poorly treated phenylketonuria have an IQ profile (lower Comprehension and higher Block Design scores on Wechsler tests) like that in high-functioning autism (Dennis, Lockyer, et al., 1999); however, it is not known whether this reflects similar or partially overlapping deficits in dopaminergic function.

Many medical conditions disrupt attention and memory. Examples of these conditions include exposure to polychlorinated biphenyls (Jacobson, Jacobson, & Humphrey, 1990; Dietrich, Chapter 9, this volume); renal encephalopathy (Fennell, Chapter 16, this volume); and brain tumors (Morris, Krawiecki, Kullgren, Ingram, Kurczynski, Chapter 4, this volume). Both implicit memory and explicit memory are impaired after medial brain tumors (Dennis, Hetherington, & Spiegler, 1998), suggesting different neuropathology in medial tumors than in conditions in which explicit but not implicit memory is impaired. Comparisons of patterns of memory impairment in different disorders may clarify both cognitive phenotype and underlying neuropathology.

Understanding of phenotypes and phenocopies requires models of constituent processes and how they are related in the expression of functions. Principled study of phenotypes in this manner may contribute to better separation of phenotypes from phenocopies in childhood medical disorders.

BIOLOGICAL RISK

Biological risk is the cumulative severity of a disorder, which is a combination of effects relating to genotype, metabolism, environmental toxicity, congenital brain dysmorphologies, the primary severity and secondary effects of acquired brain insult, and/or treatment morbidity.

Genotype

Genotype defines particular disorders and delineates subgroups within a disorder. At present, genotype appears to be related to some characteristic modal profiles, although the genetic bases of differences in modal profiles among disorders is not fully understood. Study of the phenotypic variations in biological variants may be addressed by considering heterogeneity of karyotypes. Genotype differences have been related to differences in neuropsychological function for some conditions (e.g., Turner syndrome; Berch & Bender, Chapter 11, this volume) but not for others (e.g., sickle cell disease; Ris & Grueneich, Chapter 14, this volume).

Genetic as well as etiological heterogeneity is characteristic of some conditions. For example, Dandy–Walker syndrome (a neurodevelopmental disorder associated with agenesis of the cerebellar vermis, enlarged fourth ventricle, and posterior fossa cyst) may be associated with single-gene disorders, such as the autosomal recessive Warburg and Meckel–Gruber syndromes; with chromosomal abnormalities; or with environmental factors (Murray, Johnson, & Bird, 1985). It is not known whether genetic and etiological heterogeneity is related to diversity in neuropsychological outcome.

Metabolic Disorders

A class of progressive metabolic and neurodegenerative disorders occur in children that have a characteristic course of deteriorating behavior, dementia, severe disability, and even death (Shapiro & Balthazor, Chapter 8, this volume). Study of the neuropsychological sequelae of these conditions is important, not only in revealing the natural history of the conditions, but also in providing data relevant to models of childhood medical conditions and dementia.

Environmental Toxicity

Environmental toxicity contributes to biological risk. Teratogens are transferred freely to both mature and immature brains, but the immature CNS is especially vulnerable to environmental toxicity (Rodier, 1994). Early exposure to toxins interferes with CNS development and organ formation. Later exposure carries less risk of major CNS malformations, but it still increases the risk of developmental cognitive morbidity (Dobbing, 1981; Dietrich, Chapter 9, this volume).

Brain development and cognitive development are both staged and extend over a considerable time (Rodier, 1994). The co-occurrence of extended periods of myelination and protracted cognitive development means a high sensitivity to neurotoxic substances and a high risk of cognitive disorders throughout childhood. Because toxicants can often be measured and dated, level of toxicant exposure has provided important models not only for dose–response relationships between exposure and cognitive anomalies, but also for broader issues relating to the staging of cognitive development.

Brain Dysmorphologies

Much of the business of the young brain is myelination, and a significant number of childhood medical conditions affect the white matter. Before the advent of neuroimaging procedures to identify perturbations of white matter, a range of quite different multifocal white matter disorders were dismissed as childhood diffuse brain disorders.

What is needed is a better delineation of the differences—in both brain structure and cognitive functioning—between conditions now grouped together as white matter disorders. Newer imaging procedures allow the differentiation of these disorders in terms of the type and regional distribution of brain anomalies. Neuropsychological deficit in some conditions, for instance, is related to whether white matter abnormalities are anterior or posterior (Shapiro, Balthazor, Lockman, & Krivit, 1997).

Childhood-onset cortical lesions have long intrigued neuropsychologists because of presumed parallels with adult cortical lesions producing aphasia, apraxia, agnosia, and alexia. For children, however, lesions in other brain regions are more common, more prevalent, and more representative of CNS involvement. The corpus callosum, brain stem, and cerebellum are often compromised in childhood medical disorders. Only recently have these brain regions been analyzed with respect to functional outcome. Corpus callosum dysmorphologies in hydrocephalus are related to motor and cognitive dysfunctions (Hannay, Fletcher, & Brandt, 1999). Congenital and childhood acquired cerebellar lesions are associated with motor and cognitive dysfunctions from childhood to middle adulthood (Dennis, Hetherington, et al., 1999).

Primary Severity of Acquired Conditions

Primary severity is well understood as a medical risk factor for mortality and morbidity in such conditions as brain tumors, with their staging systems based on cell types, and head injury, where severity has been assessed via metrics such as depth of coma, duration of impaired consciousness, and length of posttraumatic amnesia (Yeates, Chapter 5, this volume). For some conditions, severity is predictive of outcome (e.g., intraventricular hemorrhage in low-birthweight children produces cognitive deficits; Picard, Del Dotto, & Breslau, Chapter 10, this volume).

Primary severity is less well understood for other medical disorders, particularly those that have only recently become consistent with long-term survival, or those that are only recently being studied. For any condition, it is difficult to find severity metrics for evolving as opposed to static clinical status, or for fluctuating as opposed to constant symptoms.

Secondary Effects of Congenital and Acquired Conditions

Any disorder affecting the brain is a process of events, not a single event. For example, traumatic brain injury involves a cascade of interrelated processes (direct damage caused by calcium influx into cells, free-radical-mediated damage, receptor mediated damage, and inflammation) that contribute to delayed cellular damage (Gennarelli & Graham, 1998).

Medical conditions that affect the developing CNS are often associated with significant secondary events that exacerbate the effects of the primary injury. For example, raised intracranial pressure, sometimes accompanied by hydrocephalus, occurs secondary to a variety of medical conditions: lysosomal storage diseases, such as the mucopolysaccharidoses (Whitley et al., 1993); bacterial meningitis (Stovring & Snyder, 1980); head injury (Bruce, 1995); and subtentorial brain tumors (Raimondi & Tadanori, 1981).

Some secondary effects may be partially reversible. Repetitive sickling of red blood cells produces irreversible damage, but sickling can be reversed with reoxygenation, and this prevents vascular occlusive disease (Ris & Grueneich, Chapter 14, this volume). Shunt treatment reverses some, but by no means all, of the brain effects of hydrocephalus (Del Bigio, 1993).

Cognitive morbidity appears greater when a secondary insult is added to a primary one. For example, in identical twins with low birthweight and intraventricular hemorrhage, the twin with hydrocephalus had increased neuropsychological deficit (Dennis & Barnes, 1994b). Shunt infections are a consistent risk factor for cognitive impairment in treated hydrocephalus (Fletcher et al., Chapter 2, this volume). Seizures are a risk factor for cognitive problems in both childhood diabetes (Rovet, Chapter 15, this volume) and congenital hydrocephalus (Dennis et al., 1981). It has been suggested that the primary chromosome defects and secondary effects of Turner syndrome are responsible for different parts of the cognitive phenotype (Berch & Bender, Chapter 11, this volume).

Two recent developments have focused attention on the secondary effects of brain insult. Newer neuroimaging procedures have provided better identification of these effects. For example, perfusion-weighted imaging has revealed signs of diffuse axonal damage in cases of traumatic brain injury. In addition, animal models have suggested mechanisms by which secondary damage might act, and have demonstrated methods for examining these effects either in isolation or in combination with primary brain insult. For example, rat models have elucidated the time course of myelination delay caused by hydrocephalus (Del Bigio, Kanfer, & Zhang, 1997). Animal models of radiation effects have clarified the nature of radiation damage to the developing CNS (Mildenberger, Beach, McGeer, & Ludgate, 1990). Despite the new level of interest, the secondary effects associated with childhood medical disorders continue to be understudied.

To document cognitive outcome, it is important to establish whether biological risk is elevated by the primary damage, the secondary damage, or both. Equally important is whether secondary brain and metabolic changes across conditions contribute to similar functional impairments. For example, tumor necrosis factor, a macrophage monocyte-derived immunomediator that probably contributes to cerebral edema and myelin damage, is abnormal in pediatric HIV (Mintz et al., 1989) and head injury (Ross, Halliday, Campbell, Byrnes, & Rowlands, 1994). Better delineation of secondary effects will increase understanding of variability within conditions and help interpret commonalities across conditions. In particular, it is important to understand the mechanisms of secondary insult in conditions such as head injury, because such insult has long-term effects on behavior and may contribute to the development of neurodegenerative disease (DeKosky, Kochanek, Clark, Ciallella, & Dixon, 1998).

Treatment Morbidity

Treatments modify the level of biological risk in various ways. Effective treatment lowers mortality and morbidity (e.g., transfusions lower the stroke rate in sickle cell disease; Ris & Grueneich, Chapter 14, this volume). At the same time, many standard treatments increase the risk of sensory or functional impairment. For example, steroids are associated with reduced hearing and neurological impairments in cases of bacterial meningitis (Mertsola et al., 1991), and hypoglycemia is an iatrogenic effect of insulin therapy that increases the risk of seizures (Rovet, Chapter 15, this volume). Treatment morbidity is elucidated by animal model studies of treatment effects (e.g., Schunior et al., 1990), conducted in parallel with studies of childhood behavioral outcomes.

AGE AND DEVELOPMENT AT DISORDER ONSET

Age is a marker for level of physical, brain, and cognitive development. The impact of a medical disorder thus will vary both with a child's chronological age and with the child's level of functional skill development. More broadly, measurement of outcome requires appreciation of the child's skill level at disorder onset, the subsequent course of skill development, and the status of long-term skill maintenance (Dennis, 1988; Dennis & Barnes, 1994a).

For mature adults, functional competence is demonstrated in a context of established skills, but children must master the maturational challenges involved in moving through developmental levels. In childhood-onset disorders, children must continue to meet the challenges of development, as well as the demands of recovery. Cognitive phenotype represents the expression of previously acquired skills and the acquisition of new skills.

The extent to which medical conditions of childhood interfere with the process of skill acquisition can be determined by studying deviations from anticipated developmental trajectories. Outcome may also be viewed in terms of multiple measures over the course of development. Here the variable of interest is the slope of the curve relating function and age, and the question is whether the slope differs in individuals according to the presence of a medical disorder. When one is considering possible outcomes of childhood medical conditions, then, several indices are relevant: rate of skill acquisition; stability of skill maintenance over the course of mature, optimal performance; and rate of loss with aging or deterioration in condition (Dennis, 1988; Dennis & Barnes, 1994a).

A Historical Dissonance

How age at disorder onset is related to cognitive outcome is best understood with reference to a historical cognitive dissonance. The earliest ages at onset were always known to be associated with profound neurodevelopmental disturbance. Congenital brain malformations were understood to produce profound cognitive and other impairments (e.g., mental retardation, cerebral palsy, autism). At the same time, a linear relation between age at onset and degree of deficit was proposed for specific cognitive disorders such as aphasia (Basser, 1962; Lenneberg, 1967). Even toxic, functionally debilitating symptoms in children (e.g., serious lead exposure) were believed to dissipate in short order (McKhann, 1932). The dissonance was that a young age at disorder onset was regarded as both a risk factor (e.g., for the communicative impairments of autism) and a protective factor (e.g., for aphasia).

Recent research has reduced this cognitive dissonance by showing that a younger age is associated with greater vulnerability to a variety of medical conditions and to the cognitive morbidity that follows them. Immature organisms are more likely than mature ones to experience certain disorders, and once they experience a disorder, younger organisms are more vulnerable to cognitive deficit.

Fetal Onset

Fetal toxicity occurs at lower doses of environmental neurotoxicants than does adult toxicity, and has more widespread brain effects. Adult mercury exposure produces restricted lesions in the parieto-occipital and cerebellar regions, whereas fetal exposure produces widespread brain compromise (Takeuchi, 1968). Other fetal-origin insults produce autism and Joubert syndrome, both profound neurodevelopmental disorders with dysmorphisms of the midbrain and cerebellum (Rodier, Ingram, Tisdale, Nelson, & Romano, 1996; Maria et al., 1997).

Insult or exposure to toxins early in development can sometimes be marked by co-occurring neurodevelopmental events. Autism embryopathy coexists with developmental anomalies of the cranial nerve motor nuclei (Rodier et al., 1996). Autism and thalidomide embryopathy appear to be associated, and this finding may help identify the timing and neural circuitry of autism as involving fetal development at about 20–24 postconception days (Stromland, Nordin, Miller, Akerstrom, & Gillberg, 1994). Anatomy of brain hypoplasia may also serve as a temporal marker to identify events that damage the brain in autism; for example, the sixth and seventh lobules of the neocerebellar vermis are hypoplastic in individuals with autism, in contrast to the normal development of the ontogenetically and anatomically distinct first through fifth lobules (Courchesne, Yeung-Courchesne, Press, Hesselink, & Jernigan, 1988). For Dandy-Walker syndrome, the presence of a cardiac anomaly (ventricular septal defect) suggests a teratogenic influence before the sixth embryonic week—a time when the interventricular septum is normally established (Sautreaux, Giroud, Dauvergne, Nivelon, & Thierry, 1986).

Early Childhood Onset

Within the age range of infancy and childhood, a younger age does not protect against the morbidity of various medical conditions. Postnatally, a young age is itself a risk factor for incurring such conditions as bacterial meningitis or posterior fossa tumors. For some conditions, the peak age at onset is in early childhood; for example, the peak incidence of acute lymphoblastic leukemia occurs at 3–4 years of age (Gurney, Severson, Davis, & Robison, 1995). Children may be more likely than adults to suffer medical complications; for example, diabetic children are more likely to have seizures resulting from hypoglycemia than are adults (Rovet, Chapter 15, this volume), and children have more HIV-related neurological and behavioral deficits than do adults (Belman et al., 1988).

It has always been problematic to attribute differences between child and adult outcomes solely to age, because age and pathology are often confounded (Dennis, 1996). Within a given medical condition, age affects the type of pathology. Childhood aphasia typically has traumatic etiologies, whereas adult aphasia arises most often from cerebrovascular events. Children with sickle cell disease sustain ischemic strokes, whereas adults with the disease have hemorrhagic strokes (Platt, 1994).

For conditions involving diffuse or multifocal disorder processes, a young age at onset is associated with greater cognitive morbidity (Taylor & Alden, 1997). A younger as opposed to an older age at onset is related to poorer cognitive outcome for a range of medical conditions in children. These include congenital and infantile hydrocephalus (Hetherington & Dennis, 1999), childhood diabetes (Holmes & Richman, 1985; Rovet, Ehrlich, & Hoppe, 1988), bacterial meningitis (Anderson et al., 1997), pediatric HIV (Aylward, Chapter 17, this volume), closed-head injury (Barnes, Dennis, & Wilkinson, 1999; Ewing-Cobbs, Levin, Eisenberg, & Fletcher, 1987; Kriel, Krach, & Panser, 1989; Wrightson, McGinn, & Gronwall, 1995), heart disease (Wright & Nolan, 1994), and cranial irradiation (Anderson, Smibert, Ekert, & Godber, 1994).

Time Windows

Points in development represent time windows during which brain perturbations may be especially disruptive of skills being acquired. Disruption of phonological and orthographic development (as manifested by unprincipled spelling errors) results from leukemia treatment involving radiation and chemotherapy (Kleinman & Waber, 1992). For reading, word decoding is especially vulnerable to head injury or irradiation for leukemia before age 6

(Barnes, Dennis, & Wilkinson, 1999; Spiegler & Barnes, 1997). Study of these vulnerable periods may reveal not only the risks for particular children with medical conditions, but also the nature of normal skill acquisition during periods when postthalamic acoustic pathways are myelinating and/or when prereading and reading skills are emerging.

Older Age at Onset

Evidence suggests not only that a young age of onset elevates risk, but that an older age lowers it. Young children are at increased risk from whole-brain radiation, with the highest-risk group being those 2–3 years of age or younger. Radiation at this time in development, which affects myelination and higher cortical function, produces intellectual loss (Balestrini, Micheli, Giordani, Lasio, & Giombini, 1994; Cohen et al., 1993; Geyer et al., 1995; Moore, Ater, & Copeland, 1992). For posterior fossa medulloblastomas, the younger the age at diagnosis, the greater the neuropsychological dysfunction (Allen & Epstein, 1982; Duffner, Cohen, & Thomas, 1983; Kun, Mulhern, & Crisco, 1983). An older age at onset may even be protective: Late diagnosis of medulloblastoma in an 18-year-old boy resulted in long-term neuropsychological function similar to that of his identical twin (Silverman & Thomas, 1990).

Rate of Decline

Age at onset may influence not only the level of functioning, but the rate of its decline. Early onset in pediatric HIV is associated with a more rapid disease progression than is a later onset (Aylward, Chapter 17, this volume). In several neurological disorders, a younger age at diagnosis is associated with more rapid deterioration and dementia (Shapiro & Balthazor, Chapter 8, this volume).

TIME SINCE ONSET

The Distinction between Time and Recovery

Time since onset of disease, an important moderator of cognitive phenotype, is not a synonym for recovery. Research on outcomes of meningitis, for example, has revealed that behavior problems increase and some cognitive functions decrease as a child develops (Taylor et al., 1990; Taylor, Schatschneider, & Minich, 1999), in keeping with Kennard's (1940) observation that some cognitive deficits after early brain lesions emerge in the course of development.

Time since onset of pediatric HIV or genetic metabolic disorders (Aylward, Chapter 17, this volume; Shapiro & Balthazor, Chapter 8, this volume) involves not so much recovery as disease progression and deterioration. Time may bring no change in cognitive status; alternatively, time may reveal new deficits or exacerbate old ones.

Time since onset of medical conditions in children affects both the level of cognitive functions and their rate of acquisition, so it is important to understand the shape of the curve relating time since onset to outcome. For instance, younger head-injured children show a slower rate of change over time and more significant residual deficits after their recovery plateaus than do older children with equally severe injuries (Anderson & Moore, 1995; Ewing-Cobbs et al., 1987).

Adult Survivors of Childhood Medical Disorders

It is important to study the natural course of medical disorders, from childhood into young adulthood and on into the years in which age-related declines in neuropsychological functioning may be observed. Because time since onset is a significant moderator of outcome, studies of long-term function are especially revealing of the true cognitive morbidity of a childhood medical disorder. Particularly valuable are studies that follow large cohorts from infancy through the school-age years. For example, school-age follow-up studies of children hospitalized for bacterial meningitis (Anderson & Taylor, Chapter 6, this volume) not only document long-term outcome of medical conditions, but also describe the developmental trajectories in children with different severities of disorder.

A distinct perspective on time since onset is provided by longitudinal studies of the stability, attenuation, or exacerbation of neuropsychological deficits in older adults who are long-term survivors of medical disorders. Such information can be complicated to interpret because of changes in treatment over time; nevertheless, it is relevant not only to medical conditions, but also to broader models of disorder effects and development.

Longitudinal studies of children with early-onset hydrocephalus show that children with poor math skills develop into adults with limited academic competence in math and functional innumeracy (Dennis, Barnes, et al., 1998). This means that the original impairment is a developmental deficit and not a developmental lag (Dennis, 1988).

Co-Occurrence of Developmental Change and Recovery

Long-term follow-up studies of childhood medical disorders into adulthood provide evidence relevant to distinguishing recovery of lost functions (for which the raw score at the time of the insult provides a benchmark index) from recovery plus development (which can best be established at maturity, and which requires long-term longitudinal observations). The effects of development and of recovery plus development may be differentiated on the basis of skill acquisition (or reacquisition) gradients. It is important to attempt to understand the degree and duration of postlesion developmental acceleration produced by the combined processes of recovery and development.

RESERVE

Medical disorders occur in children in the context of a reserve that varies in quality and quantity. *Reserve* refers here to factors that are available either to buffer dysfunction or to exacerbate it. Reserve can exist in the child, in the family, or in the broader social context of peers and school. The effects of reserve in buffering or enhancing the impact of a disorder are well illustrated in the research on lead toxicity (Bellinger, 1995).

Preinsult Status

Preinsult reserves may involve demographic, cognitive (e.g., high intelligence), physical, or socioeconomic resources. At least some demographic features influence outcome; for example, sex is a preinsult factor that increases the vulnerability to leukemia treatment

(Waber & Mullenix, Chapter 13, this volume). Similarly, preinsult behavior problems are more common in children with mild head injury than in noninjured children; indeed, these problems may have increased the risk of incurring the head injury (Asarnow et al., 1995).

Physical and Mental Health

Physical health is often compromised after major medical conditions. Children may have chronic sensory loss, cranial nerve dysfunction, seizure disorders, hemiplegia, and ataxia, as well as difficulties in growth, metabolism, and sleep. Chronic health problems affect school attendance, attentiveness, and performance on neuropsychological tests. Good physical health is a resource that moderates the effects of medical disorders.

Mental health is also an important determinant of cognitive outcome. After childhood traumatic brain injury, outcome depends on neuropsychiatric factors encompassing severity of brain injury and postinjury psychiatric disorders (Max et al., 1999).

Family, School, and Rehabilitation

Family resources contribute strongly to outcome after medical disorders in children. To begin with, social disadvantage increases the probability of incurring particular medical conditions (Broome, 1987). For some disorders, such as diabetes, treatment compliance is important, and family resources may either enhance or disrupt compliance. For children with conditions overrepresented in socially disadvantaged groups, such as sickle cell disease, socioeconomic status predicts IQ after onset better than the best biological moderators (Brown et al., 1993). Family stress and socioeconomic status also predict outcome after childhood brain tumors (Carlson-Green, Morris, & Krawiecki, 1995).

The family is affected by a brain disorder, and in turn the outcome of the disorder is associated with postdisorder family characteristics. After childhood traumatic brain injury, cognitive outcome depends on both neuropsychiatric factors and psychosocial disadvantage (Max et al., 1999); furthermore, biological and family variables predict different types of outcomes (Taylor et al., 1995).

School and rehabilitation opportunities can be other important factors in moderating cognitive outcome. The resources may be either enhanced by effective teachers and good cognitive rehabilitation programs, or reduced by gaps in school attendance as a result of primary severity, secondary complications, or treatment.

INTERACTIONS AMONG RESOURCES

Resource moderators do not operate in isolation, and some of their interactions have been identified. Primary severity of the disorder interacts with socioeconomic status in meningitis, with some effects being more apparent in children of low socioeconomic status than in children from more advantaged backgrounds (Taylor, Barry, & Schatschneider, 1993).

The factors that are important at one point in time may vary with disorder severity, development, and time since onset. For mild head injury, family and environmental variables are important predictors of outcome, whereas injury-related variables are relatively more significant for the more severe forms of head injury. For at least some disorders, cognitive sequelae may be related primarily to characteristics of the disease or injury, whereas behavioral outcome may be related more closely to family and socioeconomic features. Family and resource variables may also be more salient than disorder variables as recovery time increases (Aylward, 1992).

Whether resource moderators operate directly or indirectly, additively or interactively, it is especially important to understand the nature of moderator effects on cognitive phenotype. Social and family factors influence outcome directly, but also moderate disorder effects (Taylor & Schatschneider, 1992).

DRAFTING THE OUTCOME ALGORITHM

Threshold Theory for Adults

A theory called *threshold theory* has been developed to account for the variability in cognitive outcome in adult medical disorders. In its most clearly articulated form (Satz, 1993), threshold theory argues that the likelihood of a functional impairment depends on the margin of brain reserve, the temporal onset of the disorder, the number of repeated insults, and the sensitivity of the functional assay. These concepts seem equally applicable to children, although some qualifications are needed.

A larger brain has a greater number of neurons and synapses (Haug, 1987). In adults, a larger brain size delays the onset of neurological symptoms of dementia, or lessens their severity (Schofield, Mosesson, Stern, & Mayeux, 1995); this has led to the suggestion that dementing conditions emerge after exhaustion of functional reserve, which is indexed by brain size. Arguably, children have less functional brain reserve than adults, in that their brain development is incomplete (e.g., with respect to myelination). Functional brain reserve may be a moderator of the severity of the expression of cerebral disease or insult throughout life (DiSclafani et al., 1998).

Reserve for children may also differ according to brain region. For cortical brain regions, functional representation may be broader in children, so that skill acquisition and skill maintenance are affected by different patterns of injury (Hebb, 1942; Thal et al., 1991). The cerebellum, in contrast, appears to be important for both the acquisition and the maintenance of motor and timing functions (Dennis, Hetherington, et al., 1999). For example, childhood cerebellar lesions produce enduring deficits in short-duration but not long-duration time perception (Hetherington, Dennis, & Spiegler, 1999).

The temporal onset of childhood disorders refers both to the rapidity of onset and to chronological age. In this context, a younger age is often a risk factor rather than a protective factor.

The number of repeated brain insults in children can refer to repetitions of the same insult (e.g., a second head injury, repeated red cell sickling), but also to the secondary effects of a primary insult. Biological reserve can be depleted over time, so that, for instance, repeated episodes of sickling eventually cause irreversible brain damage.

Outcome Algorithm for Children

There does not exist a comparable threshold model for children, although much of the research reviewed in this chapter is relevant to its general characteristics, which are sketched in Figure 1.2. The general idea is that there exists a bar that represents the level of biologi-

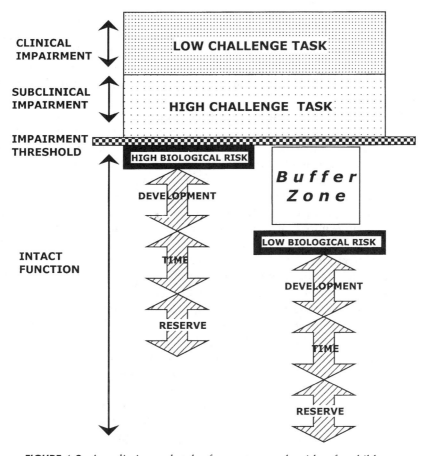

FIGURE 1.2. A preliminary sketch of an outcome algorithm for children.

cal risk as well as a floating threshold for cognitive impairment that is fixed by parameters related to development, time, and reserve.

The first postulate is that a medical condition is associated with higher or lower biological risk, determined by the parameters associated with severity and complications of each condition, and represented by the solid black bars in Figure 1.2. A high biological risk sets the bar within the range of subclinical impairment, because few children with major biological risk escape this level of cognitive morbidity. The two entailments are of the first postulate are as follows: (1) High biological risk involves at least threshold level for subclinical impairment, so that individuals with high biological risk are likely to have difficulties with high-challenge tasks, regardless of the settings of development, time, and reserve; and (2) a proportion of children with low biological risk will have neither clinical nor subclinical impairment.

The second postulate is that moderators of development, time, and reserve take positive or negative values, with the valence representing whether they buffer or exacerbate risk, and the value representing the strength of the valence. Moderators that exacerbate risk take a positive value, whereas those that buffer risk and act as a protective factor take a negative value. Moderators with no influence on cognitive phenotype take a zero value. The entailments of the second postulate are the following: (1) Almost any nonzero value for a moderator will result in placing children with high biological risk in the impairment range; (2) children with high biological risk are unlikely to move far from the impairment range unless they have one or more strong buffers in terms of development, time, or reserve; and (3) outcomes for children with low biological risk are buffered by their low-risk status, so they can tolerate modest elevations in moderator risk without showing measurable neurocognitive impairment.

The third postulate is that moderators make independent contributions to outcome. For example, age at diagnosis and time since treatment make separable contributions to cognitive outcome in radiated medulloblastoma survivors (Dennis, Spiegler, Hetherington, & Greenberg, 1996). One might assume that separable moderators would be additive in their effects, the way they are shown in Figure 1.2; however, this may not be true, or it may be true for some but not all conditions. Research indicates that at least for some conditions, moderators operate differently for children at different degrees of biological risk. To illustrate, cognitive impairments take longer to emerge after lower rather than higher doses of cranial radiation (Moore, Kramer, Wara, Halberg, & Ablin, 1991). Another example relates to interactions between biological and social factors. In children at high biological risk (e.g., those with severe hypoxic–ischemic insult), social variables have little influence, and it is the disorder that constrains the children's responsiveness to social influences; in children with lesser biological risk, by contrast, social factors may be highly salient. It is known that the level of biological risk determines how maternal interactions change social competence (Landry, Smith, Miller-Loncar, & Swank, 1998).

It would be desirable to express the condition–outcome relation as an outcome algorithm, such as a regression equation with beta weights for main effect and interaction terms. The reality is that important elements of the algorithm are only now being identified, and their separate, additive, and interactive weights for the moderator algorithm are largely unknown. For at least some medical conditions, however, we might want to begin sketching the general shape of the algorithm—in pencil, if not in ink.

ACKNOWLEDGMENTS

The writing of this chapter was supported in part by National Institute of Child Health and Human Development Grant No. P01 HD35946, "Spina Bifida: Cognitive and Neurobiological Variability"; by National Institute of Neurological Disorders and Stroke Grant No. 2R01NS 21889-16, "Neurobehavioral Outcome of Head Injury in Children"; and by project grants from the Ontario Mental Health Foundation. Caroline Roncadin, Karen Purvis, and Jennifer Archibald helped shape Figure 1.1, and Susan Inwood assisted in manuscript preparation. I also thank several colleagues for their helpful comments on words (Marcia Barnes, Gerry Taylor) and pictures (Keith Yeates).

REFERENCES

Allen, J. C., & Epstein, F. (1982). Medulloblastoma and other primary malignant neuroectodermal tumors of the CNS: The effect of patients' age and extent of disease on prognosis. *Journal of Neurosurgery, 57*, 446–451.

Anderson, V., & Moore, C. (1995). Age at injury as a predictor of outcome following pediatric head injury: A longitudinal perspective. *Child Neuropsychology, 1*, 187–202.

Anderson, V., Bond, L., Catroppa, C., Grimwood, K., Keir, E., & Nolan, T. (1997). Childhood bacterial meningitis: Impact of age at illness and acute medical complications on long term outcome. *Journal of the International Neuropsychological Society, 3*, 147–158.

Anderson, V., Smibert, E., Ekert, H., & Godber, T. (1994). Intellectual, educational, and behavioral sequelae after cranial irradiation and chemotherapy. *Archives of Disease in Childhood, 70,* 476–483.

Asarnow, R. F., Satz, P., Light, R., Zaucha, K., Lewis, R., & McCleary, C. (1995). The UCLA study of mild closed head injuries in children and adolescents. In S. H. Broman & M. E. Michel (Eds.), *Traumatic head injury in children* (pp. 117–146). New York: Oxford University Press.

Aylward, G. (1992). The relationship between environmental risk and developmental outcome. *Developmental Medicine and Child Neurology, 13,* 222–229.

Balestrini, M. R., Micheli, R., Giordano, L., Lasio, G., & Giombini, S. (1994). Brain tumors with symptomatic onset in the first two years of life. *Child's Nervous System, 10,* 104–110.

Barnes, M. A., & Dennis, M. (1992). Reading in children and adolescents after early-onset hydrocephalus and in normally-developing age peers: Comparison of phonological analysis, word recognition, word comprehension, and passage comprehension skill. *Journal of Pediatric Psychology, 17,* 445–465.

Barnes, M. A., & Dennis, M. (1996). Reading comprehension deficits arise from diverse sources: Evidence from readers with and without developmental brain pathology. In C. Cornoldi & J. A. Oakhill (Eds.), *Reading comprehension difficulties: Processes and intervention* (pp. 251–278). Hillsdale, NJ: Erlbaum.

Barnes, M. A., & Dennis, M. (1998). Discourse after early-onset hydrocephalus: Core deficits in children of average intelligence. *Brain and Language, 61,* 309–334.

Barnes, M. A., Dennis, M., & Wilkinson, M. (1999). Reading after closed head injury in childhood: Effects on accuracy, fluency, and comprehension. *Developmental Neuropsychology, 15,* 1–24.

Barnes, M. A., Faulkner, H., & Dennis, M. (1999). Word recognition speed and reading comprehension in children with spina bifida and hydrocephalus. *Journal of the International Neuropsychological Society, 5,* 149.

Basser, L. S. (1962). Hemiplegia of early onset with special reference to the effects of hemispherectomy. *Brain, 85,* 427–460.

Belman, A. L., Diamond, G., Dickson, D., Horoupian, D., Llena, J., Lantos, G., & Rubinstein, A. (1988). Pediatric acquired immunodeficiency syndrome: Neurological syndromes. *American Journal of Diseases of Children, 142,* 29–35.

Bellinger, D. C. (1995). Interpreting the literature on lead and child development: The neglected role of the "experimental system." *Neurotoxicology and Teratology, 17,* 201–212.

Broome, C. V. (1987). Epidemiology of *Haemophilus influenzae* type b infections in the United States. *Pediatric Infectious Disease Journal, 6,* 779–782.

Brown, R. T., Buchanan, I., Doepke, K., Ekman, J. R., et al. (1993). Cognitive and academic functioning in children with sickle-cell disease. *Journal of Clinical Child Psychology, 22,* 207–218.

Bruce, D. (1995). Pathophysiological responses of the child's brain following trauma. In S. H. Broman & M. E. Michel (Eds.), *Traumatic head injury in children* (pp. 40–51). New York: Oxford University Press.

Carlson-Green, B., Morris, R. D., & Krawiecki, N. (1995). Family and illness predictors of outcome in pediatric brain tumors. *Journal of Pediatric Psychology, 20,* 769–784.

Cohen, B. H., Packer, R. J., Siegal, K. R., Rorke, L. B., D'Angio, G., Sutton, L. N., Bruce, D. A., & Schut, L. (1993). Brain tumors in children under 2 years: Treatment, survival and long-term prognosis. *Pediatric Neurosurgery, 19,* 171–179.

Courchesne, E., Yeung-Courchesne, R., Press, G. A., Hesselink, J. R., & Jernigan, T. (1988). Hypoplasia of cerebellar vermal lobules VI and VII in autism. *New England Journal of Medicine, 318,* 1349–1354.

DeKosky, S. T., Kochanek, P. M., Clark, R. S. B., Ciallella, J. R., & Dixon, C. E. (1998). Secondary injury after head trauma: Subacute and long-term mechanisms. *Seminars in Clinical Neuropsychiatry, 3,* 176–185.

Del Bigio, M. R. (1993). Neuropathological changes caused by hydrocephalus. *Acta Neuropathologia, 85,* 573–585.

Del Bigio, M. R., Kanfer, J. N., & Zhang, Y. W. (1997). Myelination delay in the cerebral white matter of immature rats with kaolin-induced hydrocephalus is reversible. *Journal of Neuropathology and Experimental Neurology, 56,* 1053–1066.

Dennis, M. (1988). Language and the young damaged brain. In T. Boll & B. K. Bryant (Eds.), *Clinical neuropsychology and brain function: Research, measurement, and practice* (Master Lecture Series, Vol. 7, pp. 85–123). Washington, DC: American Psychological Association.

Dennis, M. (1996). Acquired disorders of language in children. In T. E. Feinberg & M. J. Farah (Eds.), *Behavioral neurology and neuropsychology* (pp. 737–754). New York: McGraw-Hill.

Dennis, M., & Barnes, M. (1993). Oral discourse skills in children and adolescents after early-onset hydrocephalus: Linguistic ambiguity, figurative language, speech acts, and script-based inferences. *Journal of Pediatric Psychology, 18,* 639–652.

Dennis, M., & Barnes, M. A. (1994a). Developmental aspects of neuropsychology: Childhood. In D. Zaidel (Ed.), *Handbook of perception and cognition: Vol. 15. Neuropsychology* (pp. 219–246). New York: Academic Press.

Dennis, M., & Barnes, M. A. (1994b). Neuropsychological function in same-sex twins discordant for perinatal brain damage. *Journal of Developmental and Behavioral Pediatrics, 15,* 124–130.

Dennis, M., Barnes, M. A., & Hetherington, C. R. (1999). Congenital hydrocephalus as a model of neurodevelopmental disorder. In H. Tager-Flusberg (Ed.), *Neurodevelopmental disorders: Contribution to a new perspective from the cognitive neurosciences* (pp. 505–532). Cambridge, MA: MIT Press.

Dennis, M., Barnes, M., Hetherington, C. R., Bosloy, J., Wilkinson, M., Drake, J., Gentile, F., Hoffman, H., & Humphreys, R. (1998). Adult survivors of early-onset hydrocephalus: Does mental arithmetic in childhood predict mental arithmetic and functional numeracy in adulthood? *Journal of the International Neuropsychological Society, 4,* 3.

Dennis, M., Fitz, C. R., Netley, C. T., Sugar, J., Harwood-Nash, D. C. F., Hendrick, H. B., Hoffman, H. J., & Humphreys, R. P. (1981). The intelligence of hydrocephalic children. *Archives of Neurology, 38,* 607–715.

Dennis, M., Hendrick, E. B., Hoffman, H. J., & Humphreys, R. P. (1987). Language of hydrocephalic children and adolescents. *Journal of Clinical and Experimental Neuropsychology, 9,* 593–621.

Dennis, M., Hetherington, C. R., & Spiegler, B. J. (1998). Memory and attention after childhood brain tumors. *Medical and Pediatric Oncology, 31,* 25–33.

Dennis, M., Hetherington, C. R., Spiegler, B. J., & Barnes, M. A. (1999). Functional consequences of congenital cerebellar dysmorphologies and acquired cerebellar lesions of childhood. In S. H. Broman & J. M. Fletcher (Eds.), *The changing nervous system: Neurobehavioral consequences of early brain disorders* (pp. 172–198). New York: Oxford University Press.

Dennis, M., Jacennik, B., & Barnes, M. A. (1994). The content of narrative discourse in children and adolescents after early onset hydrocephalus and in normally developing age peers. *Brain and Language, 46,* 129–165.

Dennis, M., Lockyer, L., Lazenby, A. L., Donnelly, R. E., Wilkinson, M., & Schoonheyt, W. (1999). Intelligence patterns among children with high-function autism, phenylketonuria, and childhood head injury. *Journal of Autism and Developmental Disorders, 29,* 5–17.

Dennis, M., Spiegler, B. J., Hetherington, C. R., & Greenberg, M. L. (1996). Neuropsychological sequelae of the treatment of children with medulloblastoma. *Journal of Neuro-Oncology, 29,* 91–101.

DiSclafani, V., Clark, H. W., Tolou-Shamo, M., Bloomer, C. W., Salas, G. A., Norman, D., & Fein, G. (1998). Premorbid brain size is a determinant of functional reserve in abstinent crack-cocaine and crack-cocaine-alcohol-dependent adults. *Journal of the International Neuropsychological Society, 4,* 559–565.

Dobbing, J. (1981). The later development of the brain and its vulnerability. In J. A. Davis & J. Dobbing (Eds.), *Scientific foundations of pediatrics* (pp. 744–759). London: Heinemann.

Duffner, P. K., Cohen, M. E., & Thomas, P. (1983). Late effects of treatment on the intelligence of children with posterior fossa tumors. *Cancer, 51,* 233–237.

Ewing-Cobbs, L., Levin, H. S., Eisenberg, H. M., & Fletcher, J. M. (1987). Language functions following closed-head injury in children and adolescents. *Journal of Clinical and Experimental Neuropsychology, 9,* 575–592.

Fletcher, J. M., McCauley, S. R., Brandt, M. E., Bohan, T. P., Kramer, L. A., Francis, D. J., Thorstad, K., & Brookshire, B. L. (1996). Regional brain tissue composition in children with hydrocephalus. *Archives of Neurology, 53,* 549–557.

Gennarelli, T. A., & Graham, D. I. (1998). Neuropathology of the head injuries. *Seminars in Clinical Neuropsychiatry, 3,* 160–175.

Geyer, J. R., Finlay, J. L., Boyett, J. M., Wisoff, J., Yates, A., Mao, L., & Packer, R. J. (1995). Survival of infants with malignant astrocytomas: A report from the Children's Cancer Group. *Cancer, 75,* 1045–1050.

Gurney, J. G., Severson, R. K., Davis, S., & Robison, L. L. (1995). Incidence of cancer in children in the United States. Sex-, race- and 1 year age-specific rates by histologic type. *Cancer, 75,* 2186–2198.

Hannay, H. J., Fletcher, J. M., & Brandt, M. E. (1999). The role of the corpus callosum in the cognitive development of children with congenital brain malformations. In S. H. Broman & J. M. Fletcher (Eds.), *Neurobehavioral consequences of early brain disorders* (pp. 149–171). New York: Oxford University Press.

Haug, H. (1987). Brain sizes, surfaces, and neuronal sizes of the cortex cerebri: A stereological investigation of man and his variability and a comparison with some mammals (primates, whales, marsupials, insectivores, and one elephant). *American Journal of Anatomy, 180,* 126–142.

Hebb, D. O. (1942). The effect of early and late brain injury upon test scores and the nature of normal adult intelligence. *Proceedings of the American Philosophical Society*, *85*, 275–292.

Hetherington, C. R., & Dennis, M. (1999). Motor function profile in children with early onset hydrocephalus. *Developmental Neuropsychology*, *15*, 25–51.

Hetherington, C. R., Dennis, M., & Spiegler, B. J. (1999). *Perception and estimation of time in long-term survivors of childhood posterior fossa tumors*. Manuscript submitted for publication.

Holmes, C. S., & Richman, L. C. (1985). Cognitive profiles of children with insulin-dependent diabetes. *Journal of Developmental and Behavioral Pediatrics*, *6*, 323–326.

Jacobson, J. L., Jacobson, S. W., & Humphrey, H. E. B. (1990). Effects of in utero exposure to polychlorinated biphenyls on cognitive functioning in young children. *Journal of Pediatrics*, *116*, 38–45.

Kennard, M. A. (1940). Relation of age to motor impairment in man and in subhuman primates. *Archives of Neurology and Psychiatry*, *44*, 377–397.

Kleinman, S. N., & Waber, D. P. (1992). Neurodevelopmental bases of spelling acquisition in children treated for acute lymphoblastic leukaemia. *Cognitive Neuropsychology*, *9*, 403–425.

Kriel, R., Krach, L., & Panser, L. (1989). Closed head injury: Comparison of children younger and older than six years of age. *Pediatric Neurology*, *5*, 296–300.

Kun, L. E., Mulhern, R. K., & Crisco, J. J. (1983). Quality of life in children treated for brain tumors: Intellectual, emotional and academic function. *Journal of Neurosurgery*, *58*, 1–6.

Landry, S. H., Smith, K. E., Miller-Loncar, C. L., & Swank, P. R. (1998). The relation of change in maternal interactive styles to the developing social competence of full-term and pre-term children. *Child Development*, *69*, 105–123.

Lenneberg, E. H. (1967). *Biological foundations of language*. New York: Wiley.

Maria, B. L., Hoang, K. B. N., Tusa, R. J., Mancuso, A. A., Hamed, L. M., Quisling, R. G., Hove, M. T., Fennell, E. B., Booth-Jones, M., Ringdahl, D. M., Yachnis, A. T., Creel, G., & Frerking, B. (1997). "Joubert syndrome" revisited: Key ocular motor signs with magnetic resonance imaging correlation. *Journal of Child Neurology*, *12*, 423–430.

Max, J. E., Roberts, M. A., Koele, S. L., Lindgren, S. D., Robin, D. A., Arndt, S., Smith, W. L., & Sato, Y. (1999). Cognitive outcome in children and adolescents following severe traumatic brain injury: Influence of psychosocial, psychiatric, and injury-related variables. *Journal of the International Neuropsychological Society*, *5*, 58–68.

McKhann, C. F. (1932). Lead poisoning in children: The cerebral manifestations. *Archives of Neurology and Psychiatry*, *27*, 294–298.

Mertsola, J., Kennedy, W. A., Waagner, D., Saez-Llorens, X., Olsen, K., Hansen, E. J., & McCracken, G. H., Jr. (1991). Endotoxin concentrations in cerebrospinal fluid correlated with clinical severity and neurological outcome of *Haemophilus influenzae* type b meningitis. *American Journal of Diseases of Children*, *145*, 1079–1103.

Mildenberger, M., Beach, T. G., McGeer, E. G., & Ludgate, C. M. (1990). An animal model of prophylactic cranial irradiation: Histologic effects at acute, early and delayed stages. *International Journal of Radiation Oncology, Biology, Physics*, *18*, 1051–1060.

Mintz, M., Rapaport, R., Oleska, J. M., Connor, E. M., Koenigsberger, M. R., Denny, T., & Epstein, L. G. (1989). Elevated serum levels of tumor necrosis factor are associated with progressive encephalopathy in children with acquired immunodeficiency syndrome. *American Journal of Diseases of Children*, *143*, 771–774.

Moore, B. D., Ater, J. L., & Copeland, D. R. (1992). Improved neuropsychological outcome of children with brain tumors diagnosed during infancy and treated without cranial irradiation. *Journal of Child Neurology*, *7*, 281–290.

Moore, I. M., Kramer, J. H., Wara, W., Halberg, F., & Ablin, A. R. (1991). Cognitive function in children with leukemia: Effects of radiation dose and time since irradiation. *Cancer*, *68*, 1913–1917.

Murray, J. C., Johnson, J. A., & Bird, T. D. (1985). Dandy–Walker malformation: Etiologic heterogeneity and empiric recurrence risks. *Clinical Genetics*, *28*, 272–283.

Platt, O. (1994). Membrane proteins. In S. H. Embury, R. P. Hebbell, N. Mohandas, & M. H. Seinberg (Eds.), *Sickle cell disease: Basic principles and clinical practice*. New York: Raven Press.

Raimondi, A. J., & Tadanori, T. (1981). Hydrocephalus and tumors: Incidence, clinical picture, and treatment. *Journal of Neurosurgery*, *55*, 174–182.

Reiss, A. L., Freund, L., Plotnick, L., Baumgardner, T., Green, K., Sozer, A. C., Reader, M., Boehm, C., & Denckla, M. B. (1993). The effects of X monosomy on brain development: Monozygotic twins discordant for Turner syndrome. *Annals of Neurology*, *34*, 95–107.

Rodier, P. M. (1994). Vulnerable periods and processes during central nervous system development. *Environmental Health Perspectives*, *102*(Suppl. 2), 121–124.

Rodier, P. M., Ingram, J. L., Tisdale, B., Nelson, S., & Romano, J. (1996). Embryological origin for autism: Developmental anomalies of the cranial nerve motor nuclei. *Journal of Comparative Neurology, 370,* 247–261.

Ross, S. A., Halliday, M. I., Campbell, G. C., Byrnes, D. P., & Rowlands, B. J. (1994). The presence of tumor necrosis factor in CSF and plasma after severe head injury. *British Journal of Neurosurgery, 8,* 419–425.

Rovet, J. F., Ehrlich, R. M., & Hoppe, M. (1988). Specific intellectual deficits in children with early onset diabetes mellitus. *Child Development, 59,* 226–234.

Satz, P. (1993). Brain reserve capacity on symptom onset after brain injury: A formulation and review of evidence for threshold theory. *Neuropsychology, 7,* 273–295.

Sautreaux, J. L., Giroud, M., Dauvergne, M., Nivelon, J. L., & Thierry, A. (1986). Dandy–Walker malformation associated with occipital meningocele and cardiac anomalies: A rare complex embryologic defect. *Journal of Child Neurology, 1,* 64–66.

Schofield, P., Mosesson, R., Stern, Y., & Mayeux, R. (1995). The age at onset of Alzheimer's disease and an intracranial area measurement. *Archives of Neurology, 52,* 95–98.

Schunior, A., Zengel, A. E., Mullenix, P. J., Tarbell, N. J., Howes, A., & Tassinari, M. W. (1990). An animal model to study toxicity of central nervous system therapy for childhood acute lymphoblastic leukemia: Effects on growth and craniofacial proportion. *Cancer Research, 50,* 6461–6465.

Shapiro, E., Balthazor, M., Lockman, L., & Krivit, W. (1997). Memory and dementia in white matter disease. *Journal of the International Neuropsychological Society, 3,* 16.

Silverman, C. L., & Thomas, P. R. M. (1990). Long-term neurologic and intellectual sequelae in brain tumor patients. In M. Deutsch (Ed.), *Management of childhood brain tumors* (pp. 493–500). Boston: Kluwer.

Spiegler, B. J., & Barnes, M. A. (1997). Two different forms of brain injury (ALL and CHI) before age 6 disrupt the acquisition of phonological decoding skills in reading. *Journal of the International Neuropsychological Society, 3,* 62.

Stovring, J., & Snyder, R. (1980). Computed tomography in childhood bacterial meningitis. *Journal of Pediatrics, 96,* 820–823.

Stromland, K., Nordin, V., Miller, M., Akerstrom, B., & Gillberg, C. (1994). Autism in thalidomide embryopathy: A population study. *Developmental Medicine and Child Neurology, 36,* 351–356.

Takeuchi, T. (1968). Pathology of Minamata disease. In *Minamata disease.* Minamata, Japan: Kumamoto University, Study Group of Minamata Disease.

Taylor, H. G., & Alden, J. (1997). Age-related differences in outcome following childhood brain insults: An introduction and overview. *Journal of the International Neuropsychological Society, 3,* 555–567.

Taylor, H. G., Barry, C., & Schatschneider, C. (1993). School-age consequences of *Haemophilus influenzae* type b meningitis. *Journal of Clinical Child Psychology, 22,* 196–206.

Taylor, H. G., Drotar, D., Wade, S., Yeates, K., Stancin, T., & Klein, S. (1995). Recovery from traumatic brain injury in children: The importance of the family. In S. H. Broman & M. E. Michel (Eds.), *Traumatic head injury in children* (pp. 188–216). New York: Oxford University Press.

Taylor, H. G., Mills, E. L., Ciampi, A., DuBerger, R., Watters, G. V., Gold, R., MacDonald, & Michaels, R. H. (1990). Sequelae of *Haemophilus influenzae* meningitis in school age children. *New England Journal of Medicine, 323,* 1657–1663.

Taylor, H. G., & Schatschneider, C. (1992). Child neuropsychological assessment: A test of basic assumptions. *Clinical Neuropsychologist, 6,* 259–275.

Taylor, H. G., Schatschneider, C., & Minich, N. M. (1999). *Longitudinal outcomes of Haemophilus influenzae meningitis in school-age children.* Unpublished manuscript, Case Western Reserve University, Department of Pediatrics.

Thal, D. J., Marchman, V. A., Stiles, J., Aram, D., Trauner, D., Nass, R., & Bates, E. (1991). Early lexical development in children with focal brain injury. *Brain and Language, 40,* 491–527.

Whitley, C. B., Belani, K. G., Chang, P. G., Summers, C. G., Blazar, B. R., Tsai, M. Y., Latchaw, R. E., Ramsay, N. K., & Kersey, J. H. (1993). Long term outcome of Hurler syndrome following bone marrow transplantation. *American Journal of Medical Genetics, 46,* 209–218.

Wright, M., & Nolan, T. (1994). Impact of cyanotic heart disease on school performance. *Archives of Disease in Childhood, 71,* 64–70.

Wrightson, P., McGinn, V., & Gronwall, D. (1995). Mild head injury in preschool children: Evidence that it can be associated with a persisting cognitive defect. *Journal of Neurology, Neurosurgery and Psychiatry, 59,* 375–380.

PART II

Primary Disorders of the Central Nervous System

2

HYDROCEPHALUS

JACK M. FLETCHER
MAUREEN DENNIS
HOPE NORTHRUP

Hydrocephalus is a condition in which the ventricles of the brain fill with cerebrospinal fluid (CSF) and become enlarged. Although hydrocephalus is not a disease entity, it is the final common path of several conditions that have quite specific effects on the brain. Hydrocephalus can occur at any age: In an adult, it may be associated with dementia-like conditions; in either a child or an adult, it may be associated with trauma, infections, or tumors of the brain. In all these conditions of *acquired* hydrocephalus, the age of onset will vary unsystematically, so hydrocephalus is a secondary phenomenon that is less important in determining functional outcome than is the primary traumatic, infectious, or neoplastic disorder.

In this chapter we are concerned with *early-onset* hydrocephalus, involving children in whom hydrocephalus has been identified and treated before the first birthday, often within the first days of life. The principal etiologies of early-onset hydrocephalus involve such congenital and perinatal disorders as neural tube defects (spina bifida meningomyelocele); Dandy–Walker syndrome (DWS); aqueductal stenosis (AS); and intraventricular hemorrhage (IVH), which occurs during the perinatal period in premature infants as a complication of hypoxic–ischemic encephalopathy. In these four etiologies, which have in common an early onset of hydrocephalus, the presence of hydrocephalus, its treatment, and its neurobehavioral sequelae are major factors in the development of both brain structure and cognitive function.

Early-onset disorders that affect how the brain develops provide an opportunity to study how perturbations of the brain early in life affect the development of functional outcome domains, such as those involved in motor, visual–spatial, and perceptual skills; attention and memory; language and discourse; and behavior. For a given disorder, there are three steps involved in relating brain structure to functional outcome: identification of the prototypical outcome in each of several functional domains, analysis of the sources of variability in outcome domains, and relating outcome variability in a principled manner to structural anomalies of brain development.

Over the last decade, neuropsychological studies have identified the major outcome domains affected by early-onset hydrocephalus, and have provided a picture of the prototypical impairments in children with this condition. This chapter is therefore concerned with the second and third questions posed above. We are particularly concerned with the second question—analysis of the sources of variability in outcome domains—but we also address the question of behavior–brain relationships. This discussion is preceded by a brief review of the epidemiology, pathophysiology, and neuropathology of the four classic etiologies of early hydrocephalus. Specific outcome domains are then reviewed, followed by a consideration of different influences on outcomes.

DETECTION, EPIDEMIOLOGY, PATHOPHYSIOLOGY, AND NEUROPATHOLOGY

Detection

Congenital and perinatal forms of hydrocephalus are usually detected before, at, or shortly after birth. Spina bifida meningomyelocele, DWS, and AS represent congenital problems that occur during the first trimester of gestation. There are important differences in embryological timing and neuropathology among these three congenital etiologies of hydrocephalus. In spina bifida meningomyelocele, the spinal dysraphism present at birth usually indicates the presence of a brain malformation involving the cerebellum and hindbrain (Arnold–Chiari II or ACII) as a result of a prolonged disruption of neuroembryogenesis during the first trimester (Barkovich, 1995). Hydrocephalus is typically detected shortly after birth and occurs because the ACII malformation obstructs the flow of CSF. AS and DWS are usually detected because of rapid expansion of head size in infancy to accommodate the increase in CSF pressure. In AS, obstruction is due to the narrowing of the aqueduct of Sylvius, while the cerebellar malformation and cyst characteristic of DWS leads to hydrocephalus in these children. The cerebellar malformation also leads to problems with head control in infants with DWS, resulting in detection of hydrocephalus (Tal, Freigang, Dunn, Durity, & Moyes, 1980). Children born prematurely with low birthweight may develop hydrocephalus in the perinatal period that is identified through ultrasonography of the brain, routinely completed on high-risk infants. In these cases hydrocephalus is due to IVH involving the germinal matrix, which, if sufficiently severe, leads to obstruction of CSF.

Epidemiology and Neuroembryology

It is not possible to provide estimates of the prevalence of hydrocephalus independent of specific etiologies, although figures for specific etiologies are available. Neural tube defects occur in approximately 1–2 cases per 1,000 live births in North America. Spina bifida meningomyelocele, the most common neural tube defect compatible with survival, occurs at a rate of 0.5–1.0 per 1,000 births. Spina bifida meningomyelocele is characterized by malformations of both spine and brain. The spinal dysraphism involves protrusion of the spinal cord and meninges through a defect in the spine at any point along the spinal column. The level of the spinal lesion affects functioning; at low levels, it can lead to paralysis of the lower extremities, incontinence, and other abnormalities of the body. Most children with spina bifida meningomyelocele have the ACII malformation, involving the herniation of a compressed cerebellum through the exits of the fourth ventricle, and causing obstruction of the flow of CSF in the fourth and/or third ventricles. Hydrocephalus occurs in some 80–90% of children with spina bifida meningomyelocele (Reigel & Rotenstein, 1994). Partial agenesis of the corpus callosum is commonly observed in children with spina bifida meningomyelocele, representing a congenital defect that occurs as a result of the disruption in neuroembryogenesis characteristic of neural tube defects (Barkovich, 1995).

DWS is quite rare, occurring in about 1 individual per 30,000 live births. About 70–80% of children with DWS develop hydrocephalus. The primary defining characteristic of DWS is the presence of a large cystic fourth ventricle with partial to complete agenesis of the cerebellar vermis. The posterior fossa is enlarged with substantial dilation of the fourth ventricle. Partial agenesis of the corpus callosum is common (Chuang, 1986).

AS occurs somewhat later in gestation. Children with AS develop hydrocephalus because of a congenital narrowing of the cerebral aqueduct (Barkovich, 1995; Robertson, Leggate, Miller, & Stears, 1990). AS occurs in approximately 0.5 per 1,000 live births and is generally observed only in the presence of hydrocephalus. In contrast to spina bifida meningomyelocele and DWS, the cerebellum is generally normal, although some downward extension of the cerebellum may be present because of pressure effects from hydrocephalus.

Children with IVH develop hydrocephalus because of a hemorrhage of the germinal matrix shortly after birth. The presence of IVH is clearly related to perinatal asphyxia, with the hemorrhage occurring as part of a complex sequence of events involving problems with cerebral blood flow and perfusion. The circulatory problems that lead to IVH are also associated with ischemic lesions in the white matter around the ventricles (periventricular leukomalacia), leading to bilateral loss of periventricular white matter (Volpe, 1994). In terms of hydrocephalus, the germinal matrix hemorrhage bleeds into the ventricles and can obstruct the flow of CSF. Shunting is sometimes necessary, but arrested hydrocephalus is a more common outcome in children with IVH. In arrested cases, it is often possible to control the flow of CSF with medications (e.g., diuretics) that reduce the volume of CSF. Shunting is typically reserved for those cases where the progression of hydrocephalus becomes so severe that the balance of production and absorption of CSF cannot be restored. Although IVH was once estimated to occur in about half of all preterm infants, the incidence has been declining dramatically, and it now occurs in only 20% of premature infants (Volpe, 1994). Even in these cases, the need to shunt now occurs infrequently and largely in association with other severe complications of prematurity.

Pathophysiology and Neuropathology

Although these four etiologies have in common the effects of hydrocephalus, particularly when shunting occurs, each condition has characteristic pathophysiological and neuropathological features. Regardless of etiology, hydrocephalus is always due to an obstruction that blocks the flow of CSF (Raimondi, 1994). The site of the blockage varies, depending in part on the etiology. In addition, the hydrocephalus may be progressive or arrested. *Progressive* hydrocephalus often requires aggressive neurosurgical intervention, such as the insertion of a shunt to divert the flow of CSF around the obstruction. *Arrested* hydrocephalus, also referred to as *compensated* or *nonprogressive* hydrocephalus, indicates the presence of large ventricles with pressure effects from accumulation of CSF. In arrested hydrocephalus, the relationship of CSF production and absorption is perturbed but then becomes balanced, leaving residual dilation of the ventricles, or ventriculomegaly (McCullough, 1990).

Early hydrocephalus has significant consequences for brain development (Del Bigio, 1993). The compressive effects of hydrocephalus are similar across etiologies, leading to major changes in the midbrain that are influenced primarily by severity of the condition (Raimondi, 1994). Congenital hydrocephalus also has features that are etiology-specific and that may lead to additional variability in outcomes. Table 2.1 summarizes the defining neuropathology of each of the major etiologies, and lists the commonly occurring features. As is evident in this table, there is some variability in neuropathology, but certain features are shared across etiologies (either because of primary defect or because of associated pathology).

As Table 2.1 also shows, children with congenital and perinatal hydrocephalus often have other malformations of the brain. Partial agenesis of the corpus callosum is common in all congenital forms of hydrocephalus (Barkovich, 1995). Even when all portions of the corpus callosum are present, this structure may be thinned and stretched (i.e., hypoplastic) due to the effects of hydrocephalus. The extent to which the corpus callosum is abnormal varies across cases. Cerebellar and posterior fossa abnormalities are also common in children with spina bifida meningomyelocele and DWS. The cerebellum is often displaced or shows partial agenesis, and may extend downward through the fourth ventricle. The degree and type of cerebellar dysmorphism vary within and between etiologies. The effects on the brain can include thinning of the corpus callosum, compression of the diencephalon, defects of the optic pathways, and rearrangement of the cortical architecture of the midbrain. Other pathophysiological features, such as polygyria, heterotopias, and abnormalities of the tectum and medulla, occur across etiologies and vary among children within etiologies. Finally, the brain as a whole may show reduction in the thickness of the cortical mantle, reduced overall brain mass, and selective thinning of brain areas, particularly in posterior regions (Dennis et al., 1981). Hence these three etiologies of early-onset hydrocephalus are distinct, but they also share certain pathologies.

Children with hydrocephalus due to IVH sustain additional insult to the brain because of hypoxic–ischemic encephalopathy associated with prematurity. Other brain lesions,

TABLE 2.1. Summary of Major Core and Associated Neuropathologies Associated with Different Etiologies of Early Hydrocephalus

Etiology	Disorder of:	Core neuropathology	Associated neuropathology
Spina bifida meningomyelocele	Neuroembryogenesis	Cerebellar deformation Cerebellar tonsil herniation Elongation of pons and medulla	Callosal agenesis Tectum stretched ("beaking") Aqueduct stretched
Dandy–Walker syndrome (DWS)	Neuroembryogenesis	Agenesis of cerebellar vermis Large cystic fourth ventricle	Callosal agenesis
Aqueductal stenosis (AS)	Neuroembryogenesis	Focal reduction in aqueduct Tectum stretched ("beaking")	Callosal agenesis Fusion of quadrigeminal body
Intraventricular hemorrhage (IVH)	Germinal matrix	Periventricular axonal and myelin damage	Periventricular leukomalacia Intraparenchymal bleeds Callosal hypoplasia

particularly periventricular leukomalacia, can be observed as a consequence of early hypoxic injury. Most effects on the brain are due to the hemorrhage, to the underlying pathophysiological factors producing the hemorrhage, and to the effects of ventricular expansion and pressure.

Figure 2.1 illustrates the varying morphological appearances of the brains of children with hydrocephalus, with four midsagittal slices from magnetic resonance imaging (MRI) scans. The scans depict a normal child (upper left panel) and children with spina bifida meningomyolocele (lower left panel), AS (upper right panel), and IVH (lower right panel). The image of the child with spina bifida meningomyelocele shows the changes in the cerebellum and hindbrain forming the ACII deformation. In addition, this scan shows partial agenesis of the corpus callosum, dilation of the third ventricle, and interdigitation of the gyri of the brain, which are often observed in children with spina bifida meningomyelocele. The primary defects apparent in the scan of the child with AS are partial agenesis of the corpus callosum and dilation of the third ventricle. Finally, the scan for the child with IVH shows very severe hydrocephalus in the third and fourth ventricles, hypoplasia of the corpus callosum, and periventricular leukomalacia. Periventricular leukomalacia is represented as the dark shading in the region around the third ventricle.

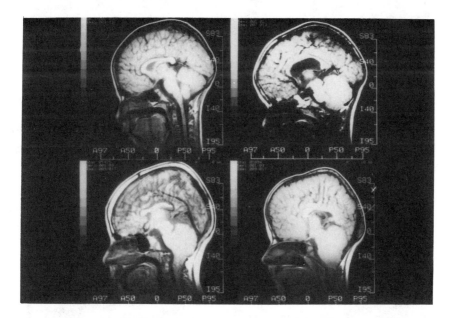

FIGURE 2.1. Midsagittal slices from MRI scans of school-age children. The upper left panel is a scan of a normal child. The upper right panel is a scan of a child with aqueductal stenosis showing partial agenesis of the corpus callosum and ventricular dilation. The lower left panel is a scan of a child with spina bifida meningomyelocele, showing abnormalities of the hindbrain and cerebellum (ACII malformation), partial agenesis of the corpus callosum, and dilation of the third ventricle. The lower right panel is a scan of a child born prematurely with IVH, showing hypoplasia (thinning) of the corpus callosum and ventricular dilation. The bright spots around the ventricle are areas of periventricular leukomalacia. All three of the children with hydrocephalus had average or above-average Verbal IQ scores and significantly lower Performance IQ scores. From Fletcher, Brookshire, Bohan, Brandt, and Davidson (1995, p. 211). Copyright 1995 by The Guilford Press. Reprinted by permission.

Figure 2.2 shows a 3-D reconstructed MRI image of a child with DWS. The gross malformations of the cerebellum are apparent. This child also has significant dilation of the fourth ventricle and partial agenesis of the corpus callosum.

EVALUATION OF NEUROBEHAVIORAL OUTCOMES OF HYDROCEPHALUS

General Considerations in Outcome Research

In the present context, the term *outcome* refers to a child's functional status in a particular area that has relevance to his or her overall adaptation. Neuropsychologists subdivide these domains into areas that would be the subject of some form of assessment, such as motor, visual–motor, and spatial abilities; language and academic skills; memory; attention; executive functions; and behavior. Research on many neurological disorders has been conducted within each of these broad and overlapping outcome domains. This research varies in quality, as well as in sample composition and methods for assessing outcomes. Group

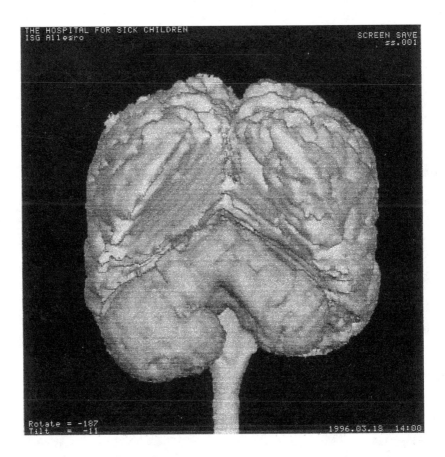

FIGURE 2.2. Reconstructed 3-D coronal MRI slice of a child with Dandy–Walker syndrome. The image is designed to highlight the significant malformation of the cerebellum. The child's brain, from which this image was made, also has hydrocephalus and partial agenesis of the corpus callosum, which cannot be seen on this image.

means are usually reported in summarizing outcome domains for special populations, together with estimates of variability around the mean. Differing factors explain outcome variability. Some of these factors are not specific to any particular population (e.g., how well the outcome domain has been measured, sampling, and other measurement factors). Other factors may be specific to the population under study.

With respect to hydrocephalus, it is useful to conceptualize neuropsychological functions in terms of a set of outcome domains. Here, however, variability in outcomes needs to be considered in relation not only to sampling and measurement issues, but also to a set of factors distinctive to the hydrocephalic condition. The latter factors include the etiology, neuropathology, treatment, and medical sequelae of hydrocephalus, as well as the environmental context in which development occurs. The goal is to understand how a specific outcome varies as a function of each of these factors.

Beginning with early reviews by Anderson (1975) and others, the literature on outcomes of hydrocephalus has developed to a point where a *general* description of sequelae in each of several outcome domains is possible (Dennis, 1996). Unfortunately, however, these descriptions continue to be limited in large part to children with spina bifida (Wills, 1993). Another problem with the existing research literature is that samples are typically made up of children with different types of spinal lesions, ranging from meningomyelocele to less severe forms of spinal dysraphism (meningocele). In addition, the status of hydrocephalus is often inadequately addressed or not specified; for example, shunted cases are often combined with arrested cases. References to children with spina bifida and no hydrocephalus are commonly made, but it is apparent from neuroimaging studies that some children with spina bifida have arrested hydrocephalus that was never documented because the hydrocephalus was nonsymptomatic (Fletcher, Brookshire, Bohan, Brandt, & Davidson, 1995). Studies of children with IVH are also fairly common (Fletcher, Levin, & Landry, 1984; Fletcher et al., 1997; Landry et al., 1984; Landry, Chapieski, Fletcher, & Denson, 1988; Landry, Fletcher, Denson, & Chapieski, 1993). However, few studies have addressed outcomes in children with rarer etiologies, such as AS and DWS.

Another limitation is that many of the studies involve relatively small samples. Outcomes tend to be quite variable in hydrocephalus populations, and firm conclusions regarding disease sequelae are precluded by inconsistent findings. Furthermore, the probability of Type II errors may be high because of low power for statistical comparisons (Schmidt, 1996). In one recent paper, the power issue has been addressed by using a methodology of sample-to-population inference with 95% confidence limits (Hetherington & Dennis, 1999).

Information about specific outcome domains associated with early hydrocephalus has been covered in several recent reviews, which summarize what is known about this condition (Baron, Fennell, & Voeller, 1995; Dennis, 1996; Dennis, Barnes, & Hetherington, 1999; Fletcher & Levin, 1988; Fletcher, Levin, & Butler, 1995; Wills, 1993). This section of the chapter considers some of the core conceptual and methodological issues, many of which arise from what is not known. These issues affect how research on children with hydrocephalus is and will be conducted.

The Importance of Studies of Variability in Outcomes

The existence of significant variability within outcome domains means that studies of averaged performance scores are of limited value in understanding neuropsychological outcomes associated with early hydrocephalus. A test average fails to provide any basis for cognitive remediation, even for the "average" child with hydrocephalus, who is probably nonexistent. Moving beyond depictions of averages toward understanding the sources of variability in outcomes is more likely to enhance the relationship between research and practice, and to have more direct application to individual children with hydrocephalus.

Psychometric IQ Scores: An Example of Variability

Studies comparing verbal and nonverbal psychometric intelligence in children with hydrocephalus show significantly lower *average* scores on performance-based measures than on verbal measures (Dennis et al., 1981; Donders, Canady, & Rourke, 1990; Fletcher, Francis, et al., 1992; Riva et al., 1994; Wills, 1993). However, the literature on psychometric IQ test scores clearly illustrates some of the difficulties associated with neurobehavioral research on children with hydrocephalus. The substantial literature that documents lower nonverbal IQ scores compared to verbal IQ scores reveals substantial variability in the number of children with shunted hydrocephalus who show these discrepancies, as well as in the probability that an individual child will reliably show this discrepancy over time. Researchers thus need to consider two types of variability: *longitudinal variability*, or stability in the same individuals over time; and *concurrent variability*, which occurs as a function of factors associated with hydrocephalus when the subject is assessed at a single time point.

Longitudinal Variability

Longitudinal variability has been studied by Brookshire, Fletcher, Bohan, Landry, Davidson, and Francis (1995). Children with shunted hydrocephalus ($n = 26$), arrested hydrocephalus ($n = 11$), and no hydrocephalus ($n = 28$) received multiple assessments of verbal and nonverbal intellectual and cognitive skills over a 5-year period, beginning when the children were 5 to 7 years of age. Longitudinal evaluations of performance were obtained on the McCarthy Scales of Children's Abilities (McCarthy, 1972), the Wechsler Intelligence Scale for Children—Revised (WISC-R; Wechsler, 1974), and composite measures of verbal and nonverbal neuropsychological skills. The verbal composite was created by averaging scores on measures of fluency and automaticity of speech (Controlled Oral Word Association; Gaddes & Crockett, 1975), Rapid Automatized Naming (Denckla & Rudel, 1974), phonological awareness (Auditory Analysis Test; Rosner & Simon, 1971), and semantics (the Vocabulary, Opposite Analogies, and Fluency subtests of the McCarthy Scales). The nonverbal composite was created by averaging scores on a visual–spatial task that minimized motor demands, the Judgment of Line Orientation Test (Lindgren & Benton, 1980), and a perceptual–motor task, the Developmental Test of Visual–Motor Integration (Beery, 1982).

Over three to four longitudinal time points, each separated by 1 to 2 years, children with shunted hydrocephalus had significantly lower nonverbal than verbal scores at each time point and on all three sets of measures. Children with arrested hydrocephalus and those without hydrocephalus did not show significant verbal–nonverbal discrepancies. Of particular interest, the children with shunted hydrocephalus had comparable levels of impairment on the motor-free and motor-based tasks, suggesting that their poorer nonverbal scores were not due to concomitant motor deficits.

Examination of Verbal–Performance discrepancies on the WISC-R within and across each of three longitudinal time points revealed that from 27% to 42% of the children with shunted hydrocephalus exhibited a statistically significant ($p < .05$) Verbal–Performance discrepancy (Performance IQ $\leq$ Verbal IQ by 12 or more points). However, only 35% of children with shunted hydrocephalus obtained a Performance IQ that was 12 points below

Verbal IQ on more than one occasion. The variability in rates of discrepancies in this group over time is easily explained in terms of variations in children's scores around the cutting score of 12 points. The effects of regression to the mean, which would tend to deflate more extreme discrepancies in multiple comparisons over time, may have been another contributing factor. Nonetheless, no more than 42% of children exhibited a statistically significant discrepancy at any single time point. At each time point, most children had Performance IQ scores that were either below or comparable with Verbal IQ scores; few had Performance IQ scores significantly higher than Verbal IQ scores. These results indicate that the group averages (which for many studies suggest lower Performance IQ scores than Verbal IQ scores) actually characterize less than half the sample of children with shunted hydrocephalus, and that this pattern varies over time. The critical question is how to explain this variability in outcomes.

Concurrent Variability

A number of studies have examined WISC-R Verbal IQ and Performance IQ scores in relation to the nature and extent of hydrocephalus (Dennis et al., 1981; Wills, 1993). These investigations have been somewhat limited because of small sample sizes. Nonetheless, lower Performance IQ scores have been associated with the presence of ocular–motor deficits, seizures, and ambulation problems in children with hydrocephalus (Dennis et al., 1981). In addition, the presence of lower Performance IQ than Verbal IQ scores has been related to asymmetrical anterior–posterior brain thinning in children with hydrocephalus (Dennis et al., 1981; Fletcher, McCauley, et al., 1996). The children in these studies with larger Performance–Verbal IQ discrepancies (Performance IQ < Verbal IQ) showed proportionately greater brain thinning in posterior brain regions relative to anterior brain regions. Children with smaller Performance–Verbal IQ discrepancies had proportionate anterior–posterior thinning. Finally, area measurements of the corpus callosum from MRI were more highly correlated with Performance IQ than with Verbal IQ (Fletcher, Bohan, et al., 1992, 1996). These several studies provide examples of associations of disease-related factors to concurrent intellectual outcomes.

SUMMARY OF RECENT FINDINGS BY OUTCOME DOMAIN

Several studies conducted in the past 5–10 years have attended to the above-noted methodological requirements and therefore represent more contemporary applications of cognitive neuroscience to developmental disorders involving hydrocephalus. These more recent studies are reviewed below. When possible, comparisons across the four etiologies of hydrocephalus are highlighted, and emphasis is placed on attempts to explain variability in outcomes in terms of the nature of hydrocephalus; CSF factors; and other disease, subject, and environmental variables.

Motor Domain

Children with early-onset hydrocephalus have difficulties with a wide range of motor skills. Both gross and fine motor abilities are poorly developed in relation to age expectations. Motor problems, moreover, occur across the etiological groups associated with early hydrocephalus.

Gross motor deficits would be expected in many children with spina bifida meningomyelocele, who have paraparesis in the lower limbs because of the spinal lesion (Anderson & Plewis, 1977). The paraparesis results in limited ambulation (often with use of leg braces or other assistive devices) or complete paraplegia (with use of wheelchairs). However, both ambulatory and nonambulatory children exhibit significant impairment on a tests of gross motor function (standard scores < 2 on scales with $M = 10$, $SD = 3$; Hetherington & Dennis, 1999). Congruent with the idea that the level of the spinal lesion per se does not determine gross motor function, gait abnormalities are extremely common in various etiological groups, occurring in 92% of children with spina bifida meningomyelocele, 36% of children with AS, and 44% of children with IVH (Fletcher, Brookshire, et al., 1995).

Fine motor skills are often deficient, in the form of upper limb and hand incoordination. Most commonly observed in children with spina bifida meningomyelocele, these fine motor deficits include both speed and dexterity limitations (Anderson & Plewis, 1977; Fletcher, Brookshire, et al., 1995; Zeiner, Prigitano, Pollay, Briscoe, & Smith, 1985). Like gross motor deficits, fine motor deficits are not restricted to a single etiology. Fletcher, Brookshire, et al. (1995) found that group means on tests of these skills fell at least two standard deviations below those of similar-age peers for children in each of three etiological groups (spina bifida meningomyelocele, IVH, and AS), with a strong trend for children with AS to have better fine motor skills than children in the other two groups.

A recent study by Hetherington and Dennis (1999) compared motor function in 42 children with hydrocephalus arising from four etiologies. Two etiologies were congenital, arising in the first trimester of gestation (spina bifida meningomyelocele, AS), and two arose from events in early postnatal development, typically shortly after birth (IVH, infections/adhesions of the brain). All children in the sample had a Verbal IQ and/or Performance IQ of 70 or above on the age-appropriate Wechsler scale. Four different motor domains were tested: balance, coordination, and kinesthetic integration; fine motor control and manual dexterity; persistence and smooth motor control; and motor strength. The results of this study supported the view that many different motor functions are disrupted in children with early-onset hydrocephalus. Motor skills were poor in all domains tested, and mean performance was between one and three standard deviations below the mean for normally developing children in the standardization sample. Motor skills were so poor, in fact, that the upper limit of 95% confidence intervals fell below one standard deviation of the mean for normally developing children on 9 of 10 subtests.

Various sociodemographic and medical factors have been shown to be correlated with motor outcome (Wills, 1993). In studies of the developmental consequences of hydrocephalus, it is clearly valuable to examine differences in motor skills as a function of some of these factors. Hetherington and Dennis (1999) found that handedness, gender, and seizures appeared to be weakly related to some motor functions, but independent effects of these variables could not be determined, given the limitations in sample size. Large samples of individuals with early-onset hydrocephalus are required to evaluate the independent and additive effects of demographic factors, factors related to the spinal lesion, and other medical sequelae.

Although children with each etiology of hydrocephalus tested thus far have shown some motor deficits, differences in motor profiles between etiological groups require further clarification. In the Hetherington and Dennis (1999) study, multivariate analyses demonstrated that the profiles of motor functions differed significantly between the congenital and infantile-onset groups, and that a test of gross motor skill (standing balance) contributed most to this difference. Evaluation of differences in motor function related to the etiology of hydrocephalus requires larger samples than have been studied to date, especially for low-incidence etiologies such as DWS and AS.

Hydrocephalus affects the development of many brain regions important for motor function, from the cerebellum and midbrain to the motor cortex. Etiology is only a marker for these different types of developmental neuropathology. Because motor deficits may arise from different neural substrates in children with hydrocephalus, it will be important in future studies to relate motor function to patterns of pathology evident in brain neuroimaging, and to make comparisons both within and across etiologies.

Visual–Motor and Spatial Outcomes

Children with hydrocephalus have problems with visual–motor and spatial ability (Dennis et al., 1981; Fletcher, Francis, et al., 1992; Fletcher, Brookshire, et al., 1995)—both on tasks that require constructional performance and on tests that minimize motor demands, such as the Judgment of Line Orientation Test (Lindgren & Benton, 1980). Differences in these outcomes between etiological groups are not readily apparent. For example, Fletcher, Brookshire, et al. (1995) compared children with hydrocephalus due to spina bifida meningomyelocele, AS, and IVH on the different subtests of the Test of Visual-Perceptual Skills (Gardner, 1988). Children with hydrocephalus showed preserved abilities on measures of facial recognition, simple visual discrimination, and spatial relationships, particularly when stimuli were presented in a matching-to-sample format. Much greater impairment was evident on complex visual–spatial tasks involving form consistency, figure–ground relationships, spatial memory, and the location of stimuli in external space. These differential effects of hydrocephalus on various aspects of spatial function did not vary across etiological groups.

Several recent studies have highlighted relationships between measures of the integrity of the central nervous system in children with early hydrocephalus and performance on nonverbal tasks. Fletcher, Bohan, et al. (1992) obtained assessments of verbal and nonverbal skills in children with shunted hydrocephalus due to AS and spina bifida meningomyelocele. The sample also included children with arrested hydrocephalus and normal controls. MRI was conducted as part of the assessment procedures and served as the basis for quantitative evaluations of the areas of the corpus callosum, internal capsules, and centrum semiovale. The volumes of the lateral ventricles in both hemispheres were also measured. For the sample as a whole, significant correlations of the verbal and nonverbal cognitive assessments with MRI measures of the cross-sectional area of the corpus callosum were observed. However, the relationship was stronger for nonverbal skills and within the group with shunted hydrocephalus. The nonverbal measures also correlated with the volume of the right ventricle (but not with the volume of the left ventricle) and with the area of the right and left internal capsules. This initial study documented robust relationships of nonverbal cognitive skills to measurements reflecting the effects of hydrocephalus on the brain.

Fletcher, Bohan, et al. (1996) subsequently replicated the findings showing a relationship between test performance and measures of the corpus callosum. The latter study included a much larger sample of children with shunted hydrocephalus (n = 42) due to AS, spina bifida meningomyelocele, and IVH, along with children with arrested hydrocephalus (n = 19), patient controls with no hydrocephalus (n = 23), and a normal, nonpatient comparison group (n = 15). As in the study by Fletcher, Bohan, et al. (1992), the area measurement of the corpus callosum was smaller in the group with shunted hydrocephalus than in the other groups. The group with shunted hydrocephalus also had larger lateral ventricle volumes and smaller internal capsule areas in both hemispheres. The correlations between measures of the corpus callosum and test performance were significant for assessments of both verbal and nonverbal cognitive skills, but the relation remained more robust for tests of nonverbal cognitive skills. No significant relationships were found for measures in the domain of executive functions. However, the corpus callosum measure did correlate significantly with a measure of motor dexterity (Grooved Pegboard Test). The latter measure also correlated significantly with lateral ventricle assessments. The internal capsule correlations were not significant in this sample, which was larger and more heterogeneous than the sample examined by Fletcher, Bohan, et al. (1992). Together, these two studies provide strong support for a relationship between the size of the corpus callosum and nonverbal cognitive and motor skills.

Other neuroimaging studies have identified potential factors that influence nonverbal cognitive skills in children with shunted hydrocephalus. When hydrocephalus occurs, the ventricles expand in a posterior-to-anterior direction, and cerebral white matter is damaged. Due to these factors, the posterior regions of the brain may be particularly susceptible to insult. Early studies that utilized air encephalograms (AEGs) found that global measures of intelligence were related to the thickness of the cortical mantle before and after treatment (Young, Nulsen, Weiss, & Thomas, 1973). Using the same AEG/ventriculogram technology, Dennis et al. (1981) examined regional patterns of cortical mantle thinning based on radiological review in a group of children with classic etiologies of shunted hydrocephalus. Those children with hydrocephalus who showed proportionately greater thinning of posterior brain regions relative to anterior brain regions had lower nonverbal IQ scores than verbal IQ scores. In contrast, children with proportionate anterior–posterior thinning had comparable verbal and nonverbal IQ scores.

Using quantitative measures from MRI, Fletcher, McCauley, et al. (1996) obtained similar findings. In this study, children with hydrocephalus were separated according to quantitative assessment of the distribution of CSF in anterior and posterior brain regions. Those with proportionately greater amounts of CSF in posterior than in anterior brain regions had much lower nonverbal and motor skill performance than did children with proportionate amounts of CSF in posterior and anterior brain regions. Correlations with the measure of anterior–posterior CSF distribution were significant for the Grooved Pegboard Test. Although the language composite described by Brookshire, Fletcher, Bohan, and Landry (1995) was only weakly related to the CSF index, this index was robustly and significantly correlated with a composite measure of visual–spatial skill.

In summary, recent studies that have incorporated current neuroimaging technology demonstrate relationships between measures of cerebral white matter integrity and nonverbal cognitive and motor skills, as well as more pervasive consequences of hydrocephalus. The variability in outcomes appears to be related to the size of the corpus callosum, and also to more global morphometric assessments of the long-observed effects of hydrocephalus on the brain.

Language, Discourse, and Reading Comprehension

Results from several recent studies of the language characteristics of children and adolescents with hydrocephalus indicate that language structure appears better preserved than language content. In an earlier, systematic study of language development in hydrocephalic children, Dennis, Hendrick, Hoffman, and Humphreys (1987) employed language tests from five different component areas (word finding, fluency and automaticity of speech, sentence memory, grammar, and metalinguistic awareness). These tests were administered to 75 hydrocephalic children and 50 normal controls. Performance of the two groups, particularly in fluency and automaticity of speech, sentence memory, and metalinguistic awareness, was quite comparable. The most consistent differences in language development occurred on tests measuring the children's ability to understand complex grammatical relationships; the children with hydrocephalus were consistently slower than the controls in comprehending grammatical structures. Another common problem was word finding in context, which was linked to intraventricular but not extraventricular hydrocephalus. A spina bifida etiology was also associated with impaired overall fluency in rapid word finding.

In a more recent study, Brookshire, Fletcher, Bohan, and Landry (1995) compared children with shunted hydrocephalus due to spina bifida, IVH, and AS to children with arrested or no hydrocephalus with spina bifida and IVH, as well as to neurologically normal children. The areas assessed included phonological awareness skills, semantic language ability, fluency and automaticity, and word-finding abilities. The children with shunted hydrocephalus had significantly lower scores in each of these domains. The etiology of shunted hydrocephalus was not significantly related to outcome, but there were only seven children with AS. An interesting pattern emerged, particularly when the sample was expanded and the data were reanalyzed (Fletcher, Brookshire, et al., 1995). Children with AS had phonological awareness, semantic, and word-finding skills that were, on average, comparable to those of normal controls; however, the group with AS had a significant deficit on a measure of rapid automatized naming. On this test, the level of performance for the group with AS was similar to that for children with hydrocephalus due to IVH or spina bifida. The latter finding suggests that a deficit in the rapid recruitment of words from semantic memory may be consistently associated with hydrocephalus, regardless of how the hydrocephalus arises. There was little difference in language outcomes for children whose shunted hydrocephalus was due to IVH as compared to spina bifida. However, Brookshire, Fletcher, Bohan, and Landry (1995) found a clear trend for children with spina bifida to have the poorest outcomes across all domains.

The profile of preserved and impaired language skills in children with hydrocephalus requires further evaluation. For now, what is important is evidence for variability in outcomes. In general, the Texas cohorts evaluated by Fletcher and associates (Fletcher, Brookshire, et al., 1995; Brookshire, Fletcher, & Landry, 1995) performed at much lower levels on these language measures than the Toronto cohort (Dennis et al., 1987); these findings suggest a possible geographic variation in outcomes, particularly for the children with spina bifida. Further study of factors contributing to this variability may provide insights on ways to influence language outcomes.

Despite this variability, rapid and accurate word finding may be a consistent problem area for many children with hydrocephalus. Recent studies of discourse, for example, show that children with several etiologies of early hydrocephalus have problems in conveying semantic content in a clear and economical manner (Barnes & Dennis, 1998; Dennis & Barnes, 1993; Dennis, Jacennik, & Barnes, 1994). Using a story-retelling format, the latter investigations found that children with hydrocephalus produced oral language that was less coherent and cohesive than the discourse production of controls. The children with hydrocephalus also communicated less of the actual content of the story, and their narratives included more ambiguous material and were more convoluted and verbose. The problems in language usage exhibited by the children with hydrocephalus involved semantic–pragmatic functions and world knowledge, and were probably cognitively derived.

Consistent with this interpretation, the textual components of the discourse were impaired (i.e., the children failed to convey content in a clear, economical manner), while the social component was generally preserved. Other studies (e.g., Murdoch, Ozanne, & Smyth, 1990) have also found that children with hydrocephalus obey the social demands of storytelling and conversations, reflecting intact interpersonal discourse skills. More recently, the findings of impoverished semantic narrative content have been demonstrated in children with hydrocephalus who have higher levels of general verbal skills (Verbal IQ > 90), showing that problems in conveying semantic content occur across all levels of verbal intelligence in children with shunted hydrocephalus (Barnes & Dennis, 1998).

The difficulties in reading comprehension evident among children with hydrocephalus are likely to be related to problems in discourse. Barnes and Dennis (1992) compared the phonological analysis, word recognition, word comprehension, and reading comprehension skills of 50 children with early hydrocephalus to those of 51 age- and education-matched controls. The two groups were equally able to recognize real words or pseudowords, but the hydrocephalus group had more difficulty understanding single words in text, even when controlling for children's single-word-decoding skills. Barnes and Dennis (1996) observed a similar dissociation between word recognition and reading comprehension skills in children with early hydrocephalus.

Difficulties in accessing text-based or knowledge-based information may be a common denominator for both oral discourse and reading comprehension problems in children with hydrocephalus. Difficulties in these abilities seem to reflect weaknesses in rapidly *accessing* diverse information during comprehension, as opposed to an inability to *integrate* the different sources of information. Study of these outcomes is a very promising area for future research, with clear implications for overall adaptive functioning. To date, there is little evidence for differences between etiological groups in these skills. Variations in the effect of hydrocephalus on the brain are thus the most likely sources of individual differences in this area of functioning.

Memory

There are few studies of memory functions in children with hydrocephalus. The studies conducted to date, moreover, have yielded inconsistent findings (Wills, 1993). Most recently, Yeates, Enrile, Loss, Blumenstein, and Delis (1995) and Scott et al. (1998) evaluated verbal learning and memory in children with hydrocephalus. Yeates et al. (1995) administered the California Verbal Learning Test—Children's Version (CVLT-C; Delis, Kramer, Kaplan, & Ober, 1994) to 33 children with spina bifida meningomyelocele with shunted hydrocephalus, 8 children with spina bifida meningomyelocele who were not shunted, and 41 control subjects obtained from the CVLT-C standardization sample. The children with shunted hydrocephalus performed more poorly than the other groups on many of the measures from the CVLT-C. Although the groups did not differ in terms of first-trial learning, children with shunted hydrocephalus acquired words more slowly across trials, and their overall recall was therefore lower. A pronounced recency effect was apparent in the children with shunted hydrocephalus, due to poor delayed recall of the original lists. In contrast, the children with shunted hydrocephalus performed well relative to controls on the recognition measure. The authors concluded that spina bifida meningomyelocele and shunted hydrocephalus were associated with significant problems in memory retrieval.

Scott et al. (1998) administered several different measures of memory functions to children with shunted hydrocephalus due to spina bifida meningomyelocele, IVH, and AS. Children with arrested hydrocephalus due to spina bifida and IVH, patient controls with spina bifida and IVH but no hydrocephalus, and normal controls were also included. Results failed to reveal differences according to etiology within the shunted group. However, the children with shunted hydrocephalus performed more poorly than the other groups on measures of encoding and retrieval from the verbal and nonverbal versions of the Selective Reminding Test (Buschke, 1974; Fletcher, 1985). Visual recognition memory was also poorer in the group with shunted hydrocephalus, and this group tended to perform more poorly on measures of prose recall and visual–constructive memory. These findings may also reflect problems at the level of discourse and motor functions, respectively.

Given the effects of hydrocephalus on the periventricular, midline, and diencephalic structures important for memory, it is not surprising that children with shunted hydrocephalus show significant problems on list-learning tasks (Yeates et al., 1995; Scott et al., 1998), apparently unrelated to etiology. Relationships of neuropathology to specific aspects of memory functioning are largely unexplored. Application of neuroimaging techniques in conjunction with assessment of memory and learning would address this issue, particularly if carried out to assess sources of individual *variations* in outcomes.

Attention and Executive Functions

As concluded by Wills (1993) in her review of literature on the neuropsychology of hydrocephalus, "one issue raised by Anderson (1975) [and] still not adequately addressed is the role of attention, concentration, 'frontal' or 'executive' processes in producing the neuropsychological profile of children with [spina bifida and hydrocephalus]" (p. 260). Several recent studies have addressed this issue. Fletcher, Brookshire, et al. (1996) administered measures of problem solving, focused attention, and selective attention to a large sample of children with shunted hydrocephalus due to spina bifida meningomyelocele, AS, and IVH, along with children with arrested hydrocephalus and no hydrocephalus. Overall, children with shunted hydrocephalus showed poorer problem-solving skills than children in the other groups. However, the poorer performance of the shunted group seemed to reflect a need for more trials to achieve a correct solution. With enough trials, children with shunted hydrocephalus were able to achieve solutions comparable to those of children with arrested and no hydrocephalus. Children with shunted hydrocephalus also performed more poorly on measures of focused and selective attention, but these findings probably reflected the motor and speed-of-processing deficits common to this condition. In support of this possibility, deficits in focused attention were not apparent when speed of motor processing was accounted for in overall performance. Similarly, on tasks that measured selective attention, children with shunted hydrocephalus simply performed more slowly, regardless of whether response selection or inhibition was required.

Like the construct of executive functions, attention is not a unitary construct. Contemporary models of attention distinguish processes involving alerting and orienting, which are more closely related to posterior and midline brain regions, from executing, which is more closely related to anterior brain regions (Posner & Raichle, 1994). The neuropsychological model proposed by Mirsky, Anthony, Duncan, Ahearn, and Kellam (1991) and Mirsky (1996) includes several component processes (Focus, Sustain, Encode, and Shift). The Focus component represents the ability to select target information from an array, while the Sustain component involves the maintenance of focus and alertness over time. Encode is a memory/learning component, whereas Shift is the ability to change the focus of attention flexibly. Some of these components, such as Focus, are viewed as the operation of an attention system in the posterior brain, while other components, such as Shift, are viewed as more anterior in origin (Mirsky, 1996).

In an application of this model, Brewer, Fletcher, and Hiscock (1999) examined the performances of children with hydrocephalus on measures from the Wisconsin Card Sorting Test (Heaton, 1981), a continuous-performance test (Halperin, Matier, Bedi, Sharma, & Newcorn, 1992), and the Visual Orientation and Detecting Test developed by Posner, Cohen, and Rafal (1987). Children with shunted hydrocephalus due to AS and spina bifida meningomyelocele were compared to groups of non-brain-injured children with attention-deficit/hyperactivity disorder (ADHD), combined type, and normal controls. The results revealed that children in the hydrocephalus and ADHD groups had different impairments in attention. Children with hydrocephalus showed an impaired ability to focus attention. In contrast, children with ADHD showed an intact capacity for focusing attention, but had difficulty sustaining attention over time, particularly when the tasks included multiple distractors. Hence, children with hydrocephalus had difficulties on tasks associated primarily with posterior attention systems, whereas children with ADHD showed problems with components of attention involving anterior attentional systems. More specifically, children with hydrocephalus tended to achieve fewer categories on the Wisconsin Card Sorting Test than the ADHD group, and made more nonperseverative errors on the Wisconsin Card Sorting Test. Children with ADHD, on the other hand, made more perseverative errors on the Wisconsin Card Sorting Test. On the Visual Orienting and Detection Test, children with ADHD had more difficulty than the other groups in sustaining attention, whereas children with hydrocephalus had difficulty with components of this task requiring them to disengage attention. The latter problems were apparent for targets presented in the left visual half-field, but not for targets in the right visual half-field. The results of the Brewer et al. (1999) study help in interpreting the findings from the Fletcher, Brookshire, et al. (1996) study by suggesting that the problems of children with hydrocephalus on measures of attention and executive functions may be related to the posterior brain abnormalities characteristic of these children.

More research is needed to understand the nature and extent of deficits in attention and executive functions in children with early hydrocephalus. Larger samples will be required, and comparisons within and across etiologies of hydrocephalus may be particularly useful. Studies of the relationship between measures of attention and executive functions on the one hand, and indices of the integrity of the corpus callosum on the other, would also be productive. Comparisons among the children with hydrocephalus who can and cannot sustain attention may be interesting. The role of the midbrain and tectum dysmorphology in visual attention remains to be explored. To restate, the goal of these studies should be to explain variations in outcomes, not simply to examine group differences.

Behavior

Children with chronic neurological or orthopedic disorders have higher rates of behavioral disorders than the general population (Wallander et al., 1989)—a finding that holds also for children with hydrocephalus (Donders, Rourke, & Canady, 1992; Fletcher, Brookshire, et al., 1995). Behavioral outcomes in children with hydrocephalus are additionally related to treatment factors such as shunting and shunt revisions, as well as to sociodemographic factors (Fletcher, Brookshire, et al., 1995; but see Donders et al., 1992). Fletcher, Brookshire, et al. (1995) found that children with shunted hydrocephalus had higher rates of both internalizing and externalizing behavior disorders. Categorical modeling analyses to predict the presence or absence of behavior problems revealed that treatment, family, and sociodemographic variables were important predictors of behavioral outcomes. Future studies should measure a broader range of these outcomes, using both rating scale and interview formats. It is also possible that the behavioral consequences of hydrocephalus may be cumulative, with more marked behavioral difficulties in adolescents than in younger children (Holler, Fennell, Crosson, Boggs, & Mickle, 1995).

CONCLUSIONS

The more recent research reviewed in this chapter reveals improvements in the quality of neurobehavioral research on children with hydrocephalus over the last few years. Most striking is the application of contemporary assessment paradigms from cognitive neuroscience to developmental disorders. The results of these studies help to sharpen hypotheses for future research, particularly in areas involving discourse and language development, memory, and attention/executive functioning. In addition, the sample sizes used in recent studies have been larger than those included in previous research, with more explicit variation in and account taken of the etiology of hydrocephalus. Even in work involving smaller samples, the subjects have been better described, and procedures have often included state-of-the-art neuroimaging. Recent studies have afforded more opportunity to examine the effects of hydrocephalus in relation to etiology, type of hydrocephalus, and other factors. New and promising findings have related medical and neuroimaging variables to outcomes, and there have been initial attempts to relate outcomes to social and age-related factors as well.

Etiology is now being considered explicitly in outcome studies of hydrocephalus. However, etiology is a marker for a complex set of developmental neuropathologies that have both unshared and shared variance across etiologies. In future studies, grouping by neuropathology should allow us to address important questions. For example, do differences in discourse abilities vary according to degree of the corpus callosum agenesis/hypoplasia, regardless of etiology of hydrocephalus?

In undertaking this research, it is important not to lose sight of some of the design features incorporated into earlier research on hydrocephalus. Dennis et al. (1981), for example, related a large number of variables to intellectual outcome. Predictors included sociodemographic variables; the presence of symptomatic disturbance of the visual system, motor system, and seizures; other medical factors, such as hypoxic–ischemic encephalopathy, periventricular leukomalacia, jaundice, and metabolic disorders; treatment factors, including the type, location, and age of shunting, as well as the number of shunt revisions; and the presence of central nervous system infections. With contemporary neuroimaging capabilities, we can now begin to relate outcomes to MRI indices that reflect both the general integrity of the brain (e.g., ratios of gray to white matter) and quantitative assessment of structures especially relevant to an outcome domain.

The developmental dysmorphologies associated with hydrocephalus are widespread in the brain but rarely studied in relation to neurobehavioral outcomes. For example, cerebellar pathology varies across different etiologies of hydrocephalus, just as corpus callosum pathology varies within and across etiologies. Study of associations between outcomes and these types of variations may be of particular value. General assessments of cortical thinning in the whole brain and in specific brain regions may also be useful (Dennis et al., 1981; Fletcher, McCauley, et al., 1996). Similarly, there is a major need to relate outcomes to social factors, such as socioeconomic status and familial resources, cultural factors, and educational interventions.

To accomplish these aims, much larger samples than those commonly studied are necessary. Even the respectable sample recruited by Fletcher, Brookshire, et al. (1995) yielded small numbers of children in some cells of the design. As work in this area proceeds, it will be important to compare children across etiologies. For example, children with DWS would be an excellent comparison group for children with spina bifida meningomyelocele and with AS. This is because DWS children, who have even more pervasive cerebellar deficits than children with spina bifida meningomyelocele, tend not to show verbal–nonverbal skill discrepancies. Variations in other features of hydrocephalus, such as the integrity of the corpus callosum, are also apparent in children with DWS. However, there are no well-controlled studies of these children—a fact reflecting the relative rarity of the condition and its lack of scrutiny by researchers. Large-scale studies of children within more common etiologies should also be undertaken. Spina bifida meningomyelocele is an obvious candidate for such an investigation. Children with this disorder show large variations in outcomes, and brain morphology is distinctive but variable. For example, the corpus callosum and cerebellum are usually abnormal, but the nature and extent of the abnormalities vary across cases. Other aspects of the central nervous system impairment are even more variable, such as midbrain changes and the level of the spinal lesion. Variability due to hydrocephalus and its treatment, ocular–motor difficulties, presence of seizures, and sociodemographic characteristics is also apparent. Mapping out the relationships of outcomes to these sources of variability may help elucidate behavior–brain relationships. Genetic factors associated with the presence of neural tube defects in some children could also be related to neurobehavioral outcomes.

Recent conceptual models for studying children with hydrocephalus have attempted to make explicit the influences on outcomes stemming from variations within and across etiological groupings (e.g., Dennis et al., 1999). To accrue the data base to confirm or disconfirm such models, a broad range of outcomes must be measured, together with a variety of neuroimaging, medical, and sociodemographic factors. With large enough samples, answers may be sought to long-standing questions regarding the sequelae of hydrocephalus, some of which have gone unanswered since the advent of shunting in children with hydrocephalus. Despite 40 years of research, questions remain with regard to the relationships of neuropsychological outcomes to the level of the spinal lesion in children with spina bifida meningomyelocele, central nervous system infections, and number of shunt revisions. These relationships have practical import in treating children, and thus should have some priority in clinical research. Recent neuroimaging studies reveal intriguing relationships between neuropsychological findings and patterns of regional brain thinning and dysmorphology of the corpus callosum (Fletcher, Bohan, et al., 1992, 1996); however, these studies need to be replicated and performed on larger samples.

Finally, children with hydrocephalus do not develop in a vacuum. The early central nervous system deficits characteristic of these children are likely to have a reciprocal effect on their ability to operate in a social environment, although we do not yet know how these environmental interactions affect subsequent development (Landry, Jordan, & Fletcher, 1994; Rourke, 1989). An obvious and common example is a child with spina bifida meningomyelocele who has limited ambulation and other motor difficulties arising from brain and spinal cord problems during the first year of development. Restricted ambulation will clearly inhibit environmental exploration, which in turn will delay the mastery of spatial skills (Abercombie, 1968; Rourke, 1989). Further research is needed to determine the extent to which the spatial deficits commonly observed in children with hydrocephalus reflect specific brain defects, as opposed to interactions between the central nervous system defects and environmental influences. Equally relevant is investigation of the relationship of these early deficits to the long-term development of these children.

No one would doubt the complexities involved in undertaking this research. Unlike the situation of 10 years ago, however, the questions are now clearer and answerable. Finding the answers, moreover, will almost certainly suggest ways to facilitate the development of children with hydrocephalus. There is a need to begin to study children with hydrocephalus earlier in their development, and to continue to monitor cognitive and behavioral outcomes at a variety of developmental levels. Such studies would help facilitate the long-term development of children with hydrocephalus by providing a fuller and truer understanding of the factors that enhance or retard cognitive maturation.

Obviously, the methodological principles we espouse apply not only to children with hydrocephalus. We would urge investigators interested in children with a variety of diffuse central nervous system disorders to begin to reconceptualize their research and move beyond simple description. Future research needs to include careful assessments of outcomes across multiple domains. Outcomes should be conceptualized not only in terms of group averages, but also in terms of questions relevant to individual children (i.e., the problem of explaining the sources of variability in outcomes). Neuroimaging studies should be included to assess the integrity of the central nervous system. Other factors related to the disorder, such as treatment effects and other medical variables (e.g., seizures), need also to be considered. Children with a comorbid seizure disorder, for example, almost always have poorer scores on cognitive and motor tests than children with hydrocephalus and no seizures (Dennis et al., 1981; Fletcher & Levin, 1988). Finally, sociodemographic and environmental factors that influence a child's development need to be incorporated in the model. The goal of studies of this sort should be to account for variability in outcomes in terms of the multiple factors suspected of influencing the development of the child with brain disorder.

ACKNOWLEDGMENTS

The writing of this chapter was supported in part by National Institute of Neurological Disorders and Strokes Grant No. R01 NS25368, "Neurobehavioral Development of Hydrocephalic Children," and National Institute of Child Health and Human Development Grant No. PO1 HD35946, "Spina Bifida: Cognitive and Neurobiological Variability," to Jack M. Fletcher; and by project grants to Maureen Dennis from the Ontario Mental Health Foundation, the Ontario Ministry of Community and Social Services, and the Spina Bifida Association of Canada. We thank Rita Taylor and Irene Desjardin for assistance with manuscript preparation.

REFERENCES

Abercombie, M. L. I. (1968). Some notes on spatial disability: Movement, intelligence quotient, and alertness. *Developmental Medicine and Child Neurology, 10,* 206–213.

Anderson, E. M. (1975). Cognitive deficits in children with spina bifida and hydrocephalus: A review of the literature. *British Journal of Educational Psychology, 45,* 257–268.

Anderson, E. M., & Plewis, I. (1977). Impairment of motor skill in children with spina bifida cystica and hydrocephalus: An exploratory study. *British Journal of Psychology, 68,* 61–70.

Barkovich, A. J. (1995). *Pediatric neuroimaging* (2nd ed.). New York: Raven Press.

Barnes, M. A., & Dennis, M. (1992). Reading in children and adolescents after early onset hydrocephalus and in normally developing age peers: Phonological analysis, word recognition, word comprehension, and passage comprehension skills. *Journal of Pediatric Psychology, 17,* 445–465.

Barnes, M. A., & Dennis, M. (1996). Reading comprehension deficits arise from diverse sources: Evidence from readers with and without developmental brain pathology. In C. Cornoldi & J. Oakhill (Eds.), *Reading comprehension difficulties: Processes and intervention* (pp. 251–278). Hillsdale, NJ: Erlbaum.

Barnes, M. A., & Dennis, M. (1998). Discourse after early-onset hydrocephalus: Core deficits in children of average intelligence. *Brain and Language, 61,* 309–334.

Baron, I. S., Fennell, E., & Voeller, K. (1995). *Pediatric neuropsychology in the medical setting.* New York: Oxford University Press.

Beery, K. E. (1982). *Revised administration, scoring, and teaching manual for the Developmental Test of Visual–Motor Integration.* Cleveland, OH: Modern Curriculum Press.

Brewer, V., Fletcher, J. M., & Hiscock, M. (1999). *Attentional skills in children with early hydrocephalus versus children with attention deficit/hyperactivity disorder.* Manuscript submitted for publication.

Brookshire, B. L., Fletcher, J. M., Bohan, T. P., & Landry, S. H. (1995). Specific language deficiencies in children with early onset hydrocephalus. *Child Neuropsychology, 1,* 106–117.

Brookshire, B. L., Fletcher, J. M., Bohan, T. P., Landry, S. H., Davidson, K. C., & Francis, D. J. (1995). Verbal and nonverbal skill discrepancies in children with hydrocephalus: A five year longitudinal follow-up. *Journal of Pediatric Psychology, 20,* 785–800.

Buschke, H. (1974). Components of verbal learning in children: Analysis by selective reminding. *Journal of Experimental Child Psychology, 18,* 488–496.

Chuang, S. (1986). Perinatal and neonatal hydrocephalus: Part 1. Incidence and etiology. *Perinatal Neonatology, 10,* 8–19.

Delis, D. C., Kramer, J. H., Kaplan, E., & Ober, B. A. (1994). *California Verbal Learning Test—Children's Version.* New York: Psychological Corporation.

Del Bigio, M. R. (1993). Neuropathological changes caused by hydrocephalus. *Acta Neuropathologica, 85,* 573–585.

Denckla, M. B., & Rudel, R. G. (1974). Rapid "automatized" naming of pictured objects, colors, letters, and numbers by normal children. *Cortex, 10,* 186–202.

Dennis, M. (1996). Hydrocephalus. In J. G. Beaumont, P. Kenealy, & M. Rogers (Eds.), *The Blackwell dictionary of neuropsychology* (pp. 406–411). Oxford: Blackwell.

Dennis, M., & Barnes, M. A. (1993). Oral discourse after early-onset hydrocephalus: Linguistic ambiguity, figurative language, speech acts, and script-based inferences. *Journal of Pediatric Psychology, 18,* 639–652.

Dennis, M., Barnes, M. A., & Hetherington, C. R. (1999). Congenital hydrocephalus as a model of neurodevelopmental disorder. In H. Tager-Flusberg (Ed.), *Neurodevelopmental disorders: Contribution to a new perspective from the cognitive neurosciences* (pp. 505–532). Cambridge, MA: MIT Press.

Dennis, M., Fitz, C. R., Netley, C. T., Sugar, J., Harwood-Nash, D. C. F., Hendrick, E. B., Hoffman, H. J., & Humphreys, R. P. (1981). The intelligence of hydrocephalic children. *Archives of Neurology, 38,* 607–715.

Dennis, M., Hendrick, E. B., Hoffman, H. J., & Humphreys, R. P. (1987). The language of hydrocephalic children. *Journal of Clinical and Experimental Neuropsychology, 9,* 593–621.

Dennis, M., Jacennik, B., & Barnes, M. A. (1994). The content of narrative discourse in children and adolescents after early-onset hydrocephalus and in normally-developing age peers. *Brain and Language, 46,* 129–165.

Donders, J., Canady, A. I., & Rourke, B. P. (1990). Psychometric intelligence after infantile hydrocephalus. *Child's Nervous System, 6,* 148–154.

Donders, J., Rourke, B. P., & Canady, A. I. (1992). Behavioral adjustment of children with hydrocephalus and of their parents. *Journal of Child Neurology, 7,* 375–380.

Fletcher, J. M. (1985). Memory for verbal and nonverbal stimuli in learning disability subgroups: Analysis by selective reminding. *Journal of Experimental Child Psychology, 40,* 244–259.

Fletcher, J. M., Bohan, T. P., Brandt, M. E., Brookshire, B. L., Beaver, S. R., Francis, D. J., Davidson, K. C., Thompson, N. M., & Miner, M. E. (1992). Cerebral white matter and cognition in hydrocephalic children. *Archives of Neurology, 49,* 818–824.

Fletcher, J. M., Bohan, T. P., Brandt, M. E., Kramer, L. A., Brookshire, B. L., Thorstad, K., Davidson, K. C., Francis, D. J., McCauley, S., & Baumgartner, J. (1996). Morphometric evaluation of the hydrocephalic brain: Relationships with cognitive abilities. *Child's Nervous System, 12,* 192–199.

Fletcher, J. M., Brookshire, B. L., Bohan, T. P., Brandt, M. E., & Davidson, K. C. (1995). Early hydrocephalus. In B. P. Rourke (Ed.), *Syndrome of nonverbal learning disabilities: Neurodevelopmental manifestations* (pp. 206–238). New York: Guilford Press.

Fletcher, J. M., Brookshire, B. L., Landry, S. H., Bohan, T. P., Davidson, K. C., Francis, D. J., Levin, H. S., Kramer, L. A., & Morris, R. D. (1996). Attentional skills and executive functions in children with early hydrocephalus. *Developmental Neuropsychology, 12,* 53–76.

Fletcher, J. M., Francis, D. J., Thompson, N. M., Brookshire, B. L., Bohan, T. P., Landry, S. H., Davidson, K. C., & Miner, M. E. (1992). Verbal and nonverbal skill discrepancies in hydrocephalic children. *Journal of Clinical and Experimental Neuropsychology, 14,* 593–609.

Fletcher, J. M., Landry, S. H., Davidson, K. C., Brookshire, B. L., Lachar, D., Kramer, L. A., Bohan, T. P., & Francis, D. J. (1997). Effects of intraventricular hemorrhage and hydrocephalus on the long-term neurobehavioral development of premature, very low birthweight children. *Developmental Medicine and Child Neurology, 39,* 596–606.

Fletcher, J. M., & Levin, H. S. (1988). Neurobehavioral effects of brain injury in children. In D. Routh (Ed.), *Handbook of pediatric psychology* (pp. 258–296). New York: Guilford Press.

Fletcher, J. M., Levin, H. S., & Butler, I. J. (1995). Neurobehavioral effects of brain injury in children: Hydrocephalus, traumatic brain injury, and cerebral palsy. In M. Roberts (Ed.), *Handbook of pediatric psychology* (2nd ed., pp. 362–383). New York: Guilford Press.

Fletcher, J. M., Levin, H., & Landry, S. H. (1984). Behavioral consequences of cerebral insult in infancy. In C. R. Almli & S. Finger (Eds.), *Early brain damage: Research orientations and clinical observations,* (Vol. 1, pp. 189–213). New York: Academic Press.

Fletcher, J. M., McCauley, S. R., Brandt, M. E., Bohan, T. P., Kramer, L. A., Francis, D. J., Thorstad, K., & Brookshire, B. L. (1996). Regional brain tissue composition in children with hydrocephalus. *Archives of Neurology, 53,* 549–557.

Gaddes, W. H., & Crockett, D. J. (1975). The Spreen–Benton Aphasia Tests: Normative data as a measure of normal language development. *Brain and Language, 2,* 257–279.

Gardner, M. F. (1988). *Test of Visual-Perceptual Skills.* San Francisco: Health.

Halperin, J. M., Matier, K., Bedi, G., Sharma, V., & Newcorn, D. M. (1992). Specificity of inattention, impulsivity, and hyperactivity to the diagnosis of attention deficit hyperactivity disorder. *Journal of the American Academy of Child and Adolescent Psychiatry, 31,* 190–196.

Heaton, R. E. (1981). *The Wisconsin Card Sorting Test manual.* Odessa, FL: Psychological Assessment Resources.

Hetherington, C. R., & Dennis, M. (1999). Motor function profile in children with early onset hydrocephalus. *Developmental Neuropsychology, 15,* 25–51.

Holler, K. A., Fennell, E. B., Crosson, B., Boggs, S. R., & Mickle, J. P. (1995). Neuropsychological and adaptive functioning in younger versus older children shunted for early hydrocephalus. *Child Neuropsychology, 1,* 63–73.

Landry, S. H., Chapieski, L., Fletcher, J. M., & Denson, S. (1988). Three year outcomes for low birth weight infants: Differential effects of early medical complications. *Journal of Pediatric Psychology, 13,* 317–327.

Landry, S. H., Fletcher, J. M., Denson, S. G., & Chapieski, M. L. (1993). Longitudinal outcomes for low birth weight infants: Effects of intraventricular hemorrhage and bronchopulmonary dysplasia. *Journal of Clinical and Experimental Neuropsychology, 15,* 205–218.

Landry, S. H., Fletcher, J. M., Zarling, C., Chapieski, L., Frances, D., & Denson, S. (1984). Differential outcomes associated with early medical complications in premature infants. *Journal of Pediatric Psychology, 9,* 385–401.

Landry, S. H., Jordan, T., & Fletcher, J. M. (1994). Developmental outcomes for children with spina bifida. In M. G. Tramontana & S. R. Hooper (Eds.), *Advances in neuropsychology* (Vol. 2, pp. 85–118). New York: Springer-Verlag.

Lindgren, S. D., & Benton, A. L. (1980). Developmental patterns of visuospatial judgment. *Journal of Pediatric Psychology, 5,* 217–225.

McCarthy, D. (1972). *McCarthy Scales of Children's Abilities.* New York: Psychological Corporation.

McCullough, D. (1990). Hydrocephalus: Etiology, pathologic effects, diagnosis and natural history. In R. M. Scott (Ed.), *Hydrocephalus* (pp. 180–199). Baltimore: Williams & Wilkins.

Mirsky, A. F. (1996). Disorders of attention: A neuropsychological perspective. In G. R. Lyon & N. A. Krasnegor (Eds.), *Attention, memory, and executive functions* (pp. 71–96). Baltimore: Paul N. Brookes.

Mirsky, A. F., Anthony, B. J., Duncan, C. C., Ahearn, B. B., & Kellam, S. G. (1991). Analysis of the elements of attention: A neuropsychological approach. *Neuropsychology Review, 2,* 109–145.

Murdoch, B. E., Ozanne, A. E., & Smyth, V. (1990). Communicative impairments in neural tube disorders. In B. E. Murdoch (Ed.), *Acquired neurological speech/language disorders in children* (pp. 216–244). London: Taylor & Francis.

Posner, M. I., Cohen, Y., & Rafal, R. D. (1987). Neural systems and the control of spatial orienting. *Philosophical Transactions of the Royal Society of London, 298,* 187–198.

Posner, M. I., & Raichle, M. E. (1994). *Images of mind.* New York: Scientific American Books.

Raimondi, A. J. (1994). A unifying theory for the definition and classification of hydrocephalus. *Child's Nervous System, 10,* 2–12.

Reigel, D. H., & Rotenstein, D. (1994). Spina bifida. In W. R. Cheek (Ed.), *Pediatric neurosurgery* (3rd ed., pp. 51–76). Philadelphia: W. B. Saunders.

Riva, D., Milani, N., Giorgi, C., Pantaleoni, C., Zorzi, C., & Devoti, M. (1994). Intelligence outcome in children with shunted hydrocephalus of different etiology. *Child's Nervous System, 10,* 70–73.

Robertson, I. J. A., Leggate, J. R. S., Miller, J. D., & Steers, A. J. W. (1990). Aqueduct stenosis: Presentation and prognosis. *British Journal of Neurosurgery, 4,* 101–106.

Rosner, J., & Simon, P. (1971). The Auditory Analysis Test. *Journal of Learning Disabilities, 8,* 24–37.

Rourke, B. P. (1989). *Nonverbal learning disabilities: The syndrome and the model.* New York: Guilford Press.

Schmidt, F. L. (1996). Statistically significance testing and cumulative knowledge in psychology: Implications for training of researchers. *Psychological Methods, 1,* 115–129.

Scott, M., Fletcher, J. M., Brookshire, B. L., Davidson, K. C., Landry, S. H., Bohan, T. P., Kramer, L., Brandt, M., & Francis, D. J. (1998). Memory functions in children with early hydrocephalus. *Neuropsychology, 12,* 578–589.

Tal, Y., Freigang, B., Dunn, H. G., Durity, F. A., & Moyes, P. D. (1980). Dandy–Walker syndrome: Analysis of 21 cases. *Developmental Medicine and Child Neurology, 22,* 189–201.

Volpe, J. J. (1994). *Neurology of the newborn* (3rd ed.). Philadelphia: W. B. Saunders.

Wallander, J. L., Varni, J. W., Babani, L., Banis, H. T., DeHaan, C. B., & Wilcox, K. T. (1989). Disability parameters, chronic strain, and adaptation of physically handicapped children and their mothers. *Journal of Pediatric Psychology, 14,* 23–42.

Wechsler, D. (1974). *Wechsler Intelligence Scale for Children—Revised.* New York: Psychological Corporation.

Wills, K. E. (1993). Neuropsychological functioning in children with spina bifida and/or hydrocephalus. *Journal of Clinical Child Psychology, 22,* 247–265.

Yeates, K. O., Enrile, B., Loss, N., Blumenstein, E., & Delis, D. C. (1995). Verbal learning and memory in children with myelomeningocele. *Journal of Pediatric Psychology, 20,* 801–812.

Young, H. F., Nulsen, F. F., Weiss, M. H., & Thomas, P. (1973). The relationship of intelligence and cerebral mantle in treated hydrocephalus. *Pediatrics, 52,* 38–44.

Zeiner, H. K., Prigitano, G. P., Pollay, M., Biscoe, C. B., & Smith, R. V. (1985). Ocular motility, visual acuity, and dysfunction of neuropsychological impairment in children with shunted uncomplicated hydrocephalus. *Child's Nervous System, 1,* 115–122.

3

EPILEPSY

JANE WILLIAMS
GREGORY B. SHARP

HISTORY

The perplexing and frightening nature of epilepsy has historically confounded our understanding of this disorder. Theories concerning the etiology of seizures have included both mystical beliefs and physiological causes, as summarized by Haynes and Bennett (1992). Hippocrates was the first to provide a physiological explanation that attributed manifestations of seizures to a brain disorder. He postulated that phlegm rushed into the vessels of the brain, filled the ventricles, and resulted in increased pressure that was relieved by the occurrence of a seizure. During the Middle Ages, theories concerning the origin of seizures were based on beliefs in demonic possession or lunar cycles. Diseases with periodic occurrences, such as epilepsy, were felt by some to be associated with the phases of the moon and were thus called "lunacies." Epilepsy was attributed by others to contagious demonic possession that could pass from person to person. The Renaissance brought a trend toward more physiological explanations. During the 17th century, Thomas Willis hypothesized that seizures were caused by the mixture of two chemicals produced by muscle activity that entered the brain via the blood, irritating the nerves. He attributed a loss of memory and intellectual function to seizures. During the 19th and early 20th centuries, the trend toward institutionalization of individuals with epilepsy resulted in increasing scientific efforts to understand, classify, and treat seizures. Epileptic vertigo was used to describe mental changes associated with epilepsy. Sir William Gowers associated alterations in consciousness with recurrence of brief disturbances in brain function, while Hughlings Jackson described epilepsy as an abnormal local discharge originating in the gray matter of the brain. Gowers noted associated deficits in attention and memory with epilepsy, and descriptions of personality changes included hyposexuality, mania, and rage.

More recently, the study of epilepsy has yielded increased knowledge of brain–behavior relationships such as the association between stimulation of motor and sensory cortex with specific behavioral responses, the role of the hippocampus and temporal lobe in memory function, hemispheric plasticity for speech in childhood, and hemispheric specialization for cognitive skills (Novelly, 1992). Although a debt of gratitude is owed to patients with epilepsy for the knowledge gained in the study of this disorder, the long-standing myths and misunderstandings associated with seizures have significantly contributed to the psychosocial difficulties experienced by these individuals.

EPIDEMIOLOGY

Epilepsy is a disorder that most often begins during childhood and adolescence. At least 75% of individuals with epilepsy experience their first seizures before the age of 20, and 50% of childhood epilepsy occurs during the first 5 years of life (Kim, 1991).

Epilepsy is the most common neurological condition in childhood, with a slightly higher occurrence in boys than in girls. Prevalence within the pediatric population is approximately 4.3 to 9.3 per 1,000 children, and there are an estimated 150,250 to 325,000 cases of active epilepsy in children between 5 and 14 years of age in the United States (Hauser & Hesdorffer, 1990a). These prevalence rates do not involve febrile seizures, as they are not considered a form of epilepsy. Febrile seizures occur in 2–5% of children, do not typically warrant treatment, generally resolve by the age of 5 years, and result in a slightly increased risk for later unprovoked seizures (Annegers, Hauser, Shirts, & Kurland, 1987; Consensus Development Conference on Febrile Seizures, 1981; Forsgren, Sidenvall, Blomquist, & Heijbel, 1990).

The course of epilepsy is highly diverse. Seizures are controlled in approximately 70–80% of children treated with antiepileptic drugs (AEDs). Remission over a 5-year period occurs in approximately 70% of individuals with epilepsy, and 75% of children who have been seizure-free for at least 2 years can be successfully withdrawn from AEDs. Children with normal neurological examination, electroencephalographic (EEG) recording, and intelligence are more likely to continue in remission following withdrawal from AEDs. There is a slight increase in mortality for children with epilepsy compared to the general population. Status epilepticus (i.e., continuous seizures lasting over 30 minutes) poses a higher risk, but mortality generally results from underlying brain pathology rather than prolonged seizures (Hauser & Hesdorffer, 1990b; Hauser & Hesdorffer, 1997).

ETIOLOGY

Epilepsy is not a specific disease, but rather a condition in which an individual has recurrent seizures resulting from abnormal electrical activity in the brain. In order to be diagnosed with epilepsy, the individual must experience more than one unprovoked seizure. The cause for recurrent seizures may be symptomatic or idiopathic. In *symptomatic* epilepsy, the origin of seizures is identified and may include structural brain anomalies, metabolic derangements, birth anoxia, cerebrovascular insults, central nervous system (CNS) infections, CNS neoplasms, or moderate to severe head trauma. Mild head trauma is rarely a cause of seizures. An underlying etiology for epilepsy is identified in only 30% of the cases, and children with symptomatic epilepsy are more likely to have seizures that are difficult to control with medications. The vast majority of children with epilepsy have *idiopathic* seizures, in which the cause is unknown (Hauser & Kurland, 1975; Annegers, 1997). The descriptor *cryptogenic* is sometimes used instead of *idiopathic*; it implies that an underlying cause exists but cannot be identified.

PATHOPHYSIOLOGY OF SEIZURES

The neurophysiological mechanism underlying seizures is not completely understood, as it is complex, multifactoral, and variable. The source of epileptic activity is at the cellular level. Under normal physiological circumstances, signals are transmitted from one neuron to the next primarily by the release of chemical neurotransmitters or by direct electrical connections. The arrival of an action potential from the neuron after it has propagated down the axon results in depolarization of the presynaptic membrane. This yields an influx of calcium (Ca) via Ca channels across the presynaptic membrane, which results in release of neurotransmitters into the synaptic cleft. The excitatory neurotransmitter binds to its specific postsynaptic receptor and induces an excitatory postsynaptic potential (EPSP). When the summation of EPSPs reaches a threshold potential, depolarization via the opening of sodium (Na) and sometimes Ca channels results in an influx of Na and Ca, respectively. This reaction is an all-or-none phenomenon. Closing of the Na channels, coupled with opening of slower potassium (K) channels, allows an efflux of K; this results in repolarization. The primary inhibitory neurotransmitter in the forebrain is gamma-aminobutyric acid (GABA). GABA release results in inhibitory postsynaptic potentials (IPSPs) that induce opening of chloride channels, thus hyperpolarizing the cell and decreasing excitation. Neuronal function is modulated by a normal "balance" between excitatory and inhibitory neurotransmitters. Glutamate and aspartate are the primary excitatory neurotransmitters in the brain, and GABA and, to a lesser extent, glycine are the primary inhibitory neurotransmitters (Knowles & Luders, 1993).

At the cellular level, numerous abnormalities that give rise to epileptogenic activity can exist or potentially coexist. Defects or abnormalities involving ion channels (Na, K, and Ca), such as prolonged opening of the Na or Ca channels, may result in a tendency for excessive depolarization and epileptiform activity. Excessive excitatory neurotransmitter (glutamate and aspartate) activity or deficient inhibitory neurotransmitter (GABA and glycine) activity may also result in seizure activity. Progressive cellular changes can occur, such as the development of recurrent excitatory pathways or synaptic reorganization, that result in an increased tendency for epileptiform discharges. Some groups of neurons may have a tendency for burst firing or repetitive rapid depolarizations that commonly result in the onset of a seizure discharge. As the rapid discharge progresses, excitatory neurotransmitter activity is enhanced and inhibitory neurotransmitter activity is inhibited, thus resulting in propagation of the seizure (Schwartzkroin, 1993).

Seizures of focal onset occur when bursts of synchronous electrical firing are generated from a group or focal population of neurons. Recruitment of other surrounding neurons and spread via cortical projections to other parts of the brain result in progression of the clinical seizure activity. Spread to the contralateral cerebral hemisphere via the corpus callosum, anterior or posterior commissures, or other anatomical pathways may result in secondary generalization and a generalized convulsion.

Generalized absence seizures are thought to arise from the thalamus due to abnormalities in Ca current via low-threshold Ca channels (Coulter, Huguenard, & Prince, 1989; Gloor, Avoli, & Kostopoulos, 1990). Studies have documented a cortical dysgenesis with misplaced neurons in some patients with primary generalized epilepsies (Meencke & Janz, 1985), but the neurochemical basis of generalized spike-wave discharges is poorly understood.

In symptomatic epilepsy, identifiable structural cerebral abnormalities are often associated with seizure occurrence. Congenital anomalies of the brain due to abnormal neural induction or neuronal migration during embryonic development result in disordered anatomical structure, neuronal placement, and synaptic organization. Cellular injury due to hypoxia and ischemia, hemorrhage, metabolic disturbance, toxic exposure, trauma, or infection can result in neuronal injury that may lead to epileptic seizures.

Status epilepticus can result in cerebral injury with potential worsening of seizure control. Clinical status epilepticus produces systemic effects, including hypoxia, hypercarbia, and respiratory and metabolic acidosis. Neurons are very sensitive to hypoxic and metabolic insults. Significant cerebral hypoxia and ischemia may result in focal or diffuse cerebral injury. Selective neuronal injury may result in the hippocampus, which is highly sensitive to the effects of status epilepticus and is potentially induced by excitatory neurotransmitters and/or Ca-mediated cell damage (Lothman, 1990; Meldrum, 1983).

Recurrent seizures are less likely to induce structural injury, but the hippocampus is again selectively sensitive. Hippocampal sclerosis has been commonly documented in patients with medically intractable temporal lobe seizures. Changes include increased axonal branching, neuronal loss, astrocytic proliferation, and synaptic reorganization (Babb & Pretorius, 1993).

CLASSIFICATION OF SEIZURES

Classification of seizures is based on the clinical description and EEG findings (Commission on Classification and Terminology of the International League Against Epilepsy, 1981). An EEG is diagnostic if it reveals an epileptiform abnormality (i.e., focal spike vs. generalized spike-wave), but a normal EEG does not exclude the possibility of seizures. EEG recordings may be confirmatory in up to 70% of cases (Ajmone-Marsan & Zivin, 1970).

Epileptic seizures have to be clinically differentiated from other paroxysmal events, such as syncope, narcolepsy, breath holding, hyperventilation, night terrors, rage, migraine, tics, vertigo, and nonepileptic seizures. Nonepilepsy seizures, often referred to as psychogenic seizures or pseudoseizures, consist of seizure-like changes in movement, sensation, or experience which involve no epileptiform activity in the brain but are caused by emotional or behavioral disorders (Lesser, 1996). Nonepileptic seizures are generally more common in adolescence and frequently associated with conversion disorders. Some pediatric patients experience both epileptic and nonepileptic events. Because of the difficulty in distinguishing between these types of events, video EEG monitoring is often necessary to make a differential diagnosis (Chabolla, Krahn, So, & Rummans, 1996).

In contrast to nonepileptic events, periods of nonconvulsive status epilepticus may be unrecognized as seizure events and may be confused with psychiatric symptomatology involving associated clouding of consciousness or unusual behavior. Subclinical electrographic seizures may not induce an apparent clinical change, but may induce transient cognitive effects.

The primary division in seizure type is based on the origin of the electrical discharge. *Partial seizures* (see Figure 3.1, left) begin within a local region of the brain and are frequently heralded by an aura or warning such as a strange feeling of fear, nausea, foul odor or taste, dizziness, or déjà vu. The clinical expression of the aura and the seizure frequently reflect the function of the involved neurons (i.e., frontal onset is accompanied by contralateral tonic posturing or clonic jerking of part of the body, occipital onset by visual phenomena, parietal onset by somatosensory changes, and temporal onset by confusion and unresponsiveness). With a *simple partial seizure*, there is no alteration of consciousness and no amnesia for events that occurred during the seizure. *Complex partial seizures*, also

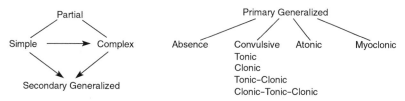

FIGURE 3.1. Classification of epileptic seizures.

known as *psychomotor seizures*, involve an alteration of consciousness. The individual commonly appears confused and frequently exhibits automatisms such as lip smacking, facial grimacing, mumbling or humming, fumbling hand movements, or picking at clothing. These seizures usually last a few minutes and are accompanied by postictal confusion and fatigue. A temporary postictal aphasia is common with involvement of the dominant cerebral hemisphere. The electrical seizure activity may spread, resulting in a *secondary generalized convulsion*.

Primary generalized seizures (see Figure 3.1), characterized by synchronous bilateral electrical epileptic discharges, have an abrupt onset without an aura and usually involve a sudden loss of consciousness. The most common generalized convulsive type is the *tonic–clonic seizure*, formerly known as *grand mal*. The generalized electrical discharge produces tonic stiffening of the trunk and extremities, which is followed by clonic rhythmical jerking of the extremities. These seizures generally last less than 5 minutes and are followed by postictal unresponsiveness. A *tonic seizure* is a brief stiffening episode without the clonic phase, and a *clonic seizure* consists of rhythmical jerking without the tonic phase. Occasionally seizures may begin with a few clonic jerks, followed by a tonic and then a clonic phase, resulting in a *clonic–tonic–clonic seizure*.

Atonic seizures are characterized by an extremely abrupt loss of muscle tone that produces a sudden fall. *Myoclonic seizures* are brief, single, symmetrical jerks of the head and upper extremities that may occur in a series or cluster, commonly after awakening. There is no loss of consciousness, as the associated burst of generalized polyspike-wave activity typically has a duration of less than 1 second.

Absence seizures, formerly known as *petit mal*, are brief staring episodes involving a sudden cessation of activity. Absence seizures are nonconvulsive. Behaviorally, there may be a simple blank stare or a rapid eye flutter. The episodes last only seconds, and there is a rapid return of consciousness without significant postictal symptoms. *Atypical absence seizures* usually begin in early childhood and are frequently accompanied by other generalized seizures, including tonic–clonic, tonic, atonic, and/or myoclonic types. These seizures are often difficult to control.

Specific classification of seizures is difficult in about 10–20% of persons with epilepsy, who have mixed seizure types.

The EEG can be a helpful tool to aid in classification of seizure types. A focal spike or a sharp wave are considered epileptiform abnormalities and may help identify the focus of epileptogenesis. Generalized spike-wave discharges are consistent with primary generalized epilepsy. More specific abnormalities are associated with certain seizure types, such as the 3-per-second generalized spike and wave discharges seen with absence seizures. Focal slowing can be associated with a focal epileptiform abnormality, an underlying structural abnormality, or a postictal state. Generalized slowing during wakefulness is abnormal but nonspecific and can be seen during the postictal period or associated with any form of encephalopathy. A single EEG recording will reveal an epileptiform abnormality in approximately 60–70% of people with epilepsy if the recording is obtained during both wakefulness and sleep (Ajmone-Marsan & Zivin, 1970). A recording obtained only during the awake state may be less productive at revealing an abnormality. Activation procedures such as photic stimulation, hyperventilation, and sleep deprivation may all be utilized to increase the possibility of detecting an epileptiform abnormality. A normal EEG does not exclude the diagnosis of epilepsy. In that circumstance, diagnosis is determined by clinical history.

SPECIFIC SYNDROMES

There are several specific epileptic syndromes that occur in childhood and generally follow a developmental course (Commission on Classification and Terminology of the International League Against Epilepsy, 1989). West syndrome (infantile spasms) has an onset in infancy and generally involves clusters of myoclonic seizures. A pattern of hypsarrhythmia is noted on the EEG. Etiology may be cryptogenic or symptomatic (e.g., CNS infections, head trauma, intrapartum asphyxia, inborn errors of metabolism, and neurodegenerative diseases). The seizures generally cease between the second and fourth years of life, only to give rise to other seizure types in 25–60% of children (Freeman, Vining, & Pillas, 1990; Murphy & Dehkharghani, 1994). Up to 10–20% of these infants will die, commonly as a result of the underlying disease or associated complications (Jeavons, Bower, & Dimitrakoudi, 1973; Lacy & Penry, 1976; Dulac, Plouin, & Schlumberger, 1997).

Lennox–Gastaut syndrome is a mixed seizure disorder that includes atypical absence, atonic, and myoclonic seizures. Onset is generally between 2 and 8 years of age. The EEG reveals background slowing and slow spike-wave discharges. Etiology may be symptomatic or cryptogenic, the seizures are frequently difficult to control, and status epilepticus is common (Gastaut, 1982).

In benign focal epilepsy of childhood, seizures begin in childhood, are typically infrequent, and spontaneously resolve before late adolescence. Onset is generally between 3 and 10 years of age. In the most common type, benign rolandic epilepsy, the seizures generally occur nocturnally and involve unilateral clonic activity of the face and upper extremity. Centrotemporal spikes are apparent on the EEG, and AEDs are often not prescribed unless the seizures occur frequently, during the day, or secondary generalized convulsions occur (Loiseau, 1993; Murphy & Dehkharghani, 1994). A less frequently occurring type, benign occipital epilepsy, involves visual symptoms such as a partial or total loss of vision, figurative hallucinations, illusions, or flashing stars. Rhythmical 2- to 3-per-second spike and wave complexes are noted unilaterally or bilaterally over the occipital and posterior temporal regions on the EEG; they are typically induced by eye closure. There appears to be a relationship to migraine, as postictal headaches with nausea and vomiting are sometimes reported (Niedermeyer, 1990).

Childhood absence epilepsy characteristically begins between the ages of 4 and 8 years, has a peak occurrence between 6 and 7 years of age, and is characterized by a pattern of 3-per-second spike and wave discharge on the EEG. This seizure disorder is usually easily treated and often resolves spontaneously, with remission rates of approximately 80% (Annegers, Hauser, & Elueback, 1979). Generalized tonic–clonic seizures may develop in 40% of patients, but are infrequent and tend to occur during adolescence (Berkovic, 1997; Charlton & Yahr, 1969; Dieterich, Baier, Doose, Toxhorn, & Fichsel, 1985; Loiseau, Pestre,

Dartiques, Barberger-Gateau, & Cohadon, 1983). There is a peak in onset of absence sei-zures near puberty in a syndrome classified as juvenile absence epilepsy. In contrast to those with childhood absence epilepsy, the majority of those with juvenile absence epilepsy will experience generalized convulsive seizures, and persistence of epilepsy into adulthood is more common (Berkovic, 1997; Gastaut, Zifken, Mariani, & Puig, 1986).

Juvenile myoclonic epilepsy has an onset in late childhood to early adolescence and involves myoclonic jerks of the upper extremities generally associated with morning wak-ening. There is no associated loss of consciousness; however, 90–95% of these patients will have generalized tonic–clonic seizures. The condition responds positively to valproate (valproic acid), but resolution of seizures is infrequent. The condition is quite common, accounting for 10% of all epilepsies, and is genetically inherited in an autosomal domi-nant fashion (Serratosa & Delgado-Escueta, 1993).

Landau–Kleffner syndrome (LKS), also referred to as acquired aphasia with convul-sive disorder, has an age of onset between 2 and 11 years (Fenichel, 1997). LKS occurs following a period of normal development and is characterized by a sudden or gradual onset of auditory agnosia. The severity of the language disturbance varies, but it may in-volve total unresponsiveness to oral communication, with a progressive deterioration of expressive speech and vocabulary (Paquier, Van Dongen, & Loonen, 1992). Although there is an absence of abnormal neurological signs, the EEG is abnormal, with typical patterns of bilateral spike and slow waves. Focal abnormalities are variable, but predominantly occur in the temporal, temporo-parietal, and parieto-occipital regions. Seizures are present in approximately 70% of these children (Murphy & Dehkharghani, 1994). Seizures may include a variety of types, but the most common are generalized motor seizures. The lan-guage deterioration is accompanied by seizures in at least two-thirds of the cases; how-ever, the seizures may occur before, during, or after the development of aphasia (Feekery, Parry-Fielder, & Hopkins, 1993). Seizures are generally responsive to anticonvulsants, and only 10–20% of the children continue to have seizures at 10 years of age, with a cessation of seizures by 15 years. Anticonvulsant treatment does not typically alleviate the language deficit, however, and it has been postulated that the seizure activity is an epiphenomenon associated with an underlying abnormality of the speech areas, rather than the cause of the aphasia (Gordon, 1990). Long-term outcome of the language deficit is unpredictable, ranging from total recovery to severe auditory agnosia. Onset prior to the age of 5 years is associated with a poorer prognosis. Behavioral changes, including hyperactivity and tem-per outbursts, are often present; these may be attributable to brain alteration or may be reactions to the loss of language (Gordon, 1990). Nonlanguage cognitive abilities are gen-erally preserved.

A similar syndrome—continuous spike-wave discharges during sleep, also referred to as electrical status epilepticus during sleep (ESES)—involves continuous spike and wave activity during more than 85% of non-rapid-eye-movement (non-REM) sleep. The etiol-ogy can be symptomatic or cryptogenic. The majority of children experience neuropsy-chological regression associated with the emergence of ESES, although some children have prior developmental delay. Seizures are often present, and partial motor seizures frequently occur prior to the recognition of ESES. Absence seizures are more prevalent during the emergence of ESES (Jayakar & Seshia, 1991). Age of onset is generally between 4 and 14 years, with discontinuation of the abnormal EEG pattern and seizures during adolescence. As continuous spike-wave activity during non-REM sleep has been reported for some chil-dren with LKS, the disorders may reflect different points on the continuum of a single syn-drome (Feekery et al., 1993). In both syndromes, recovery of language may be associated with disappearance of continuous spike waves during slow-wave sleep (Paquier et al., 1992).

Children with ESES generally demonstrate a more global neuropsychological disturbance, whereas those diagnosed with LKS typically display an isolated language disorder. Differences in predominant seizure types and EEG patterns have also been noted (Jayakar & Seshia, 1991). Both disorders are rare in occurrence.

CLINICAL MANAGEMENT

Most children diagnosed with epilepsy are effectively treated with AEDs, and complete seizure control can be established in up to 80% of the pediatric population. Treatment is initiated when the benefits outweigh the risks of medication use. In most circumstances, seizures that are prolonged or significantly recurrent indicate the need for AED therapy. The correct classification of seizures and epilepsy syndromes contributes to the selection of an appropriate AED. The initial goal is to provide adequate seizure control with a single AED. Monotherapy is more efficacious and results in fewer and less significant side effects. Polytherapy is used with greater caution and only when indicated by poor seizure control after one or more AEDs have failed individually. AED toxicity associated with higher serum concentrations is more prevalent with greater dosages and polytherapy. When indicated, plasma levels of AEDs are measured to assist in adjustment of medication dose, to monitor compliance, and to prevent toxicity. Established AED therapeutic serum concentration ranges are used as guidelines only. Some individuals treated with a specific AED dosage may have complete seizure control at a serum level below the accepted therapeutic range, while others may require a concentration greater than the norm to maintain adequate control and not demonstrate significant toxicity. Dosage is clinically adjusted for the individual patient. Traditional AEDs are typically selected first, and newer AEDs are more appropriately considered for difficult-to-control seizures or under special circumstances, such as intolerable idiosyncratic reactions or side effects in response to traditional medications. Tables 3.1 and 3.2 outline the appropriate selection, serum concentrations, and common side effects of both traditional and newer AEDs.

Although the majority of children and adolescents can be effectively treated with AEDs, approximately 20–30% of the pediatric population will have medically resistant or intractable seizures. Technological advances have resulted in improved seizure classification and patient selection, thereby increasing the use of surgical intervention (Duchowny, 1989).

TABLE 3.1. AEDs of Choice for Specific Seizure Types

	Partial	Primary generalized	Absence	Absence + primary generalized
First-choice AEDs	Carbamazepine Phenytoin Valproate	Valproate	Ethosuximide Valproate	Valproate
Second-choice AEDs	Gabapentin Lamotrigine Felbamate Phenobarbital Primidone Topiramate Tiagabine	Lamotrigine Carbamazepine Phenytoin Felbamate Topiramate Tiagabine	Lamotrigine	Lamotrigine Felbamate

TABLE 3.2. AED Side Effects and Toxicity

AED (Common brand name)	Therapeutic serum concentration (mg/liter)	Side effects	Toxicity
Phenobarbital	10–20	Sedation / Hyperactivity / Behavioral changes	Sedation
Primidone (Mysoline)	8–15	Same as phenobarbital	Same as phenobarbital
Phenytoin (Dilantin)	10–20	Gingival hyperplasia / Rash	Ataxia / Nystagmus / Vomiting
Ethosuximide (Zarontin)	40–60	GI distress / Headaches	Sedation
Carbamazepine (Tegretol)	6–12	Drowsiness / Decreased WBC count / Rash	Sedation / Blurred vision / Diplopia / Aplastic anemia
Valproate (Depakote, Depakene)	50–100	Tremor / Weight gain / Hair loss	Sedation / Thrombocytopenia / Hepatic failure / Pancreatitis
Felbamate (Felbatol)	Not established	Anorexia / Weight loss / Insomnia	Hepatic failure / Aplastic anemia
Gabapentin (Neurontin)	Not established	Sedation / Ataxia	Sedation / Ataxia
Lamotrigine (Lamictal)	Not established	Rash / Sedation / GI distress / Ataxia	Sedation / Ataxia
Topiramate (Topamax)	Not established	Sedation / Weight loss / Language disturbance	Sedation / Language disturbance
Tiagabine (Gabatril)	Not established	Dizziness / Somnolence	Somnolence / Confusion

Note. GI, gastrointestinal; WBC, white blood cell.

Earlier surgery has been urged in order to avoid the cognitive and psychosocial consequences of long-term intractable seizures and drug therapy, as well as the possibility of stopping the propagation of seizures to other areas in the brain.

In a review article by Duchowny (1989), three primary types of pediatric surgery are described. Focal resection involves ablation of a localized seizure focus, often associated with a structural lesion. This surgical intervention is most frequently employed to control complex partial seizures emanating from the anterior temporal lobe, but extratemporal resections are also performed. Approximately 80% of the children who have temporal lobectomies are seizure-free or have greatly reduced seizure frequency after surgery. Research concerning outcome does not suggest cognitive deterioration following surgery. Although significant increases in IQ scores have not generally been reported, improvements in behavior and psychosocial functioning have been suggested. In a pilot study of 9 patients, no marked changes in cognition were found with the exception of decreases in delayed verbal memory regardless of side of surgery. Positive effects on quality of life were suggested by reduced internalizing symptoms and increased social interaction (Williams, Griebel, Sharp, & Boop, 1998). Likewise, Szabo et al. (1998) reported significant postoperative decreases in delayed verbal memory scores, independent of preoperative ability or side or resection, for 14 preadolescent patients. Corpus callosotomy is used to control intractable generalized seizures, theoretically by preventing the rapid spread of seizures from one hemisphere to the other. This procedure, which involves partial anterior–posterior or complete anatomical division of the corpus callosum, stops atonic seizures in approximately 80% of the cases, thereby eliminating injuries associated with these seizures. Improved seizure control ranges from 25% to 75% when tonic, clonic, or partial seizures are involved. Since many children have seizures that are multifocal in origin, the goal is often improved control rather than complete seizure cessation. Although initial symptoms following surgery may include mutism and behavioral depression, these symptoms are typically transitory in nature. The "disconnection syndrome" noted in adults following surgery is not common in children. The majority of children who undergo a corpus callosotomy have various degrees of mental retardation and behavioral difficulties. Although cognitive abilities do not generally increase after surgery, improvements in behavior, attention, and performance of daily activities are noted. Based on findings involving 25 families in which a child experienced a corpus callosotomy, Yang et al. (1996) reported increased satisfaction and quality of life. Improvements in self care, family life, and school performance were found. Functional hemispherectomy is used to treat intractable partial seizures in children who most commonly already demonstrate hemiplegia. This surgical procedure includes partial resection of the involved hemisphere. Typically, the frontopolar and occipital areas are left vascularly intact, but the white matter connections are severed. This procedure results in control of complex partial seizures for 80–90% of the children. Improved behavioral and cognitive status is commonly reported. When the surgery is completed before 10 years of age, there is a lack of aphasia, although problems with nonverbal spatial abilities are evident. In all three types of surgery, complication rates are low.

Surgical workups for pediatric patients generally include EEG video monitoring to record ictal and interictal abnormalities. When equivocal findings concerning seizure localization are present, invasive EEG monitoring is employed to clarify the seizure origin through placement of subdural, epidural, or depth electrodes. Subdural electrode grids can also be used for brain mapping via cortical stimulation studies, to localize areas of cerebral function (e.g., speech and motor areas) to be avoided at the time of resection. Magnetic resonance imaging (MRI) and computerized tomography are utilized to identify structural abnormalities, such as mesial temporal sclerosis and other lesions. When available, other neuroimaging techniques—including positron emission tomography, single-photon emission computed tomography, MRI spectroscopy, and functional MRI (fMRI) may be used to assist in localization of the seizure focus. Neuropsychological assessment is employed for both diagnostic and prognostic purposes.

Prior to temporal lobe resections, the intracarotid amobarbital procedure (IAP) or Wada test is frequently used to determine language dominance as well as competence of memory skills in the hemisphere contralateral to the seizure focus. Sodium amobarbital is injected alternately into the internal carotid artery supplying the anterior and middle cerebral arteries of each hemisphere. Injection of the dominant hemisphere results in aphasia. Memory skills are assessed by recall of objects, pictures, verbalizations, and simple commands following dissipation of medication effects. Surgery may be contraindicated for individuals with evidence of decreased memory skills in the hemisphere contralateral to the seizure focus, due to risk of a possible amnestic syndrome following surgery. Although there has been hesitancy to use the IAP with children in the past, it is presently being employed to a greater extent in presurgical evaluations. Williams and Rausch (1992) found the IAP to be an effective tool in determining language dominance in children; however, memory results for pediatric patients under 13 years of age following injection of the left (language-dominant) hemisphere were less reliable than for older children or younger children whose seizure focus was in the right (non-language-dominant) hemisphere. Similarly, Szabo and Wyllie (1993) found that a modified pediatric IAP was effective in clarifying the language-dominant hemisphere in preadolescent children with borderline or higher intelligence, but that memory retention scores tended to be lower in children than in adults. Results from the IAP and brain mapping, which identify critical language cortex, may affect the size of the focal resection. Previous research with the IAP has suggested that individuals with epilepsy are more likely to have language skills redistributed, particularly if a child had a left-hemisphere injury prior to 5 years of age. Language dominance may be transferred to the right hemisphere or may be displaced within the left hemisphre (Abou-Khalil, 1995). There is some evidence to suggest that fMRI may be a promising tool for the noninvasive study of language organization in children and adolescents. In a study comparing IAP and fMRI results of hemispheric language dominance, perfect agreement was noted for the 6 cases examined (Hertz-Pannier et al., 1997).

In addition to surgical intervention, a ketogenic diet has also been used to increase seizure control in children with drug-resistant epilepsy. One-third of these children can experience complete control of their seizures while on this diet. A significant reduction in seizure frequency or required AED dosage is reported in about one-half of those without complete control (Freeman, Kelly, & Freeman, 1996). The ketogenic diet generally consists of greater than 80% of total calories supplied as fat, with a relatively equal amount of remaining calories from protein and carbohydrates.

EFFECTS ON GENERAL INTELLIGENCE AND GLOBAL COGNITIVE FUNCTIONING

The distribution of IQ scores in children with epilepsy is similar to that found in the general pediatric population (Hauser & Hesdorffer, 1990b), although some research has suggested a skew toward the lower end of the average range and an increased risk for mental retardation (Dodson, 1993; Singhi, Bansal, Singhi, & Pershad, 1992). In a prospective study in which neurological abnormalities and socioeconomic status were controlled for, children with epilepsy performed within the average range of intelligence and did not differ from sibling controls (Ellenberg, Hirtz, & Nelson, 1986).

Some epileptic syndromes are associated with specific cognitive outcomes. Benign rolandic epilepsy and juvenile myoclonic epilepsy do not result in any progressive deterioration and have a generally good intellectual prognosis. Lennox–Gastaut syndrome, in contrast, is associated with a high incidence of moderate to severe mental retardation even when the etiology is cryptogenic. Mental retardation is often progressive and may occur in up to 96% of these children (Gastaut, 1982). West syndrome (infantile spasms) is also associated with a high incidence (80–90%) of mental retardation. However, if the etiology is cryptogenic, 50% of these children may have a normal cognitive outcome (Murphy & Dehkharghani, 1994).

In addition, there are specific conditions that result in developmental abnormalities of the brain and are frequently associated with seizures and altered intellectual functioning. Tuberous sclerosis may be accompanied by early-onset epilepsy and neuropsychiatric disorders, particularly autism. Mental deficits are more commonly present in children with a history of associated infantile spasms or poorly controlled seizures. Mental ability ranges from average intelligence to severe retardation, with lower IQs in approximately 50% of these patients (Jambaque et al., 1991). Some chromosomal disorders, such as Angelman syndrome, have a high incidence of seizures and mental retardation. Other etiologies that may affect global cognitive function and have varying occurrences of seizures include CNS infections (e.g., meningitis and encephalitis), perinatal asphyxia, neurofibromatosis, untreated inborn errors of metabolism, Rett syndrome, and symptomatic neonatal hypoglycemia (Dodson, 1993). All of these conditions are rare and involve only a small portion of children with seizure disorders.

Epilepsy occurs in association with mental retardation (9–31%), autism (11–35%), and cerebral palsy (18–35%). There is no causative link between epilepsy and these conditions; rather, common underlying antecedents result in their co-occurrence (Hauser & Hesdorffer, 1990b).

Epilepsy is not generally associated with an intellectual decline. In one longitudinal study, children compared before and after the onset of seizures with matched controls, as well as with siblings, did not experience a significant change in overall IQ (Ellenberg et al., 1986). In a prospective study in which children with epilepsy were assessed at the initial diagnosis and at follow-up periods, the mean IQ was within the average range, did not change with time, and was not significantly different from that of siblings. Furthermore, IQ change did not differ between seizure types (Bourgeois, Presnky, Palkes, Talent, & Busch, 1983).

When IQ declines have been found, AED toxicity has often been reported. In a subset of children who demonstrated intellectual decline over time, there was a higher incidence of anticonvulsant levels in the toxic range, the epilepsy was more difficult to control, and the seizures began at an earlier age. Drug toxicity, especially phenobarbital toxicity, predicted an IQ decline more effectively than poor seizure control did in one study (Bourgeois et al., 1983). In children with epilepsy and associated neuropsychological deficits, cognitive deterioration has been related to long-term anticonvulsant therapy, particularly phenytoin and phenobarbital (Corbett, Trimble, & Nichol, 1985).

One factor that has consistently been associated with decreased cognitive functioning is a history of status epilepticus. In a review of 13 studies, Dodrill and Wilensky (1990) concluded that there was an adverse effect on mental abilities apart from underlying neurological disease. Status epilepticus accounted for the greatest amount of variance (14%) of epilepsy-related variables on IQ scores among children with idiopathic generalized epilepsy (Singhi et al., 1992).

Earlier seizure onset has also been related to lower IQ scores and poorer prognosis for intellectual outcome (Farwell, Dodrill, & Batzel, 1985). However, inclusion of children with early epileptic syndromes, such as Lennox–Gastaut and West syndrome, may have confounded this relationship (Addy, 1987). Neurological and developmental status prior to the initial seizure has been found to be a major determinant of intellectual outcome among children with nonfebrile seizures. A prospective study indicated that the higher risk for abnormal outcome in children with early-onset epilepsy was nonexistent if children were excluded who had neurological abnormalities before their seizures began (Ellenberg, Hirtz, & Nelson, 1984).

Children with symptomatic epilepsy have consistently been found to score lower on tests of intelligence (Bourgeois et al., 1983). In addition, higher IQ scores have been associated with good seizure control and negatively correlated with duration of seizures in years

(Farwell et al., 1985). Findings concerning intellectual level based on seizure type have been inconsistent. Generally, children with absence seizures have performed at the highest level, and children with atypical absence and mixed seizure types have had the lowest IQ scores (Bourgeois et al., 1983; Farwell et al., 1985).

On the whole, children with epilepsy have normal intelligence and do not experience intellectual deterioration over time (Addy, 1987). Neurological abnormalities contribute more than seizures do to lowered intellectual functioning among children with epilepsy, and the appearance of seizures in otherwise normal children does not predict reduced intelligence (Dodson, 1993). The presence of status epilepticus, early onset of seizures in combination with neurodevelopmental abnormalities, poor seizure control, and drug toxicity appear to be risk factors for altered intellectual function.

SPECIFIC COGNITIVE CORRELATES

Although children with epilepsy have intellectual functioning within the normal range, specific patterns of cognitive strengths and weaknesses may be associated with this disorder. Some researchers have indicated a lack of specific cognitive impairments in children with epilepsy, but others have reported decreased short-term memory skills and poorer concentration in such children than in age-matched controls (Blennow, Heijbel, Sandstedt, & Tonnby, 1990; Dam, 1990).

It is unclear whether the attention and memory difficulties result from the effects of abnormal discharges at a specific site, from a more generalized underlying epileptogenic factor, or from associated factors such as anticonvulsants. Evidence for the specific effects of seizures has been based on the disruption of cognitive and motor performance noted during EEG recordings. Computerized testing of verbal short-term memory and visual spatial skills indicates that cognitive functioning can be disrupted by even brief subclinical epileptiform EEG discharges (Kasteleijn-Nolst-Trenite, Smit, Velis, Willemse, & van Emde Boas, 1990). Interference with cognitive performance by subclinical discharges has been referred to as *transitory cognitive impairment* (Aarts, Binnie, Smit, & Wilkins, 1984). Complex tasks, especially those involving working memory and language, appear to be the most sensitive to disruption, and generalized spike and wave bursts lasting at least 3 seconds are the most likely to produce demonstrable changes (Binnie & Marston, 1992). Even though the cognitive impairment may be transitory, experimental evidence suggests that subclinical discharges may adversely affect a child's acquisition of educational skills (Binnie, Channon, & Marston, 1990; Henriksen, 1990).

It has been postulated that focal epileptic activity can alter the cerebral mechanisms underlying specific cognitive skills, especially in a developing brain. For example, memory deficits may reflect the effects of continued abnormal activity or damage to the underlying neurological substrate, so that children with partial seizures involving the temporal lobe and hippocampus may be particularly vulnerable. In some studies, memory deficits have been found to be more severe in children with partial epilepsy, and these deficits have been related to hemispheric specialization. Left temporal lobe epilepsy in children has been associated with decreased performance on verbal memory tasks, while right temporal lobe epilepsy has been related to decreased visual memory function (Cohen, 1992; Jambaque, Dellatolas, Dulac, Ponsot, & Signoret, 1993). Lateralized cognitive dysfunction has also been demonstrated in children with benign rolandic epilepsy who had no evidence of brain damage and were not treated with anticonvulsants. In a study by Piccirilli et al. (1994), processing of visual–spatial information was disrupted in children who had right-sided or bilateral foci, while children with a left-sided focus performed as well as control subjects. In contrast, children with a left unilateral focus demonstrated an atypical pattern of language lateralization, with more bilateral representation of speech function compared to children with a right unilateral focus or to controls (Piccirilli, D'Alessandro, Tiacci, & Ferroni, 1988).

However, other studies have failed to demonstrate focus-specific cognitive dysfunctions. Camfield et al. (1984) did not find differences between children with pure left and children with pure right temporal lobe epilepsy on verbal and performance skills. Williams et al. (1996) also failed to find decreased memory skills in children with complex partial seizures who had average IQs and no comorbid learning or emotional disorders. In the study by Jambaque et al. (1993), memory problems were found in children with temporal lobe epilepsy as well as in children with a focus outside the temporal lobe. Children with frontal lobe seizures had memory difficulties similar to those of children with temporal lobe seizures. In Cohen's (1992) study, children with right and left temporal lobe epilepsy differed from controls; however, the lateralized groups did not significantly differ from each other, suggesting more diffuse memory difficulties.

The inconsistency in findings may reflect less lateralization in brain organization during early childhood, or possible reorganization of cerebral function in children with epilepsy whose seizures resulted from an early brain insult. In addition, bilateral damage or rapid spread between the temporal lobes may be reflected in less lateralized patterns of memory performance.

Research has consistently suggested a disruption of attentional skills in children with epilepsy. This has been found both in children with normal intellectual functioning and in children with lowered IQ. In a sample of mentally retarded patients with seizure disorders, specific weaknesses were noted in attentional processes, as measured by the Coding and Digit Span subtests of the Wechsler Intelligence Scale for Children—Revised (Forceville, Dekker, Aldenkamp, Alpherts, & Schelvis, 1992). In a study using a computerized test of simple and complex reaction time, children with seizure disorders demonstrated significant inattention and slowing of reaction time when compared to normal controls. Neither seizure history nor anticonvulsant treatment resulted in differences in performance on these variables, and the authors concluded that the inattention and slowed reaction time did not result from seizures or treatment alone, but may have been caused by coexisting neurological abnormalities (Mitchell, Zhou, Chavez, & Guzman, 1992). Stores (1973) has suggested that disruption of either subcortical or cortical mechanisms may result in reduced attentional skills, which might explain the presence of attentional problems regardless of seizure type.

Children with epilepsy may demonstrate highly individualistic patterns of cognitive strengths and weaknesses during neuropsychological performance, but research findings would support a need for assessment of these children's attention and memory skills. Repetition and drill of information may be critical during the learning process for children with epilepsy.

EFFECTS ON ACHIEVEMENT

Children with epilepsy have been found to have a higher risk of learning disabilities and underachievement (Bolter, 1986; Dodson, 1993). In one study, children with seizure disorders repeated grades and were placed in special education twice as frequently as matched controls. In spite of more frequent placements with younger classmates, children with seizures also had higher rates of academic underachievement than controls (Farwell et al., 1985). Lowered educational and occupational achievement in adults whose seizures continued from childhood have been found (Dodrill, 1992b; Kokkonen, Kokkonen, Saukkonen, & Pennanen, 1997).

Specific subtypes of learning disabilities do not appear to be associated with seizure focus. In an early study, underachievement in reading was reported in association with left temporal lobe epilepsy (Stores & Hart, 1976). Camfield et al. (1984), however, failed to find different rates of school failure or need for remediation between children with left and children with right temporal lobe epilepsy. When academic areas are examined, underachievement has been found in math, spelling, writing to dictation, reading comprehension, and general knowledge (Jennekens-Schinkel, Linschooten-Duikersloot, Bouma, Peters, & Stijnen, 1987; Mitchell, Chavez, Lee, & Guzman, 1991; Seidenberg et al., 1986). School failure thus does not appear to involve reading skills alone, and problems may occur in all academic subjects (Addy, 1987; Sturniolo & Galletti, 1994).

The etiology of this generalized pattern of underachievement in children with epilepsy remains unclear. Problems with specific cognitive skills have been hypothesized to adversely affect learning. Seidenberg et al. (1988) examined correlates of academic achievement in two groups of children with epilepsy, based on their academic performance. Neuropsychological test performance and seizure characteristics were compared for the children with epilepsy who demonstrated either satisfactory or unsatisfactory academic progress. Impairments in verbal/language abilities and attention/concentration skills were noted in children with lower achievement, in comparison to the academically successful group. Visual–spatial abilities, problem-solving skills, nonverbal learning and memory, and motor skills did not differ between the groups. Other researchers contend that decreased alertness in these children results in problems with initial encoding of information and may play a significant role in underachievement, regardless of seizure type or treatment (Mitchell et al., 1991; Sturniolo & Galletti, 1994). Similarly, Jambaque et al. (1993) suggest that memory problems, which may impact learning, stem from reduced encoding of information rather than from problems with retrieval or consolidation.

Demographic and clinical seizure variables have been reported to be only modestly predictive of underachievement (Seidenberg, 1996). Mitchell et al. (1991) did not find a relationship between academic underachievement and seizure type, duration of seizure disorder, severity of seizures, or AED exposure. Low socioeconomic status and cultural variables were the major determinants of underachievement, with equal proportions of newly diagnosed children and of children with long-standing epilepsy and anticonvulsant treatment underachieving. Sturniolo and Galletti (1994) failed to find associations of underachievement with gender, age of onset, seizure type, duration, EEG findings, or treatment. Children with epilepsy who were not performing well in school had difficulties with emotional maladjustment, inattentiveness, and visual–motor impairment. However, children with adequate academic performance did not differ from peers without epilepsy on these variables. Jennekens-Schinkel et al. (1987) also failed to find any relationship between seizure variables and spelling errors made by children with seizure disorders. Substandard spelling in the latter group of children was postulated to result from emotional concomitants of epilepsy, reflected in insufficient problem-solving strategies and lack of attention to task requirements.

It would appear that the determinants of academic vulnerability are multivariate and require an approach that includes cognitive, psychosocial, seizure, and medication correlates (Seidenberg, 1996). Often ignored, the influence of socioeconomic factors and emotional variables, especially self-esteem and perceived control, need to be carefully considered when examining academic underachievement in these children. In a recent study by Austin,

Huberty, Huster, and Dunn (1998), factors related to poor academic achievement in children with epilepsy were severity of the medical condition, negative attitudes, and lower school adaptive functioning. Boys with high seizure severity were most at risk for achievement-related problems. The authors encouraged the use of a broad model for predicting academic underachievement. Considering the risk of occurrence and multivariate nature of academic problems, the importance of monitoring academic performance in children with epilepsy is critical, as well as a multidisciplinary approach to treatment that addresses cognitive, psychosocial, and medical issues.

NEUROPSYCHIATRIC AND BEHAVIORAL FUNCTIONING

Children with epilepsy have higher rates of psychiatric disturbance than children in the general population or those with chronic illness (Bolter, 1986; Corbett et al., 1985; Hoare, 1984; Kim, 1991). Epilepsy is associated with a wide range of psychiatric and behavioral disorders, rather than with any specific symptomatology (Hoare & Kerley, 1991).

Both neurological and psychosocial factors contribute to increased risk for psychological maladjustment. Neurological variables may involve underlying brain damage, localized epileptogenic activity in areas regulating emotion, or neurotransmitter and neurohormonal alterations affecting cerebral metabolism (Hermann & Whitman, 1992). Most authorities agree that behavioral difficulties result from brain dysfunction, not epilepsy (Dodson, 1993). In one study, children with epilepsy who demonstrated decreased neuropsychological performance manifested significantly more aggression and overall psychopathology with decreased social competence, compared to children with relatively good neuropsychological function (Hermann, 1982). In another study, children rated by their parents as maladjusted demonstrated significantly lower neuropsychological and cognitive functioning than normally adjusted children with epilepsy. Poor social maturation and dependent lifestyle factors in young adults who had experienced childhood onset epilepsy, were associated with neurological and cognitive impairment rather than epilepsy itself (Kokkonen et al., 1997). Behavioral and emotional disturbance appears to be closely linked to cognitive deficits (Camfield et al., 1984). Individuals with idiopathic epilepsy and normal neuropsychological abilities do not appear to be at higher risk of psychiatric disturbance than a non-neurological patient population (Fiordelli, Beghi, Boglium, & Crespi, 1993).

Some studies have suggested that children with focal EEG abnormalities and temporal lobe epilepsy, particularly left temporal lobe spikes, demonstrate a higher rate of psychiatric disorder (Hoare, 1984; Kim, 1991). However, the preponderance of research provides little empirical support for a specific behavioral syndrome, personality disorder, or increased aggression in individuals with temporal lobe epilepsy (Dodrill, 1992b; Mungas, 1992; Pliszka, 1991). Findings from studies that have controlled for relevant psychosocial factors fail to indicate a relationship between disruptive behavior disorders and epilepsy; nor is there evidence that children with temporal lobe epilepsy exhibit more interictal aggression (Pliszka, 1991). In a study involving controls who had chronic asthma, adolescents with temporal lobe epilepsy did not have a higher rate of specific psychiatric illness (Kaminer, Apter, Aviv, Lerman, & Tyano, 1988). Increased symptoms of depression were noted for both groups, and depressive symptoms were thus attributed to the presence of a chronic illness. Camfield et al. (1984) found no measurable emotional difficulties in children with unilateral temporal lobe epilepsy. Personality problems, when present, were distributed equally between left and right temporal epilepsy groups.

Family variables and seizure frequency have been found to be significant predictors of behavior problems in children with epilepsy (Austin, Risinger, & Beckett, 1992). In one study, child–parent relationships predicted the development of behavior problems to a greater extent than the influence of disease-related factors did, even for children at considerable biological risk (Pianta & Lothman, 1994). Similarly, Mitchell, Scheier, and Baker (1994) found that sociocultural factors were related to parental anxiety and negative attitudes about epilepsy even after psychosocial, behavioral, and medical risk factors were taken into account.

Epilepsy is a unique condition. Seizure events are unpredictable and are associated with a loss of control. The unpredictability of occurrence often results in hypervigilance by parents and teachers, with lowered expectations for achievement and independence (Kim, 1991). Myths and misinformation, such as the belief in "swallowing one's tongue," have been associated with poorer psychosocial adjustment. Lower self-esteem, increased depression and anxiety, and an external locus of control may therefore stem in large part from social-environmental sources of distress (Hermann & Whitman, 1992).

In brief, underlying brain damage, increased seizure frequency, and social factors all appear to be associated with increased risk for behavioral disturbance in children with epilepsy (Corbett et al., 1985). Although neurological dysfunction may predispose children to both behavior problems and epilepsy, psychosocial considerations—including family variables, sociocultural attitudes, myths and misinformation, and a child's level of self-esteem—are critical in determining overall psychological function. Thus measurements of emotional and behavioral functioning are important components of the neuropsychological assessment.

EFFECTS OF ANTICONVULSANTS

Understanding the impact of epilepsy on cognition and behavior is confounded by AED treatment. The effects of AEDs have been difficult to isolate, and findings have been inconsistent and contradictory (Bourgeois, 1998). Reynolds (1983) concluded that these drugs may interfere with attention, concentration, motor speed, memory, and mental processing speed. The underlying causes for AED side effects are difficult to determine, but they may include alteration in metabolism of cerebral monoamines, especially serotonin; alteration in endocrine function related to hormonal changes; drug-induced folate deficiency; and neuronal damage (Reynolds, 1983).

Carbamazepine has been associated with few cognitive side effects (Herranz, Armijo, & Arteaga, 1988; Trimble & Cull, 1988). Although short-term administration of carbamazepine, valproate, or phenobarbital does not appear to increase attentional difficulties in children with with epilepsy or febrile convulsions, long-term administration of carbamazepine seems to have less adverse effects on sustained attention than either valproate or phenobarbital (Hara & Fukuyama, 1989). In a study by Aman, Werry, Paxton, Turbott, and Steward (1990), carbamazepine in normal therapeutic doses not only failed to impair psychomotor function, but even led to improvement on some specific tasks. Trimble (1990) has suggested that the relationship between performance and carbamazepine serum levels varies across cognitive tests. Memory scanning at lower serum levels seems to improve, but error rates appear to rise. Mitchell, Zhou, Chavez, and Guzman (1993) found that carbamazepine monotherapy at higher dosage levels was associated with faster responses and fewer omission errors on more complex tasks. In contrast, Forsythe, Butler, Berg, and McGuire (1991) found that carbamazepine in a moderate dosage, compared to valproate and phenytoin, adversely affected memory in children randomly assigned to AED treatment.

Valproate appears to have minimal effects on cognitive function (Trimble & Cull, 1988). However, the effects of valproate may be significantly associated with dose level. For example, Trimble (1990) found that high valproate levels produced motor impairments. Similarly, Aman, Werry, Paxton, and Turbott (1987) found that lower doses of valproate were associated with higher scores on neuropsychological tests.

In a comparison study of phenobarbital, primidone, phenytoin, carbamazepine, and valproate monotherapy in children, phenytoin led to the highest rates of side effects and treatment withdrawal. The authors concluded that phenytoin may result in a progressive encephalopathy with deterioration of intellectual function, particularly in children with mental retardation or neurological problems (Herranz et al., 1988). Trimble (1990) has also noted that the side effects of phenytoin are more frequently deleterious in individuals with lowered intellectual functioning than in individuals with normal cognitive abilities. Cognitive performance appears to be particularly susceptible to high serum levels of phenytoin; children showing cognitive deterioration are often found to have higher serum concentrations of this anticonvulsant (Trimble & Cull, 1988).

Studies of the cognitive effects of phenobarbital have yielded inconsistent findings. Children in a double-blind, counterbalanced, crossover study were found to perform significantly more poorly on tasks involving short-term memory skills when on phenobarbital than when on valproate (Vining et al., 1987). In a study of children with febrile seizures randomly assigned to phenobarbital treatment or a placebo control, IQ performance was depressed for treated children. The difference remained evident several months after discontinuation of the drug (Farwell et al., 1990). In contrast, Mitchell et al. (1993) reported that phenobarbital caused minimal dose-related effects on attention, reaction time, and impulsivity, but more variability and impulsivity were noted with increasing serum levels. However, few subjects in this study received dosages within the upper levels of the therapeutic range. From the available findings, Trimble (1990) concluded that phenobarbital may have only subtle effects on cognitive functions as long as dosages fall within the therapeutic range.

Other researchers have found little evidence to suggest that AEDs have adverse effects on higher-order cognitive functions. In a review article, Bourgeois (1998) contends that the cognitive and behavioral effects of AEDs in children have been overrated in the past largely due to methodological problems in the studies. More recent research suggests that the majority of children taking AEDs do not experience clinically relevant cognitive or behavioral adverse effects from anticonvulsants. Williams et al. (1998) compared cognitive and behavioral performance for children with newly diagnosed seizures prior to treatment and 6 months following the initiation of an anticonvulsant when seizures were controlled. In a repeated measures design that included a control group of children with newly diagnosed diabetes, changes in performance on cognitive and behavioral measures were not different for children treated with AEDs and controls. Findings suggested a lack of adverse effects during the first 6 months of AED therapy. Tennison et al. (1998) retrospectively examined more chronic effects of AEDs for children who had been treated from 6 months to 6 years. The children in the study had well-controlled seizures, no AED toxicity, and placements in regular classroom settings. Results from the California Achievement Test indicated average performance at the national mean, and the authors concluded that clinically important adverse effects of AEDs on cognitive function are rare. Aldenkamp et al. (1993) compared children on monotherapy before and after withdrawal of AEDs with normal controls. The children with epilepsy had been seizure-free for at least 1 year and had blood serum levels within the therapeutic range. A neuropsychological test battery was used that included both psychomotor function and central cognitive processing skills. Significant improvement attributable to drug withdrawal was found in only one area, psychomotor speed. These researchers suggested that the impact of anticonvulsants on higher-order cognitive function was limited. However, the authors also found some evidence to suggest that phenytoin had a more negative impact on measures of psychomotor speed than carbamazepine did, and that this difference remained after drug withdrawal. The latter outcome is similar to findings by Dodrill and Temkin (1989), which failed to show adverse cognitive effects of phenytoin after motor slowing was controlled for. Motor speed may thus have been a contaminating factor in past studies reporting cognitive impairments on phenytoin.

One consistent finding concerning AED effects is the negative impact of polytherapy compared to monotherapy on cognition and mood (Aldenkamp et al., 1993; Thompson & Trimble, 1982). This effect appears to be independent of drug type (Reynolds, 1983). Monotherapy in children has been associated with improvements in both cognitive abilities and behavior (Trimble & Cull, 1988).

With regard to behavioral side effects, phenobarbital has been consistently implicated in complaints of increased hyperactivity, irritability, and sleep disruption (Herranz et al., 1988; Vining et al., 1987). Phenobarbital appears to exacerbate existing behavioral problems, particularly hyperactivity, but it may have less effect on children with normal intellectual functioning and an absence of prior behavior problems (Trimble & Cull, 1988). The fewest behavioral effects have been noted with valproate and carbamazepine (Dodrill, 1991; Trimble & Cull, 1988). Phenytoin has not been associated with either positive or negative behavioral effects (Dodrill, 1991). Berg, Butler, Ellis, and Foster (1993) did not find persisting differences in the effects of carbamazepine, phenytoin, or valproate on behavioral function in children randomly assigned to these anticonvulsants. The latter investigators also failed to find differences in behavior when the children with seizure disorders were compared to a control group.

Evidence indicates that the most negative effects of AEDs appear to be associated with higher serum levels and polypharmacy. However, findings concerning polytherapy and higher AED concentration may be confounded by the presence of an intractable seizure disorder or underlying brain pathology. Due to individual responsivity, any child may have adverse effects even when established therapeutic ranges are followed. It has been suggested that children with preexisting behavioral disorders, such as attention-deficit/hyperactivity disorder, may be more vulnerable to intensification of baseline behavioral difficulties, while children with mental retardation may be more susceptible to cognitive loss after AED treatment (Lee et al., 1996; Trimble & Cull, 1989).

METHODOLOGICAL DIFFICULTIES IN RESEARCH

Research on the cognitive and psychological effects of epilepsy has been limited by a number of factors. Subject selection bias has resulted from the evaluation of patients with intractable seizures, who are frequently seen in university-affiliated medical centers (Hermann & Whitman, 1984). Patients with uncontrolled seizures are more often on polytherapy and have symptomatic epilepsy. However, as patients with uncontrolled seizures represent only

20% of the population, generalization of findings to the remaining 80% with controlled epilepsy is questionable. Studies have repeatedly shown that uncontrolled seizures have a negative impact on cognitive and behavioral functioning in children (Farwell et al., 1985). In addition, few studies have excluded children with comorbid conditions, such as learning disabilities and attention-deficit/hyperactivity disorder, which themselves may be associated with substandard cognitive performance. An example of such sample bias is noted in a study by Jambaque et al. (1993). The children with epilepsy in this study were reported to demonstrate lower memory scores than controls. However, 30% of the children with epilepsy had repeated one or more grades, and 30% had more than one seizure per day. The mean IQ of controls, moreover, was significantly higher than that of the children with epilepsy. In light of these findings, it would be difficult to conclude that epilepsy is associated with specific cognitive impairment or to accept the epilepsy group as representative of children with seizure disorders.

A complicating factor unique to the study of epilepsy is the confounding of the effects of anticonvulsants with the effects of seizures per se. Although the effects of AEDs are unclear, their influence is frequently ignored in research designs. Ethical considerations preclude the withholding of AEDs, and the study of children after removal from treatment may reflect neuronal changes resulting from either seizures or prolonged use of AEDs. Dodrill (1992c) suggests that many AED studies are weakened by subject selection basis, the overinterpretation of a few statistically significant findings, and the possibility that adverse cognitive effects may reflect psychomotor slowing alone. In a review of studies over the past 25 years, Vermeulen and Aldenkamp (1995) indicate that methodological limitations found in past research preclude precise statements about AED effects in children. Some of these limitations include small sample sizes with multiple outcome measures, lack of a control group, inclusion of subjects on polytherapy, lack of baseline assessments, and failure to measure serum AED concentrations.

The prevailing theme in research on epilepsy has been to examine seizure history and neurobiological variables (e.g., duration of seizures, presence of brain lesions, type of seizures, and frequency of seizures) as predictors of cognitive functioning. Dodrill (1992a) contends that the majority of variance in mental abilities cannot be accounted for by these factors. Family and sociocultural variables are frequently ignored as potential predictors of cognitive outcome, and investigators fail to control for these factors in carrying out statistical analyses. Singhi et al. (1992), for example, found that socioeconomic status was one of the two best predictors of IQ in children with epilepsy. The effects of sociocultural and psychological variables on mental abilities in children with seizure disorders require further investigation.

As is the case with many other neurological disorders, research in epilepsy has often assumed that findings from adult studies can be generalized to children. However, outcomes may differ substantially, depending on whether seizures develop in adulthood or as the result of an early cerebral insult (Dikman, Matthews, & Harley, 1975). The increased likelihood of brain reorganization following early brain injury has been demonstrated in amobarbital studies of speech localization (Rasmussen & Milner, 1977). Young children may also exhibit more pervasive deficits than older children or adults, and patterns of deficits may be quite dissimilar to the lateralized findings sometimes reported in adult samples (Aram & Eisele, 1992). In addition, neuropsychological test instruments and normative data for children have been limited in the past, particularly in measuring those skills thought to be most affected by epilepsy (e.g., memory, attention span, and speed of information processing).

NEW APPROACHES

There is a growing awareness of the importance of a multietiological approach in research concerning the impact of epilepsy on neuropsychological function. Hermann and Whitman (1991) have proposed a conceptual model that examines multiple risk factors predictive of psychological and social dysfunction in individuals with epilepsy. In this model, neurobiological factors (age at onset, seizure control, presence or absence of structural damage, neuropsychological function, ictal/interictal EEG characteristics, etc.), psychosocial variables (adjustment to epilepsy, perceived stigma, financial stress, social support, parental overprotection, etc.), and medication effects (monotherapy vs. polytherapy, presence or absence of barbiturate medications, folate deficiency, medication-induced alterations in cerebral metabolism, etc.) are combined to determine their influence on patients' emotional and behavioral status. Correlations between risk factors and outcome measures of social, psychological, or behavioral functioning are calculated. Statistically significant variables are then entered into a stepwise multiple-regression analysis to identify independent, nonredundant risk factors. Using this model in a study of social competence and behavior problems in children with epilepsy, the researchers found that some neurobiological factors (good seizure control and shorter duration of epilepsy) and psychosocial variables (intact parental marriage and higher family income) were associated with increased social competence, whereas other neurobiological factors (poor seizure control and symptomatic etiology) and psychosocial variables (divorced/separated parents) were predictive of behavior problems (Hermann & Whitman, 1991; Hermann, Whitman, & Anton, 1992). Similarly, Sillanpaa and Helenius (1993) used a multivariate method involving a stepwise cumulative-regression analysis to examine a broad range of potential risk factors. They found that effective communication skills, normal intelligence, and freedom from seizures were significant predictors of social competence in a representative sample of children followed as adults 30 years after seizure onset. In the earlier-cited study by Mitchell et al. (1994), a multietiological approach was employed to determine risk factors affecting psychosocial, behavioral, and medical outcomes. Data were collected at baseline concerning medical and seizure history, cognitive functioning, behavior problems, and family functioning. Children and their families were followed longitudinally, and reassessment of medical status, parental attitudes toward epilepsy, and behavioral and cognitive functioning was completed at follow-up. Confirmatory factor analysis was used to determine baseline predictor factors, including Sociocultural Risk, Seizure Risk, and Behavior Problems; outcome factors included Medical/Seizure Problems, Parent's Negative Attitudes Toward Epilepsy, and Behavior Problems. Structural equation modeling (path analysis) was then employed to determine across-time causal effects. Seizure history was the best predictor of ongoing medical difficulties, while sociocultural factors contributed the most to ongoing parental anxiety and negative attitudes toward epilepsy. Further well-controlled, prospective, multietiological studies combining psychosocial, medication, and neurobiological variables are needed to provide a more comprehensive understanding of the etiology and treatment of psychosocial and cognitive dysfunction in epilepsy.

Recognition of the importance of determining both the medical efficacy as well as potential cognitive and behavioral side effects of anticonvulsants is apparent with the advent of the new generation of AEDs. The inclusion of neuropsychological test batteries in drug trials with children of newly developed AEDs attests to this realization. Unfortunately, newer AEDs have been tested mostly in add-on trials thus far (Bourgeois, 1998). To address previous methodological problems noted in studies concerning the effects of anticonvulsants, a number of recommendations has been made for study designs (Bourgeois, 1991; Devinsky, 1995; Legarda, Booth, Fennell, & Maria, 1996; Vermeulen & Aldenkamp, 1995; Williams et al., 1998). Assessing children with newly diagnosed epilepsy prior to being placed on AEDs with a follow-up assessment after seizures are controlled would assist in isolating the sequelae of AEDs from the consequences of the seizure disorder itself. A no-treatment control group tested at similar time periods should be included or a repeated-measures design in which each child serves as his or her own control would provide a clear view of individual variability across treatment conditions. The neuropsychological test battery should be limited in the number of outcome variables assessed and should include tasks sensitive to subtle changes in higher cortical functions critical to learning. AED levels need to be monitored at each assessment. Children with poorly controlled seizures or those requiring polytherapy need to be excluded from outcome findings.

In addition to research concerning AED efficacy and side effects, further study is needed regarding factors that may predispose children to experience negative effects of anticonvulsants, such as children with baseline behavioral and cognitive difficulties.

In any study of epilepsy's cognitive and neurobehavioral effects, possible subject selection biases need to be closely examined. Inclusion of broader samples of children, including those referred from private practitioners, is critical. Issues pertaining to subject demographics and comorbid disorders need to be carefully addressed, as cognitive outcomes may have more to do with these conditions than with epilepsy.

Further basic research on the pathophysiology of epilepsy is needed. Neurophysiological studies will enhance understanding of the neuronal mechanisms involved in the origin and propagation of seizures. Functional neuroimaging techniques may allow delineation of more specific neurochemical abnormalities within the epileptogenic zone. Increased understanding of the mechanism of epileptogenesis will aid in the development of more selectively active AEDs and will result in improved efficacy. Information with regard to both the biological and neurobehavioral aspects of epilepsy will help direct medical and psychosocial interventions and will thereby contribute to an improved quality of life for children with epilepsy.

REFERENCES

Aarts, J. H. P., Binnie, C. D., Smit, A. M., & Wilkins, A. J. (1984). Selective cognitive impairment during focal and generalized epileptiform EEG activity. *Brain, 107,* 293–308.

Abou-Khalil, B. (1995). Insights into language mechanisms derived from the evaluation of epilepsy. In H. S. Kirshner (Ed.), *Handbook of neurological speech and language disorders* (pp. 213–275). New York: Marcel Dekker.

Addy, D. P. (1987). Cognitive function in children with epilepsy. *Developmental Medicine and Child Neurology, 29,* 394–404.

Ajmone-Marsden, C., & Zivin, L. S. (1970). Factors related to the occurrence of typical paroxysmal abnormalities in the EEG records of epileptic patients. *Epilepsia, 11,* 361–381.

Aldenkamp, A. P., Alpherts, W. C. J., Blennow, G., Elmqvist, D., Heijbel, J., Niosson, H. L., Sandstedt, P., Tonnby, B., Wahlander, L., & Wosse, E. (1993). Withdrawal of antiepileptic medication in children—effects on cognitive function: The multicenter Holmfrid study. *Neurology, 43,* 41–50.

Aman, M. G., Werry, J. S., Paxton, J. W., & Turbott, S. H. (1987). Effect of sodium valproate on psychomotor performance in children as a function of dose, fluctuations in concentration, and diagnosis. *Epilepsia, 28,* 115–124.

Aman, M. G., Werry, J. S., Paxton, J. W., Turbott, S. H., & Steward, A. W. (1990). Effects of carbamazepine on psychomotor performance in children as a function of drug concentration, seizure type, and time of medication. *Epilepsia, 31,* 51–60.

Annegers, J. F. (1997). The epidemiology of epilepsy. In E. Wyllie (Ed.), *The treatment of epilepsy: Principles and practice* (2nd ed., pp. 165–172). Baltimore, MD: Williams & Wilkins.

Annegers, J. F., Hauser, W. A., & Elueback, L. R. (1979). Remission of seizures and relapse in patients with epilepsy. *Epilepsia, 20,* 729–737.

Annegers, J. F., Hauser, W. A., Shirts, S. B., & Kurland, L. T. (1987). Factors prognostic of unprovoked seizures after febrile convulsions. *New England Journal of Medicine, 316,* 493–498.

Aram, D. M., & Eisele, J. A. (1992). Plasticity and recovery of higher cognitive functions following early brain injury. In F. Boller & J. Grafman (Eds.), *Handbook of neuropsychology* (Vol. 6, pp. 73–92). Amsterdam: Elsevier.

Austin, J. K., Huberty, T. J., Huster, G. A., & Dunn, D. W. (1998). Academic achievement in children with epilepsy or asthma. *Developmental Medicine and Child Neurology, 40,* 248–255.

Austin, J. K., Risinger, M. W., & Beckett, L. A. (1992). Correlates of behavior problems in children with epilepsy. *Epilepsia, 33,* 1115–1122.

Babb, T. L., & Pretorius, J. K. (1993). Pathologic substrates of epilepsy. In E. Wyllie (Ed.),*The treatment of epilepsy: Principles and practices* (pp. 55–70). Philadelphia: Lea & Febiger.

Berg, I., Butler, A., Ellis, M., & Foster, J. (1993). Psychiatric aspects of epilepsy in childhood treated with carbamazepine, phenytoin, or sodium valproate: A random trial. *Developmental Medicine and Child Neurology, 35,* 149–157.

Berkovic, S. (1997). Childhood absence epilepsy and juvenile absence epilepsy. In E. Wyllie (Ed.), *The treatment of epilepsy: Principles and practice* (2nd ed., pp. 461–466). Baltimore, MD: Williams & Wilkins.

Binnie, C. D., Channon, S., & Marston, D. (1990). Learning disabilities in epilepsy: Neurophysiological aspects. *Epilepsia, 31*(4), S2–S8.

Binnie, C. D., & Marston, D. (1992). Cognitive correlates of interictal discharges. *Epilepsia, 33,* S11–S17.

Blennow, G., Heijbel, J., Sandstedt, P., & Tonnby, B. (1990). Discontinuation of antiepileptic drugs in children who have outgrown epilepsy: Effects on cognitive function. *Epilepsia, 31*(4), S50–S53.

Bolter, J. F. (1986). Epilepsy in children: Neuropsychological effects. In J. E. Obrzut & G. W. Hynd (Eds.), *Child neuropsychology* (Vol. 2, pp. 59–81). Orlando, FL: Academic Press.

Bourgeois, B. F. D. (1991). Relationship between anticonvulsant drugs and learning disabilities. *Seminars in Neurology, 11,* 14–19.

Bourgeois, B. F. D. (1998). Antiepileptic drugs, learning, and behavior in childhood epilepsy. *Epilepsia, 39,* 913–921.

Bourgeois, B. F. D., Prensky, A. L., Palkes, H. S., Talent, B. K., & Busch, S. G. (1983). Intelligence in epilepsy: A prospective study in children. *Annals of Neurology, 14,* 438–444.

Camfield, P. R., Gates, R., Ronen, G., Camfield, C., Ferguson, A., & MacDonald, G. W. (1984). Comparison of cognitive ability, personality profile, and school success in epileptic children with pure right versus left temporal lobe EEG foci. *Annals of Neurology, 15,* 122–126.

Chabolla, D. R., Krahn, L. E., So, E. L., & Rummans, T. A. (1996). Psychogenic nonepileptic seizures. *Mayo Clinic Proceedings, 71,* 493–500.

Charlton, G. B., & Yahr, M. D. (1969). Long term follow-up of patients with petit mal. *Archives of Neurology, 16,* 595–598.

Cohen, M. (1992). Auditory/verbal and visual/spatial memory in children with complex partial epilepsy of temporal lobe origin. *Brain and Cognition, 20,* 315–326.

Commission on Classification and Terminology of the International League Against Epilepsy. (1981). Proposal for revised clinical and electroencephalographic classification of epileptic seizures. *Epilepsia, 22,* 489–501.

Commission on Classification and Terminology of the International League Against Epilepsy. (1989). Proposal for revised classification of epilepsies and epileptic syndromes. *Epilepsia, 26,* 268–278.

Consensus Development Conference on Febrile Seizures. (1981). Proceedings. *Epilepsia, 22,* 377–381.

Corbett, J. A., Trimble, M. R., & Nichol, T. C. (1985). Behavioral and cognitive impairments in children with epilepsy: The long-term effects of anticonvulsant therapy. *Journal of the American Academy of Child Psychiatry, 24,* 17–23.

Coulter, D. A., Huguenard, J. R., & Prince, D. A. (1989). Characterization of ethosuximide reduction of low-threshold calcium current in thalamic neurons. *Annals of Neurology, 25,* 582–593.

Dam, M. (1990). Children with epilepsy: The effect of seizures, syndromes, and etiological factors on cognitive functioning. *Epilepsia, 31*(4), S26–S29.

Devinsky, O. (1995). Cognitive and behavioral effects of antiepileptic drugs. *Epilepsia, 36,* S46–65.

Dieterich, E., Baier, W. K., Doose, H., Toxhorn, I., & Fichsel, H. (1985). Longterm follow-up of childhood epilepsy with absences: I. Epilepsy with absences at onset. *Neuropediatrics, 16,* 149–154.

Dikman, S., Matthews, C. O., & Harley, J. P. (1975). The effect of early versus late onset of major motor epilepsy upon cognitive–intellectual performance. *Epilepsia, 16,* 73–81.

Dodrill, C. B. (1991). Behavioral effects of antiepileptic drugs. *Advances in Neurology, 55,* 213–224.

Dodrill, C. B. (1992a). Interictal cognitive aspects of epilepsy. *Epilepsia, 33,* S7–S10.

Dodrill, C. B. (1992b). Neuropsychological aspects of epilepsy. *Psychiatric Clinics of North America, 15,* 383–394.

Dodrill, C. B. (1992c). Problems in the assessment of cognitive effects of antiepileptic drugs. *Epilepsia, 33,* S29–S32.

Dodrill, C. B., & Temkin, N. R. (1989). Motor speed is a contaminating factor in evaluating the "cognitive" effects of phenytoin. *Epilepsia, 30*(4), 453–457.

Dodrill, C. B., & Wilensky, A. J. (1990). Intellectual impairment as an outcome of status epilepticus. *Neurology, 40,* 23–27.

Dodson, W. E. (1993). Epilepsy and IQ. In W. E. Dodson & J. M. Pellock (Eds.), *Pediatric epilepsy: Diagnosis and therapy* (pp. 373–385). New York: Demos.

Duchowny, M. S. (1989). Surgery for intractable epilepsy: Issues and outcome. *Pediatrics, 84,* 886–894.

Dulac, O., Plouin, P., & Schlumberger, E. (1997). Infantile spasms. In E. Wyllie (Ed.), *The treatment of epilepsy: Principles and practice* (2nd ed., pp. 540–572). Baltimore, MD: Williams & Wilkins.

Ellenberg, J. H., Hirtz, D. G., & Nelson, K. B. (1984). Age at onset of seizures in young children. *Annals of Neurology, 15,* 127–134.

Ellenberg, J. H., Hirtz, D. G., & Nelson, K. B. (1986). Do seizures in children cause intellectual deterioration? *New England Journal of Medicine, 314,* 1085–1088.

Farwell, J. R., Dodrill, C. B., & Batzel, L. W. (1985). Neuropsychological abilities of children with epilepsy. *Epilepsia, 26,* 395–400.

Farwell, J. R., Lee, Y. J., Hirtz, D. G., Sulzbacher, S. I., Ellenberg, J. H., & Nelson, K. B. (1990). Phenobarbital for febrile seizures: Effects on intelligence and on seizure recurrence. *New England Journal of Medicine, 322,* 364–369.

Feekery, C. J., Parry-Fielder, B., & Hopkins, I. J. (1993). Landau–Kleffner syndrome: Six patients including discordant monozygotic twins. *Pediatric Neurology, 9,* 49–53.

Fenichel, G. M. (1997). *Clinical pediatric neurology* (pp. 1–46). Philadelphia: W. B. Saunders.

Fiordelli, E., Beghi, E., Bogliun, G., & Crespi, V. (1993). Epilepsy and psychiatric disturbance: A cross-sectional study. *British Journal of Psychiatry, 163,* 446–450.

Forceville, E. J. M., Dekker, M. J. A., Aldenkamp, A. P., Alpherts, W. C. J., & Schelvis, A. J. (1992). Subtest profiles of the WISC-R and WAIS in mentally retarded patients with epilepsy. *Journal of Intellectual Disability Research, 36,* 45–59.

Forsgren, L., Sidenvall, R., Blomquist, H. K., & Heijbel, J. (1990). A prospective incidence of unprovoked seizures after febrile convulsions. *Acta Paediatrica Scandinavica, 79,* 550–557.

Forsythe, I., Butler, R., Berg, I., & McGuire, R. (1991). Cognitive impairment in new cases of epilepsy randomly assigned to carbamazepine, phenytoin, and sodium valproate. *Developmental Medicine and Child Neurology, 33,* 524–534.

Freeman, J. M., Kelly, M. T., & Freeman, J. B. (1996). *The epilepsy diet treatment: An introduction to the ketogenic diet.* New York: Demos.

Freeman, J. M., Vining, E. P. G., & Pillas, D. J. (1990). *Seizures and epilepsy in childhood: A guide for parents.* Baltimore: Johns Hopkins University Press.

Gastaut, H. (1982). The Lennox–Gastaut syndrome: Comments on the syndrome's terminology and nosological position among the secondary generalized epilepsies of childhood. *Electroencephalography and Clinical Neurophysiology, 35,* S71–S84.

Gastaut, H., Zifken, B. G., Mariani, A., & Puig, J. S. (1986). The long-term course of primary generalized epilepsy with persisting absences. *Neurology, 36,* 1021–1028.

Gloor, P., Avoli, M., & Kostopoulos, G. (1990). Thalamocortical relationships in generalized epilepsy with bilaterally synchronous spike-and-wave discharge. In M. Avoli, P. Gloor, R. Naquet, & G. Kostopoulos (Eds.), *Generalized epilepsies: Neurobiological approaches* (pp. 190–212). Boston: Birkhauser.

Gordon, N. (1990). Acquired aphasia in childhood: The Landau–Kleffner syndrome. *Developmental Medicine and Child Neurology, 32,* 270–274.

Hara, H., & Fukuyama, Y. (1989). Sustained attention during the interictal period of mentally normal children with epilepsy or febrile convulsions, and the influence of anticonvulsants and seizures on attention. *Japanese Journal of Psychiatry and Neurology, 43*(3), 411–416.

Hauser, W. A., & Hesdorffer, D. C. (1990a). *Epilepsy: Frequency, causes, and consequences.* New York: Demos.

Hauser, W. A., & Hesdorffer, D. C. (1990b). *Facts about epilepsy.* New York: Demos.

Hauser, W. A., & Hesdorffer, D. C. (1997). The natural history of seizures. In E. Wyllie (Ed.), *The treatment of epilepsy: Principles and practice* (2nd ed., pp. 173–178). Baltimore, MD: Williams & Wilkins.

Hauser, W. A., & Kurland, L. T. (1975). The epidemiology of epilepsy in Rochester, Minnesota, 1936 through 1967. *Epilepsia, 16,* 1–36.

Haynes, S. D., & Bennett, T. L. (1992). Historical perspective and overview. In T. L. Bennett (Ed.), *The neuropsychology of epilepsy* (pp. 3–16). New York: Plenum Press.

Henriksen, O. (1990). Education and epilepsy: Assessment and remediation. *Epilepsia, 31*(4), S21–S25.

Hermann, B. P. (1982). Neuropsychological functioning and psychopathology in children with epilepsy. *Epilepsia, 23,* 545–554.

Hermann, B., & Whitman, S. (1984). Behavioral and personality correlates of epilepsy: A review, methodological critique, and conceptual model. *Psychological Bulletin, 95,* 451–497.

Hermann, B., & Whitman, S. (1991). Neurobiological, psychosocial, and pharmacological factors underlying interictal psychopathology in epilepsy. *Advances in Neurology, 55,* 439–452.

Hermann, B., & Whitman, S. (1992). Psychopathology in epilepsy. *American Psychologist, 47,* 1134–1138.

Hermann, B. P., Whitman, S., & Anton, M. (1992). A multietiological model of psychological and social dysfunction in epilepsy. In T. L. Bennett (Ed.), *The neuropsychology of epilepsy* (pp. 39–57). New York: Plenum Press.

Herranz, J. L., Armijo, J. A., & Arteaga, R. (1988). Clinical side effects of phenobarbital, primidone, phenytoin, carbamazepine, and valproate during monotherapy in children. *Epilepsia, 29,* 794–804.

Hertz-Pannier, L., Gaillard, W. D., Mott, S. H., Cuenod, C. A., Bookheimer, S. Y., Weinstein, S., Conry, J., Papero, P. H., Schiff, S. J., LeBihan, D., & Theodore, W. H. (1997). Noninvasive assessment of language dominance in children and adolescents with functional MRI: A preliminary study. *Neurology, 48,* 1003–1012.

Hoare, P. (1984). The development of psychiatric disorder among school children with epilepsy. *Developmental Medicine and Child Neurology, 26,* 3–13.

Hoare, P., & Kerley, S. (1991). Psychosocial adjustment of children with chronic epilepsy and their families. *Developmental Medicine and Child Neurology, 33,* 201–215.

Jambaque, I., Cusmai, R., Curatolo, P., Cortesi, F., Perrot, C., & Dulac, O. (1991). Neuropsychological aspects of tuberous sclerosis in relation to epilepsy and MRI findings. *Developmental Medicine and Child Neurology, 33,* 698–705.

Jambaque, I., Dellatolas, G., Dulac, O., Ponsot, G., & Signoret, J. L. (1993). Verbal and visual memory impairment in children with epilepsy. *Neuropsychologia, 31,* 1321–1337.

Jayakar, P. B., & Seshia, S. S. (1991). Electrical status epilepticus during slow-wave sleep: A review. *Journal of Clinical Neurophysiology, 8,* 299–311.

Jeavons, P. M., Bower, B. D., & Dimitrakoudi, M. (1973). Long term prognosis of 150 cases of "West syndrome." *Epilepsia, 14,* 153–164.

Jennekens-Schinkel, A., Linschooten-Duikersloot, E. M. E. M., Bouma, P. A. D., Peters, A. C. B., & Stijnen, T. (1987). Spelling errors made by children with mild epilepsy: Writing-to-dictation. *Epilepsia, 28,* 555–563.

Kaminer, Y., Apter, A., Aviv, A., Lerman, P., & Tyano, S. (1988). Psychopathology and temporal lobe epilepsy in adolescents. *Acta Psychiatrica Scandinavica, 77,* 640–644.

Kasteleijn-Nolst-Trenite, D. G. A., Smit, A. M., Velis, D. N., Willemse, J., & van Emde Boas, W. (1990). On-line detection of transient neuropsychological disturbances during EEG discharges in children with epilepsy. *Developmental Medicine and Child Neurology, 32,* 46–50.

Kim, W. J. (1991). Psychiatric aspects of epileptic children and adolescents. *Journal of the American Academy of Child and Adolescent Psychiatry, 30,* 874–886.

Knowles, W. D., & Luders, H. (1993). Normal neurophysiology: The science of excitable cells. In E. Wyllie (Ed.), *The treatment of epilepsy: Principles and practices* (pp. 503–512). Philadelphia: Lea & Febiger.

Kokkonen, J., Kokkonen, E. R., Saukkonen, A. L., Pennanen, P. (1997). Psychosocial outcome of young adults with epilepsy in childhood. *Journal of Neurology, Neurosurgery and Psychiatry, 62,* 265–268.

Lacy, J. R., & Penry, J. K. (1976). *Infantile spasms.* New York: Raven Press.

Lee, D. O., Steingard, R. J., Cesena, M., Helmers, S. L., Riviello, J. J., & Mikati, M. A. (1996). Behavioral side effects of gabapentin in children. *Epilepsia, 37,* 87–90.

Legarda, S. B., Booth, M. P., Fennell, E. B., & Maria, B. L. (1996). Altered cognitive functioning in children with idiopathic epilepsy receiving valproate monotherapy. *Journal of Child Neurology, 11,* 321–330.

Lesser, R. P. (1996). Psychogenic seizures. *Neurology, 46,* 1499–1507.

Loiseau, P. (1993). Benign focal epilepsies of childhood. In E. Wyllie (Ed.), *The treatment of epilepsy: Principles and practices* (pp. 503–512). Philadelphia: Lea & Febiger.

Loiseau, P., Pestre, M., Dartigues, J. F., Barberger-Gateau, C., & Cohadon, S. (1983). Long term prognosis in two forms of childhood epilepsy: Typical absence seizures and epilepsy with rolandic (centrotemporal) EEG foci. *Annals of Neurology, 13,* 642–648.

Lothman, E. W. (1990). The biochemical basis and pathophysiology of status epilepticus. *Neurology, 40,* 13–23.

Meencke, H. J., & Janz, D. (1985). The significance of microdysgenesia in primary generalized epilepsy: An answer to the considerations of Lyon and Gastaut. *Epilepsia, 26,* 368–371.

Meldrum, B. S. (1983). Metabolic factors during prolonged seizures and their relation to nerve cell death. *Advances in Neurology, 34,* 261–275.

Mitchell, W. G., Chavez, J. M., Lee, H., & Guzman, B. L. (1991). Academic underachievement in children with epilepsy. *Journal of Child Neurology, 6,* 65–72.

Mitchell, W. G., Scheier, L. M., & Baker, S. A. (1994). Psychosocial, behavioral, and medical outcomes in children with epilepsy: A developmental risk factor model using longitudinal data. *Pediatrics, 94,* 471–477.

Mitchell, W. G., Zhou, Y., Chavez, J. M., & Guzman, B. L. (1992). Reaction time, attention, and impulsivity in epilepsy. *Pediatric Neurology, 8*(1), 19–24.

Mitchell, W. G., Zhou, Y., Chavez, J. M., & Guzman, B. L. (1993). Effects of antiepileptic drugs on reaction time, attention, and impulsivity in children. *Pediatrics, 91*(1), 101–105.

Mungas, D. M. (1992). Behavioral syndromes in epilepsy: A multivariate, empirical approach. In T. L. Bennett (Ed.), *The neuropsychology of epilepsy* (pp. 139–180). New York: Plenum Press.

Murphy, J. V., & Dehkharghani, F. (1994). Diagnosis of childhood seizure disorders. *Epilepsia, 35,* S7–S17.

Niedermeyer, E. (1990). *The epilepsies: Diagnosis and management.* Baltimore: Urban & Schwarzenberg.

Novelly, R. A. (1992). The debt of neuropsychology to the epilepsies. *American Psychologist, 47,* 1126–1129.

Paquier, P. F., Van Dongen, H. R., & Loonen, C. B. (1992). The Landau–Kleffner syndrome or acquired aphasia with convulsive disorder. *Archives of Neurology, 49,* 354–359.

Pianta, R. C., & Lothman, D. J. (1994). Predicting behavior problems in children with epilepsy: Child factors, disease factors, family stress, and child–mother interaction. *Child Development, 65,* 1415–1428.

Piccirilli, M., D'Alessandro, P. D., Sciarma, T., Cantoni, C., Dioguardi, M. S., Giuglietti, M., Ibba, A., & Tiacci, C. (1994). Attention problems in epilepsy: Possible significance of the epileptogenic focus. *Epilepsia, 35,* 1091–1096.

Piccirilli, M., D'Alessandro, P., Tiacci, C., & Ferroni, A. (1988). Language lateralization in children with benign partial epilepsy. *Epilepsia, 29,* 19–25.

Pliszka, S. R. (1991). Anticonvulsants in the treatment of child and adolescent psychopathology. *Journal of Clinical Child Psychology, 20,* 277–281.

Rasmussen, T., & Milner, B. (1977). The role of early left-brain injury in determining lateralization of cerebral speech functions. *Annals of the New York Academy of Sciences, 299,* 335–369.

Reynolds, E. H. (1983). Mental effects of antiepileptic medication: A review. *Epilepsia, 24*(2), S85–S95.

Schwartzkroin, P. A. (1993). Basic mechanisms of epileptogenesis. In E. Wyllie (Ed.), *The treatment of epilepsy: Principles and practices* (pp. 83–98). Philadelphia: Lea & Febiger.

Seidenberg, M. (1996). Academic performance of children with epilepsy. In J. C. Sackellares (Ed.), *Psychological disturbances in epilepsy* (pp. 99–107). Boston, MA: Butterworth Heinemann.

Seidenberg, M., Beck, N., Geisser, M., Giordani, B., Sackellares, J. C., Berent, S., Dreifuss, F. E., & Boll, T. J. (1986). Academic achievement of children with epilepsy. *Epilepsia, 27,* 753–759.

Seidenberg, M., Beck, N., Geisser, M., O'Leary, D. S., Giordani, B., Berent, S., Sackellares, C., Dreifuss, F. E., & Boll, T. J. (1988). Neuropsychological correlates of academic achievement of children with epilepsy. *Journal of Epilepsy, 1,* 23–29.

Serratosa, J. M., & Delgado-Escueta, A. V. (1993). Juvenile myoclonic epilepsy. In E. Wyllie (Ed.), *The treatment of epilepsy: Principles and practices* (pp. 552–570). Philadelphia: Lea & Febiger.

Sillanpaa, M., & Helenius, H. (1993). Social competence of people with epilepsy: A new methodological approach. *Acta Neurologica Scandinavica, 87,* 335–341.

Singhi, P. D., Bansal, U., Singhi, S., & Pershad, D. (1992). Determinants of IQ profile in children with idiopathic generalized epilepsy. *Epilepsia, 33,* 1106–1114.

Stores, G. (1973). Studies of attention and seizure disorders. *Developmental Medicine and Child Neurology, 15,* 376–382.

Stores, G., & Hart, J. (1976). Reading skills of children with generalised or focal epilepsy attending ordinary school. *Developmental Medicine and Child Neurology, 18,* 705–716.

Sturniolo, M. G., & Galletti, F. (1994). Idiopathic epilepsy and school achievement. *Archives of Disease in Childhood, 70,* 424–428.

Szabo, C. A., & Wyllie, E. (1993). Intracarotid amobarbital testing for language and memory dominance in children. *Epilepsy Research, 15,* 239–246.

Szabo, C. A., Wyllie, E., Stanford, L. D., Geckler, C., Kotagal, P., Comair, Y. G., & Thornton, A. E. (1998).

Neuropsychological effect of temporal lobe resection in preadolescent children with epilepsy. *Epilepsia, 39*, 814–819.

Tennison, M., Kankirawatana, P., Bowman, M. R., Greenwood, R., Lewis, D., & Burchinal, M. (1998). Effect of chronic antiepileptic drug therapy on California achievement test scores. *Journal of Epilepsy, 11*, 208–214.

Thompson, P. J., & Trimble, M. R. (1982). Anticonvulsant drugs and cognitive functions. *Epilepsia, 23*, 531–544.

Trimble, M. R. (1990). Antiepileptic drugs, cognitive function, and behavior in children: Evidence from recent studies. *Epilepsia, 31*(4), S30–S34.

Trimble, M. R., & Cull, C. (1988). Children of school age: The influence of antiepileptic drugs on behavior and intellect. *Epilepsia, 29*, S15–S19.

Trimble, M. R., & Cull, C. A. (1989). Antiepileptic drugs, cognitive function, and behavior in children. *Cleveland Clinic Journal of Medicine, 56*, S140–146.

Vermeulen, J., & Aldenkamp, A. P. (1995). Cognitive side-effects of chronic antiepileptic drug treatment: A review of 25 years of research. *Epilepsy Research, 22*, 65–95.

Vining, E. P. G., Mellits, E. D., Dorsen, M. M., Cataldo, M. F., Quaskey, S. A., Spielberg, S. P., & Freeman, J. M. (1987). Psychologic and behavioral effects of antiepileptic drugs in children: A double-blind comparison between phenobarbital and valproic acid. *Pediatrics, 80*, 165–174.

Williams, J., Bates, S., Griebel, M. L., Lange, B., Mancias, P., Pihoker, C. M., & Dykman, R. (1998). Does short-term antiepileptic drug treatment in children result in cognitive or behavioral chagnes? *Epilepsia, 39*, 1064–1069.

Williams, J., Griebel, M. L., Sharp, G. B., & Boop, F. A. (1998). Cognition and behavior after temporal lobectomy in pediatric patients with intractable epilepsy. *Pediatric Neurology, 19*, 189–194.

Williams, J., & Rausch, R. (1992). Factors in children that predict performance on the intracarotid amobarbital procedure. *Epilepsia, 33*, 1036–1041.

Williams, J., Sharp, G., Lange, B., Bates, S., Griebel, M., Spence, G. T., & Thomas, P. (1996). The effects of seizure type, level of control, and AEDs on memory and attention in non-handicapped children with epilepsy. *Developmental Neuropsychology, 12*, 239–251.

Yang, T. F., Wong, T. T., Kwan, S. Y., Chang, K. P., Lee, T. C., & Hsu, T. C. (1996). Quality of life and life satisfaction in families after a child has undergone corpus callosotomy. *Epilepsia, 37*, 76–80.

4

BRAIN TUMORS

ROBIN D. MORRIS
NICHOLAS S. KRAWIECKI
KRIS A. KULLGREN
SUE M. INGRAM
BETTY KURCZYNSKI

Children with brain tumors constitute a group at risk for neurocognitive, psychosocial, and behavioral difficulties. Given that brain tumors directly affect those areas of the developing brain in which they are located, and that many of their treatments result in additional insults to the central nervous system (CNS), neurobehavioral consequences can be diverse. Many children with brain tumors evidence significant neuropsychological and emotional difficulties, but others do not. Longitudinal studies suggest that both cognitive and psychosocial problems evident in early phases of a tumor may persist over time (Mulhern, Wasserman, Friedman, & Fairclough, 1989), although many of the neurocognitive and psychosocial problems are not clearly evident until years after diagnosis and treatment. In addition, although a brain tumor is clearly an acute life-threatening condition for many children, it can also become a chronic disease for them and their families. This heterogeneity of neurobehavioral outcomes in children with brain tumors, and the ever-changing nature and impact of associated medical treatments, complicate both the study and clinical assessment of these neurodevelopmental conditions.

The pediatric neuropsychologist is frequently involved in the ongoing care of children with brain tumors from the day of diagnosis (or sometimes before) throughout their childhood and young adult years. Ongoing neuropsychological and psychological monitoring is required to maximize children's long-term recovery and level of functioning. This chapter provides an overview of research findings on outcomes of childhood brain tumors, particularly from a neuropsychological perspective, but it also emphasizes common clinical issues that arise in working with these children. The information presented in this chapter is derived in part from our longitudinal study of over 150 children with brain tumors, some of whom have been followed for over 10 years (Buono et al., 1998; Carlson-Green, Morris, & Krawiecki, 1995; Waldrop, Davis, Padgett, Shapiro & Morris, 1998).

EPIDEMIOLOGY AND MAJOR TYPES OF TUMORS

Brain tumors and other CNS cancers account for nearly 20% of all childhood cancers and are the most common solid tumors in children (Gurney, Severson, Davis, & Robinson, 1995). Approximately 1,500 children in the United States each year will develop brain tumors (Albright, 1993), making such tumors low-incidence conditions. The infrequency of brain tumors, in fact, may have a negative impact on recovery and rehabilitation, as many pediatricians, medically related therapists, neuropsychologists, and school personnel have very little experience with the needs of these children. The risk of brain tumor development in children decreases with increasing age, with nearly 80% of childhood brain tumors occurring within the first 10 years of life (Leviton, 1994). Given the young ages of children at the time of diagnosis and the increasing survival rates for many types of brain tumors, most children experience the impact of these tumors over an extended period of their development.

The United States is fifth behind Scandinavia, New Zealand, Israel, and Canada in terms of incidence of pediatric brain tumors (Bleyer, 1990). The overall incidence of pediatric brain tumors in the United States is 23% higher among European Americans than among African Americans (Gurney et al., 1995). Incidence rates may be slightly higher in males than in females, especially for primitive neuroectodermal tumors (PNETs; Gurney et al., 1995). The etiology of national, racial, and sex differences in rates of occurrence is unknown.

Unfortunately, cancer is the second leading cause of death, after accidents, among children aged 1 to 14 years in the United States; it accounted for 10% of all childhood deaths in 1991 (Wingo, Tong, & Bolden, 1995). According to the American Cancer Society, brain tumors and other CNS cancers have the second highest mortality rates among childhood cancers, after leukemia (Wingo et al., 1995). On a more positive note, the National Cancer Institute (NCI, 1995) estimates that more than 50% of all children diagnosed with brain tumors can be expected to survive 5 years from diagnosis. A child with a brain tumor who survives for 5 years is commonly considered "cured," although such children can have later recurrences, and children with brain tumors have more frequent later recurrences than children with other types of cancer. Five-year survival rates of children with brain tumors have significantly increased over the past 30 years, most likely because of advances in detection and treatment (Bordeaux, 1986; Wingo et al., 1995). These survival rates, however, vary with a child's age at diagnosis, as well as with the type of tumor. Children under 2 years of age at the time of diagnosis have the lowest survival rates, while children between the ages of 10 and 14 have the highest rates of survival (Duffner, Cohen, Myers, & Heise, 1986).

Although numerous systems are used to classify brain tumors, most specialists in this area use a combination of pathology and location to identify tumor type in children. Astrocytomas/gliomas, PNETs, and ependymomas are the three most common types of brain tumors seen in children, accounting for approximately 97% of all pediatric brain tumors (Gurney et al., 1995).

Astrocytomas and Gliomas

The most common tumor types in children are astrocytomas and gliomas, or glial cell tumors, which together account for approximately 60% of all childhood CNS tumors (Duffner et al., 1986; Gurney et al., 1995). These tumors include anaplastic astrocytomas, glioblastomas multiformes, astrocytomas, and ependymomas. Approximately 17 children per million are diagnosed with astrocytomas and gliomas each year in the United States (Breslow & Langholz, 1983; Gurney et al., 1995). Although there is little difference in incidence rates between males and females, European American children have incidence rates 22% higher than those of African American children (Gurney et al., 1995).

Survival rates for astrocytomas and gliomas depend on the tumors' grade (of histopathological severity), as well as on their location in the brain. For children with astrocytomas located in the cerebellum, the most common location for astrocytomas, the 10-year survival rate is approximately 80% (NCI, 1995). The survival rate for children with low-grade cerebral astrocytomas is approximately 50–80% after 5 years, but less than 35% after 2 years for children diagnosed with high-grade cerebral astrocytomas (Duffner et al., 1986; NCI, 1995). Survival rates for children with brain stem gliomas are less than 25% at 2 years after diagnosis; children with optic tract gliomas have a more optimistic prognosis, with 5-year survival rates of greater than 50% (NCI, 1995).

Ependymomas are the third most common type of pediatric brain tumor, constituting approximately 10–15% of all cases (Leviton, 1994; Miller, Young, & Novakovic, 1995). Incidence rates of ependymomas are higher in children under 5 years of age, at 4 per million, but drop to 1 per million for children 5 years and older (Gurney et al., 1995). The 2-year survival rate for children with supratentorial ependymomas is approximately 40%, while those with infratentorial ependymomas have a 5-year survival rate of 25–60% (NCI, 1995).

Primitive Neuroectodermal Tumors

The second most common pediatric brain tumors are PNETs. This tumor type includes primarily medulloblastomas in the cerebellum, and accounts for 20–25% of pediatric brain tumors (Duffner et al., 1986; Leviton, 1994; Miller et al., 1995). The cellular origin of a PNET is related to the specific location of the tumor (i.e., granule cells in the cerebellum) or to undifferentiated cells of primitive CNS origin, although there is some debate in this regard. The fact that incidence rates of PNETs are reported to be 33% higher in males than in females accounts for most of the overall sex differences in rates of pediatric brain tumors (Gurney et al., 1995). Incidence rates for PNETs decline with age. Children under age 3 have an incidence of PNETs of 10 per million. Children aged 12–14 years have the lowest incidence rates, averaging approximately 3 per million (Gurney et al., 1995). Approximately 50% of children diagnosed with PNETs are expected to survive 5 years past diagnosis (NCI, 1995).

ETIOLOGIES AND RISK FACTORS

The heterogeneity of pediatric brain tumors makes it difficult to draw any generalizations with regard to etiology or risks for adverse developmental outcomes. Whereas some researchers have limited their samples to children with certain types of childhood tumors, other investigations have included children with diverse tumor types. Research in this area has focused primarily on probable genetic or familial risk factors, or on gestational or early childhood exposures to environmental toxins or other harmful events. Existing findings with regard to the factors that lead to brain tumors are limited and nonconclusive.

Molecular Biology and Genetics

Most often the cause of cancer, and in particular of a childhood brain tumor, is unknown. Rarely is there a family predisposition for cancer or a well-documented exposure to environmental toxins known to cause cancer. Cancer is nevertheless viewed as a genetic disease that results from defective genes as well as from environmental factors. The genes responsible for cell growth are called *oncogenes*, and the genes that slow down cell growth are known as *tumor suppressor genes*. The p53 gene is the gene most frequently known to be mutated in human malignancies, including some brain tumors, and it is located on the short arm of chromosome 17. It is a tumor suppressor gene whose role is to induce cell cycle arrest, allowing the repair of damaged deoxyribonucleic acid (DNA) to take place; if the DNA damage is beyond repair, the p53 gene induces programmed cell death, or *apoptosis*. Mutated p53 genes appear to be present in all grades of malignancy and seem to be an early event in the development of cancer, at least in adult patients (Pomeroy, 1994). In children, however, the incidence of this mutation is very low, as only 1–2% of children with brain tumors may have mutation in the p53 gene (Pomeroy, 1994).

Unfortunately, there are few currently known genetic causes of brain tumors in children (von Ammon & Roelcke, 1994). Deletions of the short arm of chromosome 9 can occur in intermediate and advanced malignancies. Abnormalities of the gene encoding the epidermal growth factor receptor (EGFR) can also occur in advanced malignancy. Chromosome 10 changes may be present in nearly all malignant cell lines of glioblastoma multiforme. A MYCN-gene has been discovered in association with neuroblastoma and is located on chromosome 2 (2p24.1). Both neurofibromatosis 1 and neurofibromatosis 2 are also associated with chromosome 2 oncogenes (Darlymple & Jenkins, 1994).

Familial Risk Factors

There is limited evidence that a familial history of certain neurological disorders increases risks for childhood brain tumors. Familial histories of neurofibromatosis, tuberous sclerosis, Sturge–Weber syndrome, von Hippel–Lindau disease, and the multiple-basal-cell nevus syndrome are associated with increased rates of childhood brain tumors (Leviton, 1994). Studies of the relationship between a familial history of epilepsy and risks for childhood brain tumors have yielded inconsistent findings. Gold et al. (1994) and Guiffre, Liccardo, Pastore, Spallone, and Vagnozzi (1990) failed to identify epilepsy in first-degree relatives as a risk factor. Kuijten et al. (1993), however, did find epilepsy to be a familial risk factor for children with astrocytomas. A familial history of mental retardation also appears to be more common in children with brain tumors than in the general population (Kuijten, Bunin, Nass, & Meadows, 1990). A maternal family history of birth defects appears to be associated with an increased risk, especially for infratentorial tumors (Gold et al., 1994). A family history of stroke, however, has not been found to be a risk factor in astrocytomas and medulloblastomas (Giuffre et al., 1990; Kuijten et al., 1993).

A familial history of cancer has long been suspected as a risk factor. Children with PNETs are significantly more likely than the general population or controls to have relatives with childhood cancers (Kuijten et al., 1993). Kuijten et al. (1990) found that cancer in a relative significantly increased a child's risk for astrocytoma, especially if the child was between the ages of 0 and 4 years at the time of diagnosis. Increases in tumor occurrences have also been found in paternal relatives of children with astrocytomas and infratentorial tumors (Gold et al., 1994). These studies and others suggest that familial histories of cancers may act as risk factors only for specific types of childhood brain tumors.

Environmental and Other Risk Factors

Environmental exposure to certain agents suspected to increase risks for childhood brain tumors can occur during gestation and in the first few years of life. Products containing N-nitroso compounds, which are frequently found in cured and broiled meat, beer, cosmetics, new cars, cigarette smoke, rubber baby bottle nipples and pacifiers, and incense, have been hypothesized to play a role in childhood brain tumor incidence (Bunin, Buckley, Boesel, Rorke, & Meadows, 1994; Bunin, Kuijten, Boesel, Buckley, & Meadows, 1994). Several studies that have focused on maternal diet have found that the consumption of cured and broiled meat increases brain tumor risk, especially if the foods are eaten frequently during the gestational period (Kuijten et al., 1990; Sarasua & Savitz, 1994). Mothers of children with PNETs and astrocytomas are also more likely than control mothers to report drinking beer during pregnancy (Bunin, Buckley, et al., 1994). Parental smoking, however, has not been found to influence the risk of brain tumors in children (Bunin, Buckley, et al., 1994; Gold et al., 1993).

Parental occupation has been hypothesized to pose a risk for pediatric brain tumors, since workers in many industries are exposed to dangerous chemical carcinogens. Wilkins and Sinks (1990) found that children whose fathers were employed in the agriculture, food, construction, metal, and tobacco industries were at increased risk for brain tumors. The risk was amplified when these jobs were held during the preconception period. Kuijten, Bunin, Nass, and Meadows (1992), however, failed to find associations between parental occupation and childhood astrocytomas, suggesting that astrocytomas may not be influenced by the same risk factors as other childhood tumors.

CLINICAL PRESENTATION AND NATURAL HISTORY

Symptoms

Family members frequently report a history of multiple nonspecific symptoms and trips to their pediatrician before the diagnosis of a brain tumor is made. The initial signs and symptoms of brain tumors in children depend mainly on tumor location and growth rate. Tumors located in the posterior fossa often cause obstruction to the cerebrospinal fluid flow, causing hydrocephalus and clinical manifestations of increased intracranial pressure: headaches, diplopia, papilledema, nausea, vomiting, alteration of consciousness, ataxia, posturing, and coma. Early detection of these tumors is sometimes difficult, particularly since intermittent headaches are frequently seen by pediatricians and do not imply a specific etiology. Nocturnal headaches, waking up in the middle of the night or much earlier in the morning than usual, morning nausea, and poor appetite can all be early symptoms of increased intracranial pressure. Typically, these symptoms will progress over a period of a few weeks into the more severe symptoms of increased intracranial pressure noted above.

Seizures can be the first manifestation of a supratentorial hemispheric brain tumor. Partial seizures are a more common symptom than are generalized seizures. Presenting signs can also include weakness of an extremity or a side of the body (hemiparesis), or abnormal movements or posture. Tumors involving the brain stem usually present with complex neurological signs, often pathognomonic, called *alternating syndromes*. These syndromes involve cranial nerve deficits on one side, and long-tract signs, such as hemiparesis or sensory deficits, on the other. Cerebellar dysfunction, often seen in posterior fossa tumors, may be manifested as a clumsy, unsteady gait, poor hand coordination, and difficulties with articulation. Presenting complaints rarely include cognitive deficits or related problems. A post hoc review of a child's school performance or behavior may suggest subtle changes in functioning that are only clear in hindsight.

Medical Evaluation

Once a child is suspected of having a brain tumor, neuroimaging is usually obtained immediately to confirm the diagnosis (Allen, Byrd, Darling, Tomita, & Wilczynski, 1993). Both computed tomography (CT) and magnetic resonance imaging (MRI) scans may be taken, due to their differential sensitivity to tumor margins and volume. Depending on the tumor's location, a biopsy is also obtained at this time, and a shunt is placed if necessary to relieve intracranial pressure. Our experience in evaluating children with brain tumors is that limited accurate information about neuropsychological functioning is available until the increased intracranial pressure is reduced. The negative impact of increased intracranial pressure on general arousal, and its correlated impact on general cognitive functioning, preclude meaningful assessment. If a child has not experienced increased cranial pressure, early neuropsychological evaluation may be helpful in monitoring treatment effects and recovery rate.

Pathological evaluation of the biopsy sample leads to a neuropathological classification of the tumor, which has implications both for expectations regarding survival and for treatment options. The current neuropathological classification of the World Health Organization (1979)—which is more appropriate for adults than for children, and therefore has been modified for pediatrics by various groups—includes (1) tumors of neuroepithelial tissue, (2) astrocytic tumors, (3) oligodendroglial tumors, (4) ependymal and choroid plexus tumors, (5) pineal cell tumors, (6) neuronal tumors, (7) poorly differentiated and embryonal tumors, (8) tumors of the nerve sheaths, (9) tumors of meningeal and related tissues, (10) primary malignant lymphomas, (11) tumors of blood vessel origin, (12) germ cell tumors, (13) other malformative tumors and tumor-like lesions, (14) vascular malformations, (15) tumors of the anterior pituitary, (16) local extensions from regional tumors, (17) metastatic tumors, and (18) unclassified tumors.

The distinction between benign and malignant tumors is often confusing when applied to brain tumors. Cruveilhier, a 19th-century surgeon, defined a neoplasm as "malignant" when "it recurred and killed the patient," even if the tumor "were cut and burnt out" (quoted in Zulch, 1986, p. 26). Childhood brain tumors practically never metastasize (spread) to other organs. They can progress locally and invade the spinal cord at a distance, but typically remain confined to the CNS. In contrast to other cancers, the chances of developing metastases are low in brain tumors, and thus are not used in grading them; accordingly, the difference between benign and malignant tumors takes on a somewhat different meaning.

The most critical determinant of the seriousness or severity of brain tumors is the length of survival expected after diagnosis. Two main factors contribute to survival: the location of a tumor and its histological type. A small tumor that is histologically benign, but that is located in the brain stem close to the respiratory center, can be fatal on the basis of the functions it interrupts rather than because of its type. Grades have been defined for most brain tumors, and a majority of neuropathologists use the same classification system. Grade I represents a benign tumor with a survival time of at least 5 years; grade II is a semibenign tumor with a 3- to 5-year survival; grade III is a relatively malignant tumor with a 2- to 3-year survival; and grade IV is a highly malignant tumor with survival rarely exceeding 15 months. *Anaplasia* (lesser degree of differentiation), *pleomorphism* (presence of different types and shapes of cells from a same origin), increased cellularity, disproportionate size of the nucleus, high rate of cell division (mitosis), and abnormalities of the vessels in the tumor are additional characteristics used to define the degree of malignancy. Within this framework, malignant tumors are aggressive tumors with poorly differentiated cells, whereas benign tumors are less aggressive and have better-defined cells on histopathology.

Medical Treatment

Once the tumor type has been identified, options for treatments are considered (Cohen & Duffner, 1994). Although neurosurgery and radiation therapy are the most traditional treatment options, large cooperative study groups (e.g., the Children's Cancer Group and the Pediatric Oncology Group) have developed state-of-the-art treatment protocols for children. These treatment protocols may include any combination of surgery, radiation, and/or chemotherapy. The latter treatment modalities may be linked in time or spread out over a postdiagnosis period as long as 2 years. A tumor's response to a given treatment sometimes helps determine whether additional treatment modalities will be needed. Our research suggests that the number of treatment modalities a child receives is a critical factor in predicting neuropsychological outcomes. Children in need of more modalities are at increased risk for cognitive and related deficits (Carlson-Green et al., 1995). The fact that treatment protocols are frequently confounded with tumor pathology, grade, and location may be largely responsible for this association.

Surgical Intervention

 A ventriculoperitoneal shunt or ventriculostomy is frequently performed to relieve obstruction to cerebrospinal fluid flow. Such a procedure is performed either as an initial step prior to resection, or at the time of the surgery. Some pediatric neurosurgeons prefer to reduce intracranial pressure prior to undertaking a more extensive surgery, whereas other surgeons perform both operative procedures in a single surgery (Burger, Scheithauer, & Vogel, 1991). In some instances a biopsy is the only safe procedure available to obtain tissue for histological diagnosis. The latter procedure can be performed as an MRI- or CT-scan-guided biopsy or as an open biopsy. An advantage of an open biopsy is that more tissue can be obtained and the risks of sampling error diminished.

    If the tumor is accessible surgically, the resection, or removal, can be performed with microsurgery techniques and computer-guided instrumentation. Resections can be subtotal or total, depending on the amount of the tumor that can be removed without jeopardizing critical brain functions. Surgical procedures have become increasingly accurate with improved technological advances (e.g., microscopic and laser techniques). Surgical techniques used to treat epilepsy, such as a temporal lobectomy, can also be used to resect brain tumors associated with refractory seizures. In cases of more poorly defined or malignant tumors, this type of surgery is frequently followed by radiation and/or chemotherapy.

Radiation Therapy

Radiation therapy remains an effective tool for the treatment of brain tumors. Because of the negative consequences of radiation therapy for the developing brain, children under the ages of 2–3 years typically are not radiated, or radiation therapy is delayed when possible (Jenkin et al., 1995). In this younger age group, either surgery alone, surgery plus chemotherapy, or ongoing observation is the preferred mode of treatment. In older children, external-beam radiation therapy is used to deliver 2,000 to 7,000 cGy to the tumor, the whole brain, or the spinal cord. Even in very focused treatment of a tumor, radiation's impact on brain systems may be found in distant locations (Waldrop et al., 1998). Children frequently receive daily radiation treatments until the protocol for their type of tumor is complete, which in some cases can extend over a period of several weeks. Hyperfractionated protocols deliver a smaller dose twice a day, and allow for a larger total overall dose, although their benefits have not been clearly documented. Stereotactic radiosurgery (gamma knife) uses multiple beams and allows the delivery of a high dose of radiation to a highly defined brain area. Brachytherapy introduces radioactive elements through a catheter inside the cranial cavity (Healey, Shamberger, Grier, Loeffler, & Tarbell, 1995). This method allows the delivery of radiation to the center of the tumor. The radioactive elements are removed after a given period of time, and the catheter may be left in place for further treatment.

Chemotherapy

Chemotherapeutic agents have been used for many years to treat cancer, with trial applications to brain tumors beginning in the 1960s. The efficacy of these agents is based on their ability to cross the blood–brain barrier and disrupt the normal cell cycle with minimal toxicity. There are many chemotherapy protocols, involving a variety of drugs, dosages, and frequencies of treatments. Some agents are cell-cycle-nonspecific and can act at any stage of cell reproduction. Other agents are cell-cycle-specific and even cell-phase-specific. The alkylating agents, such as nitrosoureas (BCNU, CCNU), oxazaphosphorines, cyclophosphamide, and ifosfamide, are cell-cycle-nonspecific. Mitotic inhibitors, such as vincristine and vinblastine, are cell-phase-specific agents. Antimetabolites, such as methotrexate, are cell-cycle-specific agents. Platinum compounds (cis-platin and carbo-platin) and VP-16, which are probably cell-cycle-specific, are finding increasing use in treatment of pediatric brain tumors. Steroids are also frequently used to decrease edema from the mass effect of a tumor, often providing dramatic symptom relief. Little is known about the neurocognitive impact of these agents.

Molecular and Genetic Therapy

The first approved clinical trial of genetic therapy was for adults with glioblastoma multiforme (Yung, 1994a, 1994b). In this therapy, a retroviral vector was used to carry a gene into the tumor cells. A nontoxic antiviral agent, which was designed to selectively destroy the gene-sensitized tumor cells, was then given to the patient. Other molecular genetic therapies, not typically employed in treatment of children, have included the use of herpes virus and adenovirus, instead of retrovirus, to carry genetic material into tumor cells; molecular immunotherapy using recombinant interleukin (IL)-2 and IL-4; and human interferon gamma in association with IL-2. Clinical trials involving applications of these newer treatments to children are anticipated once research has demonstrated their efficacy in treating adult patients.

DEVELOPMENTAL OUTCOMES

General Considerations

Numerous studies of long-term outcomes in pediatric brain tumor patients have been conducted over the past decade. Most of the neuropsychological work in this area is described in major reviews by Mulhern, Crisco, and Kun (1983) and Ris and Noll (1994). Due to the comprehensive nature of these reviews, the present section highlights studies of special relevance to the pediatric neuropsychologist. It is important to emphasize, however, that the heterogeneity of tumors, treatments, patient characteristics, and methods for evaluating outcomes makes it difficult to draw any special conclusions regarding neuropsychological sequelae. To complicate matters further, the immediacy of treatment following diagnosis suggests that much of what is currently known about the effects of brain tumors has come from patients who have already undergone some form of treatment, usually including radiation (Fletcher & Copeland, 1988); therefore, the impact of both the tumor and its treatment is actually being evaluated. A further limitation is that much of the literature, especially that dating back 10 to 15 years, is based on treatment protocols that are obsolete (e.g., cobalt therapy) and have little in common with current protocols.

The major focus of outcome research to date has been on the sequelae of radiation therapy (Roman & Sperduto, 1995). Radiation therapy is thought to be the most effective treatment for childhood brain tumors, and is credited for the dramatic rise in the number of survivors over the past several decades; however, outcome research has shown that pediatric brain tumor survivors, particularly the younger ones, are faced with various neurological, intellectual, neuropsychological, and behavioral problems (Brookshire, Copeland, Morrie, & Ater, 1990; Mulhern et al., 1983; Ris & Noll, 1994; Waldrop et al., 1998). Concern about possible long-term cognitive deficits following radiation therapy first arose from studies documenting the effects of CNS radiation on children with leukemia (Copeland et al., 1985; Duffner & Cohen, 1992; Gamis & Nesbit, 1991), since these patients routinely receive CNS radiation treatment. Comparisons of leukemia patients receiving CNS radiotherapy with those receiving systemic radiotherapy showed that those who received treatment to the CNS were the more cognitively impaired and differed significantly from patients who received only systemic therapy (Copeland & Moore, 1992). Cognitive skills that appear to be most affected by CNS radiotherapy are memory, attention, fine motor speed and coordination, and mathematics skills. Nevertheless, no single profile of neuropsychological impairment has been identified. Moreover, tumor location may be less critical in predicting neuropsychological outcomes than other factors, such as the amount of radiation or numbers of modalities used in treating a child.

Intellectual Functioning

A change in IQ scores is the most frequently reported effect of brain tumors. In a series of studies by Radcliffe and her colleagues, children with malignant brain tumors who were treated with cranial radiotherapy were prospectively followed 2 to 4 years after diagnosis (Packer et al., 1989; Radcliffe et al., 1992; Radcliffe, Bunin, Sutton, Goldwein, & Phillips, 1994). Intellectual testing at 2 years after diagnosis indicated a drop in Full Scale, Performance, and Verbal IQ scores from baseline testing conducted after surgical resection of the tumor but prior to the onset of radiation treatment. Patients who did not receive cranial radiotherapy demonstrated no cognitive declines at 2 years after diagnosis. The Packer et al. (1989) study also replicated results from an earlier study by Ellenberg, McComb, Siegel, and Stowe (1987). Both studies showed an inverse relationship between age at the time of treatment and later IQ scores, such that younger patients (under 7 years old) demonstrated greater cognitive loss than their older counterparts. Because the declines observed after 2 years by Packer et al. (1989) were not evident after the first year, these authors concluded that cognitive sequelae become progressively worse over time.

In an extension of the original study by Packer et al. (1989), Radcliffe et al. (1992) evaluated the sample at 3 and 4 years after diagnosis. Contrary to expectations, IQ scores were not significantly lower at this follow-up than at the previous assessment. However, because of the small number of patients available for follow-up assessments after 4 years, Radcliffe et al. (1994) followed a second set of children who had received craniospinal radiation treatments for noncortical brain tumors. As in the Packer et al. (1989) study, they observed a decrease in Full Scale IQ scores in children who were under 7 years of age at the time of treatment. Although both Verbal and Performance IQ scores also dropped over 4 years, a decline in Verbal IQ was evident by 2 years after diagnosis, whereas Performance IQ dropped more gradually over the 4-year period. The authors concluded that most of the impact of brain tumors and their treatment on intelligence is evident within 2 years after diagnosis, and they argued against a steady, progressive, or continual decline in cognitive functioning.

Although this conclusion is consistent with findings from several other studies (Ellenberg et al., 1987; Johnson et al., 1994; Lannering, Marky, Lundberg, & Olsson, 1990; Mulhern, Kovnar, Kun, Crisco, & Williams, 1988; Packer et al., 1989), Hoppe-Hirsch et al. (1990) found evidence for longer-term declines. The latter investigators completed yearly evaluations of individuals for up to 20 years following radiation treatment for childhood medulloblastoma. Their data revealed a progressive intellectual deterioration extending over 10 years after completion of radiotherapy, with the extent of decline and the final IQ score dependent on a child's age at the time of radiation treatment.

Evidence for a relationship between the dose or frequency of radiation and IQ outcome is contradictory. Silber et al. (1992) found greater declines in IQ over time for children receiving higher doses of radiation. Packer et al. (1989), however, failed to identify a relationship between radiation dose and later IQ performance.

Our clinical experience is consistent with research findings suggesting that the younger the child at the time of diagnosis, the more severe the tumor, the more treatment modalities used, and the longer the time since diagnosis, the more pronounced the cognitive sequelae of radiation treatments will be. We should emphasize, however, that many of the children we follow score in the average IQ range, particularly during the first year following diagnosis. Our interpretation of the tendency of children to maintain normal-range IQ scores during this period is that measures of intelligence and academic achievement are more sensitive to the level of children's learning prior to diagnosis and treatment than to their concurrent information-processing abilities. Neuropsychological evaluation of more specific functions is required to assess the more immediate cognitive sequelae of brain tumors and their treatment. The most important issue for the pediatric neuropsychologist is determination of the nature of the neurocognitive deficits underlying more global IQ changes. Our ongoing study suggests that such IQ changes appear to be related to changes in attention, memory, and problem-solving abilities. As Ris and Noll (1994) conclude, comprehensive batteries that steer assessment away from IQ scores, together with developmental neuropsychological models that consider changes over time (Morris, Fletcher, & Francis, 1992), are clearly needed to understand the impact of brain tumors on children's neurobehavioral growth and development.

Neuropsychological Functioning

Neuropsychological assessments of survivors of childhood brain tumors indicate that the long-term sequelae of such tumors include problems with fine motor coordination and declines in perceptual–motor, visual–constructive, and memory abilities (Dennis et al., 1991; Ris & Noll, 1994). The latter impairments are likely to contribute to the well-documented changes in IQ. Although we are aware of no longitudinal studies that have undertaken comprehensive neuropsychological follow-up of children for more than about 2 years after diagnosis, several studies have examined neuropsychological consequences at various time points following treatment. In one of the first studies to evaluate neuropsychological functioning in long-term survivors of childhood medulloblastoma, Packer et al. (1987) found significant impairments in memory, manual dexterity, verbal fluency, and mathematical ability despite average intellectual functioning. In a later study, Packer et al. (1989) also found that children suffered from deficits in visual–motor and visual–spatial skills. Similarly, Lannering et al. (1990) observed that long-term survivors had problems in cognitive, motor, visual, and psychological/emotional functioning as late as 16 years following diagnosis. More recently, Johnson et al. (1994) evaluated neuropsychological and behavioral outcomes in a group of children diagnosed with medulloblastoma who had survived more than 5 years after treatment. Motor speed and coordination were severely affected, as was perceptual organization as measured by the Benton Visual Retention Test. Visual memory, attention, and organization skills were all moderately to severely impaired, whereas performance on verbal memory and verbal fluency tasks was relatively unimpaired.

As is true of research on intellectual changes in brain tumor patients, studies have failed to assess neuropsychological functioning prior to the administration of some form of treatment. In one of the few studies that examined pretreatment abilities, Bordeaux et al. (1988) compared the pre- and posttherapy neuropsychological performances of brain tumor patients who were treated with either radiation or surgery. Both groups of patients performed within the average range on most measures prior to treatment. However, pretreatment performance on timed tests measuring fine motor coordination, psychomotor speed, and language skills was below average in both groups. After treatment, but within 1 year after diagnosis, neither group showed significant changes in performance compared to pretherapy scores. The authors concluded that neither surgery nor radiotherapy considered in isolation has neuropsychological consequences within the first posttreatment year. Similarly, Moore, Ater, Needle, Slopis, and Copeland (1994) compared the neuropsychological test performances of children with brain tumors alone to those of children with both brain tumors and neurofibromatosis. Results from their study also suggest that cognitive abilities are normal prior to treatment, and that the long-term cognitive changes seen in pediatric brain tumor survivors are due to the radiation or chemotherapy treatment, rather than to either the brain tumor itself or surgical treatment.

Academic Functioning and Quality of Life

A more practical question regarding long-term outcome in pediatric brain tumor survivors is how well they are functioning outside the hospital. Studies of functional outcomes have included measures of academic functioning, psychological adjustment, and quality of life (Carlson-Green et al., 1995, Stehbens, Kisker, & Wilson, 1983). The most comprehensive outcome study of the effects of brain tumors on later functioning, conducted by Lannering et al. (1990), revealed that children's lives were most affected by the intellectual and psychological/emotional effects of tumors. The authors speculated that these dysfunctions were the most difficult to live with and led to a poorer quality of life. In contrast, children's self-reports indicated that visual and hearing impairments, hormonal deficiencies, and disfigurement, although recognized as highly disabling, were not associated with diminished quality of life.

In their study of medulloblastoma survivors, Packer et al. (1987) defined quality of life more narrowly in terms of school performance (as determined by academic achievement scores and classroom placement). As expected, children who scored poorly on standardized academic achievement tests were more likely than higher achievers to be placed in a special education classroom or to receive tutorial help within a regular classroom. The children with academic difficulties were also more likely to have impaired mathematical abilities compared to their reading skills—a finding our research also supports (Buono et al., 1998). Later in follow-up, the majority of children receiving whole-brain radiation treatment had lower achievement scores and significant learning problems that required special help at school (Packer et al., 1989). Packer and his colleagues did not discuss the implications of these findings with respect to quality of life outside the classroom, but they emphasized that scores within the average range on IQ tests are not necessarily indicative of children's levels of adaptive functioning.

Similar educational sequelae were reported by Radcliffe et al. (1992), although these effects were demonstrated only for younger patients. Johnson et al. (1994) also determined that learning disabilities were common long-term consequences of brain tumors treated with radiation. Quality of life was assessed in terms of psychosocial interviews, such as the Vineland Adaptive Behavior Scales, and parent ratings, including the Child Behavior Checklist and the Symptom Checklist—90. Parents reported a significant number of maladaptive behaviors in children, and also acknowledged learning problems; however, there were few clinically significant levels of behavioral or psychiatric symptoms.

In a study from our research group, Carlson-Green et al. (1995) evaluated predictors of cognitive and behavioral outcomes in 63 children with brain tumors. The findings showed that contextual factors, such as family stress and socioeconomic status, were important correlates of outcomes. Results from this study also demonstrated that the predictors of noncognitive outcomes, such as behavior problems, may be different from the factors that predict neuropsychological outcomes in children with brain tumors.

Treatment Variability and Neuropsychological Effects

Of all the influences on outcome, the administration of radiation therapy has repeatedly been shown to be the most critical determinant of outcome. This generalization applies not only to pediatric brain tumors, but to other forms of pediatric cancer as well (Copeland et al., 1988; Copeland & Moore, 1992; Duffner & Cohen, 1992). Because radiation treatment has been so effective in prolonging the life of brain tumor patients, the majority of outcome studies have examined neuropsychological functioning subsequent to the implementation of radiation therapy. For this reason, deficits documented in the existing literature may reflect effects of radiation, rather than the impact of the tumor itself. However, not all children receive radiation therapy, and investigators are now involved in studies evaluating the effects of alternative treatment approaches.

A review of the literature suggests that both the acute and long-term effects of chemotherapy and surgery differ markedly from the sequelae of radiation (Copeland & Moore, 1992; Packer, 1995; Packer et al., 1989). According to the Ellenberg et al. (1987) study of intellectual outcome in pediatric brain tumor patients, neither the degree of tumor resection nor chemotherapy had significant effect on intellectual outcome 3 years after diagnosis. Similarly, Moore, Ater, and Copeland (1992) compared children's performance on a battery of neuropsychological tests 6 years after diagnosis. They found that children treated with chemotherapy and surgery performed within the average range, and significantly better than irradiated patients, in all neurocognitive domains except visual–spatial skills. Most significantly, they found no increase in mortality in the surgery/chemotherapy group.

Despite the indications from these studies that radiation is the cause of most, if not all, of the neuropsychological sequelae of brain tumors and their treatment in children, Moore et al. (1994) showed that cognitive abilities can be affected by either radiation or chemotherapy treatment. In their study, cognitive deficits emerged only after treatment with either of these therapies, and these deficits were not present in patients without any form of treatment or patients who had undergone only surgical resection. Their results also demonstrated the selective effects of chemotherapy and radiation on neurocognitive abilities.

The results of these studies suggest that long-term neuropsychological abilities are most dramatically affected by radiation, are affected to some degree by chemotherapy, and are relatively little affected by surgery only. Findings from our own studies in this area indicate that the number of different types of treatments a child undergoes may be a better predictor of later neurocognitive deficits than the presence versus absence of radiation treatment (Carlson-Green et al., 1995), although any firm conclusions in this regard before these results are replicated would be unwise.

Neuropsychological Outcome in Infants and Toddlers

Younger children are at particular risk for intellectual and neuropsychological problems after treatment with radiation therapy. As noted earlier, children younger than about 7 years of age appear to be at greater risk than older children (Packer et al., 1989); however, several studies have reported that children younger than 2 or 3 years old (infants and toddlers) are at the highest risk (Balestrini, Micheli, Giordano, Lasio, & Giombini, 1994; Cohen et al., 1993; Geyer et al., 1995; Moore et al., 1992). This is due to damage to the brain during early childhood, either from the tumor itself or from its treatment at a time of rapid growth and development of the nervous system (Spreen, 1984). In contrast to brain tumors in adult patients, whose neuropsychological skills are already well established, brain tumors in infants and toddlers have the potential to disrupt the initial acquisition of skills, the completion of myelination, and/or the development of cortical areas responsible for higher cognitive functioning. Brain tumors may thus have greater consequences for infants and toddlers.

Brain tumors in children younger than 2 years old also differ from those in older children in their location (supratentorial tumors are more common), histology, symptomatology, and medical outcome (Balestrini et al., 1993; Duffner et al., 1993). Until recently, tumors in children less than 2 years of age were preferentially treated with surgical resection followed by radiation. There is a current trend away from radiation therapy, or at least toward delaying it until children are older, and chemotherapy is increasingly the preferred form of treatment for very young children. In general, investigations of neuropsychological outcomes in children diagnosed with brain tumors in infancy or early childhood have revealed deficits similar to those seen in older children. Research in this area documents deficits in intellectual, memory, attention, motor, and visual–spatial skills (Duffner et al., 1993; Moore et al., 1992), which may be related to the distant effects of radiation treatment on cortical white matter (Waldrop et al., 1998).

Summary

Follow-up of children with brain tumors suggests several critical influences on neuropsychological, intellectual, and behavioral outcomes. Patient characteristics (e.g., age at diagnosis and treatment, tumor site and type) and characteristics of treatment (e.g., whether or not radiation was administered and the number of treatment modalities used) are the major predictors of long-term outcome. Evidence for a progressive decline in IQ suggests that some disease consequences may not be fully apparent for several years after treatment has been completed. The damaging effects of radiation have led physicians to consider alternative treatments for children, such as forms of chemotherapy previously reserved for adults, which may delay or eliminate the need for radiation.

FUTURE DIRECTIONS

Despite the increased attention being given to neuropsychological and functional outcomes for children with brain tumors, there are many unanswered questions, and much further research is needed. Because traditional between-groups univariate designs have limited utility in informing us about the nature of the neuropsychological functioning following a childhood brain tumor, it will be important to employ developmental and multivariate frameworks (Ris & Noll, 1994). The use of neuropsychological and other outcome measures that are appropriate over a child's lifespan would be helpful for monitoring and interpreting the changes that occur following diagnosis. Although an abundance of research has documented IQ changes, studies have administered different measures depending on the ages of the children being assessed, or they have altered the test protocols as the children matured. For example, the series of studies by the group at Children's Hospital of Philadelphia (Packer, 1994; Packer et al., 1989; Radcliffe et al., 1992, 1994) used an assortment of intelligence tests, including the Mental Scale of the Bayley Scales of Infant Development, the Wechsler Intelligence Scale for Children—Revised for young children, the Wechsler Adult Intelligence Scale—Revised for older children, and the Stanford–Binet Intelligence

Scale. Employing changing test protocols complicates the interpretation of performance scores, particularly when the same children are assessed on different instruments over consecutive follow-ups (Morris, Fletcher, & Francis, 1992).

An almost exclusive emphasis on IQ (Ris & Noll, 1994) has stalled the process of understanding the effects of brain tumors and their treatment on activities of daily living and adaptive functioning. Increased attention to the neuropsychological effects of tumors, as well as to the behavioral, social, emotional, and adaptive functioning of survivors, is a critical component of long-term follow-up that has been too often ignored (Kazak & Meadows, 1989; Kazak & Nachman, 1991; Koocher & O'Malley, 1991). Clearly, comprehensive evaluations that take the "whole child" into account are necessary to begin to understand the complex interplay among children's preexisting attributes, the effects of brain tumors and their treatment, and social environment (Carlson-Green et al., 1995). Although a few of the studies reviewed here address these issues, more precise definitions of *quality of life* and *disability* would also enable comparisons of outcomes across studies, and would provide a better understanding of the relationship of underlying neurocognitive abilities to these more global outcome measures.

In addition, few studies have examined the effect of school disruptions on neurocognitive outcomes. Treatment of brain tumors requires that children miss school for substantial periods of time—in some cases, for several months of every school year. Because most studies report IQ scores based on age norms, children with brain tumors are compared to children of the same age when their performance on intelligence tests is being interpreted (Morris et al., 1992). Although this procedure is necessary in documenting disease sequelae, it is not very helpful in indicating how children with brain tumors are developing, or how they compare to children who have received similar amounts of schooling. The impact of missed schooling on functioning is especially crucial in studies with limited numbers of follow-ups (e.g., one assessment at diagnosis and one at 5 years after treatment). In general, assessments of children at only one point in time have little to offer in advancing our understanding of the developmental of brain tumors in children, either clinically or conceptually. Individual variability in response to treatment strongly suggests that children will often fail to show a steady or stable change following diagnosis and treatment, and that multiple assessments are thus critical in evaluating outcome.

Finally, at a clinical level, we have been impressed with how well many of our children with brain tumors are doing many years after their diagnosis and treatment. The tendency for the neuropsychological literature to focus exclusively on deficits might lead some readers to conclude that all children with brain tumors are impaired. In fact, sample averages obscure the positive functioning of many individual children, some of whom function at exceptionally high levels (e.g., some have graduated from top-ranked private colleges). Children with brain tumors are at increased risk for developmental problems, but being at risk does not mean that all children with brain tumors have to have neuropsychological or other deficits. The individual differences in this population are striking, and any group-level description is bound to be of limited value. This heterogeneity in outcomes is the very reason why the pediatric or developmental neuropsychologist is such a critical player in both the initial and long-term care of these children.

ACKNOWLEDGMENTS

The writing of this chapter was supported by Grant No. CA 33097 from the National Cancer Institute, and by the Brain Tumor Foundation for Children, Inc.

REFERENCES

Albright, A. L. (1993). Pediatric brain tumors. *CA: A Cancer Journal for Clinicians, 43*(1), 272–288.

Allen, E. D., Byrd, S. E., Darling, C. F., Tomita, T., & Wilczynski, M. A. (1993). The clinical and radiological evaluation of primary brain tumors in children: Part I. Clinical evaluation. *Journal of the National Medical Association, 85*(6), 445–451.

Balestrini, M. R., Micheli, R., Giordano, L., Lasio, G., & Giombini, S. (1994). Brain tumors with symptomatic onset in the first two years of life. *Child's Nervous System, 10*, 104–110.

Bleyer, W. A. (1990). The impact of childhood cancer in the United States and the world. *Cancer, 40*, 355–367.

Bordeaux, J. D. (1986). Developmental consequences of brain tumors and their treatment in children. In B. F. Brooks (Ed.), *Malignant tumors of childhood* (pp. 264–268). Austin: University of Texas Press.

Bordeaux, J. D., Dowell, R. E., Copeland, D. R., Fletcher, J. M., Francis, D. J., & van Eys, J. (1988). A prospective study of neuropsychological sequelae in children with brain tumors. *Journal of Child Neurology, 3*, 63–68.

Breslow, N. E., & Langholz, B. (1983). Childhood cancer incidence: Geographical and temporal variations. *International Journal of Cancer, 32*, 703–716.

Brookshire, B., Copeland, D. R., Morrie, B. D., & Ater, J. (1990). Pretreatment neuropsychological status and associated factors in children with primary brain tumors. *Neurosurgery, 27*, 887–891.

Bunin, G. R., Buckley, J. D., Boesel, C. P., Rorke, L. B., & Meadows, A. T. (1994). Risk factors for astrocytic glioma and primitive neuroectodermal tumor of the brain in young children: A report from the Children's Cancer Group. *Cancer Epidemiology, Biomarkers and Prevention, 3*, 197–204.

Bunin, G. R., Kuijten, R. R., Boesel, C. P., Buckley, J. D., & Meadows, A. T. (1994). Maternal diet and risk of astrocytic glioma in children: A report from the Children's Cancer Group (United States and Canada). *Cancer Causes and Control, 5*, 177–187.

Buono, L. A., Morris, M. K., Morris, R. D., Krawiecki, N., Norris, F. H., Foster, M. F., & Copeland, D. R. (1998). Evidence for the syndrome of nonverbal learning disabilities in children with brain tumors. *Child Neuropsychology, 4*(1), 1–14.

Burger, P. C., Scheithauer, B. W., & Vogel, F. S. (1991). *Surgical pathology of the nervous system and its coverings.* New York: Churchill Livingstone.

Carlson-Green, B., Morris, R. D., & Krawiecki, N. (1995). Family and illness predictors of outcome in pediatric brain tumors. *Journal of Pediatric Psychology, 20*(6), 769–784.

Cohen, B. H., Packer, R. J., Siegel, K. R., Rorke, L. B., D'Angio, G., Sutton, L. N., Bruce, D. A., & Schut, L. (1993). Brain tumors in children under 2 years: Treatment, survival and long-term prognosis. *Pediatric Neurosurgery, 19*(4), 171–179.

Cohen, M. E., & Duffner, P. K. (1994). *Brain tumors in children: Principles of diagnosis and treatment* (2nd ed.). New York: Raven Press.

Copeland, D. R., Dowell, R. E., Fletcher, J. M., Bordeaux, J. D., Sullivan, M. P., Jaffee, N., Frankel, L. S., Ried, H. L., & Cangir, A. (1988). Neuropsychological effects of childhood cancer treatment. *Journal of Child Neurology, 3*, 53–62.

Copeland, D. R., Fletcher, J. M., Pfefferbaum-Levine, B., Jaffe, N., Ried, H., & Maor, M. (1985). Neuropsychological sequelae of childhood cancer in long-term survivors. *Pediatrics, 75*, 745–753.

Copeland, D. R., & Moore, B. D. (1992). Neuropsychological outcome among children treated at M. D. Anderson Cancer Center. *Cancer Bulletin, 44*, 509–517.

Dalrymple, S. J., & Jenkins, R. B. (1994). Molecular genetics of astrocytomas and meningiomas. *Current Opinion in Neurology, 7*, 477–483.

Dennis, M., Spiegler, B. J., Hoffman, H. J., Hendrick, E. B., Humphreys, R. P., & Becker, L. E. (1991). Brain tumors in children and adolescents: I. Effects on working, associative, and serial-order memory of IQ, age at tumor onset and age of tumor. *Neuropsychologia, 29*(9), 813–827.

Duffner, P. K., & Cohen, M. E. (1992). Changes in the approach to central nervous system tumors in childhood. *Pediatric Neurology, 39*(4), 859–877.

Duffner, P. K., Cohen, M. E., Myers, M. H., & Heise, H. W. (1986). Survival of children with brain tumors: SEER program, 1973–1980. *Neurology, 36*, 597–601.

Duffner, P. K., Horowitz, M. E., Krischer, J. P., Friedman, H. S., Burger, P. C., Cohen, M. E., Sanford, R. A., Mulhern, R. K., James, H. E., Freeman, C. R., Seidel, F. G., & Kun, L. E. (1993). Postoperative chemotherapy and delayed radiation in children less than three years of age with malignant brain tumors. *New England Journal of Medicine, 328*(24), 1725–1731.

Ellenberg, L., McComb, J. G., Siegel, M. D., & Stowe, S. (1987). Factors affecting outcome in pediatric brain tumor patients. *Neurosurgery, 21,* 638–644.

Fletcher, J. M., & Copeland, D. R. (1988). Neurobehavioral effects of central nervous system prophylactic treatment of cancer in children. *Journal of Clinical and Experimental Neuropsychology, 10,* 495–538.

Gamis, A. S., & Nesbit, M. E. (1991). Neuropsychologic (cognitive) disabilities in long–term survivors of childhood cancer. *Pediatrician, 18,* 11–19.

Geyer, J. R., Finlay, J. L., Boyett, J. M., Wisoff, J., Yates, A., Mao, L., & Packer, R. J. (1995). Survival of infants with malignant astrocytomas: A report from the Children's Cancer Group. *Cancer, 75*(4), 1045–1050.

Gold, E. B., Leviton, A., Lopez, R., Austin, D. F., Gilles, F. H., Hedley-Whyte, E. T., Kolonel, L. N., Lyon, J. L., Swanson, G. M., Weiss, N. S., West, D. W., & Aschenbrener, C. (1994). The role of family history in risk of childhood brain tumors. *Cancer, 73*(4), 1302–1311.

Gold, E. B., Leviton, A., Lopez, R., Gilles, F. H., Hedley-Whyte, E. T., Kolonel, L. N., Lyon, J. L, Swanson, G. M., Weiss, N. S., West, D., Aschenbrener, C., & Austin, D. F. (1993). Parental smoking and risk of childhood brain tumors. *American Journal of Epidemiology, 137*(6), 620–628.

Giuffre, R., Liccardo, G., Pastore, F. S., Spallone, A., & Vagnozzi, R. (1990). Potential risk factors for brain tumors in children: An analysis of 200 cases. *Child's Nervous System, 6,* 8–12.

Gurney, J. G., Severson, R. K., Davis, S., & Robinson, L. L. (1995). Incidence of cancer in children in the United States: Sex-, race-, and 1-year age-specific rates by histologic type. *Cancer, 75*(8), 2186–2195.

Healey, E. A., Shamberger, R. C., Grier, H. E., Loeffler, J. S., & Tarbell, N. J. (1995). A 10-year experience of pediatric brachytherapy. *International Journal of Radiation Oncology, Biology, Physics, 32*(2), 451–455.

Hoppe-Hirsch, E., Renier, D., Lellouch-Tubiana, A., Sainte-Rose, C., Pierre-Kahn, A., & Hirsch, J. F. (1990). Medulloblastoma in childhood: Progressive intellectual deterioration. *Child's Nervous System, 6,* 60–65.

Jenkin, D., Greenberg, M., Hoffman, H., Hendrick, B., Humphreys, R., & Vatter, A. (1995). Brain tumors in children: Long-term survival after radiation treatment. *International Journal of Radiation Oncology, Biology, Physics, 31*(3), 445–451.

Johnson, D. L., McCabe, M. A., Nicholson, H. S., Joseph, A. L., Getson, P. R., Byrne, J., Brasseux, C., Packer, R. J., & Reaman, G. (1994). Quality of long-term survival in young children with medulloblastoma. *Journal of Neurosurgery, 80,* 1004–1010.

Kazak, A. E., & Meadows, A. T. (1989). Families of young adolescents who have survived cancer: Social–emotional adjustment, adaptability, and social support. *Journal of Pediatric Psychology, 14*(2), 175–191.

Kazak, A. E., & Nachman, G. S. (1991). Family research on childhood chronic illness: Pediatric oncology as an example. *Journal of Family Psychology, 4*(4), 462–483.

Koocher, G. P., & O'Malley, J. E. (1981). *The Damocles syndrome: Psychosocial consequences of surviving childhood cancer.* New York: McGraw-Hill.

Kuijten, R. R., Bunin, G. R., Nass, C. C., & Meadows, A. T. (1990). Gestational and familial risk factors for childhood astrocytoma: Results of a case–control study. *Cancer Research, 50,* 2608–2612.

Kuijten, R. R., Bunin, G. R., Nass, C. C., & Meadows, A. T. (1992). Parental occupation and childhood astrocytoma: Results of a case–control study. *Cancer Research, 52,* 782–786.

Kuijten, R. R., Strom, S. S., Rorke, L. B., Boesel, C. P., Buckley, J. D., Meadows, A. T., & Bunin, G. R. (1993). Family history of cancer and seizures in young children with brain tumors: A report from the Children's Cancer Group (United States and Canada). *Cancer Causes and Control, 4,* 455–464.

Lannering, B., Marky, I., Lundberg, A., & Olsson, E. (1990). Long-term sequelae after pediatric brain tumors: Their effect on disability and quality of life. *Medical and Pediatric Oncology, 18,* 304–310.

Leviton, J. (1994). Principles of epidemiology. In M. E. Cohen & P. K. Duffner (Eds.), *Brain tumors in children: Principles of diagnosis and treatment* (2nd ed.). New York: Raven Press.

Miller, R. W., Young, J. L., & Novakovic, B. (1995). Childhood cancer. *Cancer, 75*(1), 395–405.

Moore, B. D., Ater, J. L., & Copeland, D. R. (1992). Improved neuropsychological outcome in children with brain tumors diagnosed during infancy and treated without cranial irradiation. *Journal of Child Neurology, 7,* 281–290.

Moore, B. D., Ater, J. L., Needle, M. N., Slopis, J., & Copeland, D. R. (1994). Neuropsychological profile of children with neurofibromatosis, brain tumor, or both. *Journal of Child Neurology, 9,* 368–377.

Morris, R. D., Fletcher, J. M., & Francis, D. (1992). Psychometric issues in the neuropsychological assessment of children: Measurement of ability discrepancy and change. In F. Boller & J. Grafman (Eds.), *Handbook of neuropsychology* (Vol. 6, pp. 341–352). Amsterdam: Elsevier.

Mulhern, R. K., Crisco, J. J., & Kun, L. E. (1983). Neuropsychological sequelae of childhood brain tumors: A review. *Journal of Clinical Child Psychology, 12,* 66–73.

Mulhern, R. K., Kovnar, E. H., Kun, L. E., Crisco, J. J., & Williams, J. M. (1988). Psychologic and neurologic function following treatment for childhood temporal lobe astrocytoma. *Journal of Child Neurology, 3,* 47–52.

Mulhern, R. K., Wasserman, A. L., Friedman, A. G., & Fairclough, D. (1989). Social competence and behavioral adjustment of children who are long-term survivors of cancer. *Pediatrics, 83,* 18–25.

National Cancer Institute (NCI). (1995, July). Childhood brain tumor. *CancerNet: PDQ Treatment Statements for Physicians.* Available E-mail: http://www.cancernet.nci.nih.gov

Packer, R. J. (1994). Diagnosis, treatment, and outcome of primary central nervous system tumors of childhood. *Current Opinion in Oncology, 6*(3), 240–246.

Packer, R. J. (1995). Brain tumors in children [Review]. *Current Opinion in Pediatrics, 7*(1), 64–72.

Packer, R. J., Sposto, R., Atkins, T. E., Sutton, L. N., Bruce, D. A., Siegel, K. R., Rorke, L. B., Littman, P. A., & Schut, L. (1987). Quality of life in children with primitive neuroectodermal tumors (medulloblastoma) of the posterior fossa. *Pediatric Neuroscience, 13,* 169–175.

Packer, R. J., Sutton, L. N., Atkins, T. E., Radcliffe, J., Bunin, G. R., D'Angio, G., Siegel, K. R., & Schut, L. (1989). A prospective study of cognitive functioning in children receiving whole-brain radiotherapy and chemotherapy: 2-year results. *Journal of Neurosurgery, 70,* 707–713.

Pomeroy, S. L. (1994). The p53 tumor suppressor gene and pediatric brain tumors [Review]. *Current Opinion in Pediatrics, 6*(6), 632–635.

Radcliffe, J., Bunin, G. R., Sutton, L. N., Goldwein, J. W., & Phillips, P. C. (1994). Cognitive deficits in long-term survivors of childhood medulloblastoma and other noncortical tumors: Age-dependent effects of whole brain radiation. *International Journal of Developmental Neuroscience, 12*(4), 327–334.

Radcliffe, J., Packer, R. J., Atkins, T. E., Bunin, G. R., Schut, L., Goldwein, J. W., & Sutton, L. N. (1992). Three- and four-year cognitive outcome in children with noncortical brain tumors treated with whole-brain radiotherapy. *Annals of Neurology, 32,* 551–554.

Ris, M. D., & Noll, R. B. (1994). Long-term neurobehavioral outcome in pediatric brain-tumor patients: Review and methodological critique. *Journal of Clinical and Experimental Neuropsychology, 16*(1), 21–42.

Roman, D. D., & Sperduto, P. W. (1995). Neuropsychological effects of cranial radiation: Current knowledge and future directions. *International Journal of Radiation Oncology, Biology, Physics, 31*(4), 983–998.

Sarasua, S., & Savitz, D. A. (1994). Cured and broiled meat consumption in relation to childhood cancer: Denver, Colorado (United States). *Cancer Causes and Control, 5,* 141–148.

Silber, J. H., Radcliffe, J., Peckham, V., Perilongo, G., Kishnani, P., Fridman, M., Goldwein, J. W., & Meadows, A. T. (1992). Whole-brain irradiation and decline in intelligence: The influence of dose and age on IQ score. *Journal of Clinical Oncology, 10*(9), 1390–1396.

Spreen, O. (1984). *Human developmental neuropsychology.* New York: Oxford University Press.

Stehbens, J. A., Kisker, C. T., & Wilson, B. K. (1983). Achievement and intelligence test–retest performance in pediatric cancer patients at diagnosis and one year later. *Journal of Pediatric Psychology, 8,* 47–56.

von Ammon, K., & Roelcke, U. (1994). Genetics alterations of brain tumors. *Journal of Neuro-Oncology, 22,* 245–248.

Waldrop, S. M., Davis, P. C., Padgett, C. A., Shapiro, M. B., & Morris, R. (1998). Treatment of brain tumors in children is associated with abnormal MR spectroscopic ratios in brain tissue remote from the tumor site. *American Journal of Neuroradiology, 19,* 963–970.

Wilkins, J. R., & Sinks, T. (1990). Parental occupation and intracranial neoplasms of childhood: Results of a case–control interview study. *American Journal of Epidemiology, 132*(2), 275–291.

Wingo, P. A., Tong, T., & Bolden, S. (1995). Cancer statistics, 1995. *CA: A Cancer Journal for Clinicians, 45*(1), 8–30.

World Health Organization. (1979). *Histological typing of tumors of the central nervous system.* Geneva: WHO.

Yung, A. W. K. (1994a). Molecular biology, genetics, and central nervous system neoplasms [Commentary]. *Current Opinion in Neurology, 7,* 475–476.

Yung, A. W. K. (1994b). New approaches to molecular therapy of brain tumors. *Current Opinion in Neurology, 7,* 501–505.

Zülch, K. J. (1986). *Brain tumors. Their biology and pathology, 3rd ed.* Berlin: Springer Verlag.

5

CLOSED-HEAD INJURY

KEITH OWEN YEATES

Closed-head trauma in children is a major public health problem. It is a leading cause of death among youth and results in substantial neurobehavioral morbidity for survivors. The morbidity and mortality result largely from the brain injuries with which closed-head trauma is so often associated. Indeed, closed-head trauma represents the most common source of acquired brain injury among children and adolescents. Hence it is a major source of referrals for pediatric neuropsychologists in clinical practice (Yeates, Ris, & Taylor, 1995), and also has been of long-standing interest to researchers in pediatric neuropsychology.

The research literature pertaining to the neuropsychological consequences of closed-head injuries in children is extensive and has been the subject of several previous reviews (Arffa, 1998; Baron, Fennell, & Voeller, 1995; Fletcher & Levin, 1988; Fletcher, Levin, & Butler, 1995; Levin, Ewing-Cobbs, & Eisenberg, 1995). Despite this large body of literature, a substantial amount of the variance in postinjury outcomes remains unexplained. The goal of the present chapter is to provide an overview of the current state of knowledge regarding closed-head injuries, to critique the existing literature and recommend conceptual and methodological improvements, and to suggest potentially fruitful directions for future research. The chapter is written in hopes of promoting efforts to explain more thoroughly the variability in outcomes among children with traumatic brain injuries.

EPIDEMIOLOGY

Incidence of Injury

Accurate statistics regarding the incidence and prevalence of closed-head injuries in the United States are difficult to obtain. There are few registries for head trauma at either a local, regional, or national level, and existing registries are often concerned only with injuries that require hospital admission, thereby omitting many milder injuries. Moreover, as Kraus (1995) notes, epidemiological studies have varied widely in terms of definition of injury, sources of data, data collection techniques, description of cases, and ages of the target population. Not surprisingly, incidence rates varied significantly among the nine published studies reviewed by Kraus (1995), with an average annual incidence of 180 per 100,000 children per year in children less than 15 years of age.

Incidence varies as a function of injury severity. The most common measure of injury severity is the Glasgow Coma Scale (Teasdale & Jennett, 1974), on which scores range from 3 to 15 (see Table 5.1). Scores from 13 to 15 typically represent mild injuries, scores from 9 to 12 represent moderate injuries, and scores of 8 or less represent severe injuries. Studies using the Glasgow Coma Scale as the measure of severity have found that the majority of closed-head injuries are mild (Kraus, 1995). For instance, according to the United States National Coma Data Bank (Luerssen, Klauber, & Marshall, 1988), about 85% of all injuries requiring medical treatment are mild in nature, about 8% are moderate in severity, and the remaining 6% are severe. Similarly, the National Pediatric Trauma Registry (Lescohier & DiScala, 1993) indicates that 76% of injuries are mild, 10% moderate, and 13% severe.

TABLE 5.1. Glasgow Coma Scale

Category	Score	Description
Eye Opening		
None	1	Not attributable to occular swelling.
To pain	2	Pain stimulus is applied to chest or limbs.
To speech	3	Nonspecific response to speech or shout; does not imply patient obeys command to open eyes.
Spontaneous	4	Eyes are open, but this does not imply intact awareness.
Motor Response		
No response	1	Flaccid.
Extension	2	Decerebrate posturing: Adduction, internal rotation of shoulder, and pronation of forearm.
Abnormal flexion	3	Decorticate posturing: Abnormal flexion, adduction of the shoulder.
Withdrawal	4	Normal flexor response; withdraws from pain stimulus with abduction of the shoulder.
Localizes pain	5	Pain stimulus applied to supraocular region or fingertip causes limb to remove it.
Obeys commands	6	Follows simple commands.
Verbal Response		
No response	1	No vocalization.
Incomprehensible	2	Vocalizes, but no recognizable words.
Inappropriate	3	Intelligible speech (e.g., shouting or swearing) but no sustained or coherent conversation.
Confused	4	Responds to questions in a conversational manner, but the responses indicate disorientation.
Oriented	5	Normal orientation to time, person, and place.

Note. Glasgow Coma Scale Score = Eye Opening score + Motor Response score + Verbal Response score (range 3 to 15). Adapted from Teasdale & Jennet (1974).

Causes of Injury

Data regarding the external causes of closed-head trauma can provide important information about the mechanisms of brain injuries. Despite substantial inconsistencies in the categorization of external causes, the most common causes of head trauma are transportation-related (including those involving motor vehicles and bicycles) and falls. Together, transportation-related trauma and falls typically account for between 75% and 80% of all brain injuries in published studies (Kraus, 1995).

The distribution of causes varies significantly as a function of children's ages (Kraus, 1995). Infants and young children are especially likely to be injured in falls. Among older children, sports and recreational accidents and pedestrian or bicycle collisions with motor vehicles account for an increasing proportion of head injuries. Adolescents are especially likely to be injured in motor vehicle accidents.

Demographic Variation

The incidence of closed-head injuries varies significantly according to demographic factors. Boys are at considerably higher risk for closed-head trauma than are girls. In published studies, the ratio of boys to girls rises from approximately 1.5:1 for preschool children to approximately 2:1 for school-age children and adolescents (Kraus, 1995). The change appears to reflect a sharp increase in head injuries among males and a gradual decrease among females (Kraus, Fife, Cox, Ramstein, & Conroy, 1986).

The incidence of closed-head trauma also varies with age. The incidence is relatively stable from birth to age 5, with injuries occurring in about 160 per 100,000 children in this age group. After age 5, the overall incidence gradually increases until early adolescence and then shows rapid growth, reaching a peak incidence of approximately 290 per 100,000 by age 18 (Kraus et al., 1986).

Incidence rates may also vary as a function of family socioeconomic status. In one study from San Diego County (Kraus, Rock, & Hamyari, 1990), the incidence of brain injury among children was related to median family income as determined from census tract data. The relationship with income was not affected by children's age or ethnicity. On the other hand, a telephone survey of nonfatal childhood injuries in San Diego County did not find a relationship between parental education or income and the incidence of head injury (Klauber, Barrett-Connor, Hotstetter, & Micik, 1986).

Mortality and Morbidity

Traumatic injuries are the leading cause of death among children and adolescents, and about 40–50% of the deaths resulting from trauma are associated with brain injuries (Kraus, 1995). In a study of children less than 15 years of age residing in Olmsted County, Minnesota, from 1935 to 1974, the mortality rate associated with head injuries was about 10 per 100,000 (Annegers, Grabow, Kurland, & Laws, 1980). In a more recent review, Kraus (1995) cited a mortality rate of approximately 20 per 100,000 among children in this age group, based on national health statistics.

Overall, mortality rates are lower among children than among adults (Goldstein & Levin, 1987). The mortality rate is highest among children with severe injuries, and is virtually nil among those with mild injuries. In his review of five studies, Kraus (1995) found case fatality rates among hospital admissions to range from 12% to 62% for severe injuries, but to be less than 4% for moderate injuries and less than 1% for mild injuries.

Survivors of severe closed-head trauma frequently experience adverse consequences. One gross measure of outcome that has been employed in several epidemiological studies is the Glasgow Outcome Scale (Jennett & Bond, 1975). The Glasgow Outcome Scale differentiates five outcome categories: death, persistent vegetative state, severe disability, moderate disability, and "good recovery." In his review, Kraus (1995) found that between 75% and 95% of children with closed-head injuries displayed a "good recovery," that about 10% showed a moderate disability, that 1–3% showed a severe disability, and that fewer than 1% were in a persistent vegetative state. However, a "good recovery" according to the Glasgow Outcome Scale does not preclude neurobehavioral impairment or associated functional disabilities (Koelfen et al., 1997). The latter outcomes are discussed later.

NEUROPATHOLOGY AND PATHOPHYSIOLOGY

Closed-head trauma can produce brain injuries in a variety of ways (see Table 5.2). These mechanisms include overt alterations in brain tissue—including both focal and diffuse lesions—as well as disruptions in brain function at a cellular level. The pathophysiology of head trauma begins at the time of impact, but continues over a period of days or weeks and perhaps even longer. Indeed, recent research indicates that the brain damage resulting from closed-head trauma involves more complex, prolonged, and interwoven processes than was previously recognized (Bigler, 1997).

Primary and Secondary Injuries

Observable injuries resulting from head trauma can be classified into two broad categories, primary and secondary. *Primary* injuries result directly from the trauma itself. They include skull fractures, contusions and lacerations, and mechanical injuries to nerve fibers and blood vessels. *Secondary* injuries arise indirectly from the trauma; in children, they

TABLE 5.2. Pathology of Closed-Head Injury

Type of insult	Pathology
Primary	Skull fracture Intracranial contusions and hemorrhage Shear–strain injury
Secondary	Brain swelling Cerebral edema Elevated intracranial pressure Hypoxia–ischemia Mass lesions (hematoma)
Neurochemical	Excessive production of free radicals Excessive release of excitatory neurotransmitters Disruption of cellular calcium homeostasis
Delayed	White matter degeneration and cerebral atrophy Posttraumatic hydrocephalus Posttraumatic seizures

include brain swelling and edema, hypoxia and hypotension, increased intracranial pressure, mass lesions such as epidural hematomas, and seizures (Pang, 1985).

The primary injuries that arise from head trauma reflect biomechanical forces, which can involve either impression or acceleration–deceleration. *Impression* occurs when there is direct contact between a stationary head and some physical force, as when a person sustains a blow to the head from a moving object. *Acceleration–deceleration* occurs when there is an impact with a moving head. Most of the common causes of head injuries in children, including falls and transportation-related, give rise to acceleration–deceleration injuries.

Acceleration injuries can involve both translational and rotational trauma. *Translational* injuries involve linear acceleration along an axis that passes through the center of the head. The acceleration can result in deformation of the skull or skull fractures, as well as contusions at the site of impact. Isolated translational injury is rare, however, and is usually combined with rotational injury. *Rotational* injuries occur when the axis of impact does not pass directly through the center of the head, and hence results in a combination of both linear and angular acceleration.

Rotational injuries arise when the skull is stopped by the impact, but the brain continues to move in the skull because of its angular acceleration. The movement results in the tearing or bruising of blood vessels that gives rise to focal contusions or hemorrhage, and to the shearing or straining of white matter nerve fibers. Shear and strain forces have been thought to be responsible for diffuse axonal injury, which triggers a process of wallerian degeneration in distal axonal projections and results in the diffuse loss of synaptic terminals (Povlishock, Erb, & Astruc, 1992).

Focal contusions are especially likely to occur in the frontal and temporal cortex, because of its proximity to the bony prominences in the anterior and middle fossa of the skull. In contrast, shear–strain injuries appear to be most common at the boundaries between gray and white matter. Although diffusely distributed, they occur most often around the basal ganglia, periventricular regions near the hypothalamus, superior cerebellar peduncles, fornices, corpus callosum, and fiber tracts of the brain stem. Neuroimaging consistently reveals an anterior–posterior gradient in the focal lesions associated with closed-head trauma. Focal lesions are generally larger and occur more frequently in frontal and anterior temporal regions than in posterior temporal, parietal, or occipital regions (Levin et al., 1989; Mendelsohn et al., 1992).

In most cases, medical management of closed-head injuries focuses on the secondary injuries that arise indirectly following the initial trauma, rather than on the primary injuries. Brain swelling and cerebral edema are two major secondary complications of closed-head injuries, and may be more common in children than among adults (Aldrich et al., 1992; Bruce et al., 1979, 1981; but see Lang, Teasdale, Macpherson, & Lawrence, 1994). Brain swelling and cerebral edema are thought to result from a disruption of the normal relationships among blood, brain tissue, and cerebrospinal fluid. A disruption of these relationships can result in decreased cerebral blood flow, increased cerebral blood volume, and increased intracranial pressure, which together can give rise to ischemic and hypoxic injury, as well as to brain herniation and death (Bruce, 1995). Decreases in cerebral blood flow are often exacerbated by hypotension (low blood pressure), which is a common symptom of shock. Pulmonary insufficiency can also contribute to hypoxia.

In contrast to brain swelling and cerebral edema, mass lesions are less common in children than in adults (Bruce, 1995). Mass lesions involve the accumulation of fluid, usually blood associated with contusion and hemorrhage. Hematomas are blood clots that occur in various locations in and around the brain. Epidural hematomas result from bleeding into the space between the dura and the skull, often in association with a skull fracture that disrupts the middle meningeal artery. Epidural hematomas occasionally become apparent clinically only after several days. Subdural hematomas result from bleeding into the space between the dura and the arachnoid membranes, frequently because of a tear in the bridging veins of the sagittal sinus, and are more often acute in nature. Intracerebral hematomas occur within the brain parenchyma, and often follow the same spatial distribution as contusions. They may result from shear injuries to brain tissue. Subarachnoid or intraventricular hemorrhages are also common in closed-head injuries, and may contribute to the diffuse pathology associated with head injury (Bruce, 1995).

Neurochemical Mechanisms

In recent years, the assumption that the shear forces involved in blunt trauma account for the majority of diffuse axonal injury has come under fire. Experimental research with animals has provided little supporting evidence for this assumption, and in fact has demonstrated that axonal injury can occur in brains that show no evidence of mechanical tearing or disruption (Povlishock et al., 1992). At the same time, research advances in the neurochemistry of brain injury have begun to suggest that diffuse axonal injury is mediated by a cascade of biochemical reactions that take place over an extended period of time following a brain injury (Novack, Dillon, & Jackson, 1996). Head trauma can result in a variety of neurochemical events, including the production of free radicals and excitatory amino acids and the disruption of normal calcium homeostasis. These events act in concert to exacerbate the hypoxic–ischemic insult that commonly occurs following closed-head trauma.

Free radicals are normal by-products of metabolism. Excessive production of free radicals, however, can affect cell membrane integrity and cause lipid peroxidation or attack cell organelles, such as the mitochondria. Brain tissue may be especially vulnerable to free radicals because it is rich in cholesterol and polyunsaturated fatty acid. Measurement of free radicals is difficult, and there is little direct evidence of the impact of free radicals on brain function. However, experimental research with animals has shown that treatment with radical scavengers can reduce brain injury (Novack et al., 1996).

Excitatory amino acids normally function as neurotransmitters. They can be harmful in excessive amounts, however, disrupting cell function and eventually resulting in cell death. Glutamate and aspartate are two common excitatory amino acids. These compounds have an affinity for receptors that are especially prevalent in regions including the hippocampus and thalamus. Experimental studies of animals indicate that the release of glutamate and aspartate is especially sensitive to hypoxic–ischemic events and increases dramatically after traumatic brain injury. Thus excitotoxicity helps to account for the severe effects of hypoxia–ischemia on the hippocampus, which has many glutamate receptors; it may also explain the selective vulnerability of the hippocampus in closed-head injuries. Experimental research indicates that substances that block glutamate receptors can reduce the brain damage associated with hypoxia–ischemia. Other neurotransmitters, including acetylcholine, are also thought to contribute to brain injury.

The disruption of cellular calcium homeostasis by hypoxia–ischemia is another indirect source of brain injury. Hypoxic–ischemic insults interrupt normal ion-pumping mechanisms and induce the release of intracellular calcium. The influx of calcium exacerbates the effects of hypoxia–ischemia on the normal metabolic process of oxidative phosphorylation and further reduces adenosine triphosphate, which is the major energy source for cell function. In addition, the calcium influx triggers other chemical events, including the release of free radicals and excitatory neurotransmitters. The disruption of calcium homeostasis can also result in vasoconstriction, leading to further hypoxic–ischemic insult.

Following hypoxic–ischemic insults, oxidative metabolism gives way to anaerobic glycolysis. With this shift in metabolic status comes a dramatic increase in lactate levels, with the highest levels often in the hippocampus. The increase in lactate is thought to reflect an acidosis that results from the release of lactic acid and is correlated with the severity of brain injury. The role of lactic acidosis in ischemic brain injury remains uncertain, however, because of findings suggesting that increases in lactate or lactic acid can occur without deleterious effects (Novack et al., 1996).

Late Effects

Closed-head injuries can be associated with a variety of late effects. Neuroimaging studies have indicated that severe traumatic brain injuries often result in a gradual and prolonged process of white matter degeneration, with associated cerebral atrophy and ventricular enlargement (Bigler, 1997). In some cases, ventricular dilatation results from an actual disturbance in the circulation of cerebrospinal fluid and is associated with hydrocephalus. Posttraumatic hydrocephalus, as opposed to cerebral atrophy and associated ventricular enlargement, is relatively uncommon and typically develops only after severe injuries associated with certain predisposing factors, such as subarachnoid hemorrhage (Cardoso & Galbraith, 1985; McLean et al., 1995).

Early posttraumatic seizures occur in about 3–9% of children with head trauma and often involve focal status epilepticus, sometimes associated with mass lesions (McLean et al., 1995). Younger children seem especially vulnerable to early posttraumatic seizures. The occurrence of seizures soon after injury does not clearly place children at risk for later epilepsy, which occurs in about 2% of the survivors of pediatric head injury. Posttraumatic epilepsy is more common in children with penetrating injuries or depressed skull fractures, among whom the incidence is approximately 10%. Most posttraumatic seizures occur within the first 2 years after injury.

NEUROBEHAVIORAL CONSEQUENCES

The literature on the neuropsychological consequences of pediatric closed-head injuries is extensive, and a detailed review of all individual studies is beyond the scope of this chapter. In general, research indicates that closed-head injuries, especially severe ones, can produce deficits in various domains: alertness and orientation; intellectual functioning; language skills; nonverbal skills; attention and memory; executive functions; corticosensory and motor skills; academic achievement; and adaptive functioning and behavioral adjustment. The following sections provide a selective overview of the existing literature and highlight recent research findings. The reader is encouraged to seek out pertinent primary sources, including the work of several prominent research groups (Dennis, Wilkinson, Koski, & Humphreys, 1995; Dennis, Barnes, Donnelly, Wilkinson, & Humphreys, 1996; Klonoff, Clark, & Klonoff, 1995; Knights et al., 1991; Levin, Ewing-Cobbs, & Eisenberg, 1995; Shaffer, 1995; Taylor et al., 1995).

Alertness and Orientation

Orientation and alertness are often disturbed following closed-head injuries, particularly during the initial phase of recovery. Most children with closed-head injuries, especially moderate or severe ones, experience a postinjury period of fluctuations in arousal, as well as disorientation, confusion, and memory loss. These changes in mental status occur during what is usually referred to as the period of posttraumatic amnesia (PTA), which is often used as a measure of injury severity. Investigators have developed standardized methods for measuring the presence and duration of PTA, such as the Children's Orientation and Amnesia Test (COAT; Ewing-Cobbs, Levin, Fletcher, Miner, & Eisenberg, 1990). Scores on the COAT have been found to predict posttraumatic memory function up to 12 months following a closed-head injury (Ewing-Cobbs et al., 1990).

Intellectual Functioning

Poor performance on intelligence tests is a common finding following closed-head injuries (Fletcher & Levin, 1988; Baron et al., 1995). The deficits occur whether children with closed-head injuries are compared to normal controls or to children with orthopedic injuries not involving the head, and the magnitude of the deficits is related to injury severity. IQ scores that reflect nonverbal skills are particularly likely to be depressed (e.g., Performance IQ score on the Wechsler Intelligence Scale for Children, third edition [WISC-III]). Measures of verbal intelligence appear less vulnerable to head injury (e.g., WISC-III Verbal IQ score), typically occurring only in conjunction with more severe injuries. The dissociation probably reflects the different demands associated with the two types of scales. For instance, Performance IQ subtests are more likely to require fluid problem-solving skills and to involve speeded motor output, whereas Verbal IQ subtests assess previously acquired knowledge and make few demands for speeded responses or motor control.

Prospective, longitudinal studies indicate that children demonstrate significant recovery in intellectual functioning following closed-head injuries. Thus IQ scores tend to increase over time following closed-head injuries, with the largest increases occurring among children with more severe injuries (Chadwick, Rutter, Brown, Shaffer, & Traub, 1981). IQ scores increase most rapidly immediately after injury and tend to plateau after 1 to 2 years, although improvements have been shown to occur for periods of up to 5 years (Klonoff, Low, & Clark, 1977). Despite substantial recovery, IQ scores often continue to be depressed relative to premorbid levels, particularly among children with severe injuries (Costeff et al., 1988).

Language Skills

Spontaneous mutism and expressive language deficits are common immediately after closed-head injuries (Levin et al., 1983), but overt aphasic disorders rarely persist following acute recovery. However, subtle language difficulties often persist, again most often following moderate to severe injuries. Long-term deficits have been identified on tests measuring a variety of basic linguistic skills, including syntactical comprehension, sentence repetition, confrontation naming, object description, and verbal fluency (Levin & Eisenberg, 1979; Ewing-Cobbs, Levin, Eisenberg, & Fletcher, 1987).

Children with closed-head injuries also display more pronounced difficulties with the pragmatic aspects of language (Chapman, 1995; Dennis & Barnes, 1990). Deficits have been demonstrated in various skills, such as interpreting ambiguous sentences, making inferences, formulating sentences from individual words, and explaining figurative expressions. Deficits in such skills are construed as reflecting a general impairment in *discourse*, which can be defined as the ability to convey a message by communicating a series of ideas, usually in sentences. Studies of narrative discourse, using story recall as the dependent measure, indicate that children with severe closed-head injuries use fewer words and sentences in their stories (Chapman, 1995). Moreover, their stories contain less information, are not as well organized, and are less complete than those produced by children with milder injuries or by normal controls. The differences remain significant even after word knowledge and verbal memory are controlled. Because of the importance of communicative skills for school success, discourse deficits may account for some of the academic difficulties that children with closed-head injuries often experience.

Nonverbal Skills

Long-term deficits in nonverbal skills are also relatively frequent consequences of pediatric closed-head injuries. The declines in Performance IQ reported after childhood head injuries reflect deficits in a variety of nonverbal skills, including both visual-perceptual and constructional abilities. Deficits following head injuries have been reported on a variety of other constructional tasks, including three-dimensional block construction (Levin & Eisenberg, 1979), the Tactual Performance Test (Klonoff et al., 1977), the Developmental Test of Visual–Motor Integration (Taylor et al., 1999; Thompson et al., 1994), and the Rey–Osterrieth Complex Figure (Yeates, Patterson, Waber, & Bernstein, 1993). Relatively few studies have included measures of visual-perceptual or visual–spatial skills that do not involve motor output, although children with closed-head injuries have shown deficits on tasks involving facial discrimination (Levin & Eisenberg, 1979) and picture matching (Klonoff et al., 1977).

Attention

Complaints about attention problems are very common following childhood head injuries. However, studies using objective measures of attention are relatively limited, and no studies have provided a comprehensive assessment of attention based on current theoretical models (e.g., Mirsky, Anthony, Duncan, Ahearn, & Kellam, 1991; Cooley & Morris, 1990). The studies that have included objective measures have generally focused on continuous-performance tasks (e.g., Kaufman, Fletcher, Levin, Miner, & Ewing-Cobbs, 1993; Dennis et al., 1995). Children with severe closed-head injuries generally display poorer performance on such tasks than do those with less severe injuries or normal controls. Attentional weaknesses among children with severe head injuries are evidenced by poorer response modulation, especially in the presence of distraction, as well as slower reaction times. Interestingly, compared to normative expectations, these deficits appear to be more pronounced among younger head-injured children than among their older counterparts (Dennis et al., 1995).

Memory

Childhood closed-head injuries frequently result in memory deficits, and the magnitude of the deficits is dependent upon injury severity (Donders, 1993). Deficits have been reported on a wide variety of verbal tasks, including tests of recognition memory for words (Levin, Eisenberg, Wigg, & Kobayashi, 1982), word list learning (Levin et al., 1982; Yeates, Blumenstein, Patterson, & Delis, 1995), paired-associates learning (Chadwick, Rutter, Shaffer, & Shrout, 1981), and story recall (Bassett & Slater, 1990). Fewer studies have examined nonverbal memory after closed-head injuries, although deficits have been reported on the recall of shapes from the Tactual Performance Test (Klonoff et al., 1977) and the reproduction of simple and complex geometric shapes (Berger-Gross & Schackelford, 1985; Yeates et al., 1993).

Most previous studies have not addressed the specific nature of the memory deficits observed following head trauma, in part because most of the tasks used have not permitted any differentiation among specific components of memory. Recent studies using the California Verbal Learning Test, however, suggest that deficits occur in a variety of memory components, including storage, retention, and retrieval (Roman et al., 1998; Yeates, Blumenstein, et al., 1995). For instance, we (Yeates, Blumenstein, et al., 1995) found that children with severe injuries display poorer learning, less retention over time, and better recognition than recall, when compared to matched controls. Further research is needed to delineate the specific nature of the explicit memory deficits associated with pediatric traumatic brain injury.

Future studies are also needed to examine types of memory other than those measured by tasks requiring explicit recall. In recent years, cognitive and developmental neuroscientists have drawn a crucial distinction between explicit and implicit memory (Nelson, 1995; Schacter, 1987). *Explicit* memory involves the conscious recollection of past events or experiences and is typically measured through recall or recognition, whereas *implicit* memory involves demonstrations of learning or facilitation of performance in the absence of conscious recollection. In contrast to explicit memory, implicit memory has been shown to remain relatively intact following closed-head injuries in adults (Vakil, Jaffe, Eluse, Groswasser, & Aberbuch, 1996). However, there are currently no published studies of implicit memory among children with traumatic brain injuries.

Executive Functions

Deficits in executive functions also occur frequently after childhood closed-head injuries. Studies of this domain are less numerous than those of specific verbal and nonverbal skills, or of attention and memory, in part because measurement of the complex and multifaceted construct of *executive functions* is so challenging (Denckla, 1994). In recent years, however, Levin and his colleagues have been studying executive functions extensively (Levin, Ewing-Cobbs, & Eisenberg, 1995). They have found that children with traumatic brain injuries display deficits on various tasks meant to assess executive functions, such as the Tower of London, which measures planning skills; Controlled Oral Word Association, which measures verbal fluency; and the 20 Questions Test and Wisconsin Card Sorting Test, which measure concept formation and mental flexibility. Interestingly, the magnitude of deficits on executive function tasks has been shown to correlate with the volume of lesions in the frontal lobes, but not with extrafrontal lesion volume (Levin et al., 1994,

1997). Studies of the emotional and behavioral aspects of executive functions (Cummings, 1993) are needed to complement the intense focus on cognitive tasks that characterizes the existing research.

Corticosensory and Motor Skills

Children with closed-head injuries often demonstrate deficits in corticosensory and complex motor skills. Levin and Eisenberg (1979) found that approximately 25% of children with severe injuries displayed deficits on tests of stereognosis, finger localization, and graphesthesia. Deficits in motor skills were reported by Klonoff et al. (1977), who examined performance on an array of complex psychomotor tasks. Later studies by Bawden and his colleagues (Bawden, Knights, & Winogron, 1985; Winogron, Knights, & Bawden, 1984) also showed deficits on various measures of fine-motor skills, especially those that were timed. These investigators created composite scores based on tests that varied in their demands for speeded performance, and found that the magnitude of the difference among groups with mild, moderate, and severe injuries was directly related to the demand for speeded output. The performance of children with severe injuries declined as the demand for speed increased, whereas the performance of children with mild and moderate injuries was less affected by speed demands.

Academic Performance

Given the litany of neurocognitive deficits described above, it is not surprising that pediatric closed-head injuries are often associated with reports of declines in academic performance (Fletcher, Ewing-Cobbs, Miner, Levin, & Eisenberg, 1990; Taylor et al., 1999) and with an increased risk of placement in special education (Kinsella et al., 1995). The precise nature of the declines in academic performance, however, has not been clearly elucidated. Children with head injuries do not differ consistently from children with mild injuries or those with injuries not involving the head on standardized tests of academic achievement (Kinsella et al., 1995; Taylor et al., 1999). For instance, in a recent prospective, longitudinal study of closed-head injuries in 6- to 12-year-old children, moderate and severe injuries were associated with modest deficits on the Broad Written Expression composite from the Woodcock–Johnson Tests of Achievement—Revised, but not on the Broad Reading or Broad Math composites (Taylor et al., 1999).

Studies of predictors of postinjury special education placement suggest that declines in school performance may reflect behavioral changes or neuropsychological deficits, rather than decrements in specific academic skills. Two recent studies have shown that placement in special education is related to higher ratings of behavioral disturbance and to neuropsychological functioning, as reflected on measures of memory, nonverbal skills, and fine motor speed and dexterity (Kinsella et al., 1995; Stallings, Ewing-Cobbs, Francis, & Fletcher, 1996). Special education placement was not related to performance on achievement testing (Kinsella et al., 1995); instead, achievement testing was related primarily to demographic variables such as socioeconomic status. Thus standardized achievement testing may not be sensitive to the effects of closed-head injuries. Long-term follow-up studies are needed, however, to determine whether the academic achievement of children with severe injuries gradually lags behind that of their uninjured peers.

Adaptive Functioning and Behavioral Adjustment

The last domain within which deficits are common following closed-head injury in childhood is that of adaptive functioning and behavioral adjustment. Most previous research has relied on general rating scales, such as the Vineland Adaptive Behavior Scales (Sparrow, Balla, & Cicchetti, 1984) or the Child Behavior Checklist (Achenbach, 1991), to assess adaptive functioning and behavioral adjustment. In research using such scales, children with severe head injuries demonstrate more behavior problems and poorer adaptive functioning than do children with mild injuries or those with injuries not involving the head (Barry, Taylor, Klein, & Yeates, 1996; Fletcher et al., 1990; Taylor et al., 1999). However, adaptive deficits and behavioral disturbance are also related to factors other than injury severity, including the children's premorbid functioning.

The need to control for premorbid status in studies of behavioral adjustment is especially acute among children with mild injuries. Recently, Asarnow and his colleagues (Asarnow et al., 1995; Light et al., 1998) found that children with mild head injuries displayed higher rates of preinjury behavior problems on the Child Behavior Checklist (Achenbach, 1991) than did children with no injury. In contrast, their preinjury behavioral functioning did not differ from that of children with injuries not involving the head. The latter finding is consistent with previous research suggesting that the presence of premorbid behavior problems actually increases the likelihood of traumatic injuries (Brown, Chadwick, Shaffer, Rutter, & Traub, 1981). Thus, although severe head injuries increase the risk of behavioral disturbance, it is also likely that behavioral disturbance increases the risk of head injury. Hence, in cases of mild head injury, preinjury functioning must be taken into account before postinjury behavioral disturbance is attributed to the head injury.

The use of general rating scales such as the Child Behavior Checklist (Achenbach, 1991) to study pre- or postinjury behavioral adjustment is somewhat problematic, because such scales were not designed to be sensitive to the effects of traumatic brain injury (Drotar, Stein, & Perrin, 1995; Perrin, Stein, & Drotar, 1991). Focused measures of the specific symptoms that are likely to arise as a result of traumatic brain injury may provide a more accurate portrayal. For instance, Barry et al. (1996) examined 30 specific somatic, cognitive, and behavioral symptoms in children with moderate to severe traumatic brain injuries and children with orthopedic injuries. They found that the children with brain injuries displayed more symptoms in all three domains than did children with orthopedic injuries, and that the total number of symptoms correlated positively with injury severity. Similarly, recent research focusing on postconcussive symptoms suggests that children with mild head injuries display more cognitive and somatic symptoms 3 months after injury than do children who are not injured, even after premorbid status is controlled for, but that they do not display more emotional or behavioral symptoms (Yeates et al., 1999).

Few previous studies of behavioral functioning following childhood closed-head injuries have used standardized interviews to assess specific psychiatric disorders. In a recent series of studies, Max and his colleagues (Max, Lindgren, et al., 1997; Max, Robin, et al., 1997; Max, Smith, et al., 1997) examined psychiatric outcomes in a group of children with traumatic brain injuries of varying severity. They found that the onset of a "novel" psychiatric disorder, defined as one never before present in an individual, occurred in nearly 50% of all children. The most common novel diagnoses were organic personality syndrome, major depression, attention-deficit/hyperactivity disorder, and oppositional defiant disorder. The onset of a novel psychiatric disorder was predicted by injury severity, as well as by preinjury intellectual functioning, socioeconomic status, child psychiatric history, family psychiatric history, and global family functioning. Interestingly, the explanatory power of these predictors varied over time. A child's psychiatric history and global family functioning predicted novel disorders at 3 and 6 months and 2 years after injury. In contrast, preinjury intellectual functioning, socioeconomic status, and family psychiatric history predicted these disorders at 3 months but not at 6 months or 2 years after injury.

Behavioral functioning following childhood closed-head injuries does not appear to be closely related to cognitive outcomes. Previous research has not shown a strong relationship between behavioral adjustment, adaptive functioning, or the onset of psychiatric disorders and cognitive performance in children with traumatic brain injuries (Fletcher et al., 1990; Max, Robin, et al., 1997). For instance, Fletcher et al. (1990) found small and generally nonsignificant correlations between five neuropsychological measures and measures of adaptive functioning and behavioral adjustment. They concluded that cognitive and behavioral variables were "weakly correlated and had stronger relations with coma duration than with one another" (p. 97). Thus cognitive and behavioral outcomes may be somewhat independent following closed-head injuries, and their determinants may differ considerably. For instance, my colleagues and I found in one study that cognitive outcomes were related more strongly to injury-related variables, whereas behavioral outcomes were related more strongly to measures of preinjury family functioning (Yeates et al., 1997).

PREDICTION OF OUTCOMES

The preceding summary of the neurobehavioral outcomes of pediatric closed-head injuries is based largely on the results of group comparisons (e.g., severe vs. mild injuries). Although the generalizations are valid, they must be tempered by the realization that children with closed-head injuries display substantial variation in outcomes, even when they are grouped according to injury severity. These individual differences in outcomes reflect a complex interplay among injury characteristics, environmental influences, and developmental factors.

Injury Characteristics

Injury severity has consistently proved to be a major determinant of the consequences of closed-head injuries (Oddy, 1993). Injury severity has been assessed with a variety of metrics, including depth of coma, duration of impaired consciousness, and length of PTA. The Glasgow Coma Scale (see Table 5.1) is often used to assess depth of coma. Duration of impaired consciousness is usually defined as the amount of time that elapses from an injury until a child is able to follow commands, which is equivalent to the number of days during which the Motor Response score on the Glasgow Coma Scale falls below 6. An injury is usually considered severe when the duration of impaired consciousness lasts more than 24 hours. Unlike the Glasgow Coma Scale, which is a measure of a child's neurological status at a given point in time, the duration of impaired consciousness is an indirect indicator of rate of recovery, because it reflects the speed with which a child's mental status improves acutely after injury. The length of PTA, or the time that elapses from the injury until a child is oriented and displays intact memory for daily events, also indirectly reflects the child's rate of recovery. As already noted, standardized measures, such as the COAT, have been developed to assess PTA.

The relationship between various measures of injury severity and neuropsychological outcomes has been explored in several studies (Ewing-Cobbs, Fletcher, Levin, Hastings, & Francis, 1996; McDonald et al., 1994). McDonald et al. (1994) compared 10 different measures of severity as predictors of various neurobehavioral and functional outcomes. They found that the indices that best predicted both early and 1-year outcomes were (1) days to age-adjusted 75% performance on the COAT; (2) days to a Glasgow Coma Scale score of 15; and (3) initial total Glasgow Coma Scale score. Across studies, the duration of coma, impaired consciousness, and PTA were generally better predictors of outcome than was any static measure, such as the lowest postresuscitation Glasgow Coma Scale score. The predictive utility of the duration measures might have been related to their utility as markers of recovery, rather than as measures of neurological status immediately after injury.

Injury severity has also been assessed with a variety of medical indicators, including brain stem abnormalities (e.g., pupillary reactivity), seizures, and intracranial pressure (Fletcher, Levin, & Butler, 1995). More recently, advances in neuroimaging have begun to permit the characterization of injury severity based on measures of the brain's structural integrity. In the past, closed-head injuries were often conceptualized primarily in terms of diffuse brain insults, and markers such as brain swelling, edema, and diffuse axonal injury were studied as predictors of outcome (e.g., Aldrich et al., 1992). However, magnetic resonance imaging has detected focal brain lesions in the majority of children whose injuries are defined as severe on the basis of conventional measures, such as the Glasgow Coma Scale (Levin et al., 1989, 1993; Mendelsohn et al., 1992). Moreover, the presence of focal lesions has been associated with reliable variations in outcomes, over and above those related to diffuse insults (Filley, Cranberg, Alexander, & Hart, 1987). One interesting finding is that focal lesion volume has proven to be a more consistent predictor of cognitive than behavioral outcomes (Fletcher et al., 1996). The latter finding is consistent with the notion that cognitive outcomes are related more strongly to injury characteristics than are behavioral sequelae (Fletcher et al., 1990).

Environmental Influences

Most previous studies of the prediction of recovery following childhood head injuries have emphasized injury-related variables rather than pre- and postinjury environmental factors, even though injury severity fails to account for most of the variance in postinjury outcomes (Fletcher, Ewing-Cobbs, Francis, & Levin, 1995). Recent studies, however, have begun to examine more closely the role of environmental influences as predictors of outcomes. The results from those studies indicate that the environment is a significant predictor of both cognitive and behavioral outcomes following traumatic brain injuries. General measures of socioeconomic status and family demographics are consistent predictors of outcomes, as are more specific measures of family status and the social environment (Taylor et al., 1999).

One critical issue addressed by studies of the comparative roles of injury characteristics and the environment as determinants of recovery is whether the environment simply affects the functioning of children with traumatic brain injuries in the same way that it does children without such injuries, or whether it moderates the impact of traumatic brain injury by either buffering or exacerbating the direct, neurologically based consequences of head injury. Rutter and his colleagues (Shaffer, 1995) found that injury severity and the postinjury environment had additive influences on behavior problems. More recently, in a study designed to examine the role of the family and social environment as determinants of children's recovery from closed-head injuries, measures of both pre- and postinjury family status were shown to moderate outcomes (Taylor et al., 1999; Yeates et al., 1997). For example, Figure 5.1 shows that verbal memory deficits in children with severe traumatic brain injury at 1 year after injury were a function of preinjury family functioning. Specifically, the effects of severe brain injuries relative to orthopedic injuries were more pronounced for children from dysfunctional families than for children from more functional families. Interestingly, this pattern was observed on both cognitive and behavioral measures, although the relative importance of injury severity and family environment varied across the two outcome domains.

Developmental Variation

The outcomes associated with childhood traumatic brain injuries depend not only on injury characteristics and environmental influences, but also on developmental factors. Specifically, previous studies suggest that outcomes can vary along three distinct but interrelated age-related dimensions: a child's age at the time of injury, the amount of time that has passed since the injury, and the child's age at the time of outcome assessment (Taylor & Alden, 1997).

Most studies of childhood traumatic brain injury have focused on school-age children and adolescents. Across this age range, there has not been a strong relationship between

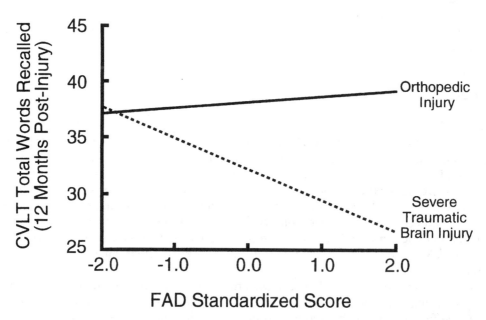

FIGURE 5.1. Relationship between the preinjury standardized score on the Family Assessment Device (FAD) General Functioning scale and total words recalled on the California Verbal Learning Test (CVLT) at 12 months after injury as a function of group membership. From Yeates et al. (1997). Copyright 1997 by the International Neuropsychological Society. Published by Cambridge University Press. Reprinted by permission.

age at injury and outcomes. Recent studies of preschool children, however, suggest that injuries sustained during infancy or early childhood are associated with more persistent deficits than are injuries occurring during later childhood and adolescence (Anderson & Moore, 1995; Anderson et al., 1997; Ewing-Cobbs et al., 1997). According to Gronwall, Wrightson, and McGinn (1997), even mild head injuries may have particularly deleterious effects for preschool children.

The effects of time since injury on the outcomes of traumatic brain injury have not been examined as closely as the effects of age at injury. However, longitudinal studies indicate that children generally display a gradual recovery over the first few years after injury, with the most rapid improvement occurring soon after the injury. The initial rate of recovery is often more rapid among children with severe injuries than among those with milder injuries, although severe injuries are also associated with persistent deficits after the rate of recovery slows (Chadwick, Rutter, Brown, et al., 1981). In the nearly complete absence of long-term follow-up studies lasting 5 or more years, we do not know whether children with severe head injuries show any progressive deterioration in functioning relative to noninjured peers after their initial recovery, despite clinical lore suggesting that this can occur. On the other hand, we do know how the rate of recovery varies as a function of factors other than injury severity, including age at injury. More specifically, younger children appear to demonstrate a slower rate of change over time and more significant residual deficits after their recovery plateaus than do older children with injuries of equivalent severity (Anderson & Moore, 1995; Anderson et al., 1997; Ewing-Cobbs et al., 1997).

Of the three age-related dimensions potentially related to injury effects, the influence of age at testing has been the focus of the least research. The effects of age at testing would be reflected in demonstrations of latent or delayed sequelae resulting from children's failure to meet new developmental demands following a head injury. One example of a possible effect of age at testing was the finding by Levin et al. (1988) of greater memory impairment in adolescents than in children following severe closed-head injuries. The investigators interpreted this finding by proposing that adolescents need to use more advanced memory strategies to perform according to normative expectations, and that such strategies are especially vulnerable to traumatic brain injuries. However, we (Yeates, Blumenstein, et al., 1995) did not find memory deficits to be more pronounced among adolescents than among children; hence such age differences require further replication. Undoubtedly, latent effects will be difficult to detect. The demonstration of such effects requires evidence that differences in the consequences of head injuries are due specifically to age at testing, as opposed to age at injury or time since injury, and it is difficult to disentangle these dimensions even in the context of longitudinal research (Taylor & Alden, 1997).

METHODOLOGICAL CRITIQUE OF EXISTING RESEARCH

Sample Selection, Recruitment, and Attrition

Many previous studies on closed-head injury suffer from shortcomings in the selection and recruitment of research participants. Children with closed-head injuries have sometimes been selected retrospectively, often on the basis of admission to a rehabilitation facility or referral for neuropsychological evaluation (e.g., Yeates, Blumenstein, Patterson, & Delis, 1995). Samples selected on this basis are likely to differ in important ways from samples that are recruited prospectively from consecutive admissions to a large hospital or trauma center. The latter method of recruitment is more likely to yield representative groups of children with closed-head injuries.

Even when samples are recruited prospectively from consecutive hospital admissions, they may not be representative of the larger population from which they are drawn, or they may become unrepresentative because of selective attrition over time. The agreement to participate in scientific research is not a random decision, nor is the decision to discontinue participation. However, relatively few studies have compared participants and nonparticipants in terms of either family demographics or child injury characteristics, to determine whether study participation introduces bias into sample selection. Similarly, few studies have compared children who are available to follow-up to those who drop out, to determine whether attrition affects the outcomes studied (Francis, Copeland, & Moore, 1994). Such comparisons are essential, however, if investigators wish to examine the generalizability of their findings.

The selection of comparison groups in research on closed-head injuries has also been problematic. In some cases, children with mild head injuries have been used as a comparison group, despite ongoing controversy regarding the outcomes associated with mild injuries (Satz, Zaucha, McCleary, Light, & Asarnow, 1997; Yeates et al., 1999). In other cases, noninjured children matched for age, gender, and other demographic variables have been used as a comparison group (Jaffe, Polissar, Fay, & Liao, 1995). Noninjured children do not constitute the best comparison group, however, because they are not equated to head-injured children in terms of the experience of a traumatic injury or ensuing medical treatment.

To the extent that traumatic injuries do not occur at random, moreover, noninjured children may also differ from head-injured children in various premorbid characteristics that are not controlled by matching on demographic factors alone. In one of the larger studies of mild head injury, for instance, the neuropsychological test performance of children with mild head injuries was significantly worse than that of children who were matched demographically but were not injured; however, the neuropsychological and behavioral functioning of children with mild head injuries did not differ from that of children with traumatic injuries not involving the head (Asarnow et al., 1995). For those reasons, a comparison group consisting of children who have sustained injuries not involving the head and who have undergone comparable medical treatment is often regarded as most desirable.

Predictors of Outcomes

Injury Characteristics

A substantial amount of the variability in the literature on closed-head injuries is attributable to differences in the characterization of injury severity. Although measures of injury severity are usually correlated, differences in how and when severity is assessed have increased the variability in results across studies. Greater uniformity in the assessment of severity would allow more meaningful cross-study comparisons.

Specific criticisms can be raised about each of the indices of injury severity described earlier. The Glasgow Coma Scale (see Table 5.1) is problematic when used with infants and young children, despite attempts to make suitable modifications (Hahn et al., 1988). The timing of assessment is also of concern when the Glasgow Coma Scale is used, because scores vary over time, and they are not always lowest at the scene of an accident or upon arrival at a hospital. The classification of injuries as mild, moderate, or severe according to this scale can vary, depending on whether decisions regarding injury severity are based on scores obtained at a specific time or on the lowest available scores.

The duration of impaired consciousness can be difficult to assess reliably, because it is often measured retrospectively, based on clinical assessments by nursing staff or physicians. Similarly, in many studies, PTA has been assessed on the basis of retrospective reports from caretakers, such as health care providers or parents. Prospective administration of standardized instruments such as the COAT (Ewing-Cobbs et al., 1990) can provide a much more reliable and objective measure of PTA.

As noted earlier, advances in neuroimaging have also begun to permit the characterization of injury severity based on underlying neuropathology. Previous studies indicate that measures of both diffuse and focal lesions both can contribute to the prediction of outcomes. However, most previous studies of the neuropsychological consequences of closed-head injuries in children have not utilized neuroimaging. In the studies that have done so, the relationship between neuroimaging variables and outcomes has depended on how the neuroimaging data were treated, when they were collected, and what outcomes were assessed (Aldrich et al., 1992; Mendelsohn et al., 1992). Future studies are likely to benefit from the use of measures of underlying neuropathology derived from neuroimaging, but they must also attend to concerns about the timing and method of neuroimaging and the specific outcomes under study.

Non-Injury-Related Factors

The literature on closed-head injuries in children has paid scant attention to the influence of non-injury-related factors on morbidity. The exclusive emphasis on injury-related factors is unfortunate, however, because outcomes such as behavioral adjustment and adaptive functioning are not strongly related to injury severity and may be more dependent on environmental factors (Fletcher et al., 1990; Taylor et al., 1999). Premorbid characteristics of the child or family are often presumed to influence postinjury behavioral adjustment or adaptive functioning, but few studies have addressed the issue directly (Taylor et al., 1995). Similarly, the postinjury family environment is likely to contribute to outcomes following closed-head injuries. Environmental factors may predict outcomes independently of injury severity, or may even exacerbate or buffer the direct effects of injury (Yeates et al., 1997). Thus future research should address the joint effects of injury characteristics and environmental factors on outcomes.

The existing literature can be further criticized for failing to assess the effectiveness of the interventions used to manage closed-head injuries. Although a substantial literature addresses the effects of neurosurgical treatment on mortality, the relationship between acute medical care and neurobehavioral morbidity is unknown, and it is possible that the treatment factors that affect survival are different from those that affect neurobehavioral outcomes. The effectiveness of postacute interventions, such as psychotropic or anticonvulsant medications, rehabilitative and educational programs, and parent education, is also unknown (Fletcher, Ewing-Cobbs, et al., 1995). Thus there is a glaring need for intervention research focusing on childhood closed-head injuries.

Measurement of Outcomes

The outcome measures used in studies of pediatric closed-head injuries often suffer from technical limitations. Most outcome measures can be classified into one of three categories: clinical judgments, psychometric tests, and rating scales and interviews (Fletcher, Ewing-Cobbs, et al., 1995). Clinical judgments, such as those reflected in the Glasgow

Outcome Scale (Jennett & Bond, 1975), often lack sensitivity to more subtle differences in outcomes. Indeed, the outcomes of childhood brain injuries are better than those of adult brain injuries when comparisons are based on the Glasgow Coma Scale (Teasdale & Jennett, 1974). In contrast, psychometric measures reveal similar or even worse outcomes in young children compared to older age groups (Anderson & Moore, 1995; Anderson et al., 1997; Ewing-Cobbs et al., 1997).

Compared to clinical judgments, psychometric tests generally provide more reliable and more sensitive outcome measures. The interpretation of psychometric results is complicated, however, by the multifactorial nature of test performance, which depends on many factors other than the integrity of brain functions (Yeates & Taylor, 1998). Another limitation is that psychometric testing often cannot be used to assess some of the most important outcomes following traumatic brain injuries, including social competence, behavioral adjustment, and adaptive functioning. The latter outcomes are generally assessed via rating scales and interviews. However, many commonly used rating scales, such as the Child Behavior Checklist (Achenbach, 1991), were not developed for use with children with brain injuries and may prove misleading or insensitive when used in that population (Drotar et al., 1995; Perrin et al., 1991).

Another shortcoming is the restricted range of outcomes assessed in studies of childhood head injuries. Outcomes that have been assessed include cognitive functioning, behavioral adjustment, and adaptive functioning. But relatively little attention has been paid to other important outcomes, such as emotional and social functioning (Nassau & Drotar, 1997), family functioning (Taylor et al., 1999), school performance (Kinsella et al., 1995), or quality of life (Klonoff, Costa, & Snow, 1986). Although the literature clearly establishes neurobehavioral morbidity in children with closed-head injuries, future studies are needed to determine the extent to which such morbidity is reflected in broader aspects of the children's daily lives.

Assessment of Recovery

Cross-sectional designs have been employed in most previous studies of traumatic brain injuries in childhood. The use of cross-sectional designs precludes investigation of the process of postinjury recovery of function. Longitudinal studies are needed to examine recovery over time, and to determine the relative importance of age at injury, age at assessment, and time since injury as predictors of outcomes (Taylor & Alden, 1997). Previous longitudinal studies, moreover, have followed children for relatively brief periods. Thus there is a need for prospective, longitudinal investigations that are of much longer duration. The study by Klonoff et al. (1995) represents one of the few attempts to date to follow children who sustained brain injuries into adulthood.

Existing longitudinal studies can also be criticized for failing to adopt a developmental approach in modeling the process of recovery. Traditional approaches to data analysis in longitudinal designs view outcomes as static endpoints. Change is conceptualized as a group phenomenon that is incremental in nature, with individual differences in change treated as error variance. Because development and recovery in children inherently involve change that is continuous and heterogeneous in nature, individual differences in developmental change should represent a major focus in studies of childhood brain injury. Fortunately, the advent of growth curve modeling and related statistical approaches permits the investigation of change (Francis, Fletcher, Steubing, Davidson, & Thompson, 1991). In this approach, intraindividual change is conceptualized in terms of growth curves that quantify the rate of development, changes in that rate over time, and the eventual level of outcome. The role of injury-related and other factors as determinants of recovery from traumatic brain injuries can be studied by analyzing rates of change and levels of outcomes separately for individual children and collectively for groups of children (Thompson et al., 1994; Yeates et al., 1997).

FUTURE DIRECTIONS

The preceding critique indicates a number of potential avenues for future research on childhood head injuries. For instance, studies are needed of outcomes in domains other than cognitive and behavioral functioning. Of particular importance will be studies examining children's general adaptation to their environment. At this time, we know very little about the implications of closed-head injuries for school placement, health care utilization, or overall quality of life. Studies are also needed that examine the link between neuropsychological abilities and these more functional outcomes, to determine the ecological validity of neuropsychological assessment in childhood head injury.

Research regarding the neural substrates of the neuropsychological deficits that occur in childhood head injury is needed as well. Studies that capitalize on advances in neuroimaging to measure underlying neuropathology, and that correlates these measures with neuropsychological functioning, will enhance our understanding of the predictors and outcomes of closed-head injuries. Such research will also provide more general insights into the nature of brain–behavior relationships in children. Moreover, the use of neuroimaging in studies of children with mild head injuries could help to resolve controversies regarding the long-term consequences of such injuries (Bijur & Haslum, 1995; Asarnow et al., 1995).

Studies of brain–behavior relationships following closed-head injuries cannot be conducted without also considering a child's family and social environment as a predictor of outcomes. Recent studies have clearly demonstrated that measures of the family and social environment are related to both cognitive and behavioral functioning following closed-head injuries, and that environmental factors often act in concert with injury-related factors to determine eventual outcomes (Taylor et al., 1995, 1999; Yeates et al., 1997). Future research is needed to clarify which aspects of the environment influence which outcomes, and to delineate the mechanisms by which the environment affects children's functioning.

Finally, future research efforts must incorporate a developmental perspective that reflects the complex interplay of age-related factors when neurobehavioral outcomes are being assessed. Studies are needed that follow children for extended periods of time after injury, and preferably into adulthood. Prospective, longitudinal studies that follow children over a period of years will allow us to move beyond the characterization of group differences in outcomes toward a better understanding of individual recovery and the influences on this process. In so doing, future studies will provide a more thorough understanding of the variability in outcomes among children with closed-head injuries.

REFERENCES

Achenbach, T. M. (1991). *Integrative guide for the 1991 CBCL/4–18, YSR, and TRF profiles.* Burlington: University of Vermont, Department of Psychiatry.

Aldrich, E. F., Eisenberg, H. M., Saydjari, C., Luerssen, T. G., Foulkes, M. A., Jane, J. A., Marshall, L. F., Marmarou, A., & Young, H. F. (1992). Diffuse brain swelling in severely head-injured children: A report from the NIH Traumatic Coma Data Bank. *Journal of Neurosurgery, 76,* 450–454.

Anderson, V., & Moore, C. (1995). Age at injury as a predictor of outcome following pediatric head injury: A longitudinal perspective. *Child Neuropsychology, 1,* 187–202.

Anderson, V. A., Morse, S. A., Klug, G., Catroppa, C., Haritou, F., Rosenfeld, J., & Pentland, L. (1997). Predicting recovery from head injury in young children: A prospective analysis. *Journal of the International Neuropsychological Society, 3,* 568–580.

Annegers, J. F., Grabow, J. D., Kurland, L. T., & Laws, E. R. (1980). The incidence, causes, and secular trends of head trauma in Olmsted County, Minnesota, 1935–1974. *Neurology, 30,* 912–919.

Arffa, S. (1998). Traumatic brain injury. In C. E. Coffey & R. A. Brumback (Eds.), *Textbook of pediatric neuropsychiatry* (pp. 1093–1140). Washington, DC: American Psychiatric Association.

Asarnow, R. F., Satz, P., Light, R., Zaucha, K., Lewis, R., & McCleary, C. (1995). The UCLA study of mild closed head injuries in children and adolescents. In S. H. Broman & M. E. Michel (Eds.), *Traumatic head injury in children* (pp. 117–146). New York: Oxford University Press.

Baron, I. S., Fennell, E. B., & Voeller, E. B. (1995). *Pediatric neuropsychology in the medical setting.* New York: Oxford University Press.

Barry, C. T., Taylor, H. G., Klein, S., & Yeates, K. O. (1996). Validity of neurobehavioral symptoms reported in children with traumatic brain injury. *Child Neuropsychology, 2,* 213–226.

Bassett, S. S., & Slater, E. J. (1990). Neuropsychological function in adolescents sustained mild closed head injury. *Journal of Pediatric Psychology, 15,* 225–236.

Bawden, H. N., Knights, R. M., & Winogron, H. W. (1985). Speeded performance following head injury in children. *Journal of Clinical Neuropsychology, 7,* 39–54.

Berger-Gross, P., & Schackelford, M. (1985). Closed head injury in children: Neuropsychological and scholastic outcome. *Perceptual and Motor Skills, 61,* 254.

Bigler, E. D. (1997). Brain imaging and behavioral outcome in traumatic brain injury. In E. D. Bigler, E. Clark, & J. E. Farmer (Eds.), *Childhood traumatic brain injury: Diagnosis, assessment, and intervention* (pp. 7–32). Austin, TX: PRO-ED.

Bijur, P. E., & Haslum, M. (1995). Cognitive, behavioral, and motoric sequelae of mild head injury in a national birth cohort. In S. H. Broman & M. E. Michel (Eds.), *Traumatic head injury in children* (pp. 147–164). New York: Oxford University Press.

Brown, G., Chadwick, O., Shaffer, D., Rutter, M., & Traub, M. (1981). A prospective study of children with head injuries: III. Psychiatric sequelae. *Psychological Medicine, 11,* 63–78.

Bruce, D. A. (1995). Pathophysiological responses of the child's brain. In S. H. Broman & M. E. Michel (Eds.), *Traumatic head injury in children* (pp. 40–51). New York: Oxford University Press.

Bruce, D. A., Alavi, A., Bilaniuk, L., Dolinskas, C., Obrist, W., & Uzzell, B. (1981). Diffuse brain swelling following head injury in children: The syndrome of "malignant brain edema." *Journal of Neurosurgery, 54,* 170–178.

Bruce, D. A., Raphaely, R. C., Goldberg, A. I., Zimmerman, R. A., Bilaniuk, L. T., Schut, L., & Kuhl, D. E. (1979). Pathophysiology, treatment, and outcome following severe head injury in children. *Child's Brain, 2,* 174–191.

Cardoso, E. R., & Galbraith, S. (1985). Posttraumatic hydrocephalus: A retrospective review. *Surgical Neurology, 23,* 261–264.

Chadwick, O., Rutter, M., Brown, G., Shaffer, D., & Traub, M. (1981). A prospective study of children with head injuries: II. Cognitive sequelae. *Psychological Medicine, 11,* 49–61.

Chadwick, O., Rutter, M., Shaffer, D., & Shrout, M. (1981). A prospective study of children with head injuries: IV. Specific cognitive deficits. *Journal of Clinical Neuropsychology, 3,* 101–120.

Chapman, S. B. (1995). Discourse as an outcome measure in pediatric head-injured populations. In S. H. Broman & M. E. Michel (Eds.), *Traumatic head injury in children* (pp. 95–116). New York: Oxford University Press.

Cooley, E. L., & Morris, R. D. (1990). Attention in children: A neuropsychologically based model for assessment. *Developmental Neuropsychology, 8,* 219–228.

Costeff, H., Abraham, E., Brenner, T., Horowitz, I., Apter, N., Sadan, N., & Najenson, T. (1988). Late neuropsychologic status after childhood head trauma. *Brain Development, 10,* 371–374.

Cummings, J. L. (1993). Frontal–subcortical circuits and human behavior. *Archives of Neurology, 50,* 873–880.

Denckla, M. B. (1994). Measurement of executive function. In G. R. Lyon (Ed.), *Frames of reference for the assessment of learning disabilities* (pp. 117–142). Baltimore: Paul H. Brookes.

Dennis, M., & Barnes, M. A. (1990). Knowing the meaning, getting the point, bridging the gap, and carrying the message: Aspects of discourse following closed head injury in childhood and adolescence. *Brain and Language, 39,* 428–446.

Dennis, M., Barnes, M. A., Donnelly, R. E., Wilkinson, M., & Humphreys, R. P. (1996). Appraising and managing knowledge: Metacognitive skills after childhood head injury. *Developmental Neuropsychology*, *12*, 77–103.

Dennis, M., Wilkinson, M., Koski, L., & Humphreys, R. P. (1995). Attention deficits in the long term after childhood head injury. In S. H. Broman & M. E. Michel (Eds.), *Traumatic head injury in children* (pp. 165–187). New York: Oxford University Press.

Donders, J. (1993). Memory functioning after traumatic brain injury in children. *Brain Injury*, *7*, 431–437.

Drotar, D., Stein, R. E. K., & Perrin, E. C. (1995). Methodological issues in using the Child Behavior Checklist and its related instruments in clinical child psychology research. *Journal of Clinical Child Psychology*, *24*, 184–192.

Ewing-Cobbs, L., Fletcher, J. M., Levin, H. S., Francis, D. J., Davidson, K., & Miner, M. E. (1997). Longitudinal neuropsychological outcome in infants and preschoolers with traumatic brain injury. *Journal of the International Neuropsychological Society*, *3*, 581–591.

Ewing-Cobbs, L., Fletcher, J. M., Levin, H. S., Hastings, P. Z., & Francis, D. J. (1996). Assessment of injury severity following closed head injury in children: Methodological issues. *Journal of the International Neuropsychological Society*, *2*, 39.

Ewing-Cobbs, L., Levin, H. S., Eisenberg, H. M., & Fletcher, J. M. (1987). Language functions following closed-head injury in children and adolescents. *Journal of Clinical and Experimental Neuropsychology*, *9*, 575–592.

Ewing-Cobbs, L., Levin, H. S., Fletcher, J. M., Miner, M. E., & Eisenberg, H. M. (1990). The Children's Orientation and Amnesia Test: Relationship to severity of acute head injury and to recovery of memory. *Neurosurgery*, *27*, 683–691.

Filley, C. M., Cranberg, L. D., Alexander, M. E., & Hart, E. J. (1987). Neurobehavioral outcome after closed head injury in childhood and adolescence. *Archives of Neurology*, *44*, 194–198.

Fletcher, J. M., Ewing-Cobbs, L., Francis, D. J., & Levin, H. S. (1995). Variability in outcomes after traumatic brain injury in children: A developmental perspective. In S. H. Broman & M. E. Michel (Eds.), *Traumatic head injury in children* (pp. 3–21). New York: Oxford University Press.

Fletcher, J. M., Ewing-Cobbs, L., Miner, M. E., Levin, H. S., & Eisenberg, H. M. (1990). Behavioral changes after closed head injury in children. *Journal of Consulting and Clinical Psychology*, *58*, 93–98.

Fletcher, J. M., & Levin, H. S. (1988). Neurobehavioral effects of brain injury in children. In D. K. Routh (Ed.), *Handbook of pediatric psychology* (pp. 258–295). New York: Guilford Press.

Fletcher, J. M., Levin, H. S., & Butler, I. J. (1995). Neurobehavioral effects of brain injury in children: Hydrocephalus, traumatic brain injury, and cerebral palsy. In M. C. Roberts (Ed.), *Handbook of pediatric psychology* (2nd ed., pp. 362–383). New York: Guilford Press.

Fletcher, J. M., Levin, H. S., Lachar, D., Kusnerik, L., Harward, H., Mendelsohn, D., & Lilly, M. A. (1996). Behavioral outcomes after pediatric closed head injury: Relationship with age, severity, and lesion size. *Journal of Child Neurology*, *11*, 283–290.

Francis, D. J., Copeland, D. R., & Moore, B. D. (1994). Neuropsychological changes in children with cancer: The treatment of missing data in longitudinal studies. *Neuropsychology Review*, *4*, 199–222.

Francis, D. J., Fletcher, J. M., Stuebing, K. K., Davidson, K. C., & Thompson, N. M. (1991). Analysis of change: Modeling individual growth. *Journal of Consulting and Clinical Psychology*, *59*, 27–37.

Goldstein, F. C., & Levin, H. S. (1987). Epidemiology of pediatric closed-head injury: Incidence, clinical characteristics, and risk factors. *Journal of Learning Disabilities*, *20*, 518–525.

Gronwall, D., Wrightson, P., & McGinn, V. (1997). Effect of mild head injury during the preschool years. *Journal of the International Neuropsychological Society*, *3*, 592–597.

Hahn, Y. S., Chyung, C., Barthel, M. J., Bailes, J., Flannery, A., & McLone, D. G. (1988). Head injuries in children under 36 months of age. *Child's Nervous System*, *4*, 34–40.

Jaffe, K. M., Polissar, N. L., Fay, G. C., & Liao, S. (1995). Recovery trends over three years following pediatric traumatic brain injury. *Archives of Physical Medicine and Rehabilitation*, *76*, 17–26.

Jennett, B., & Bond, M. (1975). Assessment of outcome after severe brain damage: A practical scale. *Lancet*, *i*, 480–484.

Kaufmann, P. M., Fletcher, J. M., Levin, H. S., Miner, M. E., & Ewing-Cobbs, L. (1993). Attentional disturbance after closed head injury. *Journal of Child Neurology*, *8*, 348–353.

Kinsella, G., Prior, M., Sawyer, M., Murtagh, D., Eisenmajer, R., Anderson, V., Bryan, D., & Klug, G. (1995). Neuropsychological deficit and academic performance in children and adolescents following traumatic brain injury. *Journal of Pediatric Psychology*, *20*, 753–767.

Klauber, M. R., Barrett-Connor, E., Hofstetter, C. R., & Micik, S. H. (1986). A population-based study of nonfatal childhood injuries. *Preventive Medicine*, *15*, 139–149.

Klonoff, H., Clark, C., & Klonoff, P. S. (1995). Outcomes of head injuries from childhood to adulthood: A twenty-three year follow-up study. In S. H. Broman & M. E. Michel (Eds.), *Traumatic head injury in children* (pp. 219–234). New York: Oxford University Press.

Klonoff, H., Low, M. D., & Clark, C. (1977). Head injuries in children: A prospective five year follow-up. *Journal of Neurology, Neurosurgery and Psychiatry, 40,* 1211–1219.

Klonoff, P. S., Costa, L. D., & Snow, W. G. (1986). Predictors and indicators of quality of life in patients with closed-head injury. *Journal of Clinical and Experimental Neuropsychology, 8,* 469–485.

Koelfen, W., Freund, M., Dinter, D., Schmidt, B., Koenig, S., & Schultze, C. (1997). Long-term follow up of children with head injuries classified as "good recovery" using the Glasgow Outcome Scale: Neurological, neuropsychological, and magnetic resonance imaging results. *European Journal of Pediatrics, 156,* 230–235.

Knights, R. M., Ivan, L. P., Ventureyra, E. C. G., Bentivoglio, C., Stoddart, C., Winogron, W., & Bawden, H. N. (1991). The effects of head injury in children on neuropsychological and behavioural functioning. *Brain Injury, 5,* 339–351.

Kraus, J. F. (1995). Epidemiological features of brain injury in children: Occurrence, children at risk, causes and manner of injury, severity, and outcomes. In S. H. Broman & M. E. Michel (Eds.), *Traumatic head injury in children* (pp. 22–39). New York: Oxford University Press.

Kraus, J. F., Fife, D., Cox, P., Ramstein, K., & Conroy, C. (1986). Incidence, severity, and external causes of pediatric brain injury. *American Journal of Diseases of Children, 140,* 687–693.

Kraus, J. F., Rock, A., & Hamyari, P. (1990). Brain injuries among infants, children, adolescents, and young adults. *American Journal of Diseases of Children, 144,* 684–691.

Lang, D. A., Teasdale, G. M., Macpherson, P., & Lawrence, A. (1994). Diffuse brain swelling after head injury: More often malignant in adults than children? *Journal of Neurosurgery, 80,* 675–680.

Lescohier, I., & DiScala, C. (1993). Blunt trauma in children: Causes and outcomes of head versus intracranial injury. *Pediatrics, 91,* 721–725.

Levin, H. S., Amparo, E. G., Eisenberg, H. M., Miner, M. E., High, W. M., Ewing-Cobbs, L., Fletcher, J. M., & Guinto, F. C., Jr. (1989). Magnetic resonance imaging after closed head injury in children. *Neurosurgery, 24,* 223–227.

Levin, H. S., Culhane, K. A., Mendelsohn, D., Lilly, M. A., Bruce, D., Fletcher, J. M., Chapman, S. B., Harward, H., & Eisenberg, H. M. (1993). Cognition in relation to magnetic resonance imaging in head-injured children and adolescents. *Archives of Neurology, 50,* 897–905.

Levin, H. S., & Eisenberg, H. M. (1979). Neuropsychological impairment after closed head injury in children and adolescents. *Journal of Pediatric Psychology, 4,* 389–402.

Levin, H. S., Eisenberg, H. M., Wigg, N. R., & Kobayashi, K. (1982). Memory and intellectual ability after head injury in children and adolescents. *Neurosurgery, 11,* 668–673.

Levin, H. S., Ewing-Cobbs, L., & Eisenberg, H. M. (1995). Neurobehavioral outcome of pediatric closed-head injury. In S. H. Broman & M. E. Michel (Eds.), *Traumatic head injury in children* (pp. 70–94). New York: Oxford University Press.

Levin, H. S., High, W. M., Ewing-Cobbs, L., Fletcher, J. M., Eisenberg, H. M., Miner, M. E., & Goldstein, F. C. (1988). Memory functioning during the first year after closed head injury in children and adolescents. *Neurosurgery, 22,* 1043–1052.

Levin, H. S., Madison, C. F., Bailey, C. B., Meyers, C. A., Eisenberg, H. M., & Guinto, F. C. (1983). Mutism after closed head injury. *Archives of Neurology, 40,* 601–606.

Levin, H. S., Mendelsohn, D., Lilly, M. A., Fletcher, J. M., Culhane, K. A., Chapman, S. B., Harward, K., Kusnerik, L., Bruce, D., & Eisenberg, H. M. (1994). Tower of London performance in relation to magnetic resonance imaging following closed head injury in children. *Neuropsychology, 8,* 171–179.

Levin, H. S., Song, J., Scheibel, R. S., Fletcher, J. M., Harward, H., Lilly, M., & Goldstein, F. (1997). Concept formation and problem solving following closed head injury in children. *Journal of the International Neuropsychological Society, 3,* 598–607.

Light, R., Asarnow, A., Satz, P., Zaucha, K., McCleary, C., & Lewis, R. (1998). Mild closed-head injury in children and adolescents: Behavior problems and academic outcomes. *Journal of Consulting and Clinical Psychology, 66,* 1023–1029.

Luerssen, T. G., Klauber, M. R., & Marshall, L. F. (1988). Outcome from head injury related to patient's age: A longitudinal prospective study of adult and pediatric head injury. *Journal of Neurosurgery, 68,* 409–416.

Max, J. E., Lindgren, S. D., Robin, D. A., Smith, W. L., Sato, Y., Mattheis, P. J., Castillo, C. S., & Stierwalt, J. A. G. (1997). Traumatic brain injury in children and adolescents: Psychiatric disorders in the second three months. *Journal of Nervous and Mental Disease, 185,* 394–401.

Max, J. E., Robin, D. A., Lindgren, S. D., Smith, W. L., Sato, Y., Mattheis, P. J., Stierwalt, J. A. G., & Castillo, C. S. (1997). Traumatic brain injury in children and adolescents: Psychiatric disorders at two years. *Journal of the American Academy of Child and Adolescent Psychiatry, 36,* 1278–1285.

Max, J. E., Smith, W. L., Sato, Y., Mattheis, P. J., Castillo, C. S., Lindgren, S. D., Robin, D. A., & Stierwalt, J. A. G. (1997). Traumatic brain injury in children and adolescents: Psychiatric disorders in the first three months. *Journal of the American Academy of Child and Adolescent Psychiatry, 36,* 94–102.

McDonald, C. M., Jaffe, K. M., Fay, G. C., Polissar, N. L., Martin, K. M., Liao, S., & Rivara, J. B. (1994). Comparison of indices of traumatic brain injury severity as predictors of neurobehavioral outcomes in children. *Archives of Physical Medicine and Rehabilitation, 75,* 328–337.

McLean, D. E., Kaitz, E. S., Kennan, C. J., Dabney, K., Cawley, M. F., & Alexander, M. A. (1995). Medical and surgical complications of pediatric brain injury. *Journal of Head Trauma Rehabilitation, 10,* 1–12.

Mendelsohn, D., Levin, H. S., Bruce, D., Lilly, M., Harward, H., Culhane, K. A., & Eisenberg, H. M. (1992). Late MRI after head injury in children: Relationship to clinical features and outcome. *Child's Nervous System, 8,* 445–452.

Mirsky, A. F., Anthony, B. J., Duncan, C. C., Ahearn, M. B., & Kellam, S. G. (1991). Analysis of the elements of attention: A neuropsychological approach. *Neuropsychology Review, 2,* 109–145.

Nassau, J. H., & Drotar, D. (1997). Social competence among children with central nervous system-related chronic health conditions: A review. *Journal of Pediatric Psychology, 22,* 771–793.

Nelson, C. A. (1995). The ontogeny of human memory: A cognitive neuroscience perspective. *Developmental Psychology, 31,* 723–738.

Novack, T. A., Dillon, M. C., & Jackson, W. T. (1996). Neurochemical mechanisms in brain injury and treatment: A review. *Journal of Clinical and Experimental Neuropsychology, 18,* 685–706.

Oddy, M. (1993). Head injury during childhood. *Neuropsychological Rehabilitation, 3,* 301–320.

Pang, D. (1985). Pathophysiologic correlates of neurobehavioral syndromes following closed head injury. In M. Ylvisaker (Ed.), *Head injury rehabilitation: Children and adolescents* (pp. 3–70). San Diego, CA: College-Hill Press.

Perrin, E. C., Stein, R. E., & Drotar, D. (1991). Cautions in using the Child Behavior Checklist: Observations based on research about children with a chronic illness. *Journal of Pediatric Psychology, 16,* 411–421.

Povlishock, J. T., Erb, D. E., & Astruc, J. (1992). Axonal response to traumatic brain injury: Reactive axonal change, deafferentation, and neuroplasticity. *Journal of Neurotrauma, 9*(Suppl. 1), S189–S200.

Roman, M. J., Delis, D. C., Willerman, L., Magulac, M., Demadura, T. L., de la Peña, J. L., Loftis, C., Walsh, J., & Kracun, M. (1998). Impact of pediatric traumatic brain injury on components of verbal memory. *Journal of Clinical and Experimental Neuropsychology, 20,* 245–258.

Satz, P., Zaucha, K., McCleary, C., Light, R., & Asarnow, R. (1997). Mild head injury in children and adolescents: A review of studies (1970–1995). *Psychological Bulletin, 122,* 107–131.

Schacter, D. L. (1987). Implicit memory: History and current status. Journal of *Experimental Psychology: Learning, Memory, and Cognition, 13,* 501–518.

Shaffer, D. (1995). Behavioral sequelae of serious head injury in children and adolescents: The British studies. In S. H. Broman & M. E. Michel (Eds.), *Traumatic head injury in children* (pp. 55–69). New York: Oxford University Press.

Sparrow, S. S., Balla, D. A., & Cicchetti, D. V. (1984). *Vineland Adaptive Behavior Scales: Survey form manual.* Circle Pines, MN: American Guidance Service.

Stallings, G. A., Ewing-Cobbs, L., Francis, D. J., & Fletcher, J. M. (1996). Prediction of academic placement after pediatric head injury using neurological, demographic, and neuropsychological variables. *Journal of the International Neuropsychological Society, 2,* 39.

Taylor, H. G., & Alden, J. (1997). Age-related differences in outcome following childhood brain injury: An introduction and overview. *Journal of the International Neuropsychological Society, 3,* 555–567.

Taylor, H. G., Drotar, D., Wade, S., Yeates, K. O., Stancin, T., & Klein, S. (1995). Recovery from traumatic brain injury in children: The importance of the family. In S. H. Broman & M. E. Michel (Eds.), *Traumatic head injury in children* (pp. 188–218). New York: Oxford University Press.

Taylor, H. G., Yeates, K. O., Wade, S. L., Drotar, D., Klein, S. K., & Stancin, T. (1999). Influences in first-year recovery from traumatic brain injury in children. *Neuropsychology, 13,* 76–89.

Teasdale, G., & Jennett, B. (1974). Assessment of coma and impaired consciousness: A practical scale. *Lancet, ii,* 81–84.

Thompson, N. M., Francis, D. J., Stuebing, K. K., Fletcher, J. M., Ewing-Cobbs, L., Miner, M. E., Levin, H. S., & Eisenberg, H. (1994). Motor, visual–spatial, and somatosensory skills after closed-head injury in children and adolescents: A study of change. *Neuropsychology, 8,* 333–342.

Vakil, E., Jaffe, R., Eluze, S., Groswasser, Z., & Aberbuch, S. (1996). Word recall versus reading speed: Evidence of preserved priming in head-injured patients. *Brain and Cognition, 31,* 75–89.

Winogron, H. W., Knights, R. M., & Bawden, H. N. (1984). Neuropsychological deficits following head injury in children. *Journal of Clinical Neuropsychology, 6,* 269–286.

Yeates, K. O., Blumenstein, E., Patterson, C. M., & Delis, D. C. (1995). Verbal learning and memory following pediatric closed-head injury. *Journal of the International Neuropsychological Society, 1,* 78–87.

Yeates, K. O., Luria, J., Bartkowski, H., Rusin, J., Martin, L., & Bigler, E. D. (1999). Post-concussive symptoms in children with mild closed-head injuries. *Journal of Head Trauma Rehabilitation, 14,* 337–350.

Yeates, K. O., Patterson, C. M., Waber, D. M., & Bernstein, J. H. (1993). Constructional and figural memory skills following pediatric closed-head injury. *Journal of Clinical and Experimental Neuropsychology, 15,* 58.

Yeates, K. O., Ris, M. D., & Taylor, H. G. (1995). Hospital referral patterns in pediatric neuropsychology. *Child Neuropsychology, 1,* 56–62.

Yeates, K. O., & Taylor, H. G. (1998). Neuropsychological assessment of older children. In G. Goldstein, A. Puente, & E. Bigler (Eds.), *Human brain function, assessment and rehabilitation: Vol. 3. Neuropsychology* (pp. 35–61). New York: Plenum Press.

Yeates, K. O., Taylor, H. G., Drotar, D., Wade, S., Klein, S., & Stancin, T. (1997). Premorbid family environment as a predictor of neurobehavioral outcomes following pediatric traumatic brain injury. *Journal of the International Neuropsychological Society, 3,* 617–630.

6

MENINGITIS

VICKI A. ANDERSON
H. GERRY TAYLOR

Meningitis is a relatively common and potentially life-threatening infectious disease involving inflammation of the meningeal membranes surrounding the brain. Incidence rates peak in infancy and decline progressively over the early childhood years (Davies & Rudd, 1994; Feigin, 1992). Mortality rates for bacterial meningitis range widely, depending in part on the specific pathogen. Davies and Rudd (1994) reported a mortality rate of 3.5% for meningococcal meningitis, 7.7% for *Haemophilus influenzae* type b (Hib) meningitis, and 30% for pneumococcal meningitis. Similar rates are reported by other investigators (Dodge, 1986; Smith, 1988). Mortality rates associated with group B *Streptococcus* infections, the most common form of neonatal meningitis, fall in the range of 17–27% (Edwards et al., 1985; Wald et al., 1986), consistent with the rates reported for tuberculous meningitis (Schoeman, 1990). Although viral meningitis—caused primarily by enteroviruses—is more common than bacterial meningitis, bacterial disease is more likely to result in death or disability (Cherry, 1992; Claesson, Trollfors, Jodol, & Rosenhall, 1984; Davies, 1989; Davies & Rudd, 1994; Dodge et al., 1984; Feldman et al., 1982; Jadavji, Biggar, Gold, & Prober, 1986; Klein, Feigin, & McCracken, 1986; Lindberg, Rosenhall, Nylen, & Ringner, 1977; Sell, 1983; Sproles, Azerrad, Williamson, & Merrill, 1972). Because of the substantial literature on bacterial meningitis and the greater likelihood that survivors will require assessment and management for neuropsychological impairments, the present chapter focuses largely on these forms of disease.

Prior to the advent of antibiotics, more than 90% of children who contracted bacterial meningitis did not survive the acute illness; as a result, there was relatively little interest in morbidity. Antibiotic treatments, introduced in the 1950s, led to a dramatic increase in survival. More recently, immunizations have been developed for Hib meningitis—previously the most common form of the disease. Vaccines for this type of meningitis have resulted in considerable reductions in disease incidence, at least in regions where the vaccines are readily available (Adams et al., 1993; Peltola, Kilpi, & Antilla, 1992).

Findings from studies conducted with prevaccine samples document neurological sequelae in approximately 20–30% of survivors. These sequelae include sensory-neural hearing loss and other cranial nerve dysfunctions, seizure disorders, hemiplegia, ataxia, and visual problems (Adams et al., 1993; Claesson et al., 1984; Dodge et al., 1984; Feldman et al., 1982; Jadavji et al., 1986; Klein et al., 1986; Lindberg et al., 1977; Sell, 1983; Sproles et al., 1972; Taylor, Schatschneider, & Rich, 1992). In the findings from prevaccine investigations, disease morbidity with respect to cognitive, linguistic, and educational outcomes is somewhat less clear. Whereas some researchers have documented pervasive impairments in cognitive functions and academic achievement in postmeningitis samples (Kresky, Buchbinder, & Greenberg, 1962; Sell, Merrill, Doyne, & Zimsky, 1972; Sell, Webb, Pate, & Doyne, 1972; Sproles et al., 1972), other reports have stressed a generally favorable disease prognosis (Emmett, Jeffery, Chandler, & Dugdale, 1980; Feldman & Michaels, 1988; Moss, 1982; Taylor et al., 1990; Tejani, Dobias, & Sambursky, 1982). Unfortunately, subtle deficits in visual–motor coordination, auditory perception, and higher cognitive functions may occur but escape detection in early childhood. As a result, children suffering from bacterial meningitis may be discharged from follow-up before problems become evident.

Despite the success of vaccines in reducing rates of Hib meningitis, immunizations are not yet available for other forms of bacterial meningitis. For this reason, there is a continued need to study disease sequelae. Appreciation of disease consequences is also relevant in following individuals who contracted Hib meningitis prior to the development of the vaccine, or who have not been successfully immunized. A further reason for continued interest in the sequelae of bacterial meningitis is the opportunity this disease provides for study of the effects of neurological insults incurred at a young age, and in children who are neurologically normal prior to disease onset. Follow-up of disease survivors allows researchers to test hypotheses regarding early neural plasticity, to study the relative contributions of organic and environmental influences on outcomes, and to explore the significance of transient neurological abnormalities for later development (Taylor et al., 1992). In light of the relative immaturity of the central nervous system (CNS) at the time of this disease, consequences may differ substantially from expectations based on adult models of recovery of function, even in cases without permanent neurological residua (Dennis & Barnes, 1994; Rutter, 1981). In contrast to adults, young children are in the process of developing many of their fundamental cognitive skills. Because the effects of brain lesions on developing abilities may be quite different from their effects on already acquired skills, patterns of impairment are likely to be unique to children (Dennis, 1988; Rourke, 1988; Taylor, 1984). Child-specific deficits have been observed in various other pediatric disorders, including head injury, hydrocephalus, cyanotic heart disease, and cranial irradiation (Anderson & Moore, 1995; Anderson, Smibert, Ekert, & Godber, 1994; Ewing-Cobbs, Miner, Fletcher, & Levin, 1989; Kriel, Krach, & Panser, 1989; Wright & Nolan, 1994). There is every reason to believe that the consequences of bacterial meningitis in children are similarly unique, and that disease sequelae have implications for processes of normal development (Dennis & Barnes, 1994).

EPIDEMIOLOGY

In the prevaccine era, 30–70 children under age 5 per 100,000 contracted bacterial meningitis annually (Feigin, 1992; Sell, 1987). Some groups have been noted to be at greater risk, with the incidence for Native Americans and for Australian aborigines cited to be up to 10 times as great as that reported for the general population (D'Angio et al., 1995; Hanna, 1990; Takala & Clements, 1992; Ward et al., 1981). Although the infection may be contracted at any age, the majority of cases occur prior to age 5. Young age continues to be the most important risk factor for this illness, with deficiencies of the immature immune system contributing to the higher rates of disease in young children. Takala and Clements (1992) suggest that psychosocial factors also increase the risk for contracting bacterial meningitis in childhood. They argue that different levels of exposure to infection, related to greater utilization of child care, may be associated with the current age distribution of this disease in the population. The presence of siblings of elementary school age or younger within the family unit is a further risk factor; the likelihood of infection doubles with each additional sibling. Constitutional risks, such as a smoker in the household, have also been identified. Breast feeding appears to be a protective factor. The incidence of meningitis in children who are breast-fed for at least 6 months, for example, is lower than that for infants who are breast-fed for shorter periods or not at all. Most studies report a slightly higher disease frequency in males (Broome, 1987; Schlech et al., 1985; Washburn, Medearis, & Childs, 1965). There is also evidence for some seasonal variation, with more cases presenting in the winter months compared to other times of the year. Hore (1992) notes that whereas the seasonal distribution of other common forms of bacterial meningitis remains relatively stable, Hib is more common in winter months.

Hib, *Neisseria meningitidis*, and *Streptococcus pneumoniae* together account for about 95% of all cases reported (Feigin, 1992). Hib meningitis is most commonly contracted between 1 month and 4 years of age, and is relatively uncommon in older children and adults. Prior to the advent of effective vaccines for children under the age of 2, this form of meningitis accounted for 70–75% of all cases in this age bracket. In contrast, there are several neonatal pathogens. Group B *Streptococcus* and *Escherichia coli* are the most common causes of meningitis in this age group (Davies & Rudd, 1994; Mustafa & McCracken, 1992). After age 5, *Neisseria meningitidis* accounts for the majority of cases of childhood meningitis (Wenger et al., 1990). Figure 6.1 provides an illustration of the relative frequency of various pathogens causing bacterial meningitis at different ages.

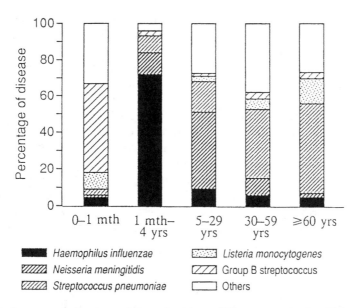

FIGURE 6.1. Pathogens causing bacterial meningitis at different ages in five U.S. states and Los Angeles County during 1986. From Wenger et al. (1990). Copyright 1990 by The University of Chicago Press. Reprinted by permission.

As noted earlier, the currently available vaccines for Hib meningitis, introduced in the mid-1980s, have reduced the rates of bacterial meningitis in countries with vaccine programs (Adams et al., 1993; Clements & Gilbert, 1990; Weinberg, Murphy, & Granoff, 1990). These vaccines are virtually free of side effects. One of the larger-scale controlled studies of vaccine efficacy was conducted in Helsinki, Finland, and its environs (Peltola et al., 1992). Initially, in 1986–1987, 50% of infants in this region were vaccinated at 3–6 months of age and again at 14–18 months. All infants received vaccinations beginning in 1989. Although the specific vaccines administered varied over time, the rate of cases admitted to hospitals with Hib meningitis dropped from 30 in 1986 to 0 in 1991. Similarly, a study in King County (the Seattle, Washington, area) found that the frequency of Hib meningitis had fallen by two-thirds from 1985 to 1990 (Anonymous, 1990). A surveillance project by the U.S. Centers for Disease Control identified 176 cases of Hib meningitis in children under 5 years of age in 1989, compared to only 50 cases in 1991 (Marwick, 1991). Cases of Hib meningitis in communities with access to vaccines appear to occur in children who are not immunized or who contract the disease prior to 2 months of age, which is the age at which children routinely receive the initial vaccination (Feigin, McCracken, & Klein, 1992).

DIAGNOSIS AND TREATMENT

Presenting Features

Researchers report a variety of presenting clinical symptoms associated with bacterial meningitis in childhood. Initial diagnosis is often difficult due to a child's age, the high frequency of preexisting infectious illness (e.g., sinusitis, otitis media), and the fact that many of the presenting symptoms (e.g., high temperature and irritability) are not specific to meningitis. Klein and Marcy (1990), in a meta-analysis of seven studies involving 225 cases of childhood meningitis, identified several common presenting symptoms: hyperthermia in 61% of cases, lethargy in 50%, anorexia or vomiting in 49%, respiratory distress in 47%, convulsions in 40%, irritability in 32%, jaundice in 28%, bulging fontanelle in 28%, diarrhea in 17%, and nuchal rigidity in 15%. Other symptoms include coma, focal neurological signs (e.g., hemiparesis), altered conscious state, raised intracranial pressure, hypotension, intracranial bleeding, and electrolyte imbalance.

The rates of various acute-phase neurological complications found in two recent studies we and our colleagues conducted (Grimwood et al., 1995; Taylor et al., 1992) are presented in Table 6.1. Both studies involved relatively large samples of school-age children who were assessed several years following recovery. The sample recruited in the Grimwood et al. (1995) study included children who had recovered from all major forms of bacterial meningitis, whereas the sample followed in the Taylor et al. (1992) study was restricted to cases of Hib meningitis. Data presented in Table 6.1, which are also comparable to figures reported by Feigin et al. (1976), show that acute neurological complications are pervasive and similar in frequency across different samples.

Diagnosis

Symptom presentation in bacterial meningitis usually follows one of two patterns. The most common pattern involves a progressive development of symptoms over several days, frequently preceded by a nonspecific febrile illness. In these cases diagnosis is often difficult,

TABLE 6.1. Acute-Phase Neurological Complications Associated with Bacterial Meningitis in Two Studies

	Taylor et al. (1992)	Grimwood et al. (1995)
Total sample	127	130
Seizures	30 (24)	41 (31)
Obtundation/coma	16 (13)	23 (18)
Hemiparesis	8 (6)	12 (9)
Sensory-neural hearing loss	15 (12)	8 (6)
Cortical blindness	1 (1)	3 (2)
Ataxia	3 (2)	9 (6)
Hydrocephalus	3 (2)	3 (2)

Note. Sample percentages are given in parentheses.

as the symptoms of the preexisting illness may overlap with those of the meningitis. The second pattern, referred to as *fulminating* meningitis, is more sudden and precipitous and is associated with poorer prognosis. The latter pattern is more common in cases of *Neisseira meningitidis*. In fulminating cases, symptoms progress very rapidly over a few hours, with severe cerebral swelling frequently noted (Klein et al., 1986).

Because of the nonspecific clinical symptoms, diagnosis is usually made on the basis of identification of bacteria in the cerebrospinal fluid (CSF), taken via lumbar puncture, in association with elevated levels of protein and decreases in glucose levels. Accurate identification of the causal agent is important, since appropriate antibiotic treatments are determined on the basis of the identified bacterial pathogen. Angiography, neuroimaging, and electroencephalograms are not routinely given, but are employed where complications arise or where clinical course is abnormal.

Treatment

Treatment is initiated promptly, often prior to the identification of the causal bacteria. The most commonly administered drugs include ampicillin alone or in combination with other drugs, such as chloramphenicol, cefuroxime, and ceftriaxone (Feigin et al., 1992). Antibiotic therapy is generally continued for 7 to 10 days, with extensions for children with complications. More recently, steroids have been used early in the course of treatment, in an attempt to reduce the spread of inflammation throughout the CNS and thus to minimize permanent cerebral injury. A number of studies have reported reduction in hearing and neurological impairments when steroids are administered (Girgis et al., 1989; Lebel et al., 1988; Mertsola et al., 1991), resulting in the common use of such therapies in pediatric centers.

The typical treatment protocol also includes careful monitoring of electrolyte balance, fluid retention, and drug levels, each of which is relevant to recovery. The occurrence of seizures, prolonged fever or obtundation, cerebral edema, or other neurological abnormalities may indicate specific pathology and require further investigation. Where such symptoms are present, additional investigations of cerebral functioning (e.g., magnetic resonance imaging [MRI] or angiography) may be performed and appropriate medications administered.

PATHOPHYSIOLOGY

Disease Processes

Bacterial meningitis causes profound disruption to the cerebrovascular and CSF dynamics. Clinical symptoms subside within weeks for the majority of children who contract the disease (Feigin, 1987; Vienny et al., 1984). However, for some children the impact of these disruptions is fatal or leads to severe residual impairment (Adams, Kubik, & Bonner, 1948; Stovring & Snyder, 1980; Thomas & Hopkins, 1972).

Bacterial meningitis results from the successful invasion of the CNS by bacterial organisms that overcome the host defense mechanisms. Quagliarello and Scheld (1992) state that the successful meningeal pathogen must first colonize the host mucosal epithelium, invade and survive within the bloodstream, cross the blood–brain barrier, and survive in the CSF. This disease sequence is illustrated in Figure 6.2.

Animal studies indicate that the release of cytokines (e.g., interleukin-1, tumor necrosis factor), which are primary mediators of the host inflammatory response (Mustafa, Ramilo, Saez-Llorens, Mertsola, & McCracken, 1989; Ramilo, Mustafa, & Saez-Llorens, 1989), is triggered by the presence of bacterial products such as lipopolysaccharides and teichoic acid (Quagliarello & Scheld, 1992; Tomasz & Saukkonen, 1989). Cytokines alter the permeability of the blood–brain barrier and precipitate other changes, such as migration of leukocytes into the CSF, penetration of the blood–brain barrier, alteration in CSF dynamics, and disruptions in cerebral blood flow (Feigin et al., 1992).

The leptomeningies (pia mater and arachnoid) and the CSF in the subarachnoid space are the primary sites of infection within the CNS in bacterial meningitis. Most early information on the pathophysiology of bacterial meningitis was derived from autopsy studies, with findings representing the most severe forms of the disease (Adams et al., 1948; Rorke & Pitts, 1963; Smith & Landing, 1960). In these cases a purulent pad of varying thickness often covered the brain and meninges. Although this purulent material tended to be widely distributed, the highest accumulations were over the convexities of the brain in the depths of the sulci, in the lateral sulcus, and along the major veins and venous sinuses. Later studies identified the region of the middle cerebral artery as being particularly vulnerable to

Mucosal colonization by bacteria
↓
Bacterial invasion of and survival within bloodstream
↓
Penetration of blood–brain barrier and into CSF
↓
Local release of inflammatory cytokines in CSF
↓
Adhesion of leukocytes to brain endothelium and diapedesis into CSF
↓
Exudation of albumin through opened intercellular junctions of meningeal venules
↓
Brain oedema, increased intracranial pressure, altered cerebral blood flow
↓
Cranial nerve injury, seizures, hypoxic–ischemic brain damage, herniation

FIGURE 6.2. Sequential steps in the pathogenesis and pathophysiology of bacterial meningitis. From Quagliarello and Scheld (1993). Copyright 1993 by The University of Chicago Press. Reprinted by permission.

infection (Pomeroy, Holmes, Dodge, & Feigin, 1990; Thomas & Hopkins, 1972). Purulent exudate has also been observed around the basal cisterns and cerebellum, in the ventricles, and around the spinal cord.

Advances in structural and functional imaging in recent years have allowed more direct investigation of the pathophysiology of meningitis. In children who have sustained acute medical complications, such methods have detected a number of associated pathologies, including inflammation and occlusion of the cerebral blood vessels throughout the CNS; cranial nerve inflammation; raised intracranial pressure and diffuse cerebral swelling; hydrocephalus (usually communicating); and hypoxic damage due to shock, poor ventilation, and seizure activity (Snyder, Stovring, Cushing, Davis, & Hardy, 1981; Stovring & Snyder, 1980). Figure 6.3 provides some examples of the cerebral abnormali-

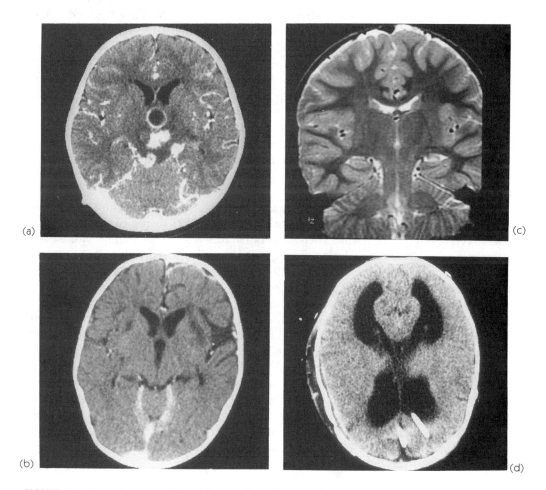

(a)   (c)

(b)   (d)

FIGURE 6.3. (a) Two-year-old child with tuberculous meningitis. Contrast-enhanced axial CT scan shows diffuse meningeal enhancement and tuberculomas in the brain stem and third ventricle. (b) Four-month-old infant with pneumococcal meningitis. Contrast-enhanced axial CT scan shows left frontal empyema and infarcts in the external capsules bilaterally. (c) Eight-year-old child with a history of Hib meningitis in infancy who subsequently developed intractable temporal lobe epilepsy. Coronal MRI scan shows atrophy and increased signal in the left hippocampus, consistent with hippocampal sclerosis. (d) Two-year-old child with a history of Hib meningitis in infancy who subsequently developed hydrocephalus, requiring insertion of ventricular shunt. Contrast-enhanced axial MRI shows evidence of hydrocephalus.

ties occurring in the acute stages of bacterial meningitis; it emphasizes the range of potential pathologies.

Biochemical changes have also been reported. Decreased concentration of glucose in CSF (resulting primarily from cerebrovascular disruption), cellular electrolyte imbalance, and inappropriate secretion of antidiuretic hormone are all common complications of meningitic infection, and have been documented as risk factors for residual impairments (Feigin et al., 1992; Taylor et al., 1990). A combination of these factors can result in focal as well as diffuse cortical insults (Dodge & Schwartz, 1965).

Vascular Changes

Cerebral angiography studies of children with bacterial meningitis have reported inflammation, narrowing, or spasm of cerebral blood vessels throughout the CNS. These vascular changes result in reduced cerebral blood flow and thrombosis, which may lead to the focal neurological signs seen in some survivors (Adams et al., 1948; Thomas & Hopkins, 1972). Occlusion of the terminal carotid arteries or their branches and prominent vasodilatation of the capillaries in the region of the middle cerebral artery have also been identified, consistent with necrosis reported in this region. Disruption of blood flow involving the middle cerebral artery may compromise the integrity of a wide cerebral area laterally, including the pre- and postcentral gyri, the superior and inferior parietal lobules, and the superior and middle temporal gyri. These areas subserve motor and sensory function, auditory processing, language, and executive functions (Dodge & Schwartz, 1965: Kandel, Schwartz, & Jessell, 1991).

Studies investigating cerebral blood flow during acute stages of infection have yielded somewhat contradictory results. McMenamin and Volpe (1984) studied the relationship between cerebral blood flow and raised intracranial pressure. Their findings indicated increases in cerebral blood flow during the acute phase of illness. Ashwal et al. (1990) studied both total and regional blood flow in 20 children suffering from bacterial meningitis. Thirteen of the children showed marked changes in blood flow at a regional level, despite normal overall blood volumes. These findings were interpreted as evidence of isolated involvement of specific blood vessels in the infectious process. Five children had significant reductions in both total and regional blood flow. Four of the five children exhibited serious sequelae, suggesting both generalized and focal vascular changes in complicated cases. Tureen, Dworkin, Kennedy, Sachdeva, and Sande (1990) have suggested that these contrasting findings with respect to cerebral blood flow may be due to loss of cerebrovascular autoregulation, which normally keeps cerebral blood flow constant. The loss of cerebrovascular autoregulation induced by bacterial meningitis may lead to changes in cerebral blood flow, either hyperperfusion or hypoperfusion (Quagliarello & Scheld, 1992). While there is clear evidence for vascular disruptions during the acute stage of illness, the long-term implications of this early pathology are less well understood.

Raised Intracranial Pressure

Evidence of raised intracranial pressure, often associated with diffuse cerebral edema, is commonly reported at autopsy in children who have died as a result of their infection (Dodge & Schwartz, 1965; Horowitz, Boxerbaum, & O'Bell, 1980). Although the exact mechanisms remain unclear, it appears that raised intracranial pressure leads to the obstruction of the flow of CSF, causing reduced cerebral blood flow and compression and herniation of the brain. Buildup of purulent exudate around the basal cisterns, cerebellum, ventricles, and spinal cord has also been documented and may contribute to communicating hydrocephalus. The latter complication occurs in a minority of cases and most frequently in younger children. While shunt insertion may relieve pressure in its most severe form, untreated raised intracranial pressure and hydrocephalus may lead to total dissolution of the cerebrum (Feigin et al., 1992).

Cranial Nerve Deficits

Abnormalities in function of the third, sixth, seventh, and eighth cranial nerves are usually thought to be related to irritation from exudate within the arachnoid sheaths enveloping those cranial nerves. Increased intracranial pressure and brain herniation may also compress the cranial nerves. As a result, deafness and vestibular disturbances are common. Visual impairment can occur as well, although less frequently. With the exception of sensory-neural hearing impairments due to damage to the eighth cranial nerve, cranial nerve abnormalities usually resolve over time. Sensory-neural hearing impairments resolve only rarely (Vienny et al., 1984) and sometimes result in severe residual deficits. These findings, in conjunction with reports of isolated sensory-neural hearing loss in children with otherwise intact neurological functioning (Grimwood et al., 1995; McIntyre, Jepson, Leeder, & Irwig, 1993; Taylor et al., 1990), imply that such deficits may be due to a specific vulnerability of the eighth nerve to primary infection (Dodge, 1986).

DISEASE SEQUELAE

Neurosensory and Other Neurological Impairments

Although the introduction of effective conjugate vaccines has led to a decline in the incidence of Hib meningitis, mortality rates for children who contract bacterial meningitis remain between 4% and 10% (Baraff, Lee, & Schriger, 1993; Feigin et al., 1992; Grimwood et al., 1995). Approximately 40% of survivors exhibit some form of acute neurological complication (Grimwood et al., 1995; Taylor et al., 1990). Many of these acute impairments resolve over time, and the majority of survivors of childhood meningitis have few residual impairments (Emmett et al., 1980; Feigin, 1987; Taylor et al., 1992). However, there is no doubt that a proportion of children suffer significant neurosensory and other neurological deficits as results of their illness. In a meta-analysis, Baraff et al. (1993) reviewed 19 prospective studies, incorporating outcome data for 1,602 children diagnosed with bacterial meningitis. These investigators found that 16% of children exhibited major long-term sequelae, including total deafness (11%), bilateral severe or profound hearing loss (5%), mental retardation (6%), spasticity or paresis (4%), and seizure disorders (4%). The risks for these sequelae differed according to disease type. Although Hib meningitis was associated with the lowest mortality rate (Hib, 4%; *Streptococcus pneumoniae*, 15%; *Neisseria meningitidis*, 8%), this form of bacterial meningitis led to greater morbidity. Similar outcomes have been reported in a retrospective, population-based survey (McIntyre et al., 1993).

Hearing loss is one of the most frequent sequelae of bacterial meningitis. In the prevaccine era, neurosensory hearing impairment due to meningitis accounted for the majority of all cases of hearing loss in infancy and childhood (Fraser, 1976). The incidence of hearing impairment reported in postmeningitis samples varies across studies, with rates ranging from 6% to 34% (Claesson et al., 1984; Dodge et al., 1984; Grimwood et al., 1995; Jadavji et al., 1986; Lindberg et al., 1977; Lutsar, Siirde, & Soopold, 1995). Hearing loss has particular significance for infants and young children: Because early childhood is a critical period for language development, reduced auditory functioning is likely to have important implications for the ongoing maturation of these skills. Follow-up studies indicate that language disorders or delays are common in children who have recovered from bacterial meningitis (Grimwood et al., 1995; Jadavji et al., 1986; Lutsar et al., 1995). Sell (1983) reported that 15% of the 50 children she followed in a prospective study had expressive and/or receptive language difficulties, while Feldman et al. (1982) observed speech delay in 34% of the children in their sample. Although postmeningitic children with hearing loss may be especially vulnerable to speech and language deficits (Taylor et al., in press), risks for these problems are also higher in children who have had meningitis without accompanying hearing impairment (Lutsar et al., 1995; Anderson et al., 1997). This is well illustrated in a recent study by Pentland, Anderson and Wrennall (in press), who evaluated 9- to 11-year-old postmeningitic children, excluding those with any history of hearing impairments. They found that these children exhibited significant language difficulties, particularly on tasks tapping expressive skills and verbal reasoning. Such findings suggest that postmeningitic speech and language deficits may be due not only to hearing loss, but also to the more generalized brain insults that can be secondary to this disease.

Cognitive, Educational, and Behavioral Deficits

Earlier Research on Disease Outcomes

The intellectual, educational, and behavioral sequelae of bacterial meningitis are less definitive than disease effects on more basic neurological functions. Early research was primarily concerned with identification of deficits in IQ, achievement, or language skills. These early studies, however, were characterized by small samples and limited outcome measures. Control groups were often lacking or inappropriate. Although the majority of these studies identified disease-related deficits in development (Feigin et al., 1976; Feldman et al., 1982; Ferry, Culbertson, Cooper, Sitton, & Sell, 1982; Jadavji et al., 1986; Kresky et al., 1962; Lawson, Metcalfe, & Pampiglione, 1965; Sproles et al., 1969; Wright & Jimmerson, 1971), such findings were not universal, and a number of researchers failed to detect disease sequelae (Emmett et al., 1980; Tejani et al., 1982).

One of the earliest comprehensive research programs investigating outcomes from childhood bacterial meningitis was conducted by Sell and her colleagues about 25 years ago (Sell, 1983; Sell, Merrill, et al., 1972; Sell, Webb, et al., 1972). Sell, Merrill, et al. (1972) initially investigated long-term outcome in an sample of 86 survivors of bacterial meningitis. Although no control group was included, the mean IQ for the 56 school-age children who returned for testing was only 84. The initial study was followed by a controlled, prospective investigation by the same research team (Sell, Webb, et al., 1972).

In the first part of this study, a group of 21 Hib meningitis survivors was compared to a sibling control group. The IQ scores of the Hib survivors were again lower than expected, and significantly lower than the IQ scores of the sibling controls (respective means of 86 and 97; $p < .05$). Inspection of the IQ scores of patient–sibling pairs, shown in Figure 6.4, revealed that 29% of the postmeningitic children scored one full standard deviation below their siblings. In contrast, no sibling scored one standard deviation below a postmeningitis child.

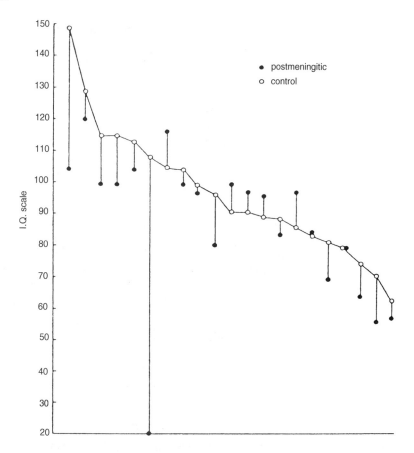

FIGURE 6.4. Representation of IQ results for postmeningitic and control pairs. From Sell, Webb, Pate, and Doyne (1972). Copyright 1972 by American Academy of Pediatrics. Reprinted by permission.

In the second part of this study, 25 survivors of various types of bacterial meningitis were compared to nonmeningitic peer controls. Disease survivors were selected to be in the first three grades of school. Only children thought to be free of disease sequelae were included (e.g., no obvious sequelae, participation in fully regular education programs). Peer matches were recruited at random from among children in the same school classroom and of the same sex and social class as the postmeningitic children. Despite the selective nature of the sample and the careful matching procedures, the meningitis survivors scored significantly lower than their peers on tests of psycholinguistic ability, vocabulary, and visual-perceptual skill.

Similar cognitive, educational, and behavioral sequelae have been reported in a number of other early studies. Cross-sectional, single-group designs were commonly utilized by researchers in their attempts to determine the frequency of residual sequelae. In 1969, Sproles et al. identified depressed IQ, educational delay, speech impairment, and/or behavioral disturbance in 27% of their sample. Consistent with these figures, Lindberg et al. (1977) reported that 27% of the 82 children they examined exhibited neurological or psychological sequelae, and Jadavji et al. (1986) found these deficits in 20% of their sample. Similarly, in a sample of 80 children followed by Kresky et al. (1962), 34% of children exhibited one or more neurological deficit. Educational difficulties were identified in 20%

of this sample and were interpreted as related to motor and sensory impairments, rather than to depressed intellectual functioning. These authors noted poorer prognosis associated with illness prior to 12 months of age, complications during acute illness, and delayed diagnosis.

Ferry et al. (1982) caution that many of the sequelae associated with bacterial meningitis may not be evident in the acute stages of recovery. They employed a prospective longitudinal design to study the recovery of 50 postmeningitic children who were considered normal at discharge. Follow-up of this group at 6 months after illness revealed a range of previously undetected early sequelae including hearing and/or language impairment ($n = 16$), mental retardation ($n = 5$), motor disability ($n = 2$), and seizure disorder ($n = 2$).

Although the matched-pairs designs used by Sell and her colleagues (Sell, Merrill, et al., 1972) and their efforts to follow total hospital cohorts represented considerable advances in research on developmental outcomes of early brain disease, the samples were relatively small. Most other studies conducted prior to the mid-1980s were subject to many additional limitations, including potential sample biases, failure to include appropriate control groups, and use of restricted outcome measures or poorly operationalized outcomes (e.g., school failure, behavior problems, and even "minimal brain dysfunction") (Kresky et al., 1962; Lawson et al., 1965; Sproles et al., 1969). While these pioneering studies utilized a variety of research designs and outcome measures, they consistently documented high rates of morbidity, involving up to 50% of survivors (Feigin et al., 1976; Feldman et al., 1982; Sell, 1983). The nature and extent of these deficits are difficult to gauge from these studies, but the findings provided a strong inpetus for further research.

Later Follow-Up Studies Conducted in Pittsburgh and in Canada

In an effort to address some of these limitations, Taylor, Michaels, Mazur, Bauer, and Liden (1984) followed a small sample of children who were treated for Hib meningitis at Children's Hospital of Pittsburgh between 1973 and 1975. Attempts were made to contact the families of all disease survivors during this period, and only one contacted family declined participation. Assessments were conducted 6 to 8 years after the children had recovered from the disease, and included evaluations of neuropsychological abilities, academic achievement, and behavior. At follow-up, 5 of the 24 postmeningitic, or index, children (21%) had frank neurological sequelae, including neurosensory hearing impairment, hemiparesis, or seizure disorders. The postmeningitic children had lower Wechsler Performance and Full Scale IQs than their siblings. The index children also performed less well on tests of auditory comprehension (Token Test, Part V), motor and perceptual–motor skills (Grooved Pegboard Test and an aggregate of "soft" neurological signs), and verbal memory (Verbal Selective Reminding Test). Despite these differences in cognitive performance, the index children did not obtain lower scores than their siblings on tests of achievement, nor were they rated by parents as having more behavior problems.

Four years after the initial assessment, Feldman and Michaels (1988) readministered achievement tests to 23 of the index cases. Their findings indicated that these children continued to progress academically over the intervening interval. Comparisons of the scores of the index children to scores obtained by siblings at a similar age (taken from the earlier assessments) failed to reveal differences on most measures of achievement. However, the index children obtained lower scores than the siblings on a measure of reading accuracy. Age-normed scores on tests of word recognition and decoding also declined in the index group across the two assessments. Interviews with parents revealed that the postmeningitic children were receiving more assistance from family members with their homework than the siblings were. The latter finding suggested that the generally favorable academic performance of the index cases may have been due in part to parental efforts to compensate for their cognitive limitations.

In a subsequent larger-scale investigation conducted at the Canadian children's hospitals (Montreal Children's Hospital, Children's Hospital of Eastern Ontario, and the Hospital for Sick Children), Taylor and his associates recruited another school-age sample of 127 children who had recovered from Hib meningitis (Taylor et al., 1990, 1992). Survivors of Hib meningitis were recruited from among consecutive admissions of children treated for this disease between the years 1972 and 1984. Nearest-aged siblings of school age again served as controls, and disease sequelae were evaluated in terms of neuropsychological, educational, and behavioral outcomes. The initial follow-up evaluation took place an average of 8 years after disease onset. Outcomes for the index group were reassessed at 1 and 2 years after the initial follow-up. A review of the medical records revealed that 53 of the index cases (42% of the sample) had neurological complications during the acute-phase illness. The distribution of acute-phase complications (described previously in Table 6.1) was similar to that reported in previous studies (Feigin et al., 1976; Lebel et al., 1988).

At the initial follow-up, 16 of the index cases (13%) had long-term neurological sequelae, including 13 children with isolated neurosensory hearing loss and three with either ongoing seizure disorders or hemiplegia. Despite these sequelae, paired comparisons of the postmeningitis children to their siblings failed to reveal group differences on most measures of outcome (Taylor et al., 1990). Although the index cases scored at lower levels on tests of reading and were receiving more special education assistance, the paired comparisons failed to reveal significant differences between the index and sibling groups in cognitive performance or behavior. Mean prorated Wechsler Full Scale IQs for the two groups were 108 and 110, respectively.

Differences were more pronounced when the index cases with acute-phase neurological complications were compared to their respective siblings. The latter comparisons yielded differences not only in reading, but also in spelling, prorated Wechsler Full Scale and Performance IQs, and adaptive communication skills. None of the differences between index cases without acute-phase neurological complications and their siblings was significant.

Subsequent comparisons of the larger group of index cases with complications (i.e., those with and without sibling controls) to index cases without complications and to siblings documented disease effects on prorated Wechsler Verbal IQ as well as Performance and Full Scale IQs, overall adaptive abilities, teacher ratings of school performance, and neuropsychological abilities (Taylor, Barry, & Schatschneider, 1993). The children with acute-phase neurological complications also had significantly higher rates of low perceptual–performance skills, weaknesses in reading and spelling achievement, and grade repetitions than the children with uncomplicated disease courses (Taylor et al., in press). These differences persisted even when age, gender, and socioeconomic status were taken into account via covariate-adjusted logistic regression analysis.

In a further study focusing on neuropsychological outcomes, Taylor, Schatschneider, Petrill, Barry, and Owens (1996) compared index children with complications, referred to as the "affected" group, to an "unaffected" group composed of both index cases without complications and siblings. Ability composites were derived from factor analysis of the neuropsychological measures. Comparisons of the two groups on the neuropsychological composites are shown in Figure 6.5. As evident in this figure, the affected group performed at significantly lower levels on both the perceptual–performance and response speed composites. Although all differences were in the predicted direction, the results support the possibility that some abilities may be particularly vulnerable to disease; they are consistent with other findings suggesting that nonverbal skills and executive functions are more clearly compromised than other abilities (Taylor, 1984; Taylor et al., 1996; Wright & Jimmerson, 1971).

The specificity of neurodevelopmental impairments in this sample of postmeningitic children was additionally explored by Taylor and Schatschneider (1992b). The latter study focused only on those index cases with prorated Wechsler Full Scale IQs of at least 80 who were free of hearing and other neurological impairments. Disease consequences were evaluated by comparing affected and unaffected index cases. According to the results of these comparisons, the affected children scored significantly below the unaffected children in prorated Wechsler Performance IQ, reading, spelling, and arithmetic skills, spatial reasoning, and perceptual–motor speed, as well as teacher ratings of school performance. One of the study's conclusions was that learning and neuropsychological sequelae of Hib meningitis can be found even in children without gross disturbances in neurological status or mentation. A further study implication was that meningitis can precipitate relatively "specific" learning problems. The nature of the neuropsychological deficits observed in the affected index group also suggested that their learning problems reflected weaknesses in executive functions and perceptual abilities, as opposed to the language-based impairments associated with more common varieties of learning disabilities.

According to preliminary analysis of the follow-up data collected by this research group, disease sequelae remained fairly stable over the 2-year follow-up period (Taylor, Schatschneider, & Minich, 1999). Differences between affected and unaffected index cases were generally unchanged across the initial and follow-up assessments. Growth modeling techniques, however, have revealed some evidence for age-related changes in cognitive functioning. Although analysis of the follow-up data is as yet incomplete, results from hierarchical linear modeling analysis suggest that the consequences of disease for certain aspects of information-processing and abstract problem-solving abilities may become more pronounced over time. Analyses are currently underway to investigate the separate effects of age at disease onset, time since disease, and age at testing as determinants of growth in cognitive abilities.

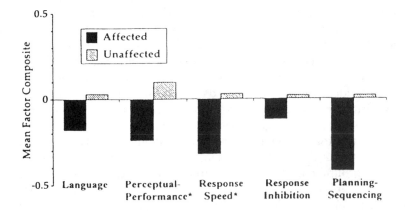

FIGURE 6.5. Differences between postmeningitic and control groups for ability factor composites. From Taylor, Schatschneider, Petrill, Barry, and Owens (1996). Copyright 1996 by Lawrence Erlbaum Associates, Inc. Reprinted by permission.

Prospective Follow-Up of Postmeningitic Children
in Melbourne, Australia

A second larger-scale study of neurodevelopmental outcomes of meningitis has been conducted by Grimwood, Anderson, and their associates in Melbourne, Australia (V. Anderson et al., 1997; Grimwood et al., 1995, 1996; Hore, 1992). The children included in this study were recruited from a cohort of 158 survivors of various forms of childhood bacterial meningitis treated at a single center (Royal Children's Hospital, Melbourne). Illness parameters and recovery course were documented, and the cohort was evaluated at hospital discharge and at 12-month and 6-year follow-ups. Sixty percent of the original cohort experienced acute neurological complications, including seizures, coma, hemiparesis, ataxia, raised intracranial pressure, and sensory impairment (see Table 6.1). Of the total sample, 29 children had computed tomography (CT) scans due to poor clinical progress, with abnormalities identified in 48% of these patients. Pathologies included hydrocephalus, cerebral edema, subdural collections, cerebritis, and ischemic lesions (Hore, 1992). At discharge 25% of the cohort exhibited neurodevelopmental abnormalities, including impairments in gross motor skills (hemiparesis, gait disturbance), fine motor skills (tremor, eye–hand incoordination), language (diminished vocalization, articulation problems, dysfluency, receptive language disorder), hearing and vision (blindness or problems in fixation or pursuit tracking), and behavior (irritability, excessive crying, aggressive behavior, anxiety) (Hore, 1992). Rates and degree of impairment for the sample are presented in Table 6.2. To obtain these data, each child was assigned a score from 0 to 4 (normal, mild, moderate, severe) in each functional area, based on results of a standard neurological examination. Results showed that gross motor problems were most common, occurring in approximately a quarter of the sample at discharge, and behavioral problems were also prevalent. Furthermore, the degree of neurdevelopmental impairment was mild in the majority of cases.

In keeping with previous studies reporting early resolution of most acute-phase neurological sequelae (Feigin, 1987; Pomeroy et al., 1990), only 15% of the sample exhibited persisting neurological and neurodevelopmental abnormalities at the 12-month follow-up, with this figure remaining constant at the 6-year follow-up (Anderson, Leaper, & Judd, 1987; Grimwood et al., 1995). None of the children with normal neurological examinations at discharge developed frank neurological disorders. On the other hand, the number of children exhibiting more subtle neurodevelopmental disorders increased with time. Based on the criteria employed at discharge, 55% of children experienced some form of neurodevelopmental problem at the 12-month follow-up, and 27% continued to exhibit diffi-

TABLE 6.2. Rates of Neurodevelopmental Abnormalities Detected at Discharge in Cohort (*n* = 160) Studied by Hore (1992)

Skill area	Degree of abnormality			Total
	Mild	Moderate	Severe	
Gross motor	14 (8.9)	9 (5.6)	14 (8.9)	37 (23.4)
Fine motor	10 (6.3)	2 (1.3)	3 (1.9)	15 (9.5)
Language	3 (1.9)	1 (0.6)	1 (0.6)	5 (3.1)
Hearing	5 (3.2)	1 (0.6)	2 (1.3)	8 (5.1)
Vision	2 (1.3)	0 (0)	4 (2.5)	6 (3.8)
Behavior	21 (13.3)	2 (1.3)	2 (1.3)	25 (15.9)

Note. Sample percentages are given in parentheses.

culties at the 6-year follow-up. The frequency of fine motor problems, impaired hearing, language difficulties, and behavioral disturbance was greater at both the 12-month and 6-year follow-ups than at discharge, as is illustrated by the data presented in Table 6.3. These results do not necessarily indicate postdischarge deterioration, but suggest that the subtle neurodevelopmental sequelae associated with bacterial meningitis may not be evident in infants and young children. Such deficits may become apparent in later childhood when these skills fail to develop as expected.

Evaluation of the predictive value of acute neurological and neurodevelopmental status at the 12-month follow-up showed that children who exhibited one or more neurodevelopmental abnormalities at discharge were more likely to achieve lower IQ scores. Furthermore, the degree of neurodevelopmental disability found at discharge (mild, moderate, severe) predicted 12-month IQ scores, regardless of the nature of the abnormality (Anderson et al., 1987; Hore, 1992).

At the 6-year follow-up, 130 children, representing 82% of the total cohort, returned for comprehensive neurological, neuropsychological, audiological, and educational evaluations (V. Anderson et al., 1997; Grimwood et al., 1995). Disease consequences were evaluated by comparing the index cases to 130 age-matched controls. The control group was formed by matching each postmeningitic child to a classmate, with matching based on teacher selection of the next same-sex child on the class roll. Comparisons of the index cases and controls revealed trends similar to those described by Taylor and his associates (Taylor et al., 1990, 1992). Group differences, however, were more pronounced. Specifically, postmeningitic children performed significantly more poorly than controls on a range of neuropsychological domains, including intelligence (Wechsler Intelligence Scale for Children—Revised [WISC-R]), language (Token Test), visual–motor coordination (Developmental Test of Visual–Motor Integration), educational ability (Neale Analysis of Reading Ability—Revised), memory and learning (Rey Auditory–Verbal Learning Test, Story Recall, Rey–Osterrieth Complex Figure—recall), and executive functions (Rey–Osterrieth Complex Figure, Controlled Oral Word Association Test). Behavioral problems were also more common in the postmeningitic group. For the most part, group differences were small. Mean scores for the postmeningitic group generally fell within the average range, indicating subtle rather than severe impairments.

Relationships of acute-phase neurological complications to outcomes were also examined. In keeping with the findings of Taylor et al. (1993), results showed that postmeningitic children experiencing such complications scored at a lower level than children without complications and controls on measures of general intellectual functioning. In this

TABLE 6.3. Rates of Neurodevelopmental Abnormalities at Discharge and at 12 Months and 6 Years after Meningitis in Follow-Up Cohort (*n* = 130) Studied by Hore (1992)

Skill area	Discharge	12 months	6 years
Gross motor	20 (15)	5 (4)	3 (2)
Fine motor	15 (11)	17 (13)	52 (40)
Language	3 (2)	13 (10)	5 (5)
Hearing	6 (5)	8 (6)	8 (6)
Vision	3 (2)	3 (2)	2 (2)
Behavior	20 (15)	27 (21)	39 (30)

Note. Sample percentages are given in parentheses.

study, however, both groups of postmeningitic children performed significantly more poorly than controls on measures of educational competence, fine motor and visual–motor coordination, auditory discrimination, and executive functions (see Table 6.4). These results suggest disease consequences regardless of a child's acute-phase neurological status, and argue that even the less severe forms of brain insult associated with this disease can result in long-term sequelae.

Comparison of the results from the large-scale studies of Taylor et al. (1990) and Grimwood et al. (1995) suggests a similar pattern of behavioral findings, but with more significant disease sequelae documented in the latter investigation. The two studies employed similar research designs, including large samples, adequate control groups with subjects enrolled during similar time periods, and equivalent test procedures. Differences in methodology, however, may help explain these discrepant results. First, sample selection procedures differed. Taylor et al. (1990) recruited children who were diagnosed with Hib meningitis only, whereas the Grimwood et al. (1995) design included all forms of bacterial meningitis. Furthermore, Taylor at al. (1990) used a retrospective design. The sample recruited may not have been representative of the population of children with this disease, and collection of medical data was dependent on whatever information was recorded in the hospital charts. In contrast, Grimwood et al. (1995) recruited subjects during initial hospital admission and used a standardized protocol to record illness variables for all children. The latter procedures may have yielded a more representative sample and more accurate documentation of acute illness data. The two studies also used different methods for recruiting control children. Taylor et al. (1990) employed sibling controls, who were on average 2 years older and perhaps adversely affected by the presence of a child with a life-threatening illness within the family. The classmate controls recruited by Grimwood et al. (1995) may not have matched the postmeningitic children so closely for

TABLE 6.4. Comparison of Outcomes for Children with Acute Complications, No Complications, and Controls

Test/measure	Cases with complications ($n = 56$)	Cases without complications ($n = 74$)	Controls ($n = 130$)
WISC-R			
Verbal IQ[a]	92.4 (2.4)	99.9 (2.1)	101.6 (1.6)
Performance IQ	97.4 (2.6)	101.3 (2.4)	105.5 (1.7)
Full Scale IQ[b]	95.4 (1.9)	101.0 (1.7)	104.3 (1.5)
Rey–Osterrieth Complex Figure			
Copy[a]	21.8 (1.0)	22.9 (0.9)	25.6 (0.8)
Recall[c]	9.7 (1.0)	10.7 (0.9)	12.5 (0.8)
Neale Analysis of Reading Ability			
Accuracy (%)[a]	46.0 (4.2)	45.0 (3.7)	55.1 (3.3)
Comprehension (%)[a]	41.6 (4.0)	48.9 (3.4)	56.9 (3.1)
Developmental Test of Visual–Motor Integration (%)[a]	47.9 (4.1)	54.7 (3.5)	62.5 (3.2)

Note. Standard errors of mean scores are given in parentheses. Data from Grimwood et al. (1995).

[a]Significant difference between cases without complications and controls.

[b]Significant differences between cases with and cases without complications.

[c]Significant differences between cases with complications and controls only.

family variables, but were more closely matched on age and not subject to potential disease-related family burden. Finally, mean age was slightly greater for the children in the Taylor et al. study (9.6 years vs 8.4 years). If postmeningitic children were experiencing a developmental delay rather than a fixed deficit, as suggested in a recent study by Pentland et al. (in press), it could be that an older sample would present with fewer deficits.

NEUROPSYCHOLOGICAL CONSEQUENCES OF OTHER FORMS OF MENINGITIS

In contrast to the considerable research literature on the developmental consequences of childhood bacterial meningitis, studies of the longer-term effects of neonatal forms of this disease are sparse. In one of the few studies in this area, Haslam et al. (1977) followed children with group B streptococcal meningitis for 3–9 years and found major neurological sequelae in 2 of 15 survivors (13%). In another study that included assessments of developmental skills at a mean age of 6 years, Edwards et al. (1985) found that half of a sample of 38 survivors of this disease had either neurological disorders or delays in language or cognitive abilities. The latter study, however, did not include a control group.

In the most comprehensive follow-up study of this disease to date, Wald et al. (1986) found a 12% rate of major neurological sequelae in children with group B streptococcal meningitis. Sequelae included cerebral palsy, mental retardation, seizure disorders, deafness, and cortical blindness. These researchers also administered a battery of neuropsychological tests to 34 index cases who were between 3 and 18 years of age at the time of the evaluations and who were judged capable of psychometric evaluation. Twenty-one siblings without histories of neurological disorder were recruited as a comparison group. Results revealed that the postmeningitis groups scored more poorly than their siblings on measures of adaptive behavior and visual–motor performance. However, there were no differences in IQ or academic achievement, and all differences were nonsignificant when the children with persistent neurological sequelae were excluded from analysis. The authors concluded that the disease sequelae can be recognized early in life and that children without frank neurological disorders are not likely to sustain long-term consequences. However, given that deficits in achievement and neuropsychological skills have been discovered in children who survive childhood bacterial meningitis without acute-phase neurological complications (Grimwood et al., 1995), the latter conclusion may be premature. Further follow-up studies are needed to determine whether the findings by Wald et al. (1986) can be replicated, and to examine associations between early disease severity and longer-term developmental outcomes.

The sequelae of viral meningitis, if any, have been more elusive than the consequences of bacterial meningitis. Several earlier studies found significant residual deficits following viral meningitis in children less than 1 year of age at disease onset (Farmer, MacArthur, & Clay, 1975; Sells, Carpenter, & Ray, 1975; Wilfert et al., 1981). The disease sequelae reported in these studies included lower IQ and speech and language deficits. Interpretation of these findings, however, is difficult because of small sample sizes and questions regarding the comparability of control groups. Documentation of viral infection in the CSF was also lacking in some cases.

Using improved methodology, Baker, Kummer, Schultz, Ho, and Gonzalez del Rey (1996) recently conducted a 3-year follow-up study of 16 children who contracted enteroviral meningitis within the first 3 months of life. Disease consequences were evaluated by comparing index cases to a group of control children on tests of cognitive and language development at 12, 24, and 36 months of age. The control children were matched to cases of similar age, sex, race, and socioeconomic status. Results revealed that the cases performed at lower levels than the controls on language testing at 24 and 36 months of age.

Other studies, however, have been unable to document long-term sequelae of early viral meningitis. Bergman et al. (1987) administered a battery of neuropsychological tests to a group of 31 children who had contracted this disease within the first year of life. Comparison of the index children (mean age 8½ years) to sibling controls (mean age 10½ years) failed to reveal any group differences. Rorabaugh et al. (1993) also failed to find disease sequelae in a study of children who contracted viral meningitis prior to 2 years of age, even when children with neurological complications with their illness were compared to children with an uncomplicated disease course.

The reason for the discrepancy between these findings and those of Baker et al. (1996) is difficult to ascertain. Despite matching on socioeconomic status, the control group selected by Baker et al. may have been more socially advantaged than their index cases. On the other hand, the disease effects discovered by these investigators may have been real, with children who are youngest at disease onset being most vulnerable, or with disease effects perhaps being more apparent in the preschool age range than in older children. Although further follow-up studies will be needed to resolve the issue of whether viral meningitis has long-term developmental consequences, it seems clear that these consequences, if any, are less pronounced than those associated with bacterial meningitis.

PREDICTORS OF OUTCOME

Follow-up studies of children with bacterial meningitis demonstrate that some survivors are at higher risk than others for developmental sequelae. Knowledge of these risks is important in guiding plans for longer-term follow-up and intervention, but it can also have implications for medical management. For example, medical procedures that may limit the extent of acute-phase neurological complications have the potential to reduce longer-term sequelae as well. Administration of dexamethasone early in the disease course is one such treatment possibility (Gary, Powers, & Todd, 1989; Lebel et al., 1988). Principles of brain–behavior relationships suggest that factors predisposing a child to either cerebral insult or transient disruption in cerebral functions may be associated with residual neurobehavioral impairment. Research, however, underscores the importance of taking both medical and subject-related factors into account (Taylor et al., 1992). The latter factors include age at disease onset, time since disease, age at testing, and gender (V. Anderson et al., 1997; Anderson, Godber, Smibert, & Ekert, 1997; Dennis, 1988; Waber et al., 1990). Social and family background factors have also been considered, both as direct influences on outcomes and as moderators of disease effects (Taylor & Schatschneider, 1992b; Taylor et al., 1993).

Disease Factors

The highest death rates from meningitis appear to occur when this disease is contracted during the neonatal period, with mortality rates higher in this age range than in later infancy or childhood (Davies & Rudd, 1994; Thomas, 1992). Pneumococcal meningitis is the most common pathogen in these cases. Delayed diagnosis and treatment, coma, and high levels of protein in the CSF have also been associated with heightened mortality rates (Bortolussi & Seeliger, 1990; Davies & Rudd, 1994; Jadavji et al., 1986). In a prospective study of 168 admissions for bacterial meningitis, Hore (1992) found that longer duration of illness prior to treatment, age less than 12 months, and pneumococcal meningitis were all associated with higher mortality. Seizures during the acute illness were observed in all of the children who died from their disease. Other factors associated with mortality included unconsciousness on admission or diminishing consciousness from 4 to 72 hours after initiation of therapy, and severe biochemical abnormalities (e.g., low serum sodium concentration and reduced CSF total leukocyte and neutrophil counts).

Illness factors have also been associated with neurological and developmental sequelae among the survivors of this disease. As noted earlier, the presence of acute-phase neurological complications is one important predictor of outcome (Grimwood et al., 1995; Taylor et al., 1992; Feigin, 1992). Studies by Pomeroy et al. (1990) and Taylor et al. (in press) have examined relationships of specific types of neurological complications to disease morbidity. In a study of 185 children with various forms of bacterial meningitis, Pomeroy et al. (1990) found that neurological complications that failed to resolve within a year after the illness, other than hearing loss, predicted which children would have seizure disorders after the initial hospitalization. Seven of the eight children who had these complications also had abnormalities on CT scan. Similarly, Taylor et al. (in press) found that rates of school-age developmental problems, including cognitive weaknesses, poor spelling ability, and grade repetition, were significantly higher in children who had persistent neurological complications other than hearing loss than in children without acute-phase neurological complications. In the latter study, even transient neurological complications were associated with adverse developmental outcomes. Specific complications that were predictive of disease sequelae included seizures, hemiparesis, coma, and bilateral hearing loss.

Additional disease factors that have been associated with unfavorable neurological or developmental outcomes include *Streptococcus pneumoniae* meningitis, late diagnosis, focal neurological symptoms, seizures later in treatment, deteriorating state of consciousness in the hospital, extended hospitalization or fever duration, and shock. Unfavorable laboratory findings include elevations in protein or antigen levels, as well as decreases in CSF glucose or CSF–blood glucose ratio, CSF white cell count, hemoglobin, or serum sodium concentration (Herson & Todd, 1977; Feldman et al., 1982; Feigin, 1992; Grimwood et al., 1996; Kaplan, Smith, Wills, & Feigin, 1986).

Age-Related Factors

Previous research has identified younger age at illness as a specific risk factor, although this variable is commonly confounded with such factors as type of meningitis, severity of illness, or socioeconomic status (Davies & Rudd, 1994; Feigin, 1992; Franco, Cornelius, & Andrewes, 1992; Herson & Todd, 1977). Anderson, Grimwood, and colleagues (V. Anderson et al., 1997; Grimwood et al., 1996) recently reported age at illness to be an independent risk factor for cognitive and behavioral sequelae of bacterial meningitis. Specifically, children who contracted one of the several forms of bacterial meningitis prior to 12 months of age performed more poorly on measures of language and reading skills than children who became ill later in infancy or in childhood. Similar differences were found in comparing the early-onset postmeningitis children to age-matched controls. These results are consistent with a wealth of data suggesting that the first year of life is a particularly critical period in language development (Gardner, 1979). A disease such as bacterial meningitis may serve to interrupt this development, leading to delays or even persisting deficits in language skills.

The fact that Anderson et al. (1997) did not find an association between age at illness and nonverbal abilities or short-term memory capacity is contrary to findings from previous research on outcomes following early brain insults (Anderson et al., 1997; Anderson & Moore, 1995; Ewing-Cobbs et al., 1989; Kriel et al., 1989). It is important to emphasize, however, that the sample of children followed by V. Anderson et al. (1997) was somewhat younger at the time of illness/insult (median age 17 months) than the samples included in these other studies. For example, Anderson et al. (1997) report consequences of cranial irradiation, which is administered only after 2 years of age, and Anderson and Moore (1995), Ewing-Cobbs et al. (1989), and Kriel et al. (1989) each describe outcomes in samples in which children's ages were distributed evenly between birth and school age. Differences in outcomes may also reflect different critical periods for verbal and nonverbal functions or cumulative language deficits over time (Dennis, Spiegler, Hetherington, & Greenberg, 1996).

More generally, evidence that language sequelae are more pronounced among children who are younger at the time of brain insult is contrary to traditional "plasticity" theories (Lenneberg, 1967; Teuber, 1962). Although neural plasticity may mediate recovery in cases of early focal insults, such as those related to tumors or hemispherectomy (Dennis, 1980; Rankur, Aram, & Horwitz, 1980), this mechanism is probably less applicable to diffuse brain insults, such as those associated with meningitis or traumatic brain injury (Levin, Benton, & Grossman, 1982).

The relative vulnerability of the immature CNS to generalized insult has been demonstrated in a number of patient groups, including children with head injuries (Anderson & Moore, 1995; Ewing-Cobbs et al., 1989; Kriel et al., 1989; Wrightson, McGinn, & Gronwall, 1995) and cranial irradiation (Anderson et al., 1994; Eiser, 1978; Rubenstein, Varni, & Katz, 1990). A common explanation for these findings is that cerebral insult in infancy and early childhood interrupts ongoing development.

Another possibility emphasized by Dennis and Barnes (1994) is that deficits will not be evident immediately, but will emerge over time as functions that the damaged areas would normally have subserved fail to develop. Limited support for this possibility was provided in the follow-up study by Taylor et al. (1990), in which differences between Hib meningitis survivors and their siblings in parent ratings of behavior problems varied with the age of the index child. More specifically, the number of behavior problems on the Child Behavior Checklist reported for postmeningitis children relative to sibling controls increased with the age of the index children. As noted earlier, more recent but as yet preliminary analysis of the data from this study suggest similar age-related declines in cognitive performance (Taylor et al., 1996).

Dennis (1988) has further hypothesized that established skills may be less vulnerable than developing skills to disruption by brain insults. According to this hypothesis, children who contract bacterial meningitis in the first year of life will be particularly susceptible to linguistic deficits. The ultimate impact of disease, moreover, may be to alter the rate of acquisition, the sequence of acquisition, or the final mastery level of the skill (Dennis, 1988).

Social Factors

Although there is some evidence for increased risk of bacterial meningitis in certain ethnic groups and in families at greater social disadvantage (Broome, 1987; Feigin, 1992), risks may not be related to socioeconomic status per se, but rather to more proximal social factors such as child-rearing practices and family size. Few studies, however, have investigated such proximal social risks as determinants of disease outcomes. There is little doubt that social factors influence the development of children with early neurological diseases (Taylor et al., 1992). The more critical issue is whether social factors exercise more or less influence on outcomes than is the case in children without brain insults. Despite the suggestion that brain insults may be more devastating for children at social disadvantage than for socially advantaged children (Escalona, 1982), findings from several follow-up studies of very-low-birthweight children suggest that disease effects are less marked in children at greater social disadvantage (Bendersky & Lewis, 1994). The reason is not that disadvantaged children are more immune to brain insults, but simply that biological risks make less of a difference for children who are already disadvantaged by social circumstances.

Taylor et al. (1993) are the only investigators to date who have explored possible interactions between disease severity and socioeconomic status in children with meningitis. Although the results of this study generally failed to demonstrate such effects, the researchers discovered that the effects of meningitis on auditory comprehension, as measured by the Token Test, did in fact vary with children's socioeconomic status. As shown in Figure 6.6, the ef-

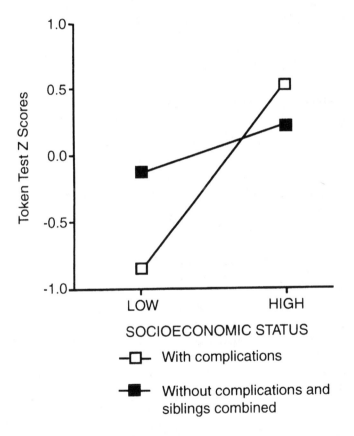

FIGURE 6.6. Example of interaction effect: Token Test performance for postmeningitis children at two socioeconomic levels. Postmeningitis children with complications are compared to a combined group of postmeningitis children without complications and siblings. From Taylor, Barry, and Schatschneider (1993). Copyright 1993 by Lawrence Erlbaum Associates, Inc. Reprinted by permission.

fects of Hib meningitis on this outcome were observed in children of lower socioeconomic status only. The latter finding indicates that some disease consequences may be moderated by social factors, and it encourages further exploration of the conditions under which such synergistic effects may be found.

Gender

Taylor and associates have also examined male–female differences in disease effects. In a study of matched pairs of index cases and siblings, Taylor et al. (1990) found that gender was related to paired differences in both teacher ratings of school adjustment and adaptive behavior. Specifically, differences on these measures in favor of the index child were greater for male than for female index children. Furthermore, this effect was independent of the sex of the sibling control. Although subsequent group analyses of interactions between gender and disease effects failed to substantiate this finding (Taylor et al., 1993), the paired analyses may have provided a more precise assessment of interaction effects. Follow-up studies of school-age children at neurological risk due to very low birthweight have also documented greater effects of this condition on the behavior of boys compared to girls (Breslau, Klein, & Allen, 1988; Ross, Lipper, & Auld, 1990; Sommerfelt, Ellertsen, & Markestad, 1993; Taylor, Klein, Schatschneider, & Hack, 1999). Sex-related sociocultural influences on internalizing and externalizing behaviors may be responsible for these findings (Breslau et al., 1988). Further study is needed to determine whether emotional functioning in girls is less affected by disease, or whether girls' behavior is affected in ways that are not well measured by the parent and teacher ratings commonly employed in follow-up research.

METHODOLOGICAL ISSUES

In a study that examined a subset of 22 research papers addressing outcome from bacterial meningitis, Radetsky (1992) identified a range of methodological limitations including incomplete data, poor study design, lack of specification of outcome measures, and inappropriate data analysis. Radetsky also noted that studies varied widely in terms of the age range of children followed and the length of follow-up. Inconsistencies in reports of disease sequelae may thus be attributed in large part to the methodological failings of much of the research in this area. Methodological limitations are particularly problematic in studies of more subtle neurobehavioral sequelae, where demarcations between normal and abnormal findings are less clear-cut than is the case for neurological abnormalities. Measurement of developmental change also presents special challenges, given the fact that many tests are applicable over only relatively narrow age spans.

Of particular importance in studies of the sequelae of bacterial meningitis, which may be relatively small in magnitude, are two factors: establishment of a sufficiently large and representative clinical sample, and comparison with an appropriate control group. Most research in this area has involved follow-up of small samples of children, limiting statistical power for detection of disease effects (Emmett et al., 1980; Feldman & Michaels, 1988; Tejani et al., 1982). Estimates of disease consequences may also be distorted by biased sample selection, overinclusion of children with significant deficits, or exclusion of those with the most serious sequelae. The possibility of sampling bias is especially acute in retrospective studies, where samples are established via perusal of medical records, where judgments of medical factors are based on unstandardized recording practices, and/or where participating centers may have unrepresentative referral patterns. Many of these limitations may be overcome through prospective study of consecutive admissions and the use of standard protocols for assessing illness and outcome variables. Prospective data collection also permits assessment of potential biases due to selective attrition, as well as inclusion of measures of direct relevance to study hypotheses (Rutter, 1988).

The recruitment of control groups has been relatively common in recent research in this area, although the manner in which these groups are formed is likely to be critical in detecting more subtle disease sequelae. Many studies have employed sibling comparison groups (Sell, Webb, et al., 1972; Taylor et al., 1990; Tejani et al., 1982) as a means of controlling for social and family background factors. Children matched in this manner, however, will necessarily differ in age. In addition, siblings may be disadvantaged because of stresses on families imposed by the index children's disease per se or disease-related developmental sequelae. An alternative strategy is to have healthy age-matched peers serve as controls (Grimwood et al., 1995). The latter comparison group provides for more optimal control of age, but makes it imperative to match groups carefully on socioeconomic factors and ethnicity.

Although time since illness may play a critical role in determining the outcome of early neurological insults (Dennis, 1988), many studies have failed to provide data on the interval between disease onset and testing. To the extent that children fall increasing further behind age expectations over time, or experience latent disease effects, both age at testing and time since insult must be taken into consideration (Anderson & Moore, 1995; Dennis, 1988, 1996; Dennis & Barnes, 1994; Godber, Smibert, Anderson, & Ekert, 1995; Taylor et al., 1992). Longitudinal studies are needed to clarify the relationship of these factors to long-term disease consequences. There is also a need to follow children prospectively from hospital discharge, in order to determine early manifestations of sequelae and to explore factors that contribute to recovery of function. Those studies that have followed post-meningitic children from time of acute illness support the existence of a range of acute disease consequences, and they document an association between the consequences and later outcomes (Anderson et al., 1987; Ferry et al., 1982; Hore, 1992). Further work is required to investigate the natural history of recovery from the infection, to separate transient from more persisting effects, to determine whether sequelae vary with a child's age and developmental stage, and to identify conditions that may promote or retard ongoing development and recovery.

A further shortcoming of many past studies relates to test selection. Much of the early research on outcomes of bacterial meningitis employed only limited assessments of potential cognitive and educational sequelae, most often restricted to tests of overall IQ and selected measures of language skills and academic competence. Furthermore, the high degree of structure inherent in IQ-type tests may mask many of the more subtle executive dysfunctions that can occur secondary to pediatric brain insults. Neuropsychological assessment can be more sensitive than IQ testing to disease sequelae. Neuropsychological procedures, however, are often poorly standardized or may have uncertain reliability or validity. Although there is no substitute for rigorous psychometric development of these procedures, large samples of control children can help to overcome some of these limitations (Taylor et al., 1992).

A final and especially critical methodological limitation is the failure of researchers to investigate outcomes in relation to indices of brain insult. Studies to date have graded the likelihood of brain damage based on the presence versus absence of acute-phase neurological complications (Grimwood et al., 1995; Taylor et al., 1992). Although this approach represents a significant advance over previous methods, further efforts are needed to examine the implications of specific neurological complications and to enhance measurement of neuropathology (Taylor et al., in press). Although few studies have examined the prognostic significance of electroencephalograms and CT scans, the lack of correspondence between findings from MRI and disease sequelae is also disappointing (Lebel et al., 1989) and suggests a need for more sophisticated measurement techniques.

CONCLUSIONS AND FUTURE DIRECTIONS

Childhood bacterial meningitis is a disease that is most commonly contracted by infants and young children. Although improvements in treatments have reduced mortality, and more recent vaccinations have led to decreases in the incidence of some forms of the disease, research suggests that considerable morbidity remains. Approximately 40% of those contracting the disease will experience acute neurological complications, such as seizures, hydrocephalus, hemiplegia, and visual and auditory impairments. In many cases these acute sequelae resolve over time; however, studies consistently find that about 20% of survivors experience ongoing neurological consequences.

More subtle neurobehavioral sequelae, including cognitive, educational, and behavioral problems, are found in many survivors. However, the percentage of children affected and the nature of their deficits vary considerably across studies. Early studies identified deficits in global IQ measures. Studies completed in the last decade and involving efforts to recruit total hospital samples have revealed more specific neuropsychological sequelae, with relatively little impairment in IQ scores (Grimwood et al., 1995; Taylor et al., 1990). Deficits have included language impairment, motor incoordination, perceptual weaknesses, memory problems, executive dysfunctions, and academic difficulties.

Recent research suggests that some of the inconsistencies in disease outcomes across studies may reflect the changing nature of problems experienced by postmeningitic children as they move through the different developmental stages. For example. gross motor deficits appear to be most evident in the postdischarge phase, whereas fine motor incoordination, perceptual deficits, and language and behavioral difficulties may become more discernible as children with early-onset disease enter their preschool years (Anderson et al., 1987; Anderson, Grimwood, Keir, Nolan, & Catroppa, 1992; Hore, 1992). Educational difficulties are commonly documented in studies employing elementary-school-age children, with evidence that such problems are less apparent in adolescent samples. However, high-level language and executive deficits have emerged in this older age group (P. Anderson et al., 1997; Pentland et al., in press).

This shifting pattern of sequelae is consistent with the model Dennis (1988) has proposed to explain the impact of early cerebral insult. According to this model, skills that were well established prior to neurological insult are less affected than is the acquisition of new skills. Even transient disruptions in brain functioning may thus interfere with learning processes that are underway at the time of insult. To the extent that samples vary in age of onset, Dennis's model would predict variability in disease sequelae. Further longitudinal studies are needed to plot the natural history of the disease into adulthood, and to investigate age-related changes in sequelae. Because meningitis occurs at varying ages early in life and in children who were neurologically normal prior to the disease, follow-up of the survivors of this disease may shed new light on the effects of the three age-related factors: age at insult, time since insult, and age at assessment (Taylor & Alden, 1997).

The interaction between disease factors and psychosocial and environmental factors also deserves further study. The relative predictive value of disease-related variables may depend on how outcomes are assessed, and even on time since illness. Some abilities may be highly vulnerable to environmental modification and thus amenable to intervention. In contrast, academic achievement, verbal knowledge, and behavioral adjustment may be more susceptible to social influences, with disease factors more closely related to fluid intelligence or processing efficiency (Taylor & Schatschneider, 1992a). Over time environmental factors, such as family functioning, socioeconomic status, and access to remedial resources, may contribute more critical determinants of outcome than illness-related variables may (Aylward, 1992). A more complete understanding of the conjoint influences of social and biological factors will require large-scale, longitudinal research.

Recent research findings indicate that many survivors of meningitis have a favorable prognosis (Taylor et al., in press). Children who experience acute neurological complications do more poorly than those with an uneventful recovery course. Persisting or focal neurological signs and younger age at illness represent additional risk factors. However, even children without acute-phase complications may experience deficits, and it is unlikely that we have identified all critical predictor factors. Current indices of disease severity have limited predictive validity, due in large part to our incomplete understanding of the neural mechanisms responsible for brain insults and of the ways in which neurological derangement (even if transient) may affect the developing CNS. More powerful predictions may be possible with the application of advanced neuroimaging techniques and monitoring of neuropsychological functioning from the point of hospital discharge.

Although neurological outcomes of childhood bacterial meningitis are usually readily apparent, documentation of subtle neurobehavioral sequelae will require both larger sample sizes and attempts to evaluate outcomes in selected subgroups of children, such as children with different types of transient neurological complications or those with persisting neurological disorders. IQ measures are likely to be less sensitive to the consequences of early brain insult than measures of more specific skills, such as tests of memory and learning, attention, and executive abilities (Taylor et al., 1993). Appraisal of the impact of meningitis on a child's level of functioning at home and at school also requires inclusion of measures of behavior, academic achievement, and adaptive abilities. Appreciation of neuropsychological deficits, moreover, may help guide educational and behavioral programs designed to enhance learning abilities and day-to-day functioning. A child with perceptual or attentional problems, for example, may have different special educational needs than a child with a language-based learning problem (Taylor & Schatschneider, 1992a).

Finally, documentation of disease sequelae suggests the need for ongoing follow-up of postmeningitic children, at least until school entry. In this manner, subtle deficits may be identified and treated early. Although children who experience neurological complications are at greater risk for sequelae, reports of disease consequences in children without complications argue for developmental monitoring of all survivors. Equally important is the need to work closely with parents, to ensure awareness of the potential problems and an openness toward early treatment and intervention.

REFERENCES

Adams, R. D., Kubik, C. S., & Bonner, F. J. (1948). The clinical and pathological aspects of influenzal meningitis. *Archives of Pediatrics, 65*, 354–376.

Adams, W. G., Deaver, K. A., Cochi, S. L., Plikaytis, B. D., Zell, E. R., Broome, C. V., & Wenger, J. D. (1993). Decline of childhood *Haemophilus influenzae* type b (Hib) disease in the Hib vaccine era. *Journal of the American Medical Association, 269*, 221–226.

Anderson, P., Anderson, V., Grimwood, K., Nolan, T., Catroppa, C., & Keir, E. (1997). Neuropsychological consequences of bacterial meningitis: A prospective study. *Journal of the International Neuropsychological Society, 3,* 47–48.

Anderson, V., Bond, L., Catroppa, C., Grimwood, K., Keir, E., & Nolan, T. (1997). Childhood bacterial meningitis: Impact of age at illness and medical complications on long term outcome. *Journal of the International Neuropsychological Society, 3,* 147–158.

Anderson, V., Godber, T., Smibert, E., & Ekert, H. (1997). Neurobehavioral sequelae following cranial irradiation and chemotherapy in children: An analysis of risk factors. *Pediatric Rehabilitation, 1,* 63–76.

Anderson, V., Grimwood, K., Keir, E., Nolan, T., & Catroppa, C. (1992). Long-term sequelae of bacterial meningitis in childhood. *Journal of Clinical and Experimental Neuropsychology, 14,* 387.

Anderson, V., Leaper, P. M., & Judd, K. (1987). Bacterial meningitis in childhood: Neuropsychological sequelae. In G. R. Gates (Ed.), *Developmental neuropsychology: Proceedings of the 12th Annual Brain Impairment Conference, ASSBI, Melbourne* (pp. 153–168).

Anderson, V., & Moore, C. (1995). Age at injury as a predictor of outcome following pediatric head injury: A longitudinal perspective. *Child Neuropsychology, 2,* 187–202.

Anderson, V., Smibert, E., Ekert, H., & Godber, T. (1994). Intellectual, educational, and behavioural sequelae following cranial irradiation and chemotherapy. *Archives of Disease in Childhood, 70,* 476–483.

Anonymous. (1990). Decline in *Haemophilus influenzae* type b meningitis—Seattle–King County, Washington, 1984–1989. *Morbidity and Mortality Weekly Report, 39,* 924–925.

Ashwal, S., Stringer, W., Tomass, L., Schneider, S., Thompson, J., & Perkin, R. (1990). Cerebral blood flow and carbon dioxide reactivity in children with bacterial meningitis. *Journal of Pediatrics, 117,* 523–530.

Aylward, G. (1992). The relationship between environmental risk and developmental outcome. *Developmental Medicine and Child Neurology, 13,* 222–229.

Baker, R. C., Kummer, A. W., Schultz, J. R., Ho, M., & Gonzalez del Rey, J. (1996). Neurodevelopmental outcome of infants with viral meningitis in the first three months of life. *Clinical Pediatrics, June,* 295–301.

Baraff, L. J., Lee, S. I., & Schriger, D. L. (1993). Outcomes of bacterial meningitis in children: A meta-analysis. *Pediatric Infectious Disease Journal, 12,* 389–394.

Bendersky, M., & Lewis, M. (1994). Environmental risk, biological risk, and developmental outcome. *Developmental Psychology, 30,* 484–494.

Bergman, I., Painter, M. J., Wald, E. R., Chiponis, D., Holland, A. L., & Taylor, H. G. (1987). Outcome of children with enteroviral meningitis during the first year of life. *Journal of Pediatrics, 110,* 705–709.

Breslau, N., Klein, N., & Allen, L. (1988). Very low birthweight: Behavioral sequelae at nine years of age. *Journal of Behavioral and Developmental Pediatrics, 27,* 605–612.

Broome, C. V. (1987). Epidemiology of *Haemophilus influenzae* type b infections in the United States. *Pediatric Infectious Disease Journal, 6,* 779–782.

Bortolussi, S., & Seeliger, H. D. (1990). Listeriosis. In J. S. Reminngton & J. O. Klein (Eds.), *Infectious diseases in the fetus and newborn infant* (3rd ed., pp. 812–833). Philadelphia: W. B. Saunders.

Cherry, J. D. (1992). Aseptic meningitis and viral meningitis. In R. D. Feigin & J. D. Cherry (Eds.), *Textbook of pediatric infectious diseases* (3rd ed., Vol. 1, pp. 439–445). Philadelphia: W. B. Saunders.

Claesson, R., Trollfors, B., Jodol, U., & Rosenhall, U. (1984). Incidence and prognosis of *Haemophilus influenzae* meningitis in children in a Swedish region. *Pediatric Infectious Disease Journal, 3,* 35–39.

Clements, D. A., & Gilbert, G. L. (1990). Immunization against *Haemophilus influenzae*. *Medical Journal of Australia, 152,* 397–398.

D'Angio, C. T., Froehlke, R. G., Plank, G. A., Meehan, D. J., Aguilar, C. M., Lande, M. B., & Hugar, L. (1995). Long-term outcome of *Haemophilus influenzae* meningitis in Navajo Indian children. *Archives of Pediatrics and Adolescent Medicine, 149,* 1001–1008.

Davies, P. A. (1989). Long term effects of meningitis. *Developmental Medicine and Child Neurology, 31,* 398–400.

Davies, P. A., & Rudd, R. T. (1994). *Neonatal meningitis* (Clinics in Developmental Medicine No. 132). Cambridge, UK: Cambridge University Press.

Dennis, M. (1980). Capacity and strategy for syntactic comprehension after left or right hemidecortication. *Brain and Language, 10,* 287–317.

Dennis, M. (1988). Language and the young damaged brain. In T. Boll & B. Bryant (Eds.), *Clinical neuropsychology and brain function: Research, measurement, and practice* (pp. 85–123). Washington, DC: American Psychological Association.

Dennis, M. (1996). Acquired disorders of language in children. In T. E. Feinberg & M. J. Farah (Eds.), *Behavioral neurology and neuropsychology* (pp. 1109–1134). New York: McGraw-Hill.

Dennis, M., & Barnes, M. (1994). Developmental aspects of neuropsychology: Childhood. In D. Zaidel (Ed.), *Handbook of perception and cognition: Vol. 15. Neuropsychology* (pp. 219–246). New York: Academic Press.

Dennis, M., Spiegler, B. J., Hetherington, C. R., & Greenberg, M. L. (1996). Neuropsychological sequelae of the treatment of children with medulloblastoma. *Journal of Neuro-Oncology, 29,* 91–101.

Dodge, P. R. (1986). Sequelae of bacterial meningitis. *Pediatric Infectious Disease Journal, 5,* 618–620.

Dodge, P. R., Davis, H., Feigin, R. D., Holmes, S. J., Kaplan, S. L., Jubelirer, D. P., et al. (1984). Prospective evaluation of hearing impairment as a sequela of acute bacterial meningitis. *New England Journal of Medicine, 311,* 869–874.

Dodge, P. R., & Schwartz, M. N. (1965). Bacterial meningitis: A review of selected aspects. II. Special neurological problems: Post meningitis complications and clinicopathological correlations. *New England Journal of Medicine, 272,* 945–960.

Edwards, M. S., Rench, M. A., Haffar, A. A. M., Murphy, M. A., Desmond, M. M., & Baker, C. J. (1985). Long-term sequelae of group B streptococcal meningitis in infants. *Journal of Pediatrics, 106,* 717–722.

Eiser, C. (1978). Intellectual abilities among survivors of childhood leukemia as a function of CNS irradiation. *Archives of Disease in Childhood, 53,* 391–395.

Emmett, M., Jeffery, H., Chandler, D., & Dugdale, A. E. (1980). Sequelae of *Haemophilus influenzae* meningitis. *Australian Paediatric Journal, 16,* 90–93.

Escalona, S. (1982). Babies at double hazard: Early development of infants at biologic and social risks. *Pediatrics, 70,* 670–676.

Ewing-Cobbs, L., Miner, M. E., Fletcher, J. M., & Levin, H. (1989). Intellectual, language, and motor sequelae following closed head injury in infants and preschoolers. *Journal of Pediatric Psychology, 14,* 531–547.

Farmer, K., MacArthur, B. A., & Clay, M. M. (1975). A follow-up study of 15 cases of neonatal litis due to Coxsackie virus B5. *Journal of Pediatrics, 87,* 568–571.

Feigin, R. D. (1987). Bacterial meningitis beyond the neonatal period. In R. D. Feigin & J. D. Cherry (Eds.), *Textbook of pediatric infectious diseases* (2nd ed., Vol. 1, pp. 439–465). Philadelphia: W. B. Saunders.

Feigin, R. D. (1992). Bacterial meningitis beyond the neonatal period. In R. D. Feigin & J. D. Cherry (Eds.), *Textbook of pediatric infectious diseases* (3rd ed., Vol. 1, pp. 401–428). Philadelphia: W. B. Saunders.

Feigin, R. D., McCracken, G. H., & Klein, J. O. (1992). Diagnosis and management of meningitis. *Pediatric Infectious Disease Journal, 11,* 785–814.

Feigin, R. D., Stechenberg, B. W., Chang, M. J., Dunkle, L. M., Wong, M. L., Palkes, H., Dodge, P. R., & Davis, H. (1976). Prospective evaluation of treatment of *Haemophilus influenzae* meningitis. *Journal of Pediatrics, 100,* 209–212.

Feldman, H., & Michaels, R. (1988). Academic achievement in children 10 to 12 years after *Haemophilus influenzae* meningitis. *Pediatrics, 81,* 339–344.

Feldman, W. E., Ginsburg, C. M., McCracken, G. H., Allen, D., Ahmann, P., Graham, J., & Graham, L. (1982). Relation of concentration of *Haemophilus influenzae* type b in cerebrospinal fluid to late sequelae of patients with meningitis. *Journal of Pediatrics, 100,* 209–212.

Ferry, P., Culbertson, J., Cooper, J., Sitton, A., & Sell, S. (1982). Sequelae of *Haemophilus* meningitis: Preliminary report of a long-term follow-up study. In S. Sell & P. Wright (Eds.), *Haemophilus influenzae: Epidemiology, immunology, and prevention of disease* (pp. 111–116). New York: Elsevier Biomedical.

Franco, S. M., Cornelius, V. E., & Andrewes, B. F. (1992). Long-term outcome of neonatal meningitis. *American Journal of Diseases of Children, 146,* 567–571.

Fraser, G. R. (1976). *The causes of profound hearing loss in childhood.* Baltimore: John Hopkins University Press.

Gardner, M. (1979). *Expressive One-Word Picture Vocabulary Test.* Nocata, CA: Academic Therapeutic.

Gary, N., Powers, N., & Todd, J. K. (1989). Clinical identification and comparative prognosis of high-risk patients with *Haemophilus influenzae* meningitis. *American Journal of Diseases of Children, 143,* 307–311.

Girgis, N. I., Farid, Z, Mikhail, I. A., Farray, I., Sultan, Y., & Kilpatrick, M. (1989). Dexamethasone treatment for bacterial meningitis in children and adults. *Pediatric Infectious Disease Journal, 8,* 848–851.

Godber, T., Anderson, V., Smibert, E., & Ekert, H. (1995). Cranial irradiation for the treatment of acute lymphoblastic leukemia: Long-term sequelae. In C. Haslam, J. Ewing, R. Farnbach, U. Johns, & B. Weekes (Eds.), *Cognitive dysfunction in health, disease and disorder: Proceedings of the 17th Annual Brain Impairment Conference* (pp. 1–22). Canberra: Academic Press.

Grimwood, K., Anderson, V. A., Bond, L., Catroppa, C., Hore, R. L., Keir, E. H., & Nolan, T. (1995). Adverse outcomes of bacterial meningitis in school-age survivors. *Pediatrics, 95,* 646–656.

Grimwood, K., Nolan, T., Bond, L., Anderson, V., Catroppa, C., & Keir, E. (1996). Risk factors for adverse outcomes of bacterial meningitis. *Journal of Pediatric Child Health, 32,* 457–462.

Hanna, J. N. (1990). The epidemiology of invasive *Haemophilus influenzae* infections in children under five years of age in the Northern Territory: A three year study. *Medical Journal of Australia, 152,* 234–240.

Haslam, R. H., Allen, J. R., Dorsen, M. M., & Kanofsky, D. (1977). The sequelae of group B streptococcal meningitis in early infancy. *American Journal of Diseases of Children, 131,* 845–849.

Herson, V. C., & Todd, J. K. (1977). Prediction of morbidity in *Haemophilus influenzae* meningitis. *Pediatrics, 59,* 35–39.

Hore, R. (1992). *Bacterial meningitis in childhood.* Unpublished doctoral dissertation, University of Melbourne, Parkville, Victoria, Australia.

Horowitz, S. J., Boxerbaum, B., & O'Bell, J. (1980). Cerebral herniation in bacterial meningitis in childhood. *Annals of Neurology, 7,* 534–528.

Jadavji, T., Biggar, W. D., Gold, R., & Prober, C. G. (1986). Sequelae of acute bacterial meningitis in children treated for seven days. *Pediatrics, 78,* 21–25.

Kandel, E. R., Schwartz, J. H., & Jessel, T. M. (1991). *Principles of neuroscience* (3rd ed.). New York: Elsevier.

Kaplan, S. L., Smith, E., Wills, C., & Feigin, R. D. (1986). Association between preadmission oral antibiotic therapy and cerebrospinal fluid findings and sequelae caused by *Haemophilus influenzae* type b. *Pediatric Infectious Disease Journal, 5,* 626–632.

Klein, J. O., Feigin, R. D., & McCracken, G. H. (1986). Report of the task force on diagnosis and management of meningitis. *Pediatrics, 78*(Suppl.), 959–982.

Klein, J. O., & Marcy, S. M. (1990). Bacterial sepsis and meningitis. In J. S. Remington & J. O. Klein (Eds.), *Infectious diseases of the fetus and newborn infant* (3rd ed., pp. 601–656). Philadelphia: W. B. Saunders.

Kresky, B., Buchbinder, S., & Greenberg, I. (1962). The incidence of neurological residua in children after recovery from bacterial meningitis. *Archives of Pediatrics, 79,* 63–71.

Kriel, R., Krach, L., & Panser, L. (1989). Closed head injury: Comparison of children younger and older than six years of age. *Pediatric Neurology, 5,* 296–300.

Lawson, D., Metcalfe, M., & Pampiglione, G. (1965). Meningitis in childhood. *British Medical Journal, i,* 557–562.

Lebel, M. H., Freij, B. J., Syrogiannopoulos, G. A., Chrane, D. F., Hoyt, M. J., Stewart, S., Kennard, B. D., Olsen, K. D., & McCracken, G. H. (1988). Dexamethasone therapy for bacterial meningitis: Results of two double-blind placebo-controlled studies. *New England Journal of Medicine, 319,* 964–971.

Lebel, M. H., Hoyt, M. J., Waagner, D. C., Rollins, N. K., Finitzo, T., & McCracken, G. H., Jr. (1989). Magnetic resonance imaging and dexamethasone therapy for bacterial meningitis. *American Journal of Diseases of Children, 143,* 301–306.

Lenneberg, E. H. (1967). *Biological foundations of language.* New York: Wiley.

Levin, H. S., Benton, A. L., & Grossman, R. (1982). *Neurobehavioral consequences of closed head injury.* New York: Oxford University Press.

Lindberg, J., Rosenhall, U., Nylen, O., & Ringner, A. (1977). Long term outcome of *Haemophilus influenzae* meningitis related to antibiotic treatment. *Pediatrics, 60,* 1–6.

Lutsar, I., Siirde, T., & Soopold., T. (1995). Long term follow-up of Estonian children after bacterial meningitis. *Pediatric Infectious Disease Journal, 14,* 624–625.

McIntyre, P., Jepson, R., Leeder, S., & Irwig, I. (1993). The outcome of childhood *Haemophilus influenzae* meningitis: A population based study. *Medical Journal of Australia, 159,* 766–772.

McMenamin, J. B., & Volpe, J. J. (1984). Bacterial meningitis in infancy: Effects of intracranial pressure and cerebral blood flow velocity. *Neurology, 34,* 500–504.

Marwick, C. (1991). *Haemophilus influenzae* declining among young? *Journal of the American Medical Association, 266,* 3398–3399.

Mertsola, J., Kennedy, W. A., Waagner, D., Saez-Llorens, X., Olsen, K., Hansen, E. J., & McCracken, G. H., Jr. (1991). Endotoxin concentrations in cerebrospinal fluid correlated with clinical severity and neurological outcome of *Haemophilus influenzae* type b meningitis. *American Journal of Diseases of Children, 145,* 1079–1103.

Moss, P. D. (1982). Outcome of meningococcal group b meningitis. *Archives of Disease in Childhood, 57,* 616–621.

Mustafa, M. M., & McCracken, G. H., Jr. (1992). Perinatal bacterial diseases. In R. D. Feigin & J. D. Cherry (Eds.), *Textbook of pediatric infectious diseases* (3rd ed., Vol. 1, pp. 891–924). Philadelphia: W. B. Saunders.

Mustafa, M. M., Ramilo, O., Saez-Llorens, X., Mertsola, J., & McCracken, G. H. (1989). Role of tumor necrosis factor alpha (cachectin) in experimental and clinical bacterial meningitis. *Pediatric Infectious Disease Journal*, 8, 907–908.

Peltola, H., Kilpi, T., & Antilla, M. (1992). Rapid disappearance of *Haemophilus influenzae* type b meningitis after routine childhood immunizations with conjugate vaccines. *Lancet*, 340, 592–594.

Pentland, L., Anderson, V., & Wrennall, J. (in press). Bacterial meningitis: Implications of age at illness for language development. *Journal of the International Neuropsychological Society*.

Pomeroy, S. l., Holmes, S. J., Dodge, P. R., & Feigin, R. D. (1990). Seizures and other neurological sequelae of bacterial meningitis in children. *New England Journal of Medicine*, 323, 1651–1657.

Quagliarello, V., & Scheld, W. M. (1992). Bacterial meningitis: Pathogenesis, pathophysiology, and progress. *New England Journal of Medicine*, 327, 864–872.

Radetsky, M. (1992). Duration of symptoms and outcome in bacterial meningitis: An analysis of causation and the implications of a delay in diagnosis. *Pediatric Infectious Disease Journal*, 11, 694–698.

Ramilo, O., Mustafa, M. M., & Saez-Llorens, X. (1989). Role of interleukin 1-beta in meningeal inflammation. *Pediatric Infectious Disease Journal*, 8, 909–910.

Rankur, J., Aram, D., & Horowitz, S. (1980). *A comparison of right and left hemiplegic children's language ability*. Paper presented at the meeting of the International Neuropsychological Society, San Francisco.

Rorabaugh, M. L., Berlin, L. E., Heldrich, F., Roberts, K., Rosenberg, L. A., Dorin, T., & Modlin, J. F. (1993). Aseptic meningitis in infants younger than two years of age: Acute illness and neurological complications. *Pediatrics*, 92, 206–211.

Rorke, L. B., & Pitts, F. W. (1963). Purulent meningitis: The pathological basis of clinical manifestations. *Clinical Pediatrics*, 2, 64–71.

Ross, G., Lipper, E., & Auld, P. (1990). Social competence and behavior problems in premature children at school age. *Pediatrics*, 86, 391–397.

Rourke, B. P. (1988). The syndrome of nonverbal learning disabilities: Developmental manifestations in neurological disease, disorder, and dysfunction. *Clinical Neuropsychologist*, 2, 293–330.

Rubenstein, C. L., Varni, J. W., & Katz, E. R. (1990). Cognitive functioning in long-term survivors of childhood leukemia: A prospective analysis. *Journal of Developmental and Behavioral Pediatrics*, 11, 301–305.

Rutter, M. (1981). Psychological sequelae of brain damage in children. *American Journal of Psychiatry*, 138, 1533–1534.

Rutter, M. (1988). Longitudinal data on the study of causal processes: Some uses and some pitfalls. In M. Rutter (Ed.), *Studies of psychosocial risk* (pp. 1–28). New York: Cambridge University Press.

Schlech, W. F., Ward, J. I., Band, J. D., Hightower, A., Fraser, D. W., & Broome, C. V. (1985). Bacterial meningitis in the United States, 1978 through 1981: The National Bacterial Meningitis Surveillance Study. *Journal of the American Medical Association*, 253, 1749–1754.

Schoeman, C. J. (1990). The epidemiology and outcome of childhood tuberculosis meningitis. *South African Medical Journal*, 78, 245–247.

Sell, S. (1983). Long-term sequelae of bacterial meningitis in children. *Pediatric Infectious Disease Journal*, 2, 90–93.

Sell, S. (1987). *Haemophilus influenzae* type b meningitis: Manifestations and long term sequelae. *Pediatric Infectious Diseases Journal*, 6, 775–778.

Sell, S., Merrill, R. E., Doyne, E. O., & Zimsky, E. P. (1972). Long term sequelae of *Haemophilus influenzae* meningitis. *Pediatrics*, 49, 206–211.

Sell, S., Webb, W. W., Pate, J. E., & Doyne, E. O. (1972). Psychological sequelae to bacterial meningitis: Two controlled studies. *Pediatrics*, 49, 212–217.

Sells, C. J., Carpenter, R. L., & Ray, C. G. (1975). Sequelae of central nervous system enterovirus infections. *New England Journal of Medicine*, 293, 1–4.

Smith, A. L. (1988). Neurologic sequelae of meningitis. *New England Journal of Medicine*, 319, 1012–1014.

Smith, J. F., & Landing B. H. (1960). Mechanisms of brain damage of *H. influenzae* meningitis. *Journal of Neuropathology and Experimental Neurology*, 19, 248–265.

Snyder, R. D., Stovring, I., Cushing, A. H., Davis, L. E., & Hardy, T. L. (1981). Cerebral infaction in childhood bacterial meningitis. *Journal of Neurology, Neurosurgery and Psychiatry*, 44, 581–585.

Sommerfelt, K., Ellertsen, B., & Markestad, T. (1993). Personality and behaviour in eight-year-old children with birth weight under 1500 g. *Acta Paediatrica*, 82, 723–728.

Sproles, E. T., Azerrad, J., Williamson, C., & Merrill, R. E. (1969). Meningitis due to *Haemophilus influenzae*: Long term sequelae. *Pediatrics*, 75, 782–788.

Stovring, J., & Snyder, R. (1980). Computed tomography in childhood bacterial meningitis. *Journal of Pediatrics*, 96, 820–823.

Takala, A. K., & Clements, D. A. (1992). Socioeconomic risk factors for invasive *Haemophilus influenzae* type b disease. *Journal of Infectious Diseases, 165*(Suppl. 1), S11–S15.

Taylor, H. G. (1984). Early brain injury and cognitive development. In C. Almli & S. Finger (Eds.), *Early brain damage: Research orientations and clinical observations* (pp. 325–345). New York: Academic Press.

Taylor, H. G., & Alden, J. (1997). Age-related differences in outcome following childhood brain insults: An introduction and overview. *Journal of the International Neuropsychological Society.*

Taylor, H. G., Barry, C., & Schatschneider, C. (1993). School-age consequences of *Haemophilus influenzae* type b meningitis. *Journal of Clinical Child Psychology, 22,* 196–206.

Taylor, H. G., Klein, N., Schatschneider, C., & Hack, M. (1999). *Predictors of early school age outcomes in very low birthweight children.* Manuscript submitted for publication.

Taylor, H. G., Michaels, R. H., Mazur, P. M., Bauer, R. E., & Liden, C. B. (1984). Intellectual, neuropsychological, and achievement outcomes in children six to eight years after recovery from *Haemophilus influenzae* meningitis. *Pediatrics, 74,* 198–205.

Taylor, H. G., Mills, E. L., Ciampi, A., DuBerger, R., Watters, G. V., Gold, R., MacDonald., & Michaels, R. H. (1990). The sequelae of *Haemophilus influenzae* meningitis in school age children. *New England Journal of Medicine, 323,* 1657–1663.

Taylor, H. G., & Schatschneider, C. (1992a). Child neuropsychological assessment: A test of basic assumptions. *Clinical Neuropsychologist, 6,* 259–275.

Taylor, H. G., & Schatschneider, C. (1992b). Academic achievement following childhood brain disease: Implications for the concept of learning disabilities. *Journal of Learning Disabilities, 25,* 630–638.

Taylor, H. G., Schatschneider, C., & Minich, N. (1999). *Longitudinal outcomes of haemophilus influenzae meningitis in school-aged children.* Manuscript submitted for publication.

Taylor, H. G., Schatschneider, C., Petrill, S., Barry, C. T., & Owens, C. (1996). Executive dysfunction in children with early brain disease: Outcomes post-*Haemophilus influenzae* meningitis. *Developmental Neuropsychology, 12,* 35–51.

Taylor, H. G., Schatschneider, C., & Rich, D. (1992). Sequelae of *Haemophilus influenzae* meningitis: Implications for the study of brain disease and development. In M. Tramontana & S. Hooper (Eds.), *Advances in child neuropsychology* (Vol. 1, pp. 50–108). New York: Springer-Verlag.

Taylor, H. G., Schatschneider, C., Watters, G. V., Mills, E. L., Gold, R., MacDonald, N., & Michaels, R. H. (in press). Acute-phase neurological complications of *Haemophilus influenzae* type b meningitis: Association with developmental problems at school age. *Journal of Child Neurology.*

Tejani, A., Dobias, B., & Sambursky, J. (1982). Long term prognosis after *H. influenzae* meningitis: Prospective evaluation. *Developmental Medicine and Child Neurology, 24,* 338–343.

Teuber, M. L. (1962). Behaviour after cerebral lesions in children. *Developmental Medicine and Child Neurology, 4,* 3–20.

Thomas, D. G. (1992). Outcome of pediatric bacterial meningitis 1979–1989. *Medical Journal of Australia, 157,* 519–520.

Thomas, V. H., & Hopkins, I. J. (1984). Arteriographic demonstrations of vascular lesions in the study of neurological deficit in advanced *Haemophilus influenzae* meningitis. *Developmental Medicine and Child Neurology, 14,* 783–787.

Tomasz, A., & Saukkonen, K. (1989). The nature of cell wall derived inflammatory components of pneumococci. *Pediatric Infectious Disease Journal, 8,* 902–903.

Tureen, J. H., Dworkin, R. J., Kennedy, S. L., Sachdeva, M., & Sande, M. A. (1990). Loss of cerebrovascular autoregulation in experimental meningitis in rabbits. *Journal of Clinical Investigation, 85,* 577–581.

Vienny, H., Despland, P. A., Lutschg, J., Deonna, T., Dutoit-Marco, M. L., & Gander, C. (1984). Early diagnosis and evaluation of deafness in childhood bacterial meningitis: A study using brainstem auditory evoked potentials. *Pediatrics, 73,* 579–586.

Waber, D., Urion, D. K., Tarbell, N., Niemeyer, C., Gelber, R., & Sallan, S. (1990). Late effects of central nervous system treatment of acute lymphoblastic leukemia in children are sex-dependent. *Developmental Medicine and Child Neurology, 32,* 238–248.

Wald, E. R., Bergman, I., Taylor, H. G., Chiponis, D., Porter, C., & Kubek, K. (1986). Long-term outcome of Group B streptococcal meningitis. *Pediatrics, 77,* 217–221.

Ward, J. J., Margolis, H. S., Lum, M. K., Fraser, D. W., Bender, T. R., & Anderson, P. (1981). *Haemophilus influenzae* disease in Alaskan Eskimos: Characteristics of a population with an unusual incidence of invasive disease. *Lancet, i,* 1281–1284.

Washburn, T. C., Medearis, D. N., & Childs, B. (1965). Sex differences in susceptibility to infection. *Pediatrics, 35,* 57–64.

Weinberg, G. A., Murphy, T. V., & Granoff, D. M. (1990). *Haemophilus influenzae* type b polysaccaride–

diptheria toxoid conjugate vaccine in vaccinated children who developed *Haemophilus* disease. *Pediatrics, 86,* 617–620.

Wenger, J. D., Hightower, A. W., Facklam, R. R., Gaventa, S., Broome, C. V., & the Bacterial Meningitis Study Group. (1990). Bacterial meningitis in the United States, 1986: Report of a multistate surveillance study. *Journal of Infectious Disease, 162,* 1316–1323.

Wilfert, C. M., Thompson, R. J., Saunder, T. R., O'Quinn, A., Zeller, J., & Blacharsh, J. (1981). Longitudinal assessment of children with enteroviral meningitis during the first three months of life. *Pediatrics, 67,* 811–815.

Wright, L., & Jimmerson, S. (1971). Intellectual sequelae of *Haemophilus influenzae* meningitis. *Journal of Abnormal Psychology, 77,* 181–183.

Wright, M., & Nolan, T. (1994). Impact of cyanotic heart disease on school performance. *Archives of Disease in Childhood, 71,* 64–70.

Wrightson, P., McGinn, V., & Gronwall, D. (1995). Mild head injury in preschool children: Evidence that it can be associated with a persisting cognitive defect. *Journal of Neurology, Neurosurgery and Psychiatry, 59,* 375–380.

7

NEUROFIBROMATOSIS

BARTLETT D. MOORE, III
MARTHA B. DENCKLA

HISTORICAL OVERVIEW

Neurofibromatosis (NF), also known as von Recklinghausen disease, was first depicted in literature and art during the 16th century, but not until the late 1800s was it described clinically and scientifically by the German pathologist Friedrich Daniel von Recklinghausen (Crump, 1981). NF is often mistakenly referred to as the "Elephant Man's" disease, after the "Elephant Man," Joseph Merrick, whose story has been dramatized on screen and stage. Merrick actually had Proteus syndrome, a disorder that has clinical characteristics (cutaneous pigmentation, subcutaneous nodules, and brain tumors) similar to those of NF, but is genetically distinct from it (Mulvihill, 1990). Despite the inaccurate association, these dramatizations have probably done more than anything else to publicize the plight of those with NF.

NF is actually a collection of diseases that have in common autosomal dominant inheritance and several clinical features. As many as eight different variants of NF have been postulated to exist (Riccardi & Eichner, 1986), but by far the most commonly described are NF-1 and NF-2. These two diseases are genetically and clinically distinct, however. NF-2 (also called central or acoustic NF) is an autosomal dominant genetic disease resulting from a mutation on chromosome 22 (Rouleau et al., 1990). It is characterized by bilateral vestibular schwannoma (also called acoustic neuroma) and has an incidence of approximately 1 in 40,000 persons (Zoller, Rembeck, Akesson, & Agrvall, 1995). This chapter emphasizes the cognitive manifestations of NF-1 rather than NF-2, which has a much lower incidence and is not associated with cognitive impairment. Therefore, the term "NF" refers to NF-1 from this point on unless otherwise noted.

From a neuropsychological standpoint, NF is an exceptionally interesting medical disorder. As we describe later, in comparison with the general population, persons with NF have higher incidences of learning disabilities (LDs), neuropsychological dysfunction, behavioral impairment, and brain tumors. In addition, intriguing and unusual "bright" areas in the brain are observed on magnetic resonance imaging (MRI) scans of persons with NF. This chapter examines the characteristics, natural history, and relationship of the neuropsychological, learning, and neuroanatomical factors associated with NF in children and adolescents.

EPIDEMIOLOGY, GENETICS, AND NATURAL HISTORY

NF is an autosomal dominant genetic disorder associated with a mutation on chromosome 17; its incidence is approximately 1 in 3,500. It is thus more common than muscular dystrophy, Tay–Sachs disease, and Huntington disease combined (Texas Neurofibromatosis Foundation, 1996). Approximately 80,000–100,000 individuals in the United States today have NF.

Approximately half of the new cases of NF are spontaneous mutations with no family history of the disease. A positive family history of the disorder is found in the remaining cases. Offspring of a parent who has NF have about a 50% chance of being born with the disorder, and there is almost complete penetrance of the inherited form of NF, with all races and both genders equally affected. The clinical expression of NF varies considerably however, even within families (von Deimling, Krone, & Menon, 1995), and many people with NF lead normal lives and experience relatively little impact from the disease. Others have chronic, progressive, and debilitating morbidity, including severely disfiguring physical stigmata, or significant and even life-threatening medical complications. At present there is no cure or effective treatment for NF. Moreover, medical complications of the disease become more prevalent and severe with advancing age (Riccardi, 1981); consequently, NF is also associated with a somewhat shortened lifespan. In a survey of 70 adults with NF in Gothenberg, Sweden, Zoller et al. (1995) reported that the mean age at death was 61.6 years, approximately 15 years less than population standards. Over a 12-year period, the mortality rate for persons with NF was approximately four times the rate for the general population. The majority of these deaths (55%) were due to malignancies. Brain tumors and other types of malignancies (e.g., neurofibrosarcoma) were more common than in the general population. Other complications of NF, such as hypertension, were also associated with increased mortality (Zoller et al., 1995).

MEDICAL AND DIAGNOSTIC FACTORS

The diagnosis of NF is based on the occurrence of criteria developed as a result of a consensus conference sponsored by the National Institutes of Health (NIH) in 1988 (NIH Consensus Development Conference, 1988). These criteria are outlined in Table 7.1, and were reaffirmed in 1997 after a review of recent scientific and medical developments in the understanding of the disease (Gutmann et al., 1997). A definitive diagnosis requires two of the seven criteria to be present.

In addition to the diagnostic criteria outlined in Table 7.1, several other clinical features are associated with NF, including vascular abnormalities, cosmetic disfigurement, seizures, headaches, macrocephaly, and speech disturbances. Hypertrophy within single or multiple segments of the body, short stature, headaches, and constipation are also common (Riccardi & Eichner, 1986). A four-level rating scale developed to quantify the severity of these clinical features (Riccardi, 1982) is widely used. Level 1 represents "minimal" or no obvious stigmata; level 2 represents symptoms rated as "mild," such as cosmetic stigmata, short stature, headaches, or school underachievement; and level 3 is character-

TABLE 7.1. Diagnostic Criteria for NF-1

1. Six or more cafe-au-lait spots greater than 5 mm in diameter in prepubertal children or greater than 15 mm in diameter postpubertal.
2. Two or more neurofibromas of any form or one plexiform neurofibroma.
3. Freckling in the axillary or inguinal regions.
4. Optic glioma.
5. Two or more Lisch nodules (iris hamartomas).
6. A distinctive osseous lesion such as sphenoid dysplasia or thinning of long bone cortex with or without pseudarthrosis.
7. A first-degree relative with NF-1 by the above criteria.

Note. A definitive diagnosis requires two or more of these criteria to be met. From NIH Consensus Development Conference (1988).

ized by "moderate" morbidity, with obvious cosmetic impact, stature at or below the 3rd percentile, seizures controllable with medication, or moderate school underachievement. Level 4 is "severe" NF, characterized by frank mental retardation, severe psychosocial burden, intracranial tumors, or intractable pain. These features are thought to be aggravated or accelerated during adolescence and pregnancy. In fact, NF is often first discovered during puberty or pregnancy, possibly because of the hormonal changes taking place at those times.

Many of the disfiguring lesions, such as plexiform and nodular neurofibromas, are not treated surgically because their progressive nature cannot be halted, only delayed. However, when a neurofibroma impinges upon a vital organ or structure (e.g., the spinal cord or the renal artery), surgery may be necessary and helpful. Other associated features of NF, such as optic gliomas (which occur in 15–20% of cases), are normally treated only if they increase in size or cause progressive visual abnormality. In those cases, standard brain tumor therapy—consisting of some combination of surgery, chemotherapy, and cranial radiation therapy (CRT)—is often considered. CRT, which frequently leads to cognitive impairment, is thought to disrupt myelin formation in the developing brain. The resulting cognitive deficits are similar to those of traumatic brain injury, which also results in damage primarily to cerebral white matter. Interestingly, some children with NF (even without optic gliomas) have cognitive profiles similar to those of both CRT-treated populations and children with traumatic brain injury populations (nonverbal deficits and difficulty in visual–spatial processing). Verbal and reading deficits have also been described in children with NF (Mazzocco et al., 1995).

NEUROPSYCHOLOGICAL FEATURES

Mental Retardation and Intellectual Profile

Early studies reported that mild to moderate mental retardation was common in persons with NF, with prevalence estimates ranging as high as 43% (Samuelsson & Riccardi, 1989; Samuelsson & Samuelsson, 1989). Although recent studies using random NF patient samples and standardized intelligence tests have reported only slight (if any) elevations in the rate of mental retardation (Eldridge et al., 1989; Eliason, 1988; Wadsby, Lindehammar, & Eeg-Olofsson, 1989), many people, including physicians, continue to associate NF with mental retardation. North (1993) reported a 3.5% incidence of moderate to severe intellectual delay in a sample of 200 pediatric and adult patients with NF (age range = 0–68 years). Moore, Ater, Needle, Slopis, and Copeland (1994) reported that approximately 6% of 65 children (age range = 5–16 years) had IQ scores within the mentally deficient range (<70). These estimates are slightly greater than the expected incidence in the general population (~2%). The shape of the IQ distribution has also been described. North (1993) observed a bimodal distribution, whereas others have reported that the distribution of IQ is skewed slightly to the left of the normal distribution, with the mean Full Scale IQ equal to approximately 94 (Eldridge et al., 1989; Moore et al., 1994; Wadsby et al., 1989).

Learning Disabilities

Although frank mental retardation is rare, difficulty in school performance may be the most pervasive problem faced by children with NF. LDs are reported in approximately 40–50% of children with NF. By contrast, in the general (non-NF) population, the incidence of LDs has been reported to be 2–15% (Fletcher, Satz, & Morris, 1986; Hynd, Obrzut, Hayes, & Becker, 1986; Rutter, Tizard, & Whitmore, 1970). Academic underachievement and behaviors characteristic of attention-deficit/hyperactivity disorder (ADHD; i.e., hyperactivity, distractibility, and impulsivity) occur much more frequently in children with NF than in the general population (Eliason, 1986; North, 1993; North et al., 1997; Stine, & Adams, 1989; DeWinter, Moore, Slopis, Jackson, & Leeds, in press). Most studies have used a discrepancy between IQ and academic achievement as the criterion to define LDs, but often LDs are not defined on the basis of strict objective criteria, or details related to their diagnosis are omitted. Speech impairment and disorders of motor coordination are other frequently reported clinical features (Eldridge et al., 1989; Varnhagen, Lewin, Das, & Bowen, 1988; Wadsby et al., 1989).

North (1993) reported on a large group of patients with NF in Australia, ranging in age from 0 to 68 years (mean = 17.4 years). In that study, LDs were defined in terms of delays in reaching developmental milestones or reports of poor school performance. The author found that 45% of the sample, which included children and adults, met these criteria for LDs—an incidence rate similar to rates reported by other researchers.

Although it is widely accepted that children with NF are at higher risk for LDs than the general population, the cognitive deficits in these children are thought to be different from those found in most other children with LDs. Children with NF, for example, frequently have deficits in visual–spatial processing, language, and motor coordination. However, no specific neuropsychological or learning profile has been universally accepted as characteristic of children with NF.

Several studies have found Wechsler Verbal IQ to be lower than Performance IQ in NF patients (Eldridge et al., 1989; Moore et al., 1994), suggesting the possibility of language-based difficulties. However, because visual–spatial and other nonverbal processing deficits are common findings in this population (Bawden et al., 1996; Eldridge et al., 1989; Eliason, 1986; Moore, Slopis, Schomer, Jackson, & Levy, 1996; Stine & Adams, 1989), the possibility of nonverbal LDs has also been explored (Hofman, Harris, Bryan, & Denckla, 1994). Eliason (1986, 1988) and Wadsby et al. (1989), for example, reported lower Performance IQ than Verbal IQ in samples of children with NF. However, only a few studies have focused on the types of LDs that children with NF have.

Eliason (1986, 1988) has conducted several studies examining the pattern of LDs in children with NF. In an early report of 23 children with NF who were referred to a learning disorders clinic (Eliason, 1986), she found three subtypes of LDs: a primarily verbal type, a primarily visual-perceptual type, and a mixed type. In her sample, 56% of the children were found to have isolated visual-perceptual impairment, 4% had primarily verbal impairment, and 30% had mixed deficits. These findings contrasted with a larger group of children without NF who were referred for LDs to the same clinic, who had a high rate of language impairment (62%) and a low rate of visual-perceptual impairment (6%). However, a 28% rate of mixed visual-perceptual and language deficits in this non-NF group closely matched that found in the smaller NF sample. Eliason (1988) reported similar results in a later study comparing the neuropsychological performances of children with NF to those of a matched sample of children with LDs but without NF. Although these studies teach us a great deal about the nature of learning problems in children with NF *who present* with LDs, the nature of participant referral raises the possibility of ascertainment bias and thus limits the ability to generalize the findings to the entire population of children with NF. In addition, Eliason's sample included some with brain tumors.

Mazzocco et al. (1995) assessed neuropsychological and academic achievement skills in 19 children with NF and their non-NF siblings, in an effort to characterize the precise nature of LDs in the NF population. The children ranged from 5 to 16 years at the time of the assessments. The investigators hypothesized that children with NF have deficits in both visual–spatial and verbal abilities, and that their neuropsychological profile is distinct from that associated with other forms of LDs. Children with NF scored lower in tests of IQ (particularly Verbal IQ) and of reading and math skills than did their siblings without NF. The presence of verbal deficits led the investigators to examine the incidence of discrepancy-based reading disability. Although there was a higher incidence of reading disability in the children with NF than in their siblings, the difference was not statistically significant. As reported in previous studies (Eldridge et al., 1989; Eliason, 1986; Hofman et al., 1994; Moore et al., 1994, 1996; North et al., 1997), children with NF also performed more poorly on tests of visual–spatial ability than did their siblings. Mazzocco et al. (1995) speculated that verbal and nonverbal LDs coexist in children with NF, and that these children thus do not display more classic and isolated forms of nonverbal LDs. This hypothesis was supported by the fact that there were significant correlations between verbal and visual–spatial test scores for the children with NF, but not for their non-NF siblings. Therefore, the profile of LDs in the children in Mazzocco et al.'s study (1995) did not fit more classic patterns of LDs associated with either specific reading disability or nonverbal LDs.

In another study, Brewer, Moore, and Hiscock (1997) used advanced statistical methods in an attempt to minimize ascertainment bias in documenting LD subtypes in a sample of 105 children with NF. These children represented consecutive referrals to an established NF clinic for routine evaluation of the usual medical sequelae associated with the disorder. No child was referred solely for LDs, and 75% were diagnosed with NF before they even entered school. Classification of LD subtypes was accomplished in five steps via cluster analysis. These steps involved selection of classification variables, selection of a robust clustering method, determination of clusters, selection of psychometric variables, and validation of the clusters. A total of 10 clusters emerged. Two of these clusters contained only one child each and thus were excluded as outliers. Six of the clusters contained 74 children (72% of the sample) who met the criterion of low academic achievement scores in at least one subject (one standard deviation or more below normative means). An additional 29 children in the two remaining clusters (28%) were not academically deficient. Most of the 74 academically deficient children performed poorly on all three subtests (Reading, Spelling, and Arithmetic) of the Wide Range Achievement Test—Revised (Jastak & Wilkinson, 1984), suggesting that the group was relatively homogeneous in terms of academic deficiencies. However, a small subset of these children performed poorly only on the Spelling subtest.

Brewer et al. (1997) then continued the clustering process with the 74 academically deficient children, using neuropsychological instead of academic achievement variables. Three clusters emerged from this analysis: a neuropsychologically intact group, a generally impaired group, and a group with specific deficits in visual–spatial/constructional skills (Figure 7.1). Despite differences in their profiles, the two neuropsychologically deficient groups (*n* = 44) had similar problems in academic achievement. Even more surprising was the finding that only 10 children fell into the visual–spatial/constructional subgroup. These 10 represented only about 10% of the total sample (*n* = 105), 14% of those with academic deficiencies, and 23% of those with academic deficiencies *and* neuropsychological impairment. All three of these figures are surprisingly low, given the impression that visual–spatial deficits are "hallmarks" of NF in children (see "Neuropsychological Profile," below; see also Eliason, 1986, 1988; Eldridge et al., 1989; Hofman et al., 1994; Moore et al., 1996). A possible explanation for the Brewer et al. (1997) finding is that the tasks used to measure visual–spatial ability had a significant motor component and hence did not constitute tests of pure visual–spatial ability. The Judgment of Line Orientation test (JLO; Lindgren & Benton, 1980), a motor-free visual–spatial test, was not used. Of additional note was the finding that the two neuropsychologically deficient groups had both verbal and visual–spatial deficits relative to the intact group (see Figure 7.1). In this respect, the results were similar to those reported by Mazzocco et al. (1995).

The estimated rate of academic deficiency in this sample, 72%, is high compared to those from other studies (which generally range from 45% to 60%) and is well above the incidence rate of 2–15% for the general population (Fletcher et al., 1986; Hynd et al., 1986;

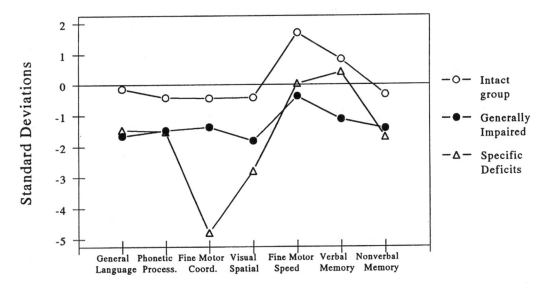

FIGURE 7.1. Clustering of LD subgroups on neuropsychological variables (Process., processing; Coord., coordination). From "Learning Disability Subtypes in Children with Neurofibromatosis" by V. R. Brewer, B. D. Moore, and M. Hiscock, 1997, *Journal of Learning Disabilities*, 30(5), 521–533. Copyright 1997 by PRO-ED, Inc. Reprinted by permission.

Rutter et al., 1970). Furthermore, 28 of the 72 academically deficient children in the Brewer et al. (1997) sample had normal neuropsychological profiles. The authors attributed this high rate of "unexplained academic underachievers" to deficits in attention or possibly to psychosocial or behavioral factors.

Neuropsychological Profile

As mentioned earlier, visual–spatial impairment has been reported so often in children with NF that it is almost considered an identifying feature of the disorder (Eldridge et al., 1989; Eliason, 1986; Hofman et al., 1994; Moore et al., 1994, 1996; North et al., 1997).

Eliason (1986, 1988) and Wadsby et al. (1989) found that visual-perceptual deficits were common in children with NF, and that Performance IQ was generally lower than Verbal IQ. Varnhagen et al. (1988) and associates also reported poor visual–spatial performance in children with NF; this was related to the severity of disease characteristics, but not necessarily to visual acuity. In a study using nonaffected siblings of children with NF, Eldridge et al. (1989) reported that those with NF had a greater incidence and severity of visual–spatial impairment than did their unaffected siblings. The Eldridge et al. study was notable for its efforts to minimize selection bias by excluding children in whom the presence of developmental disabilities led to the diagnosis of NF, together with children with a history of epilepsy or brain tumor. In addition, a comprehensive battery of neuropsychological, intellectual, and academic achievement tests was used. Although the often-reported pattern of higher Verbal than Performance IQ was not found in this study, the JLO (Lindgren & Benton, 1980) successfully discriminated patients from unaffected siblings. NF-related deficiencies in JLO performance have been reported in a number of other studies as well (Denckla et al. 1996; Moore et al., 1996).

Difficulties with speech articulation and motor incoordination are also frequently reported in children with NF (Dunn & Roos, 1989; Moore et al., 1994; North, Joy, Yuille, Cocks, & Hutchins, 1995). Moore et al. (1994) observed that as a group, children with NF had above-average fine motor speed on a finger-tapping task, but that they performed well below average on a task requiring fine motor coordination in addition to speed. Impairment in motor coordination often occurs in conjunction with deficits in visual–motor integration, resulting in an obvious classroom disadvantage (poor handwriting and difficulty copying schoolwork from the board).

Natural History of Neuropsychological Deficits

Often parents of a child with NF are aware of and concerned about the possibility of cognitive and learning deficits in their child. A typical question is "When will we know if my 3-year-old will have a learning disability?" Or, if a child is already having learning problems, "Will my child improve [grow out of it] or develop even more problems over time?" These are difficult questions to answer, because there have been no longitudinal studies of the natural history of cognitive status in this group of children. Reports of outcomes in cross-sectional samples of children with NF have yielded inconsistent findings. On the one hand, Riccardi (1992) reported higher IQ in adults than in children and adolescents younger than 17 years of age. In another study, Ferner, Hughes, and Wenman (1996) found no significant differences in IQ between children and adults with NF. Moore and Slopis (1994), however, reported *lower* IQ and neuropsychological test scores in older than in younger age groups. Their cross-sectional sample consisted of 90 children and adolescents between the ages of 4 and 16 years, who were administered a comprehensive battery of intellectual, academic achievement, and neuropsychological tests. Significant negative correlations between age and cognitive test scores were obtained in the areas of Verbal IQ, academic achievement, memory, and attention. However, longitudinal follow-up of a smaller subsample ($n = 23$) of these same children who had completed two annual follow-up exams (for a total of three evaluations) failed to reveal significant evidence for age-related declines in standard scores over time. Clearly, further longitudinal work is needed to explore the natural history of this disease, with follow-up extending well beyond the 2-year span examined in the Moore and Slopis (1994) study. A restricted age range (e.g., 6 to 16 years) would also be desirable, in order for the same tests to be applicable to all sample participants.

BEHAVIORAL MANIFESTATIONS

The psychosocial and emotional status of persons with NF has not been well studied, although there is certainly potential for difficulty in these areas in light of the physical, medical, and neuropsychological morbidity of the disorder (Riccardi, 1981). Most research on the psychosocial status of persons with NF has focused on adults. Benjamin et al. (1993) found low degrees of social support in adults, with reports of specific problems in forming relationships, restrictive choice of careers, LDs, and issues related to physical disfigurement. Study participants also recalled anxiety caused by teasing they received earlier in life because of their physical disfigurement. In another study, Varnhagen et al. (1988) reported that children and adolescents with greater numbers of physical stigmata had higher degrees of anxiety and preoccupation with potential disasters than did those with fewer physical symptoms. The latter difference, however, was not accompanied by differences on other, more clinically significant dimensions of adjustment (e.g., on mood or personality measures). In one of the few studies of psychosocial outcomes in children, Wadsby et al. (1989) used parent and teacher questionnaires to assess behavior in 25 children with NF between the ages of 4 and 16 years. Questionnaires were also completed for a comparison group of 22 siblings of the children with NF. The results indicated that the children with NF were more likely to have sleeping disturbances, episodes of "acting out," hyperactivity, and distractibility than were their siblings.

Although a high prevalence of ADHD has been mentioned repeatedly in studies of children with NF (Eliason, 1986; Moore et al., 1996; North, 1993; North et al., 1997; Stine & Adams, 1989), the actual incidence of clinically diagnosed ADHD and its accompanying characteristics has not been formally investigated. Spaepen, Borghgraef, and Fryns (1992) administered the Child Behavior Checklist (Achenbach & Edelbrock, 1983) to 15 children with NF. Symptoms of hyperactivity were reported in 6 of the 15 children. Other behavior domains in which ratings were elevated into the clinically significant range for at least one child in the sample were social withdrawal ($n = 3$), immaturity ($n = 2$), aggressiveness ($n = 2$), anxiety ($n = 4$), obsessive–compulsive behavior ($n = 2$), somatic complaints ($n = 2$), and uncommunicativeness ($n = 2$). Although this sample was relatively small and there was no control group, the results indicate that behavior problems are prevalent in children with NF. In almost half the sample (7 children), the total Behavior Problem score was at a level similar to that commonly observed in children referred to psychiatric clinics.

BRAIN TUMORS

Prevalence and Treatment Effects

Tumors of the central nervous system (CNS) are common in NF (Blatt, Jaffe, Deutsch, & Adkins, 1986; Riccardi, 1982). Estimates of the prevalence of CNS tumors range from 15% to 50% (Duffner, Cohen, Seidel, & Shucard, 1989; Mulvihill, 1990; Riccardi & Eichner, 1986). However, the contribution of CNS tumors to neuropsychological status is not well known. Most of these tumors are gliomas of the optic chiasm and tracts; if these tumors are nonprogressive and do not cause visual abnormality, they are often left untreated (Cohen, Kaplan, & Packer, 1990–1991; Roos & Dunn, 1992). Many tumors are not even biopsied, but are diagnosed and followed solely with periodic neuroimaging. More serious brain tumors in different anatomical areas may require some combination of surgery, chemotherapy, or CRT, with the accompanying risk of cognitive sequelae. Many brain tumors, however, are not accompanied by neurobehavioral deficits. In children without NF who have brain tumors, most have cognitive abilities within the normal range when assessed prior to receiving CRT (Brookshire, Copeland, Moore, & Ater, 1990; Moore et al., 1994). Intensive treatment with CRT seems to be the major contributor to cognitive decline in children with brain tumors (Bleyer, 1981; Copeland et al., 1985; Fletcher & Copeland, 1988), but fortunately few children with NF require this sort of treatment.

Impact on Neuropsychological Functioning

It is not yet clear whether an untreated optic glioma in a child with NF has consequences for cognitive functioning above and beyond the effect of having NF. For this reason, consensus is lacking to whether children with optic gliomas should be included or excluded from neuropsychological studies of children with NF. One study reported that most of the cognitive morbidity in children with a brain tumor and NF is associated with NF itself, rather than with the brain tumor (Moore et al., 1994). In that study, the neuropsychological functioning of 14 children with NF and a brain tumor was compared to that of 14 children with NF only. An additional comparison group consisted of children without NF but with brain tumors in locations similar to those found in the NF-plus-brain-tumor group. The three groups were also matched as closely as possible for socioeconomic status, age, race, and gender. The mean scores in Verbal and Performance IQ, academic achievement, language, memory, and visual–spatial domains were highest in the brain-tumor-only group. The NF-only group had the next highest means, and means were lowest for the NF-plus-brain-tumor group. Both NF groups' mean scores were significantly lower than the brain tumor group's mean scores in Full Scale IQ and academic achievement. In addition, the NF brain tumor group's mean scores were significantly lower than the brain tumor group's mean scores in memory and visual–spatial abilities and in freedom from distractibility. There were no statistically significant differences between the two NF groups, however. It was concluded that the most common types of brain tumors seen in children with NF are associated with only minimal additional cognitive impact above and beyond that related to the NF diagnosis itself. It is important to note, however, that no child in any of these groups had received CRT. A more recent study by De Winter et al. (in press) studied an additional 22 children with NF plus a brain tumor (total $n = 36$), including nine subjects who had been treated with CRT. De Winter et al. (in press) concluded that the severity of neuropsychological deficits in the child with NF is not exacerbated when a brain tumor is present unless treatment with CRT is required.

Is Visual–Spatial Impairment Related to Optic Pathway Tumors?

Although visual–spatial impairment is frequently reported in children with NF, it is possible that tumors of the optic nerve, chiasm, or retrochiasmic pathways could be responsible for deficient test performance, even if cognition is not directly affected or is affected only minimally (see above). Visual–spatial problems may simply result from an impairment in visual acuity due to an optic glioma. Impaired visual acuity may in turn contribute to poor school performance and diminished performance on specific cognitive tests. This possibility, however, does not seem likely. Listernick, Darling, Greenwald, Strauss, and Charrow (1995) found clinical symptoms of visual abnormality in only 20% of their NF sample with optic gliomas, and Roos and Dunn (1992) found these symptoms in only 33% of their sample. In the Moore et al. (1994) study discussed earlier, only 28% of the sample had clinical abnormalities of the second, third, fourth, or sixth cranial nerves, even though most children had optic gliomas. In that study, visual–spatial abilities were not any more affected by the presence of the brain tumor than were other cognitive abilities. These findings suggest that visual–spatial disability in children with NF is *not* simply a primary sensory deficit resulting from lesions of the optic pathway. It is nevertheless important to separate the contribution of distractibility and fine motor incoordination to performance on visual–spatial tasks from that of deficits in visual–spatial abilities per se, especially given the weaknesses of children with NF in the attention and fine motor domains. Although impairment of visual processing skills may be due to abnormalities in the optic radiation or association areas of the occipital cortex, abnormalities of this sort have not as yet been documented.

OTHER BRAIN ABNORMALITIES: BRAIN HYPERINTENSITIES

Nature of Hyperintensities

Focal or diffuse areas of brain abnormality are frequently visualized as non-contrast-enhancing areas of increased signal intensity, particularly on T_2-weighted MRI scans (see Figure 7.2). These hyperintensities occur in as many as 60–70% of children with NF—primarily in the basal ganglia, cerebellum, and white matter tracts, and less often in the

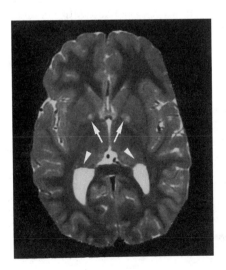

FIGURE 7.2. Brain T_2-weighted MRI scan showing hyperintensities in the basal ganglia (arrows) and CSF, cerebrospinal fluid (arrowheads).

cerebral hemispheres. Although their exact nature is unknown (see "Pathology/Histology of Hyperintensities," below), they are thought to be the result of delayed or abnormal myelination (Itoh et al., 1994) or chemically abnormal myelin (Sevick et al., 1992). Because of their uncertain origin and their appearance, these hyperintensities have been termed *unidentified bright objects*, or UBOs. UBOs are not neoplastic lesions and do not require medical intervention other than periodic radiological monitoring. In some cases, UBOs have "transformed" into malignancies; some doubt exists, however as to whether the latter cases actually involved UBOs. With continuing advances in radiological technology, it may become possible to distinguish between benign hyperintensities (or UBOs) and similar-appearing but premalignant neoplasms, and to do so earlier in their course than is presently possible. Although a significant percentage of children with NF have hyperintensities, their occurrence in other populations of children is not known. For this reason, it has been recommended that hyperintensities *not* be considered a diagnostic criterion for NF (Gutmann et al., 1997).

Relationship of Hyperintensities to Neuropsychological Status and LDs

It is enticing to presume that these brain anomalies are the cause of the LDs often found in children with NF. At this time, however, the relationship of these anomalies to cognitive and learning abilities remains unclear. Most early studies report no association between the presence or number of these hyperintensities and general measures of intellectual functioning. More recent studies, however, have found that hyperintensities are associated not only with IQ, but also with more specific areas of neuropsychological functioning.

Dunn and Roos (1989) examined the association of MRI hyperintensities with "school problems" and "poor coordination" in 31 patients ranging in age from 6 to 20 years. The group was divided according to the presence or absence of any reported or observed neurological anomalies or scholastic problems relative to normal expectations. MRI-derived status was simply categorized as "UBO-positive" or "UBO-negative." There were no consistent, standardized test data, and LDs were not specifically defined. For example, if a child was reported to be academically functioning 2 or more years below grade placement or to have an IQ below 70, those reports were all categorized as "cognitive deficits." The design thus provided a limited test of the possible relationship between cognition and UBO status. Chi-square analysis was used to relate "neurocognitive yes–no" to "UBO yes–no" status, and the results failed to reveal a statistically significant relationship between these variables.

Duffner et al. (1989) addressed the same issue in a study of 46 children with NF, ranging in age from 9 months to 18 years. For some of the children, NF was complicated by tumors or seizure disorders (30% had seizures and 25% had assorted lesions visualized on computed tomography). Again, data regarding learning problems were limited to historical information on special education placement. IQ scores were available for one-third of the children, but in some cases they were obtained as part of previous clinical assessments. Hyperintensities were simply recorded as "present" or "absent," with no account taken of the number or location of the hyperintensities. As in the Dunn and Roos (1989) study, a chi-square analysis failed to demonstrate any association between neurocognitive deficits and hyperintensities. In a similar study that included direct contemporaneous psychometric testing of 20 children with NF, Legius et al. (1995) also found no significant difference in IQ between participants whose brain scans showed hyperintensities and participants who were free of hyperintensities.

Ferner, Chaudhuri, Bingham, Cox, and Hughes (1993) examined the time course of the appearance of hyperintensities in a cross-sectional/longitudinal design with 38 patients with NF. These investigators found hyperintensities to be far more common in individuals under 18 years of age than in older individuals. Lesions seemed to be stable at 3-year follow-up. However, no correlation was found between the presence of a single hyperintensity or multiple hyperintensities and measures of cognitive functioning. Twenty-eight patients were given cognitive tests as part of the study; the level of cognitive functioning in the other 10 was estimated from the history of occupational status or school performance.

In contrast to the negative findings of the studies mentioned above, North et al. (1994) reported a strong association between hyperintensities and neuropsychological functioning in a sample of 40 children with NF who were 8–16 years old (25 had hyperintensities and 15 did not). Although these researchers did not quantify the number or the volume of hyperintensities, they collected detailed cognitive, language, and academic test data. Deficits were present in all areas of testing in the majority of children who had hyperintensities. By contrast, mean scores for the smaller subset of hyperintensity-negative children were not significantly different from those of the normal population in any test domain (IQ, motor, language, or academic skills). The authors concluded that the hyperintensity-positive group scored significantly below population norms in Wechsler Verbal, Performance, and Full Scale IQ, all language measures, a test of visual–motor integration, and a test of motor coordination. They further concluded that the presence of hyperintensities was a marker for a more developmentally disabled group within the population of those with NF. Eighteen of the total group of 40 children with NF studied by North et al. (1994) were receiving special education services; 17 of these 18 children were hyperintensity-positive. Although the mean IQ scores in this sample of hyperintensity-positive children were low compared to those in the general population and were lower than the scores of children without hyperintensities, these means were nevertheless within normal limits (Wechsler Full Scale IQ = 93). IQ scores were bimodally distributed, with scores for children who did not show a single hyperintensity indistinguishable from normal means. No distinction was made between hyperintensity signal along optic pathways related to optic glioma and signal related to involvement of locations within the substance of the brain itself. The relevance of this distinction in relation to developmental outcomes has yet to be determined.

Hofman et al. (1994) published the first study of children with NF that involved the use of a sibling control design. These investigators recruited 12 families, each of which had one child who met NIH criteria for NF and one unaffected sibling. All children ranged in age from 6 to 16 years. Intelligence measures and standardized academic, language, and neuropsychological tests were administered to the sibling pairs and their parents. MRI studies included measures of the location and volumes of hyperintensities. In contrast to the study of North et al. (1994), optic tract involvement with glioma(s) was an exclusionary criterion. The results revealed that scores on tests of IQ and of visual–spatial ability (specifically, the JLO; Lindgren & Benton, 1980) were associated with the number of brain locations in which hyperintensities were seen. The correlation between pairwise differences in Wechsler Full Scale IQ scores and the number of occupied brain locations was significant. For scores on the JLO, the measure on which the children with NF showed the greatest impairment relative to their siblings, the corresponding correlation was also significant.

In a subsequent publication using an enlarged sample of 19 sibling pairs, Denckla et al. (1996) employed a multiple-regression model to examine both the number of locations and the total hyperintensity volume as predictors of Wechsler IQ scores. The dependent measures in these analyses were scores for the children with NF relative to scores for their respective siblings. Independent or predictor variables included a child's age, whether the disease was inherited or spontaneous (familial vs. sporadic), total volume of brain tissue occupied by the hyperintensity signal, and number of locations in the brain occupied by hyperintensity signal. The number of hyperintensity-occupied brain locations was the *only* significant predictor, accounting for 42% of the variance in NF-associated reduction in IQ (pairwise difference). None of the other variables, including total volume of hyperintensity signal in relation to total brain volume, added significantly to this variable in predicting the pairwise differences.

Denckla et al. (1996) reported that if any hyperintensity signal was present at all, it was always present in the basal ganglia. The second and third most frequent locations for hyperintensities were the brain stem and the cerebellum, respectively. In most cases, a bilateral distribution of hyperintensities was noted. It is important to emphasize, however, that no cases with optic tract involvement were included in this study. Sixteen subjects had basal ganglia hyperintensities, 11 had additional brain stem hyperintensities, and 7 had cerebellar hyperintensities. A few subcortical (cerebral-peduncular and thalamic) hyperintensities were visualized. In agreement with results published by Moore et al. (1996), the few children with hyperintensities in the thalamic region were among those in the NF group with the most severe impairments in intelligence relative to their siblings. As further support for the conclusion that hyperintensities play a role in lowering of cognitive functioning, the IQs of two boys who were hyperintensity-negative were virtually identical to those of their brothers. Equally illustrative of this conclusion is the case of a boy with sporadic NF whose MRI showed hyperintensities in four separate brain regions and who had only average intelligence, whereas the rest of the family (both parents, unaffected sibling) had superior IQ scores.

Denckla et al. (1996) concluded that without data from which to derive family-based expectations for IQ, the impact of hyperintensities on cognition is likely to be obscured. Comparison with population means would not fully reveal the impact of the hyperintensities. In particular, the subtle effects of the number of brain-occupying locations on cognitive outcomes may not be apparent without suitable sibling controls. Although North et al. (1994) did suggest that hyperintensity-positive children with NF score lower than population norms on IQ and other cognitive tests, these results may vary substantially across samples (Legius et al., 1995; Moore et al., 1996). Sampling differences may reflect not only the polygenetic IQ factors contributing to cognitive heterogeneity among persons with NF, but also variability in the distribution of hyperintensity-occupied brain locations across samples.

In another recent report, Moore et al. (1996) used a comprehensive battery of tests of intelligence, academic achievement, language, memory, fine motor skills, visual–spatial skills, and attention skills to assess outcomes in 84 children and adolescents with NF (age range = 8–16 years). Twenty patients had been diagnosed with brain tumors, usually optic gliomas, but none had been treated with chemotherapy or CRT. In two cases the tumors were surgically resected, and one additional child had a biopsy. Three sets of analyses were conducted to examine how cognitive status was influenced by (1) presence or absence of hyperintensity, (2) the number of hyperintensities, and (3) the anatomical location of hyperintensities. Analyses were conducted both with and without inclusion of the brain tumor patients.

Forty-six subjects (55%) had at least one area of hyperintensity, and 38 (45%) did not. In contrast to the North et al. (1994) study, analysis failed to reveal significant differences between children with and without hyperintensities on any of the outcome measures. The number of hyperintensities, when present, ranged from one to five (the approximate mean number for children with hyperintensities was two). In contrast with the conclusions reached by Hofman et al. (1994) and Denckla et al. (1996), the number of distinct hyper-intensities was not correlated with any of the outcomes. The latter studies, however, employed somewhat different designs involving sibling controls, whereas the Moore et al. (1996) study referred scores to population means. In the Moore et al. (1996) study, boys had a slightly greater number of hyperintensities than girls. When correlations were performed separately by gender, greater numbers of hyperintensities were associated with poorer performance on language tests for boys but not girls.

Most of the hyperintensities were located in the basal ganglia, but they were also found in the cerebral hemispheres, brain stem, cerebellum, optic pathways, and thalamus. According to analyses of anatomical location, mean scores on Wechsler Performance IQ and on tests of memory, fine motor skills, and attention were significantly lower for children with hyperintensities in the thalamus than for those with hyperintensities elsewhere. No other effect of location on cognitive performance was noted (Moore et al., 1996). These results do not imply that all children who have hyperintensities in the thalamus will have cognitive difficulties, or that all children who have hyperintensities elsewhere or who are hyperintensity-negative will be immune to neuropsychological problems. The role of the thalamus in cognition, primarily memory and learning, is well documented (Gentilini, De Renzi, & Crisi, 1987; Kahn & Crosby, 1972; Slopis, Ater, Copeland, Moore, & Leeds, 1994; Squire & Butters, 1984, Chapter 13, pages 123–132). Although no child in the Moore et al. (1996) study who had a hyperintensity in the thalamus was grossly amnestic, weaknesses in verbal and visual learning may have contributed to NF-associated academic difficulties. Kaplan et al. (1997), using positron emission tomography (PET) scans, recently reported thalamic hypometabolism in 10 children with NF. Nine children and adults were used as a comparison group. Although no cases had focal hyperintensities within the thalamus, and there were no significant correlations between psychometric test results and regional glucose metabolic rate, Kaplan et al. (1997) concluded that there is a potential relationship between the thalamus and neuropsychological dysfunction in children with NF.

Pathology/Histology of Hyperintensities

The biological nature of T_2-weighted hyperintensities is not firmly established. Radiology reports often use the descriptor *hamartoma* for each area of hyperintensity (Aoki et al., 1989; Bognanno et al., 1988). A hamartoma is a benign tumor-like clustering of brain cells, almost a "birthmark" in the brain. DiPaolo et al. (1995) suggest that the hyperintense T_2-weighted signal corresponds to pathological findings of spongiform or vacuolar changes, which, in one case for which the pathology report was available, were associated with aberrant gliosis. A popular school of thought builds on the apparent similarities of hyperintensities to demyelinating or dysmyelinating conditions (multiple sclerosis for demyelinating, adrenoleukodystrophy for dysmyelinating), which all look alike on MRI scans. According to this view, the hyperintensities present in NF may represent developmental myelin hypoplasia (Sevick et al., 1992). The disappearance of the hyperintensities with age lends credence to this theory (DiMario & Ramsby, 1998; Ferner et al., 1993; Itoh et al., 1994). Itoh et al. (1994) found that more than half of the 13 children in their study who were under 18 years of age at initial assessment had decreases in the size of their hyperintensities at a mean follow-up of 2 years. Ferner et al. (1993) reached a similar conclusion. DiMario and Ramsby (1998) found that hyperintensities in 19 patients (age range = 1–53 years, mean age = 12.5 years) decreased in both total number (29% fewer) and size

(33% smaller) over a mean MRI follow-up time of 2.3 years (range 0.5–4.5 years). This finding was dependent on anatomical location, however. Brain stem hyperintensities actually increased in number and size, whereas hemispheric and cerebellar hyperintensities showed the opposite effects. DiMario and Ramsby (1998) did not, however, analyze their data to determine whether there was a relationship between age of their patients or interval between MRI scans on the one hand, and change in size or number of hyperintensities on the other. Clearly, the coevolution of hyperintensities and of cognitive status in children with NF deserves further study. Magnetic resonance spectroscopy (which permits the study of the *in vivo* chemistry of myelin), or PET studies (e.g., Kaplan et al., 1997), may help to answer questions regarding the nature and evolution of hyperintensities in individuals with NF.

Histological reviews of hyperintense areas are rare for three reasons. First, the opportunity for autopsy in children with NF is probably no higher than in children without NF. Second, hyperintensities typically do not warrant biopsy. Third, hyperintensities are not found in adults with NF. In an autopsy study of two pediatric patients, Zimmerman et al. (1992) reported that areas of hyperintensity were associated with glia infiltrated with abnormal hyperchromatic nuclei, demyelination, and a spongy appearance of the white matter at the edges of the hyperintensities. In an unpublished personal observation by Moore of a single case, an MRI scan of a 4½-year-old child with NF revealed an area of focal hyperintensity in the cerebellar vermis. On the basis of radiography, the area was suspected of being a glioma, and the child was referred for surgery. Biopsy of the suspicious tissue was negative for neoplastic disease or necrosis and was interpreted as mild demyelination.

North et al. (1994) postulated that hyperintensities may be a radiological marker for aberrant cellular differentiation and dysplastic brain development that signal a more extensive, albeit subtle, abnormality in white matter. If hyperintensities are an indication of abnormal white matter in general, then the corpus callosum, a structure that connects homologous regions of the cortex, may also be abnormal and may contribute to neuropsychological problems. The development of sophisticated MRI volumetric techniques may help characterize the relationship of corpus callosum morphology to cognitive functions, as has been the case in studies of ADHD and other disorders (Filipek et al., 1997; Giedd et al., 1994; Hynd et al., 1991; Semrud-Clikeman, Filipek, & Biederman, 1994).

Although in the past hyperintensities have best been visualized on T_2-weighted MRI scans, the recent development of a new imaging sequence, T_2-weighted fluid-attenuated inversion recovery (FlAIR) pulse sequences, provides even better resolution. Hyperintensities have signal characteristics similar to cerebrospinal fluid (CSF); consequently, it is often difficult to differentiate the two (Figure 7.3). FlAIR consists of pulse sequences with very long echo times to suppress signal from CSF. Yamanouchi et al. (1995) used the FlAIR technique in examining 14 children and adolescents with NF and concluded that it was superior to standard T_2-weighted images for visualizing hyperintensities. Studies were performed with a 1.0-tesla MRI. T_1-weighted spin echo sequences were performed with repetition time of 500 ms and echo time of 20 ms. T_2-weighted sequences were performed with repetition time of 2,000 ms and echo time of 90 ms. FlAIR sequences were performed with repetition time of 6,000 ms, echo time of 150 ms, and inversion time of 1,600 ms. This sequence produced heavily T_2-weighted images with attenuated CSF signal, rendering the distinction between CSF and hyperintensity less ambiguous. FlAIR has been particularly helpful in investigating the cerebellum, but has also improved the visualization of hyperintensities throughout the brain (Moore, personal observation). The technique holds great potential to improve our ability to determine the association of hyperintensities and cognition in children with NF.

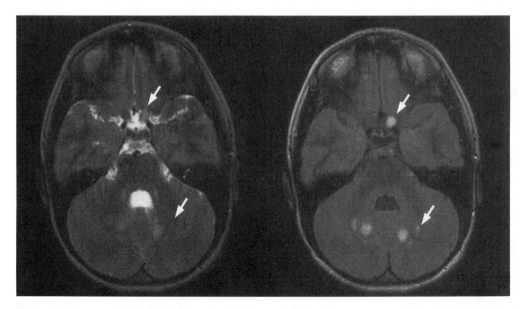

FIGURE 7.3. Brain MRI scans showing hyperintensities in the cerebellum and an optic tract glioma of a child with NF. Left image is a T_2-weighted MRI, whereas the right image uses the FlAIR protocol (Fluid Attenuation by Inversion Recovery). Note the improved visualization of hyperintensities with FlAIR, including one not visible in the T_2 image (lower arrow). Visualization of the child's optic glioma is also improved with FlAIR, as indicated by the upper arrow.

COGNITIVE PROFILE COMPARED TO THOSE OF OTHER SINGLE-GENE DISORDERS

Ten years ago, NF was portrayed as one of a large group of single-gene-based disorders falling into the category of nonverbal LDs (Mazzocco et al., 1995). This designation was based in large part on observations that children with NF often had lower Performance IQ compared to Verbal IQ or were impaired on tests of "visual processing." Closer study of NF, however, has revealed a profile in which select language impairments are, if anything, more dramatic than are visual–spatial deficits (Denckla, 1996; Mazzocco et al., 1995). It is entirely possible that closer scrutiny of several other conditions currently described as instances of nonverbal LDs will also reveal weaknesses in psycholinguistic skills.

The profile of cognitive strengths and weaknesses associated with NF, however, appears to be distinct from those found in individuals with other single-gene-based disorders. The disorder closest in nature to NF is another neurocutaneous syndrome, tuberous sclerosis. But mental retardation and/or seizures figure prominently in tuberous sclerosis, and the severity of this condition has made it difficult to carry out elegant analyses of cognitive function. Autism also occurs more often with tuberous sclerosis than with other neurocutaneous syndromes (Hunt & Dennis, 1987). Other conditions with features distinct from those associated with NF are Williams syndrome and Down syndrome. The characteristics of these conditions, well described by Bellugi, Wang, and Jernigan (1994), are not found in children with NF. Children with Williams syndrome and Down syndrome, moreover, generally score at much lower levels on intelligence testing, whereas children with NF generally score near the average range.

The cognitive abilities of individuals with disorders involving the sex chromosomes have been studied in some detail. Studies of supernumerary sex chromosome in males (i.e., those with at least one Y chromosome) report a prominence of language and reading difficulties (Bender, Linden, & Robinson, 1989). Interest in the XYY genotype has also focused on the possible developmental relationship between aggressiveness and language disorder (Rovet, Netley, Keenan, Bailey, & Stewart, 1996). This pattern of language and behavior anomalies is not characteristic of NF.

Two disorders of the X chromosome in females, fragile X (FraX) and Ullrich–Turner syndrome (UTS), have been the subject of intensive study at the Learning Disabilities Research Center at Kennedy Krieger Institute/Johns Hopkins University (Denckla is the principal investigator in this research). FraX in males results in mental retardation, and in autistic features in a substantial minority. FraX in females is associated with borderline to average IQs, with relative strengths in the verbal domain. Distinctive features of females with FraX are social avoidance and social anxiety (Reiss, Freund, Baumgardner, Abrams, & Denckla, 1995). Girls with FraX do relatively well on language tasks, including reading, but have difficulty with mathematical skills. In this respect, FraX comes as close to exemplifying the syndrome of nonverbal LDs as any type of single-gene disorder. However, the relationship of FraX girls' anxiety-like state to their cognition seems reversed from that proposed by Rourke in his many formulations of the pathogenic pathway in nonverbal LDs. The volumetric brain MRI data derived from girls with FraX are complex, with evidence for prominent abnormalities in the vermis of the cerebellum, hippocampus, and caudate nucleus (Reiss, Lee, & Freund, 1993).

UTS is the single-gene disorder with the longest history of neuropsychological investigation. Girls with UTS have been described as verbally intact but otherwise impaired. Although UTS continues to be associated with spatial impairment (Ross, Kushner, & Zinn, 1997), weaknesses in executive functions appear to be an even more striking feature of their disorder (Johnson & Ross, 1994; Ross et al., 1997). Generally of higher intelligence than are girls with FraX, those with UTS differ most clearly from "no-diagnosis" control groups on tasks involving executive functioning, and not only on tasks that would be described as exclusively "nonverbal" in nature. For example, deficits in word fluency and reading comprehension deficits have been reported (Ross et al., 1997). Impairment in mathematics is frequently described in girls with UTS (Rovet, Szekely, & Hockenberry, 1994). More recent analysis of deficiencies in mathematics in girls with UTS reveals a surprising normality of geometry and math fact knowledge, with greater difficulties in the procedural and algorithmic components of mathematical problem solving (Ross et al., 1997). Neither FraX nor UTS girls have profiles of neuropsychological skills similar to those found in individuals with NF.

CURRENT KNOWLEDGE AND FUTURE DIRECTIONS

NF is a unique disorder with a number of neuropsychological and behavioral features and associated neuroanatomical anomalies that continue to hold the clinical and research interests of neuropsychologists, neurologists, geneticists, pediatricians, and educators. During the past 5 to 10 years, a great deal has been learned about the neuropsychological and behavioral manifestations of this disorder. The primary reasons for these advances have been refinements in research methodology and technology coupled with increased scientific rigor. Contemporary investigations employ well-standardized batteries of intellectual, neuropsychological, and academic achievement skills, rather than gross estimates of IQ.

In addition, the use of nonaffected siblings as comparison subjects has helped avoid potential bias in selection of controls and has increased the sensitivity of research designs to subtle impairments in functioning. The diagnosis of LDs is a highly complex and controversial topic (Lyon, Gray, Kavanagh, & Krasnegor, 1993), and one should not be lulled into complacency with descriptions of the learning style in this highly complex disorder that are based solely on discrepancies between IQ and academic scores. Several studies have begun to use subtyping procedures and newer conceptualizations of learning problems to examine the nature of LDs in NF, rather than relying solely on more simplistic definitions or summarizing outcomes in terms of the overall prevalence of LDs (Brewer et al., 1997; Eliason, 1986, 1988; Lyon et al., 1993; North et al., 1997). That NF is associated with elevated rates of LDs has been readily accepted, but questions remain as to whether there are unique aspects of LDs in children with NF that require a novel educational approach. Sometimes parents and teachers tend to "dismiss" the children's LDs because they have a medical or neurological condition, and therefore a reason for substandard school performance. However, children with NF and LDs can and do benefit from resurce placement, language, speech, and occupational therapy, as well as standard school approaches to remediation.

Researchers have also begun to undertake rigorous investigations of relationships of brain anomalies to cognitive and learning status in NF. The anatomical location and number of hyperintensities appear relevant in predicting neurobehavioral outcomes, and it is generally believed that these hyperintensities gradually diminish in size or disappear completely with advancing age. The cognitive correlates of those changes remain largely unknown.

Future directions for research on the developmental implications of NF in children include the following:

- Further characterization of the nature of the LDs associated with this condition.
- Longitudinal studies of neuropsychological and learning status across the lifespan.
- Utilization of more advanced neuroimaging techniques (e.g., FlAIR) to determine the neuropsychological significance of brain hyperintensities. These methods should include volumetric measures of the total (and regional) "burden" of hyperintensities, and functional MRI techniques to investigate activation patterns in children with learning or neuropsychological impairment. Longitudinal studies of brain MRI will also clarify the natural history of hyperintensities, thus strengthening our understanding of their coevolution with neuropsychological and learning status.
- Genetic studies linking specific mutations within the NF gene to neuropsychological and behavioral status. Studies of this type may, for example, help elucidate genetic and physiological bases for the LDs or cognitive impairments observed in this population as well as other populations.
- More complete and accurate characterization of the psychosocial and emotional aspects of NF, with an emphasis on improving the quality of life for these individuals.

Children with NF, like those with many other genetic disorders, present with an intriguing profile of neuropsychological strengths and weaknesses. Because hyperintensities, when present, are almost always seen in the basal ganglia and cerebellum, it is likely that dysfunction of these anatomical structures may underlie linguistic deficits in children with NF (Denckla, 1996). The same may be true for visual–spatial and attention deficits as well, given the evidence that cerebellum and basal ganglia are involved in these cognitive functions also (Botez, Botez, Elie, & Attig, 1989; Schmahmann, 1991). If this turns out to be the case, then unrealized basal ganglia or cerebellar dysfunction may also underlie LDs in children without NF. We know that hyperintensities, thought to represent delayed myelination, are not typically seen in adults, but there is no consensus on the evolution of their LDs. Therefore, what we learn about the neuroanatomical and neuropsychological profile of children with NF will undoubtedly help us understand more about the characteristics, and possibly the neurological basis, of LDs in the general population as well.

ACKNOWLEDGMENTS

Some of the work reported in this chapter was supported by Grant No. P50 NS35359 from the National Institute of Neurological Disorders and Stroke (NINDS), Grant No. P30-HD 24061 from the National Institute of Child Health and Human Development, and the Batza Family Foundation Endowed Chair to Martha B. Denckla. Further support was provided by Grant No. R01 NS 31950 from the National Institute of Neurological Disorders and Stroke, the Texas Neurofibromatosis Foundation, and the T. L. L. Temple Foundation to Bartlett D. Moore, III. We acknowledge Pamula D. Yerby and Mark Brandt for their help in manuscript preparation.

REFERENCES

Achenbach, T. M., & Edelbrock, C. (1983). *Child Behavior Checklist*. Burlington: University of Vermont, Department of Psychiatry.

Aoki, S., Barkovich, A. J., Nishimura, K., Kjos, B. O., Machida, T., Cogen, P., Edwards, M., & Norman, D. (1989). Neurofibromatosis types 1 and 2: Cranial MR findings. *Radiology, 172*, 527–534.

Bawden, H., Dooley, J., Buckley, D., Camfield, P., Gordon, K., Riding, M., & Llewellyn, G. (1996). MRI and nonverbal cognitive deficits in children with neurofibromatosis 1. *Journal of Clinical and Experimental Neuropsychology, 18*, 784–792.

Bellugi, U., Wang, P. P., & Jernigan, T. L. (1994). Williams syndrome: An unusual neuropsychological profile. In S. H. Broman & J. Grafman (Eds.), *Atypical cognitive deficits in developmental disorders: Implications for brain function* (pp. 23–56). Hillsdale, NJ: Erlbaum.

Bender, B. G., Linden, M. G., & Robinson, A. (1989). Verbal and spatial processing efficiency in 32 children with sex chromosome abnormalities. *Pediatric Research, 25*, 577–579.

Benjamin, C. M., Colley, A., Donnai, D., Kingston, H., Harris, R., & Kerzin-Storrar, L. (1993). Neurofibromatosis type 1 (NF1): Knowledge, experience, and reproductive decisions of affected patients and families. *Journal of Medical Genetics, 30*, 567–574.

Blatt, J., Jaffe, M., Deutsch, M., & Adkins, J. (1986). Neurofibromatosis and childhood tumors. *Cancer, 57*, 1225–1229.

Bleyer, W. A. (1981). Neurologic sequelae of methotrexate and ionizing radiation: A new classification. *Cancer Treatment Response, 65*(Suppl. 1), 89–98.

Bognanno, J. R., Edwards, M. K., Lee, T. A., Dunn, D. W., Roos, K. L., & Klatte, E. C. (1988). Cranial MR imaging in neurofibromatosis. *American Journal of Roentgenology, 151*, 381–388.

Botez, M. I., Botez, T., Elie, R., & Attig, E. (1989). Role of the cerebellum in complex human behavior. *Italian Journal of Neurological Science, 10*, 291–300.

Brewer, V. R., Moore, B. D., & Hiscock, M. (1997). Learning disability subtypes in children with neurofibromatosis. *Journal of Learning Disabilities, 30*(5), 521–533.

Brookshire, B., Copeland, D. R., Moore, B. D., & Ater, J. L. (1990). Pretreatment neuropsychological status and associated factors in children with primary brain tumors. *Neurosurgery, 27*(6), 887–891.

Cohen, B. H., Kaplan, A. M., & Packer, R. J. (1990–91). Management of intracranial neoplasms in children with neurofibromatosis type 1 and 2: The Children's Cancer Study Group. *Pediatric Neurosurgery, 16*, 66–72.

Copeland, D. R., Fletcher, J. M., Pfefferbaum-Levine, B., Jaffe, N., Ried, H., & Maor, M. (1985). Neuropsychological sequelae of childhood cancer in long-term survivors. *Pediatrics, 75*, 745–753.

Crump, T. (1981). Translation of case reports in Ueber die in multiplen Fibrome der Haut und ihre Beziehung zu den multiplen Neuromen. In J. J. Mulvihill, V. M. Riccardi, & W. M. Wade (Eds.), *Genetics, cell biology, and biochemistry: Vol. 29. Neurofibromatosis (von Recklinghausen disease)* (pp. 259–275). New York: Raven Press.

Denckla, M. B. (1996). Neurofibromatosis type 1: A model for the pathogenesis of reading disability. *Mental Retardation and Developmental Disabilities Research Reviews, 2*, 48–53.

Denckla, M. B., Hofman, K., Mazzocco, M. M., Melhem, E., Reiss, A. L., Bryan, R. N., Harris, E. L., Lee, J., Cox, C. S., & Schuerholz, L. J. (1996). Relationship between T_2 weighted hyperintensities (unidentified bright objects) and lower IQs in children with neurofibromatosis-1. *American Journal of Medical Genetics, 67*(1), 98–102.

De Winter, A. E., Moore, B. D., Slopis, J. M., Ater, J., & Copeland, D. R. (in press). Brain tumors in children with neurofibromatosis: Additional neuropsychological morbidity? *Neuro Oncology.*

De Winter, A. E., Moore, B. D., Slopis, J. M., Jackson, E. F., & Leeds, N. E. (in press). Quantitative morphology of the corpus callosum in children with neurofibromatosis and attention-deficit/hyperactivity disorder. *Journal of Child Neurology.*

DiMario, F. J., & Ramsby, G. (1998). Magnetic resonance imaging lesion analysis in neurofibromatosis type 1. *Archives of Neurology, 55*, 500–505.

DiPaolo, D. P., Zimmerman, R. A., Rorke, L. B., Zackai, E. H., Bilaniuk, L. T., & Yachnis, A. T. (1995). Neurofibromatosis type 1: Pathologic substrate of high-signal intensity foci in the brain. *Radiology, 195*, 721–724.

Duffner, P. K., Cohen, M. E., Seidel, G., & Shucard, D. W. (1989). The significance of MRI abnormalities in children with neurofibromatosis. *Neurology, 39*, 373–378.

Dunn, D. W., & Roos, K. L. (1989). MRI evaluation of learning difficulties and incoordination in children with neurofibromatosis type 1. *Neurofibromatosis, 2*, 1–5.

Eldridge, R., Denckla, M. B., Bien, E., Myers, S., Kaiser-Kupfer, M. I., Pikus, A., Schlesinger, S. L., Pany, D. M., Dambrosia, J. M., & Zasloff, M. A. (1989). Neurofibromatosis type 1 (Recklinghausen's disease): Neurologic and cognitive assessment with sibling controls. *American Journal of Diseases of Children, 143*(7), 833–837.

Eliason, M. J. (1986). Neurofibromatosis: Implications for behavior and learning. *Journal of Developmental and Behavioral Pediatrics, 7*(3), 175–179.

Eliason, M. J. (1988). Neuropsychological patterns: Neurofibromatosis compared to developmental learning disorders. *Neurofibromatosis, 1*(1), 17–25.

Ferner, R. E., Chaudhuri, R., Bingham, J., Cox, T., & Hughes, R. A. C. (1993). MRI in neurofibromatosis 1: The nature and evolution of increased T_2 weighted lesions and their relationship to intellectual impairment. *Journal of Neurology, Neurosurgery and Psychiatry, 56*, 492–495.

Ferner, R. E., Hughes, R. A. C., & Wenman, J. (1996). Intellectual impairment in neurofibromatosis 1. *Journal of Neurological Science, 138*, 125–133.

Filipek, P. A., Semrud-Clikeman, M., Steingard, R. J., Renshaw, P. F., Dennedy, D. N., & Biederman, J. (1997). Volumetric MRI analysis comparing subjects having attention-deficit hyperactivity disorder with normal controls. *Neurology, 48*, 589–601.

Fletcher, J. M., & Copeland, D. R. (1988). Neurobehavioral effects of central nervous system prophylactic treatment of cancer in children. *Journal of Clinical and Experimental Neuropsychology, 10*, 495–538.

Fletcher, J. M., Satz, P., & Morris, R. (1986). The Florida longitudinal project: A review. In S. A. Mednick, M. Harway, & K. M. Finello (Eds.), *Handbook of longitudinal research* (Vol. 1, pp. 280–304). New York: Praeger.

Gentilini, M., De Renzi, E., & Crisi, G. (1987). Bilateral paramedian thalamic artery infarcts: Report of eight cases. *Journal of Neurology, Neurosurgery and Psychiatry, 50*, 900–909.

Giedd, J. N., Castellanos, F. X., Casey, B. J., Kozuch, P., King, A. C., Hamburger, S. D., & Rapoport, J. L. (1994). Quantitative morphology of the corpus callosum in attention deficit hyperactivity disorder. *American Journal of Psychiatry, 151*(5), 665–669.

Gutmann, D. H., Aylsworth, A., Carey, J. C., Korf, B. R., Marks, J., Pyeritz, R. E., Rubenstein, A., & Viskochil, D. (1997). The diagnostic evaluation and multidisciplinary management of neurofibromatosis 1 and neurofibromatosis 2. *Journal of the American Medical Association, 278*, 51–57.

Hofman, K. J., Harris, E. L., Bryan, R. N., & Denckla, M. B. (1994). Neurofibromatosis type 1: The cognitive phenotype. *Journal of Pediatrics, 124*, S1–S8.

Hunt, A., & Dennis, J. (1987). Psychiatric disorder among children with tuberous sclerosis. *Developmental Medicinie and Child Neurology, 29*, 190–198.

Hynd, G. W., Obrzut, J. E., Hayes, F., & Becker, M. G. (1986). Neuropsychology of childhood learning disabilities. In D. Wedding, A. M. Horton, & J. Webster (Eds.), *The neuropsychology handbook: Behavioral and clinical perspectives* (pp. 456–485). New York: Springer.

Hynd, G. W., Semrud-Clikeman, M., Lorys, A. R., Novey, E. S., Eliopulos, D., & Lyytinen, H. (1991). Corpus callosum morphology in attention-deficit hyperactivity disorder (ADHD): Morphometric analysis of MRI. *Journal of Learning Disabilities, 24*, 141–146.

Itoh, T., Magnaldi, S., White, R. M., Denckla, M. B., Hofman, K., Naidu, S., & Bryan, R. N. (1994). Neuro-fibromatosis type 1: The evolution of deep gray and white matter MR abnormalities. *American Journal of Neuroradiology, 15*, 1513–1519.

Jastak, S., & Wilkinson, G. S. (1984). *Manual for the Wide Range Achievement Test—Revised.* Wilmington, DE: Jastak Associates.

Johnson, R., Jr., & Ross, J. L. (1994). Event-related potential indications of altered brain development in Turner syndrome. In S. H. Broman & J. Grafman (Eds.), *Atypical cognitive deficits in developmental disorders: Implications for brain function* (pp. 217–242). Hillsdale, NJ: Erlbaum.

Kahn, E., & Crosby, E. (1972). Korsakoff's syndrome associated with surgical lesions involving the mamillary bodies. *Neurology, 22*, 317–325.

Kaplan, A. M., Chen, K., Lawson, M. A., Wodrich, D. L., Bonstelle, C. T., & Reiman, E. M. (1997). Positron emission tomography in children with neurofibromatosis-1. *Journal of Child Neurology, 12*, 499–506.

Legius, E., Descheemaeker, M. J., Steyaert, J., Spaepen, A., Vlietinck, R., Casaer, P., Demaerel, P., & Fryns, J. P. (1995). Neurofibromatosis type 1 in childhood: Correlation of MRI findings with intelligence. *Journal of Neurology, Neurosurgery and Psychiatry, 59*, 638–640.

Lindgren, S. D., & Benton, A. L. (1980). Developmental patterns of visual spatial judgment. *Journal of Pediatric Psychology, 5*, 217–225.

Listernick, R., Darling, C., Greenwald, M., Strauss, L., & Charrow, J. (1995). Optic pathway tumors in children: The effect of neurofibromatosis type 1 on clinical manifestations and natural history. *Journal of Pediatrics, 127*(5), 718–722.

Lyon, G. R., Gray, D. B, Kavanagh, J. F., & Krasnegor, N. A. (Eds.). (1993). *Better understanding learning disabilities.* Baltimore: Paul H. Brookes.

Mazzocco, M. M., Turner, J. E., Denckla, M. B., Hofman, K. J., Scanlon, D. C., & Vellutino, F. R. (1995). Language and reading deficits associated with neurofibromatosis type 1: Evidence for a not-so-non-verbal learning disability. *Developmental Neuropsychology, 11*, 503–522.

Moore, B. D., Ater, J. L., Needle, M. N., Slopis, J. S., & Copeland, D. R. (1994). Neuropsychological profile of children with neurofibromatosis, brain tumor, or both. *Journal of Child Neurology, 9*(4), 368–377.

Moore, B. D., Slopis, J. M., Schomer, D., Jackson, E. F., & Levy, B. (1996). Neuropsychological significance of areas of high signal intensity on brain magnetic resonance imaging scans of children with neurofibromatosis. *Neurology, 46*, 1660–1668.

Moore, B. D., & Slopis, J. S. (1994). Stability of cognitive status in children with neurofibromatosis, type I [Abstract]. *Pediatric Research, 35*(4), 25.

Mulvihill, J. J. (1990). Neurofibromatosis 1 (Recklinghausen disease) and neurofibromatosis 2 (bilateral acoustic neurofibromatosis): An update. *Annals of Internal Medicine, 113*, 39–52.

National Institutes of Health (NIH) Consensus Development Conference. Neurofibromatosis: Conference statement. (1988). *Archives of Neurology, 45*(5), 575–578.

North, K. (1993). Neurofibromatosis type 1: Review of the first 200 patients in an Australian clinic. *Journal of Child Neurology, 8*, 395–402.

North, K., Joy, P., Yuille, D., Cocks, N., & Hutchins, P. (1995). Cognitive function and academic performance in children with neurofibromatosis type 1. *Developmental Medicine and Child Neurology, 37*, 427–436.

North, K., Joy, P., Yuille, D., Cocks, N., Mobbs, E., Hutchins, P., McHugh, K., & de Silva, M. (1994). Specific learning disability in children with neurofibromatosis type 1: Significance of MRI abnormalities. *Neurology, 44*(5), 878–883.

North, K., Riccardi, V., Samango-Sprouse, C., Ferner, R., Moore, B. D., Legius, E., Ratner, N., & Denckla, M. B. (1997). Cognitive function and academic performance in neurofibromatosis 1: Consensus statement from the NF Cognitive Disorders Task Force. *Neurology, 48*, 1121–1127.

Reiss, A. L., Freund, L. S., Baumgardner, T. L., Abrams, M. J., & Denckla, M. B. (1995). Contribution of the FMRI gene mutation to human intellectual dysfunction. *Nature Genetics, 11*, 331–334.

Reiss, A. L., Lee, J., & Freund, L. (1993). Neuroanatomy of fragile X syndrome. *Neurology, 44*, 1317–1324.

Riccardi, V. M. (1981). Neurofibromatosis: An overview and new directions in clinical investigations. *Advances in Neurology, 29*, 1–9.

Riccardi, V. M. (1982). The multiple forms of neurofibromatosis. *Pediatrics in Review, 3*, 293–298.

Riccardi, V. M. (1992). Type 1 neurofibromatosis and the pediatric patient. *Current Problems in Pediatrics, 22*, 66–107.

Riccardi, V. M., & Eichner, J. E. (1986). *Neurofibromatosis: Phenotype, natural history and pathogenesis* (2nd ed.). Baltimore: Johns Hopkins University Press.

Roos, K., & Dunn, D. (1992). Neurofibromatoses. *CA. A Cancer Journal for Clinicians, 42*, 241–254.

Ross, J. L., Kushner, H., & Zinn, A. (1997). Discriminant analysis of the Ullrich–Turner syndrome neurocognitive profile. *American Journal of Medical Genetics, 72*, 275–280.

Rouleau, G. A., Seizinger, B. R., Wertelecki, W., Haines, J., Superneau, D., Martuza, R., & Gusella, J. F. (1990). Flanking markers bracket the neurofibromatosis type 2 (NF2) gene on chromosome 22. *American Journal of Human Genetics, 46*, 323–328.

Rovet, J., Netley, C., Keenan, M., Bailey, J., & Stewart, D. (1996). The psychoeducational profile of boys with Klinefelter syndrome. *Journal of Learning Disabilities, 29*, 180–196.

Rovet, J., Szekely, C., & Hockenberry, M. N. (1994). Specific arithmetic calculation deficits in children with Turner syndrome (clinical trial). *Journal of Clinical and Experimental Neuropsychology, 16*(6), 820–839.

Rutter, M., Tizard, J., & Whitmore, K. (Eds.). (1970). *Education, health and behavior.* London: Longmans.

Samuelsson, B., & Riccardi, V. M. (1989). Neurofibromatosis in Gothenburg, Sweden: II. Intellectual compromise. *Neurofibromatosis, 2*, 78–83.

Samuelsson, B., & Samuelsson, S. (1989). Neurofibromatosis in Gothenburg, Sweden: I. Background, study design and epidemiology. *Neurofibromatosis, 2*, 6–22.

Schmahmann, J. D. (1991). An emerging concept: The cerebellar contribution to higher function. *Archives of Neurology, 48*, 1178–1187.

Semrud-Clikeman, M., Filipek, P. A., & Biederman, J. (1994). Attention deficit hyperactivity disorder: Differences in the corpus callosum by MRI morphometric analysis. *Journal of the American Academy of Child and Adolescent Psychiatry, 33*, 875–881.

Sevick, R. J., Barkovich, A. J., Edwards, M. S. B., Koch, T., Berg, B., & Lempert, T. (1992). Evolution of white matter lesions in neurofibromatosis type 1: MR findings. American *Journal of Roentgenology, 159*, 171–175.

Slopis, J., Ater, J. L., Copeland, D. R., Moore, B. D., & Leeds, N. (1994, May). *Neurobehavioral and cognitive syndromes in hypothalamic astrocytomas of childhood.* Paper presented at the Sixth International Symposium on Pediatric Neuro-Oncology, Houston, TX.

Spaepen, A., Borghgraef, M., & Fryns, J. (1992). Von Recklinghausen-neurofibromatosis: A study of the psychological profile. In G. Evers-Kiebooms, J. Fryns, J. Cassiman, & H. Van den Berghe (Eds.), *Psychosocial aspects of genetic counseling: Birth defects* (pp. 85–91). New York: Wiley–Liss.

Squire, L. R., & Butters, N. (Eds.) (1984). *Neuropsychology of memory* (Chapter 13, pp. 123–132). New York: Guilford Press.

Stine, S., & Adams, W. (1989). Learning problems in neurofibromatosis patients. *Clinical Orthopedics, 245*, 43–48.

Texas Neurofibromatosis Foundation. (1996). *Neurofibromatosis.* Dallas: Author.

Varnhagen, C. E., Lewin, S., Das, J. P., & Bowen, P. (1988). Neurofibromatosis and psychological processes. *Journal of Developmental and Behavioral Pediatrics, 9*(5), 257–265.

von Deimling, A., Krone, W., & Menon, A. G. (1995). N.F. type 1: Pathology, clinical features and molecular genetics. *Brain Pathology, 5*, 153–162.

Wadsby, M., Lindehammar, H., & Eeg-Olofsson, O. (1989). Neurofibromatosis in childhood: Neuropsychological aspects. *Neurofibromatosis, 2*, 251–260.

Yamanouchi, H., Kato, T., Matsuda, H., Takashima, S., Sakuragawa, N., & Arima, M. (1995). MRI in neurofibromatosis type I: Using fluid-attenuated inversion recovery pulse sequences. *Pediatric Neurology, 4*, 286–290.

Zimmerman, R. A., Yachnis, A. T., Rorke, L. B., Rebsamen, S. L., Bilaniuk, L. T., & Zackai, E. (1992). Pathology of findings of high signal intensity findings in neurofibromatosis type 1 [Abstract]. *Radiology, 186*, 123.

Zoller, M., Rembeck, B., Akesson, H. O., & Agrvall, L. (1995). Life expectancy, mortality and prognostic factors in neurofibromatosis type 1. *Acta Dermato-Venereologica, 75*, 136–140.

8

METABOLIC AND NEURODEGENERATIVE DISORDERS

ELSA SHAPIRO
MICHAEL BALTHAZOR

In children, the trajectory of cognitive, behavioral, and physical development can be altered by various environmental and inborn agents that affect the central nervous system (CNS). Acquired lesions from head trauma, brain tumors, neurotoxins (e.g., lead), effects of treatment of CNS cancer, infection, or sequelae from emotional trauma can alter the pace of cognitive development so that a child does not acquire abilities and knowledge at his or her premorbid rate. Disruption of children's cognitive growth can also be caused by a wide range of inborn abnormalities. Disorders such as dyslexia, language disorders, epilepsy, attention-deficit/hyperactivity disorder, fragile X syndrome, neurofibromatosis, tuberous sclerosis, spina bifida, and countless others result in altered development of specific CNS pathways and functions. These disorders are characterized by relatively constant abnormalities, frequently resulting in specific neurobehavioral and neurocognitive deficits. Some of these disorders show subtle alterations in severity over time and may change phenotypically in concert with neural development. However, in most cases these disorders are not neurodegenerative and do not represent active disease processes. In contrast, there are metabolic and neurodegenerative disorders that involve deterioration of function beginning at a defined time and in association with active disease processes. The latter disorders are the topic of this chapter.

Progressive metabolic and neurodegenerative disorders are characterized by cognitive and behavioral deterioration resulting in dementia and ultimately in death or severe incapacitation. Neuropsychologists traditionally have not evaluated such children, largely because their prognosis was so poor and nothing could be done beyond providing symptomatic relief. As a result, the natural history of their cognitive and behavioral difficulties has not been not well defined or quantified. Recently, however, dietary, medical, and genetic treatments for such disorders have been developed. The advent of these new treatments has led to studies of disease outcomes involving comparisons of treated and untreated children. As pediatric neuropsychologists, we need to be better acquainted with these disorders in order to identify children early for more effective treatment and for participation in clinical trials. Another reason for interest in these disorders is that they offer a "natural laboratory" to study specific and often localized abnormalities in cognitive and behavioral functions.

The purpose of this chapter is to review the characteristics of childhood dementia and of specific degenerative syndromes in childhood. As examples of the latter, we discuss two general disease categories, the leukodystrophies and mucopolysaccharidoses (MPS disorders). The disorders in both categories arise from inborn errors of metabolism that result in neurodegeneration. Disease presentation, pathophysiology, neuropsychological manifestations, and treatment are reviewed for disorders in each group. Research needs and future directions are also considered.

CHILDHOOD DEMENTIA

In adults, *dementia* refers to decline from a previous intellectual level and compromise in specific domains of mental activity (Cummings & Benson, 1992). However, in children, the opposing vectors of deterioration from disease and the forces of development (Dyken & McCleary, 1986; Rapin, 1976; Shapiro & Klein, 1993) make it more difficult to detect early stages of dementia. Depending on the stage of the disease, decline in IQ can reflect slowing of mental development, plateauing, or loss of skill or knowledge. In many cases, a child's premorbid level of functioning is obscured by the early and insidious nature of disease onset. Although school and parental history can provide some information, many of these diseases are present from birth and alter cognitive growth from the outset; the premorbid state thus may not be entirely "disease-free."

The rate of cognitive and neurological deterioration in childhood degenerative diseases varies across different diseases and frequently according to age of disease onset. Some diseases progress with a gradual downward trajectory, beginning with slowing of mental development. Other diseases show a sudden loss of function with a rapid downhill course. Still other disorders progress sporadically, with periods of stability interspersed with episodes of loss of function.

We have previously described various patterns of dementia in childhood that arise from differing effects of disease on the trajectory of cognitive growth (Shapiro & Klein, 1993; Shapiro, Lockman, Balthazor, & Krivit, 1995). One pattern is typical of the progressive dementia associated with metabolic and degenerative diseases. In diseases that follow this pattern, initial slowing of the developmental process is followed by plateauing of function and then, in the final stages of the disease, by loss of mental function. The first stage of the process is often difficult to detect because no actual loss of cognitive milestones is observed. As the disease progresses and a downward decline is noted, these diseases appear to progress in fits and starts, in a manner reminiscent of a stepwise decline. Following children over intervals of weeks and months, we often see periods of no change followed by periods of rapid loss of function, and then by another plateau in functioning. Following children over longer intervals of months to years precludes observation of this stepwise pattern of disease progression and leads to the impression of a continuous, gradual decline.

Another pattern of decline is that of increasingly slowed development without actual loss of skills. Children conforming to this pattern continue to acquire new skills, but at a rate that is significantly slower than that anticipated from premorbid cognitive trajectories. Pediatric HIV and AIDS, and treated metabolic diseases such as galactosemia and maple syrup urine disease, are examples of disorders associated with early encephalopathy and gradual slowing of mental development. Some children with Hurler syndrome also show this pattern after bone marrow transplantation (BMT) (Peters et al., 1996; Peters, Shapiro, Anderson, et al., 1998).

A third pattern of dementia involves rapid loss of cognitive function and subsequent cessation of development or minimal mental growth. An arrest of development occurs, with loss of ability to encode new information resulting in a decline of IQ over time. Some cases of severe head injury, severe epileptic syndrome, and brain tumor follow this pattern of dementia. Rett syndrome may also fall into this category, as the development of children with Rett syndrome frequently comes to a halt late in the first year of life.

The fourth pattern of decline is also characterized by a sudden loss of skills. In this instance, however, development is not fully arrested, and a child is able to learn (albeit at a slower than premorbid rate). Inflammatory disease, trauma, infections, and toxins can result in this pattern.

Figure 8.1 graphically portrays hypothetical growth trajectories corresponding to each of these four types of childhood dementia. These developmental pathways are only theo-

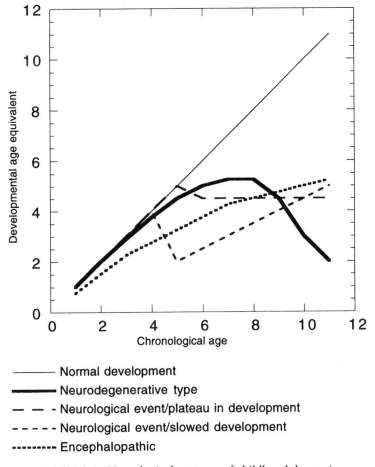

FIGURE 8.1. Hypothetical patterns of childhood dementia.

retical; patterns of progression are quite variable. Also, there may well be diseases that follow other patterns of progression. The pattern of dementia associated with the diseases discussed in this chapter, which involve actual neural degeneration, is the one labeled *neurodegenerative type*.

NEURODEGENERATIVE DISEASES

In many neurodegenerative diseases, a relationship between age of disease onset and rate of deterioration exists, with earlier onset associated with a more rapid downhill course (Shapiro, Lockman, et al., 1995). Often a relationship may also be found between age of onset and pattern of neuropsychological decline. Presumably the same pathological process has different effects at different stages of the child's development. Each disease has a characteristic course and effect on cognition and behavior, although some diseases have more variable phenotypes than do others.

Neuropsychological manifestation of metabolic and neurodegenerative diseases vary with the pathophysiology and locus of disease. In adults, distinctive neuropsychological characteristics are associated with cortical dementias (e.g., Alzheimer disease) as contrasted with subcortical dementias. Patterns of neuropsychological performance in subcortical dementias can be further subdivided into those that are due to insults to subcortical white matter and those reflecting damage to extrapyramidal deep gray matter (Cummings & Benson, 1992). Childhood neurodegenerative diseases affect white matter more than gray matter. The negative effects of white matter disease on cognitive development may be heightened in childhood by the concurrence of myelination and cognitive development, and the resultant increased sensitivity of the child's brain to neurotoxic substances. Many conditions, such as hydrocephalus, late effects of radiation in childhood cancer, leukodystrophies, and metabolic disorders, affect myelin development. Although many symptoms found in children with white matter diseases are associated with the "nonverbal learning disability syndrome" (Rourke, 1987), patterns of deficit vary greatly according to locus of the disease and age of onset (Shapiro, Lipton, & Krivit, 1992). For example, profiles of neuropsychological deficit are related to whether abnormality in white matter is anterior or posterior; research to date suggests that anterior lesions are more likely to have behavioral manifestations (Shapiro, Balthazor, Lockman, & Krivit, 1997).

In the most common adult neurological disorders, Alzheimer disease and stroke, deterioration of cognitive function results from damage to gray matter. Verbal memory and aphasia are primary symptoms of these conditions. In contrast, few childhood neurological diseases present with aphasia and selective memory impairments. Batten disease (neuronal ceroid lipofuscinosis) and dementias associated with epilepsy are among the few disorders that primarily affect the cells rather than the myelinated fibers connecting cells. Diseases of the striatum, such as Parkinson and Huntington diseases, are primarily adult conditions. These diseases rarely occur in children, with the exception of Hallervorden–Spatz syndrome and juvenile-onset Huntington disease. As in adult diseases of the deep gray matter, neuropsychological findings in children with these disorders include motor deficits, decreased speed of processing, and executive dysfunctions.

The subset of childhood neurodegenerative disorders of central interest in this chapter is characterized by abnormalities that interfere with enzyme or protein synthesis, resulting in the buildup of neurotoxic substances in the developing child's brain. Each of these "storage" diseases is caused by an inherited deficiency of a specific enzyme. Neurotoxic substances accumulate in the CNS and sometimes in other parts of the body, because the enzyme that breaks down these substances is deficient or absent. The gradual accumulation of abnormal material interferes with brain function. Storage diseases can be classified by the location of the structures within the neuron (lysosomes or peroxisomes) containing the enzymes that degrade and digest material within or outside of the cell. Such neurotoxic substances accumulate because of the absence of these lysosomal or peroxisomal enzymes.

Storage diseases fall into two major categories: the leukodystrophies and the MPS disorders. The former diseases affect the white matter and are characterized by demyelination. The leukodystrophies include the lysosomal storage diseases metachromatic leukodystrophy (MLD) and globoid cell leukodystrophy (GLD, sometimes called Krabbe disease), and a peroxisomal storage disease, adrenoleukodystrophy (ALD). In the MPS disorders, accumulation of glycosamineglycans (GAGs) damages multiple body organs, including heart, lungs, eye, liver, spleen, skeletal system, and connective tissue. These substances also accumulate in the neurons and other brain tissues. Although demyelination can occur in the MPS disorders, it is not a primary feature of this category of diseases.

Childhood neurodegenerative diseases have received limited attention in the neuropsychological literature. Our group at the University of Minnesota, together with other members of the Storage Disease Collaborative Study Group, has established a national data base on children with leukodystrophies and MPS disorders. Although we describe the course and neuropsychological features of several storage diseases in this chapter, 500 diseases are listed in the on-line Mendelian Inheritance in Man (*sic*!) data base (http://www3.ncbi. nlm.nih.gov/Omim/). Many metabolic and neurodegenerative diseases have received only incidental comment or have only been the subjects of single-case studies. Other diseases of this type have been reviewed more extensively. Because we cannot address all neurodegenerative diseases here, we have prepared a table (Table 8.1) that describes current knowledge regarding inheritance, onset, neurological and neuroradiological findings, and the neuropsychological profiles of 10 additional metabolic and genetic diseases. The diseases chosen for presentation were selected to serve as examples of a given type of disorder. We have also described some of the more common diseases, and have focused on diseases for which there is a reasonable body of information and with which we have direct experience. Due to space limitations, we have omitted discussion of several important disorders, including juvenile Huntington disease; Williams, Angelman, and Prader–Willi syndromes; and Rasmussen encephalitis. We have mentioned several disorders that have received scant attention in the neuropsychological literature (mitochondrial encephalopathies, Rett syndrome), in the hope that neuropsychologists will begin to follow children with these diseases more systematically.

INCIDENCE AND IMPORTANCE OF NEURODEGENERATIVE DISEASES

Metabolic and neurodegenerative diseases are rare by epidemiological standards. Incidence in the normal population ranges from 1 in 10,000 to 1 in 200,000 persons for each disease. Although most neuropsychologists will not encounter many of these diseases over a lifetime of practice, it behooves practitioners to know the diseases' important signs, in order to aid early diagnosis for effective treatment and to be able to follow children over time to assess their progress. Centers that study these diseases are emerging, because sufficient numbers of cases for research purposes can only be collected through a coordinated effort at the national or international level. However, funds are often not available to bring

TABLE 8.1. Additional Metabolic and Genetic Diseases

Disease	Etiology/pathophysiology	Cognitive/behavioral/neuropsychological findings	Neurological/medical/neuroimaging findings	Treatment
Maple syrup urine disease Presents as an acute, critical neurotoxic condition often prior to age 2 weeks, with lethargy, seizures, and vomiting.	Incidence: 1 in 290,000. Gene location: 19q13. Disorder of amino acid metabolism. Branched-chain amino acids (BCAAs) are normally transaminated to branched-chain keto acids (BCKAs). The enzyme required to metabolize BCKAs is deficient. Resulting elevations of BCAAs and BCKAs are associated with clinical symptoms.	Cognition varies from normal to severe retardation. Early diagnosis and metabolic control contribute to IQ outcome, especially Performance IQ (Kaplan et al., 1991; Hilliges, Awiszus, & Wendel, 1993) Verbal > Performance IQ ($n = 9$). Severity of neonatal symptoms correlated with severity of cognitive deficits (Nord, van Doorninck, & Greene, 1991). Deficits in motor and visual analytic tasks. Familial IQ depressed.	MRI does not reveal consistent major abnormalities, although it demonstrated bilateral high-intensity periventricular signals on T_2-weighted images in 4 of 10 patients (Taccone, Schiaffino, Cerone, Fondelli, & Romano, 1992). The presence of dysmyelination is still not clear (Muller, Kahn, & Wendel, 1993).	Apart from dietary therapy, which does not always result in good outcomes, liver transplantation has been shown to be effective in a few cases in correcting the metabolic disorder (Jan et al., 1994).
Galactosemia Presents as failure to thrive, along with hepatomegaly and cataracts. Poor physical and mental growth, speech abnormality, and ovarian failure in females are the long-term outcomes.	Incidence: 1 in 35,000–60,000. Gene location: 9p13. Autosomal recessive disorder of carbohydrate metabolism. Toxic syndrome resulting from exposure to galactose (through milk) shortly after birth.	On neuropsychological testing, despite dietary restrictions, increasing intellectual deficits, with 83% of children over 12 having IQs below 85 (Schweitzer, Shin, Jakobs, & Brodehl, 1993). Verbal apraxia is very frequent, and verbal deficits appear to predominate over nonverbal or motor (Nelson, Waggoner, Donnell, Tuerck, & Buist, 1991; Nelson, 1995). Cognitive deficits are unrelated to genotype	MRI abnormalities have been found in the majority of cases, with cerebral and cerebellar atrophy and multiple hyperintense lesions, as well as abnormal peripheral myelination (Nelson, Wolff, Cross, Donnell, & Kaufman, 1992; Kaufman et al., 1995; Moller, Ullrich, Vermathen, Schuierer, & Koch, 1995). On neurological examination, increasing ataxia, tremor, dysarthria, and hypotonia have been found	Rapid improvement may occur with early treatment with a strict lactose-free diet. Until recently, long-term prognosis was thought to be good. However, evidence points to continuing and even progressive disease (lack of myelination) even with strict lactose restriction (Koch et al., 1992).

Disorder	Genetics / Etiology	Developmental Outcome	Neurological / Imaging Findings	Treatment
Ornithine transcarbamylase deficiency Encephalopathic symptoms occur, usually in first week of life; cyclic vomiting, excessive sleepiness, and protein avoidance may develop.	Incidence: 1 in 70,000–100,000. X-linked deficiency: Xp21.1. One of five urea cycle disorders. Results from a failure of the urea cycle to rid the body of excess ammonia. This causes hyperammonemia, with potent toxic effects on the CNS.	(Kaufman, McBride-Chang, Manis, Wolff, & Nelson, 1995). About three-fourths of cases have developmental disabilities, and average IQ is below 50. Cognitive outcome is related to the number of episodes (Msall, Batshaw, Suss, Brusilow, & Mellits, 1984). Male children are very retarded. Female carriers show a wide spectrum of cognitive ability (Maestri, Brusilow, Clissold, & Bassett, 1996). Neuropsychological pattern found is typical of white matter disease (Shapiro, 1997)	(Kaufman et al., 1995; Koch, Schmidt, Wagstaff, Ng, & Packman, 1992). Types of symptoms relate to age of onset (Bachmann, 1992). Delayed diagnosis resulting in hyperammonemic coma in infant boys often leads to death or severe mental retardation and cerebral palsy. There is evidence of stroke-like lesions (Christodoulou, Qureshi, McInnes, & Clarke, 1993). On MRI, increased ventricular size, areas of focal necrosis, and areas of deficient demyelination are seen. In females, attenuation and abnormal signal in white matter are found (Pridmore, Clarke, & Blaser, 1995).	Chronic therapies for urea cycle diseases involve protein restrictions, which produce a lowering of the blood ammonia level and dietary arginine. Liver transplantation has been effective in some cases (Hasegawa et al., 1995).
Cobalamin (vitamin B12) deficiency Infants present with developmental delay, failure to thrive, megaloblastic anemia, and pigmentary retinopathy. Onset in infancy also usually involves lethargy, recurrent vomiting, dehydration, and respiratory distress. Hypotonia and hyperreflexia can be present,	Deficiencies in vitamin B12 are characterized by the presence of methylmalonic acidemia and homocystinuria, which result in clinical symptoms. There are many different metabolic causes, most autosomal recessive. Deficiencies may also arise from inadequate amounts of vitamin B12 in breast milk if the maternal	Long-term follow-up studies of treated infants find variable outcome, with intellectual impairment present in some cases (van der Meer et al., 1994). Early onset of methylmalonic acid deficiency results in less favorable outcomes than late onset. Two forms can be identified on the basis of residual enzyme activity,	MRI often shows widening of sulci and fissures with some delay in myelination, as well as symmetrical involvement of the basal ganglia (Brismar & Ozand, 1994). There may be cortical atrophy on CT scans, and EEG often shows diffuse slowing.	Treatment with cobalamin in some cases can correct biochemical findings, but neurological findings, once developed, appear irreversible. Rare cobalamin metabolic defects emerging late in childhood have normal development followed by loss of acquired skills; these defects respond well to treatment. Prenatal

(continued)

TABLE 8.1. (*continued*)

Disease	Etiology/pathophysiology	Cognitive/behavioral/neuropsychological findings	Neurological/medical/neuroimaging findings	Treatment
often with choreoathetoid movements. In adults, B12 deficiency effects are milder, with peripheral neuropathy, subacute degeneration of the spinal cord, psychosis, and dementia.	diet is deficient in vitamin B12 intake (vegan diet, severe starvation) or if the mother has unrecognized pernicious anemia (Kuhne, Bubl, & Baumgartner, 1991).	which is related to cognitive and neurological outcome (Shevell, Matiaszuk, Ledley, & Rosenblatt, 1993). In adults, psychosis and dementia have been observed.		treatment with large doses of vitamin B12 during the last trimester of pregnancy has been successful.
Glutaric acidemia Macrocephaly seen at birth, followed by progressive dystonia and athetosis, opisthotonus, and dyskinesia. Mental retardation is variable.	Gene location: 19p13.2. Autosomal recessive disorder of organic acid metabolism. Glutaric aciduria type I is an inborn error in the degradation of lysine, hydroxylysine, and tryptophan due to a deficiency of glutaryl-CoA dehydrogenase. Glutaric, 3-OH-glutaric, and glutaconic acids are excreted in the urine, particularly during illness.	Mental function is less affected than motor. Not all patients suffer from encephalopathy (Hoffmann et al., 1995). Choreoathetosis and other motor impairments are characteristic. Eight patients received neuropsychological testing, and receptive language function was found to be superior to expressive; cognitive functions were less affected than motor (Kyllerman et al., 1994).	On CT, frontotemporal atrophy, dilated sylvian fissures, and hypodensity of lenticular nuclei were found (Mandel, Braun, El-Peleg, Christensen, & Berant, 1991); also, gliosis and neuronal loss in the basal ganglia (Merinero et al., 1995).	Dietary treatment. Avoidance of illness: Illness exacerbates this disorder.
Mitochondrial encephalopathies A heterogeneous and phenotypically variable group of disorders. • Leigh syndrome: Cranial nerve dysfunction, encephalopathy, ophthalmoplegia, optic atrophy, and dysphagia.	Defect in mitochondrial DNA No incidence data. Caused by abnormalities of oxidative metabolism that affect tissue reliant upon mitochondrial energy supply. These disorders are transmitted through maternal	Delay of motor development as well as mental retardation may occur. Strokes may be the source of progressive deterioration, but encephalopathy also occurs without stroke. No neuropsychological studies are done. Cognitive regression reflects	Progressive encephalopathy and neuromuscular symptoms, with weakness, hypotonia, exercise intolerance, ataxia, ophthalmoplegia, cardiomyopathy, myoclonus, choreoathetosis, dystonia, seizures, stroke-like episodes, and headache.	Symptomatic treatment only.

• MELAS syndrome: Mitochondrial myopathy and encephalopathy, lactic acidosis, and stroke-like episodes.

• MERRF syndrome: Myoclonic epilepsy associated with ragged red fibers and cerebellar ataxia.

• NARP syndrome: Neuropathy, ataxia, retinitis pigmentosa, and variable dementia.

inheritance, caused by defects in the mitochondrial DNA, as distinct from the usual inheritance through nuclear DNA.

MERRF characterized by ragged red fibers in muscle biopsy.

disease progression (Koo et al., 1993).

Case study of an adult with MELAS revealed prosopagnosia, topographic disorientation, and EEG abnormalities with a lesion in the left occipital lobe. Authors state that because occipital cortex is a common location for MELAS attacks, neuropsychological symptoms of prosopagnosia and topographic disorientation may be commonly associated with MELAS (Funakawa, Mukai, Terao, Kawashima, & Mori, 1994)

Leigh syndrome: Frontal and basal ganglia lesions are seen on CT and MRI (Fujii et al., 1995).

MERRF: CT shows atrophy and ventricular dilatation; MRI reveals abnormalities of periventricular subcortical white matter (Huang et al., 1995).

MELAS: On MRI focal abnormalities vary in location, but there are more in periventricular subcortical white matter (Huang et al., 1995). Gray matter in the deep cerebral nuclei is also involved (Barkovich, Good, Koch, & Berg, 1993).

Symptomatic treatment only. Two children have had BMT, but outcomes are uncertain.

Neuronal ceroid lipofuscinosis

• Juvenile Batten disease: Onset at 5–9 years of age; slowly progressive visual symptoms, seizures, and dementia developing over a period of years.

• Jansky–Bielschowsky disease: Late infantile onset; acute, rapidly progressive seizure disorder; severe deterioration of visual, motor, and mental function over months, followed by a

Incidence: 0.71 per 100,000
Gene locations: 11p15 (Batten disease), 1p32 (Santavuori–Haltia disease). Autosomal recessive inheritance.

This is a group of progressive gray matter diseases rather than a single entity. Loss of cerebral neurons, and abnormal accumulation of lipopigments in neurons and non-neuronal cells inside and outside of the CNS, have been shown. Recently a

Batten disease's progression can be followed with a scoring system (Kohlschutter, Laabs, & Albani, 1988). Deterioration of intellect starts at about age 9, with language and motor functioning intact until adolescence. Visual symptoms occur between ages 5 and 10; motor symptoms, seizures, psychosis, and eventual dementia occur by adolescence (Kohlschutter et al., 1988; Bruun, Reskel-Nielsen, & Oster, 1991;

• Batten disease: CT and MRI reveal cerebral or cerebellar atrophy when disease duration is longer than 4 years; normal results in many (Nardocci et al., 1995).

• Jansky–Bielschowsky disease: MRI has paranchymal abnormalities, hyperintense periventricular white matter (especially around lateral ventricles), and a significant decrease in signal intensity in the

(continued)

TABLE 8.1. (*continued*)

Disease	Etiology/pathophysiology	Cognitive/behavioral/neuropsychological findings	Neurological/medical/neuroimaging findings	Treatment
vegetative function that can last for years. • Santavuori–Haltia disease: Onset at 8–18 months of age; an acute psychomotor deterioration and myoclonia with seizures. Death at 8–14 years of age.	single protein has been identified that is absent in the late infantile form.	Sørensen & Parnas, 1979). Memory domain is particularly impaired (Kristensen & Lou, 1983).	thalami and/or putamen (Autti, Raininko, Launes, Nuutila, & Santavuori, 1993). • Santavuori–Haltia disease: CT and MRI reveal cerebral atrophy within 3 years of onset (Nardocci et al., 1995).	
GM2 gangliosidoses • Tay–Sachs disease (infantile form): Cherry-red spot in the macula; motor weakness; irritability; sensitivity to noises with massive startle reflex; decreasing responsiveness and voluntary movement. Blindness, myoclonic seizures, and macrocephaly follow. Death at 2 to 4 years of age. • Sandhoff disease (juvenile form): Ataxia and incoordination between ages 2 and 10, with regression and dementia. Spasticity and seizures occur late. Blindness varies. Vegetative state by age 10–15 years; death in 2–4 years.	Incidence: 1 in 300,000 in each, except that Tay–Sachs has 100 times the incidence in Ashkenazic Jews. Autosomal recessive disorder. Chromosome 15 encodes subunit a of the hexosaminidase A enzyme. Gangliosides accumulate in nerve cells because of missing hexosaminidase A enzyme.	• In infantile form, decreasing responsiveness and movement after 8–10 months. • In juvenile form, speech and language difficulties occur along with ataxia and incoordination; behavioral problems and dementia occur later (Specola, Vanier, Goutieres, Mikol, & Alcardi, 1990). • In adult patients, psychiatric manifestations associated with GM2 gangliosidoses are relatively common and affect as many as 40% of patients; they include agitation, hallucinations, delusions, and paranoia, and are typically unresponsive to antipsychotic or antidepres-	• Tay–Sachs: CT and/or MRI reveals three phases, with initial involvement of the cerebral white matter and basal ganglia. Second phase involves enlargement of caudate nucleus, which protrudes into the lateral ventricles; also, white matter changes. In the third phase, the entire brain becomes atrophic. • Late-onset forms: CT and MRI often show cerebellar atrophy, particular of the vermis. A majority of patients do not show cerebral abnormalities on imaging studies (Streifler, Gornish, Hadar, & Gadoth, 1993).	Genetic screening has decreased incidence among Ashkenazic Jews. Symptomatic treatment only.

Disorder	Incidence/Genetics/Pathology	Clinical features/Neuropathology	Treatment
• GM2 gangliosidoses, adult type: Variable age of onset, with dystonia and extrapyramidal signs.	sant pharmacotherapies (Rosebush et al., 1995; Hurowitz, Silver, Brin, Williams, & Johnson, 1993).		Symptomatic treatment only.
Hallervorden–Spatz syndrome Presents with dystonia, tics, and other motor symptoms. Seizures are common. Onset is in the first two decades but is very variable. Changes in mental status usually follow motor abnormalities but occasionally are the initial complaints. Rate of mental and physical deterioration is variable.	No incidence data. Possible gene location: 20p12.3–20p13. Possibly an autosomal recessive disorder affecting deep grey matter. Many cases seem to be sporadic. Abnormal cytosomes in circulating lymphocytes and sea-blue histiocytes in bone marrow are found. May be a disorder of iron metabolism. Iron plays a role in the modulation of dopamine binding to postsynaptic receptors, as well as in myelination and oxidation reactions involving membranes and DNA (Swaiman, 1991). Pathology shows neuroaxonal swellings and large amounts of iron deposited in the globus pallidus, the pars reticulata of the substantia nigra, and red nuclei.	Optic atrophy is an early sign (Casteels et al., 1994). Cognitive deterioration progresses slowly. Behavioral/personality changes can occur later. Neuropsychological abnormalities typical of subcortical dementia include increasing fine motor difficulties, movement disorders, memory problems, calculation difficulties, deterioration of overall mental capacity, and executive dysfunctions (including inattentiveness, poor judgment, and sequential ability) (Shapiro, 1997). Progressive dystonia, complex tics, stereotypies, compulsive behaviors, unsteady gait, choreoathetosis, dysarthria, and rigidity. Hyperreflexia, extrapyramidal and corticospinal tract dysfunction, myoclonus, and tremor are also seen. Optic atrophy present, with visual evoked response and electroretinographic abnormalities (Swaiman, 1991). MRI abnormalities found in the basal ganglia; symmetrical low signal over globus pallidi (and substantia nigra), with an area of high intensity over the central zone called the "eye of the tiger" sign (Angelini et al., 1992; Casteels et al., 1994). Decreased signal areas are thought to be iron deposit; high-intensity areas are thought to be areas of "loose" tissue with vacuolization.	
Rett syndrome Progressive dementia and encephalopathy in girls after	Incidence: 1 in 15,000 to 20,000.	Profound mental retardation, with preintentional level of communication (Kerr, 1995). Neuropathology: Disruption of the growth of axonodendritic connections (Johnston,	Symptomatic treatment only.

(continued)

TABLE 8.1. (*continued*)

Disease	Etiology/pathophysiology	Cognitive/behavioral/ neuropsychological findings	Neurological/medical/ neuroimaging findings	Treatment
7–18 months of age, with autistic behavior, loss of purposeful hand use, truncal ataxia, spastic paraparesis, acquired microcephaly, and seizures. No subsequent cognitive development occurs, and physical growth is decreased.	The genetics and pathophysiology of this disorder have thus far not been delineated.	High prevalence of behavioral and emotional problems, including episodes of anxiety, low mood, and self-injurious behavior, which may diminish with age. No association of seizures with behavioral and emotional problems (Sansom, Krishnan, Corbett, & Kerr, 1993).	Hohmann, & Blue, 1995). Imaging studies show no focal findings. Volumetric analysis of MRI finds evidence of loss of gray matter, with the frontal regions showing the largest volume decrease, followed by caudate nucleus and midbrain (Reiss et al., 1993).	

children to a designated center for testing. Thus neuropsychologists may be in partnership with collaborative groups to collect data over time on children in a given geographic region. The neuropsychologists at these facilities can also be informed about a disease by investigators from the centers that are coordinating data collection. Our Storage Disease Collaborative Study Group has a data base of neuropsychological and medical information on the leukodystrophies and MPS disorders from many centers that extends beyond information on the effects of BMT per se; there is a similar consortium in Europe. Centers of this type can provide individual clinicians with the most up-to-date information in their field. The large sample sizes afforded by multisite studies also enhance the validity of findings and thus contribute to a better understanding of the natural history of these rare diseases.

THE MUCOPOLYSACCHARIDOSES

The MPS disorders are lysosomal storage diseases in which toxic substances accumulate in the body and in the CNS because the enzymes that normally degrade this material are missing. All of these disorders are characterized by deposits of these neurotoxic substances in the brain, which result in slowing of development and then progressive deterioration in cognitive abilities; the specific effects vary with the disease and genetic defect. Neuroradiological abnormalities usually begin with perivascular deposits throughout the brain. Hydrocephalus also occurs, with resultant white matter abnormalities. Finally, brain atrophy develops along with significant mental deterioration. The storage material is also deposited in the liver, heart, spleen, and other tissues and organs in the body.

Hurler Syndrome

Background and Pathophysiology

Hurler syndrome, the best-known of the MPS disorders (MPS I), is an autosomal recessive disease with deficiency of the enzyme α-L-iduronidase. The lysosomes fail to degrade normally produced GAGs and heparan and dermatan sulfate accumulate in almost all cells and organs of the body. Damage results in multiple body organs, including the brain, heart, lungs, liver, eye, spleen, skeletal system, and connective tissue. Symptoms include hepatosplenomegaly, dysostosis multiplex, corneal clouding, coarse facial features, macrocephaly, hearing loss, enlarged tongue, respiratory insufficiency, valvular heart disease, coronary artery disease, kyphosis, thoracolumbar gibbus, hip flexion contractures, carpal tunnel syndrome, and hydrocephalus due to obstruction. Lowry, Applegarth, Toone, MacDonald, and Thunem (1990) reported an incidence of this disease in British Columbia of 1 in 144,000 live births.

Sensory deficits are almost always evident as the disease progresses; these include corneal clouding, optic atrophy, glaucoma, and hearing impairment. Clinically children with Hurler syndrome may look fairly normal at birth, but the worsening of various symptoms with age brings them to medical attention. Until recently, the diagnosis was usually made in the second year of life on the basis of hepatosplenomegaly, hydrocephalus, and/or skeletal abnormalities. Due to increased physician and parent awareness, infants are now being diagnosed during the first year of life (Shapiro, Lockman, et al., 1995).

For children with severe mutations, Hurler syndrome is uniformly fatal, with such children dying at a median age of 5 years and survival rarely extending beyond 10 years of age (Krivit, Henslee-Downey, et al., 1995). In severe Hurler disease, gradual CNS deterioration begins during the first year of life. Acute hydrocephalus due to obstruction of cerebrospinal fluid (CSF) may contribute to further brain damage. Hydrocephalus may thus require shunting. Accumulation of storage material in the perivascular Virchow–Robin spaces is apparent on magnetic resonance imaging (MRI), along with enlarged ventricles (Johnson, Desai, Hugh-Jones, & Starer, 1984; Whitley et al., 1993). As the disease progresses, atrophy occurs. Both fluid accumulation in the middle ear with resultant conductive hearing loss and sensorineural hearing loss (Schachern, Shea, & Paparella, 1984) may affect language development. Visual difficulties result from corneal clouding. Gross and fine motor coordination becomes increasingly poor as skeletal abnormalities progress (Taccone et al., 1993; Tandon, Williamson, Cowie, & Wraith, 1996). Coronary artery disease occurs early in Hurler syndrome, and cardiac failure is a common cause of death in untreated children (Braunlin et al., 1992).

The gene for Hurler syndrome has been identified and is on the long arm of chromosome 4. Several alleles have been identified, W402X and Q70X being common in severe forms of the disease (Bunge et al., 1994; Scott, Litjens, Hopwood, & Morris, 1992; Scott et al., 1992). Milder forms, formerly classified as Scheie or Hurler–Scheie syndrome, have also been identified and are associated with normal intelligence, less severe physical problems, later onset, and longer life expectancy. Controversy surrounds the distinction between Hurler and Scheie syndromes, as the same enzyme deficiency is present in both syndromes, along with evidence for cognitive deterioration. The P533R mutation (Clarke & Scott, 1993) has been implicated in some cases of rare late-onset Hurler syndrome.

Neuropsychological Characteristics

Neuropsychological testing of children with Hurler syndrome shows normal development in most cases during the first year of life. Because children with Hurler syndrome are at risk for hydrocephalus and other neurological complications, cognitive decline is seen in a few children during their first year. Motor development is also slightly delayed, and some physical symptoms are evident such as hepatosplenomegaly and coronary artery disease. Development slows during the second year of life, and by the end of the second year, few children have a Mental Development Index (MDI) over 100 on the Bayley Scales of Infant Development (Bayley, 1969). Mean scores shift downward by one standard deviation by the end of the second year (Peters et al., 1996; Peters, Shapiro, Anderson, et al., 1998; Shapiro, Balthazor, Lockman, & Krivit, 1994). By age 3, almost all children with untreated Hurler syndrome have an MDI under 70. Correlation of age with MDI is –.82, reflecting a steady slowing of development (Shapiro, Lockman, et al., 1995).

Apart from language delay secondary to hearing loss, children with Hurler syndrome do not have language difficulties. Hurler syndrome is a good example of the type of childhood dementia that is characterized by a general slowing, plateauing, and then loss of function. By age 3, loss of previously acquired developmental milestones has occurred and most children have severe motoric handicap and life-threatening physical symptoms. The most common cause of death is respiratory and cardiac failure.

CNS deterioration is universal and is sometimes accompanied by hydrocephalus. Hydrocephalus is caused by poor absorption of CSF and obstruction in flow. Ventriculomegaly is the most common finding on MRI scans (Johnson et al., 1984: Lee, Dineen, Brack, Kirsch, & Runge, 1993). Periventricular white matter changes on MRI are also associated with hydrocephalus. The storage of GAGs is evident on the MRI in the perivascular Virchow–Robin spaces (Johnson et al., 1984). A "Swiss cheese" appearance in the white matter, especially the corpus callosum, results from these engorged spaces.

Magnetic resonance spectroscopy studies of children with Hurler syndrome have failed to find abnormal metabolites in either gray or white matter examinations (Shapiro, Balthazor, & Rajanayagam, 1995). At this time we do not fully understand the underlying etiology of the cognitive decline in Hurler syndrome. Cognitive decline occurs even in children without hydrocephalus, and children with this complication may do relatively well. Children with many Virchow–Robin spaces may likewise do well, even if these spaces are in the corpus callosum. Although cerebral atrophy is observed on MRI, no quantitative or volumetric studies have been done to examine the extent of atrophy, the number and location of Virchow–Robin spaces, or the age of onset and severity of hydrocephalus. One of the objectives of ongoing work in this area at the University of Minnesota is to quantify MRI abnormalities and to correlate them with neuropsychological measures.

In contrast to other forms of MPS, children with Hurler syndrome generally show normal emotional development until late stages of the disease. Unless they have neurological complications or are physically uncomfortable, these children are uniformly pleasant, with positive affect and social interests. Formal evidence in this regard was obtained in a study conducted by our research group of 16 children with Hurler syndrome (Shapiro, Salter, Balthazor, Lockman, & Krivit, 1995). At the time of the study, the children had not yet been treated for the disease. All participants were between 12 and 24 months of age and obtained scores of greater than 70 on the Mental Development Index (MDI) of the Bayley Scales of Infant Development. To assess emotional status, a videotaped measure of affect, the Minnesota Preschool Affect Rating Scale (Shapiro, McPhee, Abbott, & Sulzbacher, 1994), was administered to the 16 cases and to an age-matched control group. Group comparisons failed to reveal differences on measure of positive or negative affect or affect regulation. Comparison of a larger sample of 67 children with Hurler syndrome between the ages of 5 and 36 months to age-matched controls also failed to reveal differences on the Activity Level and Emotional Response factors of the Infant Behavior Rating of the Bayley Scales of Infant Development. A small but significant difference was found on the Infant Behavior Rating Attention factor. This factor was also correlated with age in children with Hurler syndrome: Older children were rated as more inattentive than younger children (Shapiro, Salter, et al., 1995). Although poor attention span is not a defining sign of the disease, attentional functions appear to deteriorate as the disease progresses.

Treatment

Research by our own group and other investigators (Peters et al., 1996; Peters, Shapiro, Anderson, et al., 1998; Vellodi et al., 1997) indicates that in the short term, BMT results in amelioration of life-threatening physical symptoms and alters the downhill course of the syndrome (Krivit, Shapiro, et al., 1996). After engraftment of the bone marrow, the enzymatic activity in white cells is at the donor level. The accumulated GAGs disappear from marrow, lungs, liver (Resnick, Whitley, Leonard, Krivit, & Snover, 1994), the vascular system (du Cret et al., 1994), and the CNS (Krivit, Shapiro, et al., 1996; Whitley et al., 1993). Hearing loss, which is common in the disease, improves (Krivit, Lockman, Watkins, Hirsch, & Shapiro, 1995), and improved brain status as reflected in MRI is also noted (Krivit, Shapiro, et al., 1996; Whitley et al., 1993). However, the skeletal abnormalities do not improve, and children with Hurler syndrome who have had BMT have significant skeletal deformities that require ongoing surgical intervention (Field, Buchanan,

Copplemans, & Aichroth, 1994; Tandon et al., 1996; van Heest, House, Krivit, & Walker, 1997).

BMT is most effective in preventing cognitive deterioration if carried out prior to age 2. Developmental growth curves based on Bayley scores indicate that children continue to gain cognitive skills after BMT, although at a somewhat slower rate than prior to BMT. However, children transplanted after age 2 show a somewhat slower development of cognitive skills (Peters et al., 1996; Peters, Shapiro, Anderson, et al., 1998; Shapiro, Balthazor, et al., 1994). One to two years after transplant, the pre-BMT developmental course is resumed and appears stable thereafter, as documented in several children we have followed for more than 10 years. Mild attentional problems may constitute one of the long-term consequences of the disease, but behavioral problems are infrequent.

Although BMT seems to preserve cognitive skills, resolve upper-airway obstruction and hepatosplenomegaly, and improve hearing problems, skeletal abnormalities may have a negative impact on a child's quality of life (QOL). The long-term orthopedic problems caused by dysostosis multiplex are particularly difficult for these children. Progressive hip dislocation requires surgical intervention, such as acetabulum reconstruction. Recurring spinal cord problems, such as kyphosis, spinal cord compression, and odontoid hypoplasia, have also been treated surgically but not always successfully. These problems result in decreased mobility over time (Field et al., 1994). Although surgical interventions are often successful for carpal tunnel syndrome (van Heest et al., 1997), skeletal deterioration associated with this condition may affect long-term life adjustment and QOL by interfering with the acquisition of adaptive skills, requiring repeated surgeries, and decreasing mobility.

Quantification of specific health outcomes in Hurler syndrome is important for a number of reasons. It can allow examination of change over time within each health domain, correlation of severity among domains, and prediction from baseline to specific health outcomes. Defining the baseline variables that contribute to BMT outcomes may contribute to better risk–benefit analysis for BMT decision making. Also, health outcome profiles can be correlated with parent and child ratings of QOL, as well as with neuropsychological and adaptive behavior scores.

We have developed a 4-point rating scale of functional status within each of five health domains: orthopedics, audiology, cardiology, ophthalmology, and neurology. In a recent study (Shapiro, Thrall, Peters, Ziegler, Lockman, & Krivit, 1999), medical data for 19 children with Hurler syndrome were examined and assigned a rating. These children had all had BMT at least 3 years previously. Baseline, 3-year post-BMT, and most recent evaluations were coded in these five health domains by a rater who did not know the children. Results from 3-year follow-up visits documented deterioration of orthopedic and ophthalmological function, improvement in cardiac function, and stability of neurological and audiological function. Furthermore, insignificant correlations were found between health outcome scores within each patient. Thus health domains were differentially affected by disease progression but were unrelated to each other. An overall severity score would not have been justified at either baseline or follow-up. Overall neuropsychological function as measured by MDI or IQ correlated only with neurological function and not with any of the other health outcomes; however, a correlation was found between audiological function and receptive language at baseline. Future research will focus on how health outcome profiles and neuropsychological status relate to QOL measures.

Knowledge of the factors that contribute to QOL in long-term survivors with Hurler syndrome will assist parents, physicians, and others in deciding whether to perform BMT. This disease is being diagnosed at earlier ages than was the case only a few years ago, and increased numbers of parents are seeking BMT treatment. New methods of BMT are being developed, and outcomes are improving. Gene therapy (Fairbairn et al., 1997) and intravenous enzyme replacement with genetically engineered α-L-iduronidase (Kakkis et al., 1996; Shull et al., 1994) may occur in the next several years. Studies of QOL and long-term neuropsychological outcomes following these treatments will provide information on the comparative efficacy of different methods of intervention (Peters, Shapiro, & Krivit, 1998).

Hunter Syndrome

Background and Pathophysiology

Hunter syndrome (MPS II) is an X-linked inherited disease. The disease is attributable to the deficiency of the enzyme iduronate sulfatase, resulting in tissue deposits of normally produced GAGs. The resultant accumulation of GAGs causes cellular and organ failure, and results in excretion of large amounts of chondroitin sulfate B and heparan sulfate.

The gene responsible for Hunter syndrome has been located to Xq28. There are two primary forms of the disease: a severe form resulting in progressive dementia and death by age 15, and a milder form associated with normal life expectancy and mental development. Incidence in the United Kingdom is about 1 in 132,000, with the severe form being 3.38 times as frequent as the mild form (Young & Harper, 1983). In British Columbia, the incidence is about 1 in 110,950 live births (Lowry et al., 1990). Rates are much higher in the Israeli population, where the incidence is 1 in 34,000 (Schaap & Bach, 1980).

Clinical findings include coarse facies, progressive hearing loss, hepatosplenomegaly, cardiomyopathy, dysostosis multiplex, macrocephaly, and CNS deterioration. Signs of the severe form of Hunter syndrome are usually apparent in the first year of life, but the disease is often not diagnosed until a child is 2 or 3 years of age. Phenotypically, children with Hunter syndrome look much like those with Hurler syndrome. However, corneal clouding is usually absent, and the progression of the severe form of the disease is slightly slower.

As in Hurler syndrome, cribriform (multicystic) changes reflecting storage material in the perivascular Virchow–Robin spaces have been found, particularly in white matter, corpus callosum, and basal ganglia (Lee et al., 1993). The disease is also associated with general atrophy; ventriculomegaly; increased signal in basal ganglia, thalamus, and brain stem; and increased periventricular signal in white matter in the mild variant (Parsons, Hughes, & Wraith, 1996).

Neuropsychological Characteristics

Neuropsychological consequences of the severe form of Hunter syndrome are similar to those found in Hurler syndrome, except that many behavioral abnormalities are also present. A study utilizing questionnaires sent to parents documented both hyperactivity and aggressive behaviors (Bax & Colville, 1995). Differential language delays have also been described, in conjunction with general progressive cognitive impairment and resultant mental retardation. However, systematic studies are lacking.

Treatment

BMT does not appear to alter the downward course of Hunter syndrome (McKinnis, Sulzbacher, Rutledge, Sanders, & Scott, 1996), although there are a few contradictory reports. Of the cases followed as part of the Storage Disease Collaborative Study Group data base, all children with severe Hunter syndrome have been treatment failures, as defined by a child's IQ falling below 50 a year or more after BMT. In contrast, arrest of neuropsychological and physical decline was described in a severe case of Hunter syndrome (Coppa et al., 1995) and in two cases with the mild form of the disease (Bergstrom, Quinn, Greenstein, & Ascensao, 1994; Imaizumi et al., 1994). No alternative treatment is currently available. However, several ongoing studies are examining the feasibility of gene therapy for individuals with this disorder (Braun et al., 1996; Whitley et al., 1996).

Sanfilippo Syndrome

Background and Pathophysiology

Sanfilippo syndrome (MPS III) is an autosomal recessive disorder with four variants, occurring in 1 of 24,000 births. A different enzyme deficiency is responsible for the four variants of this disease (A, B, C, and D), each of which results in storage of GAGs. All forms are characterized by heparin sulfaturia. The phenotypes are indistinguishable, although Sanfilippo A patients evidence the most severe presentation, with earlier onset and death. Most children with this disorder die by their late teens.

Children with Sanfilippo syndrome usually look normal prior to the second year of life. Macrocephaly and hepatomegaly are the first symptoms of the disease. Nidiffer and Kelly (1983) reported an average age at diagnosis of 6½ years. The somatic features of MPS III are milder than those associated with other MPS disorders, although storage of material in heart and lungs results in heart failure and pneumonia. Corneal clouding is rare, and the skeletal abnormalities are not as severe in MPS III as in these other disorders. The severity of the progressive mental deterioration differs across variants, with mental decline being the most severe in Sanfilippo A and perhaps the least severe in Sanfilippo D. As noted above, Sanfilippo A is associated with more severe illness and earlier death than the other variants, although the earlier-onset cases of Sanfilippo C are only slightly less severe than Sanfilippo A. Sanfilippo B appears to have both a severe and a mild variant (van de Kamp, Niermeijer, von Figura, & Giesberts, 1981). The gene for type A is located on chromosome 17q25, and that for type B on 17q21. Genes have not yet been identified for types C and D.

Neuropsychological Characteristics

Parent reports of memory and language difficulties are often the first signs of the cognitive symptoms of Sanfilippo syndrome. These difficulties are usually first reported when a child reaches about 5½ years of age. Gradual worsening of behavior with age is typical of Sanfilippo syndrome. We have noticed that this worsening occurs in conjunction with deterioration of language. Abnormal behaviors include hyperactivity, aggressive and oppositional behavior, limited attention span, and temper tantrums (Bax & Colville, 1995). Sleep disturbances are common (Colville, Watters, Yule, & Bax, 1996). Our experience confirms that these children exhibit excessive levels of irritability, attentional problems, and overactivity. Significant behavior problems are found even in children with mild variants who have extended survival; mild retardation and dementia occur in later life (van Schrojenstein-de Valk & van de Kamp, 1987; Wraith, Danks, & Rogers, 1987).

Ozand et al. (1994) present an interesting case of a girl with Sanfilippo D syndrome who presented with a fluctuating verbal auditory agnosia and slowly progressive dementing encephalopathy. We have seen a similar child in our group of patients.

Treatment

Children with Sanfilippo syndrome are major management problems. Medications are usually needed for behavioral control, although stimulants are generally ineffective for treatment of inattention, hyperactivity, and aggressive behavior in these children.

BMT for Sanfilippo syndrome has not been effective in preventing the mental deterioration (Klein et al., 1995). Although some improvement in somatic symptoms has been described in response to BMT (Vellodi, Young, New, Pot-Mees, & Hugh-Jones, 1992), this treatment does not prevent cognitive deterioration or disease progression (Klein et al., 1995).

Other MPS Disorders

In contrast to the MPS disorders discussed above, Maroteaux–Lamy syndrome (MPS VI) and Morquio syndrome (MPS IV) do not invariably result in CNS deterioration and are associated with much longer lifespans. Neuropsychological testing of two young adult siblings with MPS VI followed in our center, both of whom were highly intelligent prior to BMT, revealed decline of mental function in one member of the pair. Mental decline was documented by the patient's self-report, her parent's report, and neuropsychological testing. Memory and language functions seemed most impaired. This case contradicts claims in the literature that individuals with MPS VI have no CNS disease, although few if any formal investigations have been undertaken to assess patient outcomes. BMT is helpful for the treatment of the visceral disease associated with this disorder.

General Comments

The reasons for variations in cognitive functioning among individuals with MPS disorders are largely unknown. Language is selectively impaired in some individuals, frequently with accompanying behavioral abnormalities. Motor development is uniformly impaired, primarily because of orthopedic difficulties. Perception and spatial ability are relatively preserved. However, unlike patients with most gray matter diseases, these patients do not have seizures. Disease effects on memory functions have not been investigated, although studies of these outcomes are currently underway.

Hurler syndrome is the most common of the MPS disorders. At this time, the majority of children with Hurler syndrome are undergoing BMT; therefore, few untreated children are available for further study of the natural history of this disease. Two important objectives of current research on children with Hurler disease are to identify the factors that lead to better QOL outcomes after BMT, and to seek new treatments to ameliorate or prevent the severe orthopedic and other late complications that impair long-term QOL.

An important research goal in further studies of children with Hunter syndrome is to refine our understanding of the natural history of the disorder, and in particular of the pattern of decline in neuropsychological abilities. In this manner, we will be able to assess efficacy of new treatments relative to a historical control group.

MPS VI, a very rare disorder, appears to be amenable to BMT; however, we do not have information regarding the untreated course of this disease. Although the popular lore is that cognitive function is normal in this disorder, examination of a half dozen patients at our center in Minnesota indicate that this may not be a universal finding. We have observed at least subtle cognitive deficits in all MPS VI patients seen thus far. Studies of the natural history of cognitive functioning in these patients are clearly required. Cognitive and behavioral abnormalities have been better defined in children with Sanfilippo syndrome, but no effective treatments are yet available for any variants of this syndrome.

Systematic study of the course of MPS disorders is needed to assist researchers in establishing a baseline against which the effects of future treatments can be compared. Investigations of the natural history of these disorders should include repeated assessments of cognitive functions, language functions, and neurobehavioral status. Orthopedic problems in these patients may make it difficult to evaluate children's motor skills accurately. However, studies of hearing problems and their impact on language development are needed. We are convinced that language delays in children with MPS disorders are not solely due to conductive or sensory-neural hearing loss. Further investigation is needed to separate effects of CNS disease from the effects of hearing impairment on language functions.

LEUKODYSTROPHIES

Each of the leukodystrophies has a characteristic neurological and neuropsychological profile. The profile reflects the pathophysiology and loci of demyelination unique to each disease, as well as factors such as age of the patient and stage of the disease.

Adrenoleukodystrophy

Background and Pathophysiology

ALD is an X-linked disorder of the peroxisomes and is biochemically characterized by elevations in plasma very-long-chain fatty acids (VLCFAs). The incidence of this biochemical abnormality is approximately 1 in 20,000 (Mosser et al., 1993). Laboratory techniques permit identification of the abnormality in boys who have not yet developed symptoms (Moser, Smith, & Moser, 1995). Phenotypes of this disorder include Addison disease, late-onset adrenomyeloneuropathy, and childhood-onset cerebral ALD (COCALD). COCALD is a rapidly progressive and devastating form of the disease (Moser et al., 1992; Krivit, Sung, Shapiro, & Lockman, 1995). A few boys have the biochemical defect (elevated VLCFAs) only, with no neurological or neuropsychological symptoms.

Although our discussion of the leukodystrophies focuses on the cerebral forms of this disease, it is important to note that there is phenotypic variability and that multiple types of disease occur in any given family. In patients who have ALD, neither the genotype nor biochemical abnormality predicts the clinical course. An investigation by our research group, for example, failed to reveal correlations between plasma VLCFA levels and IQ or ratings of dementia (Shapiro, Lockman, Balthazor, & Krivit, 1995).

The ALD gene, X28, shows deletions and point mutations in most patients (Braun et al., 1995; Fanen et al., 1994; Feigenbaum et al., 1996; Fuchs et al., 1994; Kok et al., 1995; Ligtenberg et al., 1995; Mosser et al., 1993). This gene codes for a 75-kDa protein named ALDP (Mosser et al., 1994). ALDP is located in the peroxisomal membrane (Contreras, Sengupta, Sheikh, Aubourg, & Singh, 1996; Mosser et al., 1994; Watkins et al., 1995) and probably transports the activated VLCFA-CoA esters into peroxisomes (Hettema et al., 1996; Shani & Valle, 1996). A genetic analysis by Kok et al. (1995) revealed 4 patients of 112 with deletions of a significant part of the 3' half of the gene. Mutations were identified in 24 of 25 patients with intact genes. Mutations were distributed throughout the gene and did not correlate with the phenotype. Due to the lack of relationship between genotype and phenotype, one would assume that mutations would also fail to predict outcome after treatment.

MRIs of children with active disease indicate that areas of increased signal show enhancement with gadolinium, suggesting an inflammatory component of the disease. A recent study of ALD in a monozygotic twin pair, only one member of which had the cerebral form of the disease, suggests that an external factor (perhaps environmental) may contribute to the onset of the cerebral form (Korenke et al., 1996). The trigger that activates the cerebral disease has not yet been identified.

Depending on ascertainment method, estimates indicate that 25–50% of patients diagnosed with ALD will go on to develop the cerebral form of the disease (Moser, Moser, Naidu, & Bergin, 1991; Moser et al., 1992). COCALD occurs in the first decade, with a peak onset at 7 years of age (Moser et al., 1992). Cerebral disease onset is often preceded by adrenal insufficiency. Follow-up of children with ALD shows that younger age of onset is associated with faster rate of disease progression (Shapiro, Lockman, et al., 1995).

Currently there is no method for identifying the presymptomatic children who will develop COCALD (Krivit, Watkins, Hirsch, & Shapiro, 1995). MRIs are often normal prior to development of COCALD. Although early changes in neuropsychological and neuroradiological status signal the onset of COCALD, some boys demonstrate these changes and then stabilize for a period before deteriorating. This pattern of decline makes it difficult to decide to initiate invasive treatments such as BMT. Recent findings indicate that most individuals will show later disease progression even after a rather long period of remission. However, no longitudinal natural history studies have as yet followed these patients through adulthood to determine who develops adrenomyeloneuropathy, cerebral disease, or no disease at all.

Because no biochemical test exists for the cerebral disease, boys must be monitored every 6 months with neuropsychological tests and MRIs to determine whether changes have occurred that indicate deterioration. Guidelines (Shapiro, Lockman, Balthazor, & Krivit, 1995) have been developed for eligibility for BMT; these include degree of MRI abnormality on the Loes scale (Loes et al., 1994) and deterioration over time in neuropsychological testing.

Neuropsychological Characteristics

Patients with ALD exhibit three patterns of neuropsychological and neuroradiological abnormality (Shapiro, Lockman, et al., 1995). Eighty percent of these patients show signs of visual processing abnormality associated with demyelination of visual pathways and posterior white matter. Poor performance on measures of visual–spatial perception and simple visual processing precede loss of visual-associative ability and of object recognition (Krivit, Lockman, & Shapiro, 1996a). From 10% to 15% of patients show increased MRI signal in anterior regions, especially in the corpus callosum. These abnormalities are associated with signs of attentional, behavioral, memory, and organizational difficulties, often misdiagnosed as attention-deficit/hyperactivity disorder. Five percent of patients have brain stem, pyramidal tract, and internal capsule abnormalities associated with diffuse behavioral and motor problems (Shapiro, Lockman, et al., 1995).

Performance IQ on the Wechsler scales appears to be particularly sensitive to the degree of progression of ALD, probably due to the relationship of this measure to the status of cerebral white matter. Verbal IQ, in contrast, is insensitive to disease severity, particularly when MRI involvement is localized to posterior areas of subcortical white matter

(Balthazor, Shapiro, et al., 1996; Shapiro, Lockman, et al., 1997). In a study of measures predictive of dementia in boys with ALD, Performance IQ accounted for 83% of the variance in clinical status (as measured by the ALD Dementia Rating Scale [A-DRS]). A metabolite ratio on magnetic resonance spectroscopy predicted an additional 6% of the variance in PIQ (Balthazor, Rajanayagam, et al., 1996). When the Loes et al. (1994) method of scoring ALD severity was used, neither MRI or Verbal IQ was predictive of clinical status as measured by the A-DRS.

In a study of the validity of various measures in predicting BMT outcome, baseline Performance IQ correctly classified the A-DRS outcome with 100% accuracy (Shapiro, Lockman, et al., 1997). All patients with Performance IQs of 80 or more were clinically stable, and all patients who deteriorated after BMT had baseline Performance IQs of less than 80. For the MRI, when a cutoff score of 10 points on the 0–34 Loes et al. (1994) scale was used, 18% were misclassified with regard to BMT outcome. The sensitivity to clinical status and to BMT outcome can be attributed to the content of the Wechsler Performance scales, which combine diverse visual problem-solving tasks, the need to deal with novelty, and the requirement for visual speed and efficiency (Shapiro, Lockman, et al., 1997). These functions are compromised in boys with the posterior form of ALD because of demyelination of visual pathways.

Magnetic resonance spectroscopy, a magnetic resonance sequence that detects a spectra of brain metabolites in a specified voxel, shows special promise in early identification of cerebral ALD (Kruse et al., 1994; Rajanayagam et al., 1996; Tsika et al., 1993). ALD patients show abnormality in several metabolites in brain regions in which MRI abnormalities are present, and in which pathology would be suggested by neuropsychological deficits. Associations of impairment on neuropsychological testing with the degree of metabolite abnormality in regions of interest (ROIs) in which MRI pathology is not evident are even more intriguing (Rajanayagam et al., 1997). Correlations have been found, for example, between impairment on the Test of Variables of Attention (Greenberg, 1996) and metabolites in frontal ROIs, and between the Judgment of Line Orientation Test (Benton, Hamsher, Varney, & Spreen, 1983) and metabolites in posterior ROIs.

Treatment

Therapy for COCALD has included treatment with Lorenzo's oil, which, combined with a diet of restricted intake of saturated VLCFAs, reduces or even normalizes the plasma VLCFA levels. There is general agreement that once a child develops COCALD, Lorenzo's oil will do little to halt the progression of the disease (Shapiro, Aubourg, et al., 1997). For those individuals who are neurologically intact, it is unclear whether Lorenzo's oil can slow or alter the onset of COCALD (Moser et al., 1994).

The first report of positive effects of BMT on children with ALD indicated major neuropsychological improvement following this therapy, as well as normalization of the MRI abnormality (Aubourg et al., 1990). Short-term outcomes of BMT in a larger number of patients were also positive (Krivit & Shapiro, 1994; Lockman, Shapiro, & Krivit, 1993). The degree of improvement reported in the Aubourg et al. paper has not been replicated. However, Shapiro, Aubourg, et al. (1997) found that 12 patients in the United States and France demonstrated generally stable cognitive functioning 5 years after BMT. One boy (with a carrier donor) showed a decline in cognitive abilities during the second year after BMT, with no evidence of subsequent decline (Shapiro, Lockman, et al., 1997). All the other boys exhibited age-appropriate gains in cognition throughout follow-ups. Visual processing problems evident early in the disease course remained constant over this period, or may even have become slightly less severe. Reaction times were slow in all the boys, and attentional problems were present in some cases after BMT.

Metachromatic Leukodystrophy

Background and Pathophysiology

MLD is an autosomal recessive lysosomal storage disease caused by the deficiency of the enzyme arylsulfatase A. This deficiency results in an accumulation of sulfatides, leading to progressive demyelination in the CNS. An earlier age at onset of MLD correlates with more rapid deterioration and more severe peripheral nervous system involvement. The neuro-psychological profiles of children with early-onset (before age 6) and late-onset MLD differ markedly (Shapiro, Lockman, et al., 1995). Incidence is consistently reported to be about 1 in 100,000 births. There are at least three forms of MLD, defined according to age of onset: late infantile, juvenile, and adult forms. The age at onset of MLD is usually concordant within families.

Children with late infantile MLD, whose onset is before age 6, present with motor deterioration. They are often misdiagnosed with cerebral palsy. Early-onset MLD is characterized by a rapid downhill course, with children being bedridden within months of diagnosis. Following this acute symptom onset, children may survive for years in a vegetative state.

Neuropsychological Characteristics of Late Infantile MLD

Neuropsychological profiles for 21 untreated children assessed between the ages of 2.3 and 7.2 are described by Shapiro, Lockman, et al. (1995). The findings of this study indicate that motor symptoms predominate in the initial phases of early-onset MLD, followed by difficulties with verbal learning and perception. Auditory processing, language, and reading skills are relatively spared until later in the disease. Behavioral problems are also absent in the earlier phases of early-onset MLD. The pattern of neuropsychological deficits present in children with MLD is akin to the "nonverbal learning disability syndrome" (Rourke, 1987), but without the social and emotional components of the latter condition (Shapiro et al., 1992). The lack of social and emotional deficits in children with MLD may be due to the fact that disease onset occurs after initial acquisition of these skills, in contrast to other cases of nonverbal learning disabilities caused by congenital or developmental defects.

Treatment of Late Infantile MLD

Once motor abnormality is apparent on neurological examination, BMT is not effective in preventing disease progression in children with late infantile MLD. In children identified biochemically as a result of an older sibling's diagnosis, and transplanted prior to symptom presentation, BMT arrests or slows the course of the cerebral disease; however, it does not affect motor symptoms due to peripheral demyelination (Pridjian, Humbert, Willis, & Shapiro, 1994). In a case described by Krivit et al. (1990) and Shapiro et al. (1992), a 17-year-old woman who had undergone BMT 13 years previously for late infantile MLD failed to display signs of dementia. However, she had little motor function due to peripheral demyelination, and she used a wheelchair. Four other patients with early BMT showed continued progression of motor difficulty 2 to 5 years after transplant, but had relatively normal cognitive ability (Krivit, Lockman, & Shapiro, 1996b; Sulzbacher, McKinnis, Sanders, & Scott, 1994).

Neuropsychological Characteristics of Late-Onset MLD

Compared to the late infantile form of MLD, the course of the juvenile and adult forms is more protracted, and behavioral symptoms are more evident. Individuals with these forms of the disorder often have a distinctive behavioral profile typical of patients with frontal lobe syndrome (Shapiro, Lockman, Knopman, & Krivit, 1994). Most late-onset patients receive psychiatric treatment until dementia is recognized, with diagnoses that range from attention-deficit/hyperactivity disorder to schizophrenia, affective disorders, and personality disorders. Shapiro, Lockman, et al. (1995) described neuropsychological profiles in 11 patients from 10 to 35 years of age. Findings revealed severe abnormalities on continuous-performance measures of attention span and verbal learning, with slightly less severe impairments in executive functions and visual memory. Motor abnormalities, though common, were not present in all cases. Preservation of auditory processing, language, and reading skills was also documented.

Treatment of Late-Onset MLD

BMT appears to halt the progression of late onset MLD (Krivit et al., 1996b; Navarro et al., 1995; Navarro et al., 1996). Diagnosis of an individual in the early stages of the disease is possible when there is an affected older sibling. However, a post-BMT period of approximately 1 year is required before sufficient enzyme can be delivered to the CNS to halt progression of the disease. Thus the patient must be able to withstand a year of continued deterioration after BMT until the decline is interrupted. Follow-up of three patients beyond 1 year after BMT revealed borderline intelligence with continuing attentional and executive function deficits, but with no further disease progression (Shapiro, Lockman, et al., 1995).

Although biochemical and neuroimaging studies do not distinguish the late infantile and late-onset forms of MLD, the two forms are associated with different neuropsychological deficits. In younger patients with late infantile MLD, motor symptoms are the most salient; in older patients with late-onset MLD, executive dysfunction and behavioral disinhibition prevail. On MRI, all patients with MLD have widespread demyelination, with greater involvement of the frontal areas than of other regions.

Globoid Cell Leukodystrophy

Background and Pathophysiology

GLD is the rarest of the leukodystrophies. The incidence of the early-onset form of GLD is 1 in 50,000 births in Sweden, but the disease is much rarer elsewhere. Suzuki, Suzuki, and Suzuki (1995), for example, report an incidence of early-onset GLD of 1 per 150,000, and an incidence of only 1 per 2,000,000 for the later-onset form. The gene for GLD, an autosomal recessive disease, is on chromosome 14 (Oehlmann, Zlotogora, Wenger, & Knowlton, 1993). GLD is caused by a deficiency of galactocerebrosidase activity and an accumulation of psychosine, a toxic metabolite of galactocerebroside, in the brain. The buildup of psychosine results in progressive loss of central and peripheral myelin. The most common infantile form, often called Krabbe disease, is characterized by very rapid disease progression to death before the child's second birthday. Late-onset forms are insidious, with the disease progressing over several years prior to death. The course and presentation of late-onset forms are variable (Barone et al., 1996). MRI findings associated with late-onset disease are also variable, but often include focal, asymmetrical hyperintense signals in the early stages of the disorder. These signals may occur anywhere in the brain, but are slightly more prevalent in posterior areas. Because the onset and course of symptoms of GLD are not always concordant within families (Kolodny, Raghavan, & Krivit, 1991), young children may experience symptom onset before their older siblings.

Neuropsychological Characteristics

Although data on neuropsychological outcomes of GLD are sparse, motor and visual symptoms are common at presentation (Lyon et al., 1991). Assessment at our center of nine late-onset GLD patients ranging in age from 2 to 19 years indicated that the patients typically presented with progressive motor difficulties (Shapiro, Lockman, et al., 1995). Mathematics difficulties and specific visual impairments were also present. Language skills and auditory processing were intact. Behavioral difficulties or executive dysfunction were uncommon. Individual neuropsychological profiles revealing perceptual and language problems were associated with the specific areas of demyelination. Visual agnosia of an apperceptive type was present in one patient (Shapiro et al., 1991). Cognitive impairment was not as severe in these cases as in patients with other leukodystrophies, perhaps because motor abnormalities brought the patients to medical attention early in the disease course.

Treatment

Treatment with BMT has been reported in five cases (Krivit et al., 1998), with neuropsychological outcomes described for three of these patients. Two older children demonstrated improved nonverbal skills after BMT, with increased Performance IQ and resolution of visual agnosia. A younger child, transplanted prior to any impairment, was cognitively normal at follow-up, although his perceptual skills failed to keep pace with his superior verbal ability (Krivit et al., 1998).

FUTURE RESEARCH DIRECTIONS

There is clearly a need for more longitudinal studies of children with neurodegenerative disorders. Following children over time is both clinically beneficial and informative with regard to the course of these diseases. A single assessment is often inadequate for identification of the stage a disease has reached, whereas longitudinal assessments yield information about the rapidity and changing nature of the disease process. Serial neuropsychological studies at regular intervals are necessary in order to characterize the pattern of developmental changes associated with each type of disorder. Analysis methods such as hierarchical linear modeling are particularly appropriate for studies of childhood dementia, especially in view of the need to examine changes in raw scores over time (Francis, Fletcher, Stuebing, Davidson, & Thompson, 1991). Sole reliance on standard and/or scaled scores makes it difficult to discern whether a child is experiencing (1) a slowing in development, (2) an arrest in development, or (3) an actual loss of function. Each of these scenarios will result in a decline in standard or scaled scores over time, but for markedly different reasons.

Examination of raw scores results in a more accurate portrayal of the progression of the child's deficits; it also permits the use of measures that may be helpful in characterizing disease effects that are not well normed.

The choice of tests for children with cognitive impairment due to progressive disease is dictated by several factors. First, longitudinal assessment demands that a given test measure the same construct over time, and that differences in test scores have the same meaning at different points on the scale. Second, because the performances of children with neurodegenerative diseases range from demented to normal, tests must be capable of measuring widely disparate abilities. Third, tests should be repeatable. Tests that are subject to large practice effects are not appropriate. Fourth, the tests must measure areas of skill affected by a particular disease. For example, assessments of children with ALD must include measures of visual processing, and evaluations of children with MLD must include tests of executive functions. Finally, due to the rarity of these diseases, standard batteries should be developed for use in multiple centers.

Measurement of social and emotional outcomes of neurodegenerative disorders also deserves stronger emphasis in research. Few studies of children with these diseases have used measures of emotional or behavioral functioning. Systematic, multimethod approaches that incorporate parent ratings, self-ratings, and behavioral observations are needed. Efforts are required to assess both the direct effects of brain insults on socioemotional functioning and the psychological factors related to difficulties in adjusting to disease effects and loss of functioning, as well as to intrusive treatments such as BMT and orthopedic surgeries.

One of the major methodological pitfalls of research in this area is failure to obtain information on the staging of the disease progression. Information of this sort is essential in characterizing research samples and in examining the neuropsychological correlates of the disease process. Defining disease stage will require the development of rating scales that incorporate assessments of, for example, neurological status, sensory status, adaptive functioning, socioemotional functioning, and school performance. We have constructed dementia rating scales of this type for use in staging disease progression for children with ALD and MLD (Shapiro, Lockman, et al., 1995). These scales are completed by an independent clinician such as a neurologist, without the input of the neuropsychology staff or consideration of test results. Similarly, Swift, Dyken, and DuRant (1984), have generated a dementia rating scale called the Psychological Disability Rating Scale for patients with subacute sclerosing panencephalitis. This scale involves assignment of scores from 0 to 6 in each of several areas of functioning: gross motor skills, self-care, social skills, language and Verbal IQ, visual–motor skills and Performance IQ, and academic skills. The investigators did not find that progression of the disease differentially affected any one skill area, although a characteristic pattern of performance across domains was defined in individuals with the disease. Kohlschutter, Laabs, and Albani (1988), in their studies of juvenile neuronal ceroid lipofuscinosis, assessed five outcomes on a 0–3 scale, including vision, intellect, language, motor function, and epilepsy. Each patient's progress on these dimensions was monitored over time. Although IQ was factored into the Swift et al. (1984) rating, no mention was made of the relationship of the Kohlschutter et al. (1988) scale to other neuropsychological measures.

Dementia rating scales provide a reliable method for assessing global functioning, at least if the items are carefully constructed and behaviorally anchored. Because symptoms vary considerably across diseases, a different rating scale will be required for each disorder, based on the unique progression of that disease. If a dementia rating is not based on neuropsychological test results and is completed by an independent clinician, correlation of clinician-perceived progression of disease with neuropsychological outcomes can yield information about the sensitivity of the neuropsychological tests to disease progression.

Correlations of neuropsychological measures with medical, neurological, and neuroradiological findings are also important in understanding these diseases and in furthering our knowledge about brain–behavior relationships. Correlations between neuropsychological findings and biochemical measures (e.g., enzyme levels) and other markers of disease and treatment status have the potential to enhance our understanding of disease effects on brain function. As an example, studies of ALD fail to reveal correlations between plasma VLCFA levels, a marker for presence of the disease, and any cognitive measure. This finding suggests that plasma VLCFA levels do not reflect patients' cerebral status.

MRIs have been invaluable in identifying the locus and severity of the disease process in these disorders. A method of scoring MRIs in patients with ALD developed in our center has allowed quantification of both locus and severity, and has demonstrated a significant correlation between disease severity and extent of neuropsychological abnormality (Balthazor, Shapiro, et al., 1996). We found, for example, that MRI severity scores correlated .82 with IQ in boys with ALD. In those ALD cases with frontal demyelination, both Verbal and Performance IQs were decreased relative to scores for the sample as a whole, whereas patients with posterior demyelination showed only Performance IQ decrements (Balthazor, Shapiro, et al., 1996). In a study currently in progress, we are examining the relationship of quantified MRI variables with neuropsychological status in children with Hurler syndrome.

Magnetic resonance spectroscopy (MRS) holds special promise in improving our understanding of metabolic and neurodegenerative diseases. MRS is used to identify levels of cerebral metabolites in specified regions of cerebral white matter (Rajanayagam et al., 1996); these metabolites reflect specific disease processes and are abnormal in many neurodegenerative diseases. Our preliminary work (Rajanayagam, Balthazor, et al., 1997) has revealed correlations between neuropsychological tests and levels of cerebral metabolites in specific brain regions. Functional imaging—namely, MRI and positron emission tomography—also holds promise for investigations of brain–behavior relationships in children with metabolic and neurodegenerative disorders, although studies utilizing these techniques have yet to be completed.

Evaluation of the efficacy of new treatments for these disorders will require information regarding the natural history of the untreated diseases. Treatment effects can then be examined by comparing outcomes for treated patients to outcomes in untreated individuals. Because neurodegenerative diseases are ultimately fatal, parents and physicians are understandably reluctant to forgo treatment, even if chances are slim for a positive benefit. For this reason, contemporary control groups are rarely an option. Thus neuropsychologists are obligated to collect data quickly regarding the natural history of metabolic and neurodegenerative genetic diseases whenever possible, even if comparisons to a treated group are left for the future.

With the advent of new treatments, it will also be important to extend measurement of outcomes to include QOL variables. One question to address in this research is whether treatment effects include better long-term QOL, as well as improved cognitive status. A second goal will be to identify pretreatment variables that predict enhanced QOL outcomes. Information regarding predictors of treatment response will help physicians to better inform their patients regarding risks and benefits of treatment. Neuropsychologists are well equipped to carry out such research, especially given the likelihood of a strong relationship between cognitive outcome and QOL in these patients.

The paucity of longitudinal studies of children with metabolic and neurodegenerative disorders most probably reflects the fact that neuropsychologists have not been involved in their care. Many of the physicians who treat these children are specialists in genetics or metabolic disorders, who have not been accustomed to collaborating with neuropsychologists. These physician groups may also fail to appreciate the importance of the information that neuropsychologists can provide with respect to the conduct of clinical trials. Neuropsychologists themselves may have underestimated the contributions they can make in furthering understanding of brain–behavior relationships. Many neurodegenerative disorders have specific and localized effects on the brain, which can be correlated with neuropsychological functions. Studies of children with these diseases may also yield information regarding the impact of insults incurred in infancy and early childhood on the developing brain. Follow-up investigations of neuropsychological outcomes and QOL will be particularly critical in determining the efficacy of new treatments for these devastating diseases.

REFERENCES

Angelini, L., Nardocci, N., Rumi, V., Zorzi, C., Strada, L., & Savoiardo, M. (1992). Hallervorden–Spatz disease: Clinical and MRI study of 11 cases diagnosed in life. *Journal of Neurology, 239*(8), 417–425.

Aubourg, P., Blanche, S., Jambaqué, I., Rocchiccioli, F., Kalifa, G., Naud-Saudreau, C., Rolland, M.-O., Debré, M., Chaussain, J.-L., Griscelli, C., Fischer, A., & Bougnères, P.-F. (1990). Reversal of early neurological and neuroradiologic manifestations of X-linked adrenoleukodystrophy by bone marrow transplantation. *New England Journal of Medicine, 322,* 1860–1866.

Autti, T., Raininko, R., Launes, J., Nuutila, A., & Santavuori, P. (1992). Jansky–Bielschowsky variant disease: CT, MRI, and SPECT findings. *Pediatric Neurology, 8*(2), 121–6.

Bachmann, C. (1992). Ornithine carbamoyl transferase deficiency: findings, models and problems. *Journal of Inherited Metabolic Disease, 15*(4), 578–591.

Balthazor, M., Rajanayagam, V., Shapiro, E., Loes, D., Stillman, A., Lockman, L., & Krivit, W. (1996). Predicting dementia in white matter disease: Magnetic resonance imaging, magnetic resonance spectroscopy, and neuropsychology [Abstract]. *Annals of Neurology, 40,* 290.

Balthazor, M., Shapiro, E., Loes, D., Lockman, L., Cox, C., Moser, H., & Krivit, W. (1996). Adrenoleukodystrophy: The relationship between MRI findings and neuropsychological functioning [Abstract]. *Journal of the International Neuropsychological Society, 2,* 41.

Barkovich, A. J., Good, W. V., Koch, T. K., & Berg, B. O. (1993). Mitochondrial disorders: Analysis of their clinical and imaging characteristics. *American Journal of Neuroradiology, 14*(5), 1119–1137.

Barone, R., Bruhl, K., Stoeter, P., Fiumara, A., Pavone, L., & Beck, M. (1996). Clinical and neuroradiological findings in classic infantile and late-onset globoid-cell leukodystrophy (Krabbe disease). *American Journal of Medical Genetics, 63*(1), 209–217.

Bax, M. C., & Colville, G. A. (1995). Behaviour in mucopolysaccharide disorders. *Archives of Disease in Childhood, 73*(1), 77–81.

Bayley, N. (1969). *Bayley Scales of Infant Development.* New York: Psychological Corporation.

Benton, A. L., Hamsher, K., Varney, N., & Spreen, O. (1983). *Contributions to neuropsychological assessment.* New York: Oxford University Press.

Bergstrom, S. K., Quinn, J. J., Greenstein, R., & Ascensao, J. (1994). Long-term follow-up of a patient transplanted for Hunter's disease type IIB: A case report and literature review. *Bone Marrow Transplantation, 14*(4), 653–658.

Braun, A., Ambach, H., Kammerer, S., Rolinski, B., Stockler, S., Rabl, W., Gartner, J., Zierz, S., & Roscher, A. A. (1995). Mutations in the gene for X-linked adrenoleukodystrophy in patients with different clinical phenotypes. *American Journal of Human Genetics, 56*(4), 854–861.

Braun, S. E., Pan, D., Aronovich, E. L., Jonsson, J. J., McIvor, R. S., & Whitley, C. B. (1996). Preclinical studies of lymphocyte gene therapy for mild Hunter syndrome (mucopolysaccharidosis type II). *Human Gene Therapy, 7,* 283–290.

Braunlin, E. A., Hunter, D. W., Krivit, W., Burke, B. A., Hesslein, P. S., Porter, P. T., & Whitley, C. B. (1992). Evaluation of coronary artery disease in the Hurler syndrome by angiography. *American Journal of Cardiology, 69*(17), 1487–1489.

Brismar, J., & Ozand, P. T. (1994). CT and MR of the brain in disorders of the propionate and methylmalonate metabolism. [Review]. *American Journal of Neuroradiology, 15*(8), 1459–1473.

Bruun, I., Reske-Nielsen, E., & Oster, S. (1991). Juvenile ceroid-lipofuscinosis and calcifications of the CNS. *Acta Neurologica Scandinavica, 83*(1), 1–8.

Bunge, S., Kleijer, W. J., Steglich, C., Beck, M., Zuther, C., Morris, C. P., Schwinger, E., Hopwood, J. J., Scott, H. S., & Gal, A. (1994). Mucopolysaccharidosis type I: Identification of 8 novel mutations and determination of the frequency of the two common alpha-L-iduronidase mutations (W402X and Q70X) among European patients. *Human Molecular Genetics, 3*(6), 861–6.

Casteels, I., Spileers, W., Swinnen, T., Demaerel, P., Silberstein, J., Casaer, P., & Missotten, L. (1994). Optic atrophy as the presenting sign in Hallervorden-Spatz syndrome. *Neuropediatrics, 25*(5), 265–267.

Christodoulou, J., Qureshi, I. A., McInnes, R. R., & Clarke, J. T. (1993). Ornithine transcarbamylase deficiency presenting with strokelike episodes. *Journal of Pediatrics, 122*(3), 423–425.

Clarke, L. A., & Scott, H. S. (1993). Two novel mutations causing mucopolysaccharidosis type I detected by single strand conformational analysis of the alpha-L-iduronidase gene. *Human Molecular Genetics, 2*(8), 1311–1312.

Colville, G. A., Watters, J. P., Yule, W., & Bax, M. (1996). Sleep problems in children with Sanfilippo syndrome. *Developmental Medicine and Child Neurology, 38*(6), 538–544.

Contreras, M., Sengupta, T. K., Sheikh, F., Aubourg, P., & Singh, I. (1996). Topology of ATP-binding domain of adrenoleukodystrophy gene product in peroxisomes. *Archives of Biochemistry and Biophysics, 334*(2), 369–379.

Coppa, G. V., Gabrielli, O., Zampini, L., Pierani, P., Giorgi, P. L., Jezequel, A. M., Orlandi, F., Miniero, R., Busca, A., & De Luca, T. (1995). Bone marrow transplantation in Hunter syndrome (mucopolysaccharidosis type II): Two-year follow-up of the first Italian patient and review of the literature. *Pediatria Medica e Chirurgica, 17*(3), 227–235.

Cummings, J. L., & Benson, D. F. (1992). *Dementia: A clinical approach.* Boston: Butterworth–Heinemann.

du Cret, R. P., Weinberg, E. J., Jackson, C. A., Braunlin, E. A., Boudreau, R. J., Kuni, C. C., Carpenter, B. M., Hunter, D. W., Krivit, W., & Bodeau, G. (1994). Resting Tl-201 scintigraphy in the evaluation of coronary artery disease in children with Hurler syndrome. *Clinical Nuclear Medicine, 19*(11), 975–978.

Dyken, P., & McCleary, G. E. (1986). Dementia in infantile and childhood neurological disease. In J. E. Obrzut & G. W. Hynd (Eds.), *Child neuropsychology* (Vol. 2, pp. 175–189). Orlando, FL: Academic Press.

Fairbairn, L. J., Lashford, L. S., Spooncer, E., McDermott, R. H., Lebens, G., Arrand, J. E., Arrand, J. R., Bellantuono, I., Holt, R., Hatton, C. E., Cooper, A., Besley, G. T., Wraith, J. E., Anson, D. S., Hopwood, J. J., & Dexter, T. M. (1997). Towards gene therapy of Hurler syndrome. *Casopis Lekaru Ceskych, 136*(1), 27–31.

Fanen, P., Guidoux, S., Sarde, C. O., Mandel, J., Goossens, M., & Aubourg, P. (1994). Identification of mutations in the putative ATP-binding domain of the adrenoleukodystrophy gene. *Journal of Clinical Investigation, 94*, 516–520.

Feigenbaum, V., Lombard-Platet, G., Guidoux, S., Sarde, C. O., Mandel, J. L., & Aubourg, P. (1996). Mutational and protein analysis of patients and heterozygous women with X-linked adrenoleukodystrophy. *American Journal of Human Genetics, 58*(6), 1135–1144.

Field, R. E., Buchanan, J. A., Copplemans, M. G., & Aichroth, P. M. (1994). Bone-marrow transplantation in Hurler's syndrome: Effect on skeletal development. *Journal of Bone and Joint Surgery—British Volume, 76*(6), 975–981.

Francis, D. J., Fletcher, J. M., Stuebing, K. K., Davidson, K. C., & Thompson, N. M. (1991). Analysis of change: Modeling individual growth. *Journal of Consulting and Clinical Psychology, 59*, 27–37.

Fuchs, S., Sarde, C. O., Wedemann, H., Schwinger, E., Mandel, J. L., & Gal, A. (1994). Missense mutations are frequent in the gene for X-chromosomal adrenoleukodystrophy (ALD). *Human Molecular Genetics, 3*(10), 1903–1905.

Fujii, T., Okuno, T., Ito, M., Hattori, H., Mutoh, K., Go, T., Shirasaka, Y., Shiraishi, H., Iwasaki, Y., & Asato, R. (1995). 123I-IMP SPECT findings in mitochondrial encephalomyopathies. *Brain and Development, 17*(2), 89–94.

Funakawa, I., Mukai, K., Terao, A., Kawashima, S., & Mori, T. (1994). [A case of MELAS associated with prosopagnosia, topographical disorientation and PLED]. *Rinsho Shinkeigaku—Clinical Neurology, 34*(10), 1052–1054.

Greenberg, L. (1996). *The Test of Variables of Attention (T.O.V.A.).* Los Alamitos, CA: Universal Attention Disorders.

Hasegawa, T., Tzakis, A. G., Todo, S., Reyes, J., Nour, B., Finegold, D. N., & Starzl, T. E. (1995). Orthotopic liver transplantation for ornithine transcarbamylase deficiency with hyperammonemic encephalopathy. *Journal of Pediatric Surgery, 30*(6), 863–865.

Hettema, E. H., Vanroermund, C. W. T., Distel, B., Vandenberg, M., Vilela, C., Rodriguespousada, C., Wanders, R. J. A., & Tabak, H. F. (1996). The ABC transporter proteins Pat1 and Pat2 are required for import of long-chain fatty acids into peroxisomes of *Saccharomyces cerevisiae. EMBO Journal, 15*(15), 3813–3822.

Hilliges, C., Awiszus, D., & Wendel, U. (1993). Intellectual performance of children with maple syrup urine disease. *European Journal of Pediatrics, 152*(2), 144–147.

Hoffmann, G. F., Bohles, H. J., Burlina, A., Duran, M., Herwig, J., Lehnert, W., Leonard, J. V., Muntau, A., Plecko-Starting, F. K., Superti-Furga, A., Trefz, F. K., & Christensen, E. (1995). Early signs and course of disease of glutaryl-CoA dehydrogenase deficiency. *Journal of Inherited Metabolic Disease, 18,* 173–176.

Huang, C. C., Wai, Y. Y., Chu, N. S., Liou, C. W., Pang, C. Y., Shih, K. D., & Wei, Y. H. (1995). Mitochondrial encephalomyopathies: CT and MRI findings and correlations with clinical features. *European Neurology, 35*(4), 199–205.

Hurowitz, G. I., Silver, J. M., Brin, M. F., Williams, D. T., & Johnson, W. G. (1993). Neuropsychiatric aspects of adult-onset Tay–Sachs disease: Two case reports with several new findings. *Journal of Neuropsychiatry and Clinical Neurosciences, 5,* 30–36.

Imaizumi, M., Gushi, K., Kurobane, I., Inoue, S., Suzuki, J., Koizumi, Y., Suzuki, H., Sato, A., Gotoh, Y., & Haginoya, K. (1994). Long-term effects of bone marrow transplantation for inborn errors of metabolism: A study of four patients with lysosomal storage diseases. *Acta Paediatrica Japonica, 36*(1), 30–36.

Jan, D., Poggi, F., Laurent, J., Rabier, D., Jouvet, P., Lacaille, F., Beringer, A., Hubert, P., Revillon, Y., & Saudubray, J. M. (1994). Liver transplantation: New indications in metabolic disorders? *Transplantation Proceedings, 26*(1), 189–190.

Johnson, M. A., Desai, S., Hugh-Jones, K., & Starer, F. (1984). Magnetic resonance imaging of the brain in Hurler syndrome. *American Journal of Neuroradiology, 5,* 816–819.

Johnston, M. V., Hohmann, C., & Blue, M. E. (1995). Neurobiology of Rett syndrome. *Neuropediatrics, 26*(2), 119–122.

Kakkis, E. D., McEntee, M. F., Schmidtchen, A., Neufeld, E. F., Ward, D. A., Gompf, R. E., Kania, S., Bedolla, C., Chien, S. L., & Shull, R. M. (1996). Long-term and high-dose trials of enzyme replacement therapy in the canine model of mucopolysaccharidosis I. *Biochemical and Molecular Medicine, 58*(2), 156–167.

Kaplan, P., Mazur, A., Field, M., Berlin, J. A., Berry, G. T., Heidenreich, R., Yudkoff, M., & Segal, S. (1991). Intellectual outcome in children with maple syrup urine disease. *Journal of Pediatrics, 119*(1), 46–50.

Kaufman, F. R., McBride-Chang, C., Manis, F. R., Wolff, J. A., & Nelson, M. D. (1995). Cognitive functioning, neurologic status and brain imaging in classical galactosemia. *European Journal of Pediatrics, 154*(7, Suppl. 2), S2–S5.

Kerr, A. M. (1995). Early clinical signs in the Rett disorder. *Neuropediatrics, 26*(2), 67–71.

Klein, K., Krivit, W., Whitley, C., Peters, C., Cool, V. A., Fuhrman, M., de Alacron, P., Klemperer, M., Miller, L., Nelson, R. P., Henslee-Downey, J., Chang, P., Wraith, J. E., Lockman, L., & Shapiro, E. (1995). Poor cognitive outcome of nine children with Sanfilippo syndrome following bone marrow transplantation and successful engraftment. *Bone Marrow Transplantation, 15*(Suppl.), S176–S181.

Koch, T. K., Schmidt, K. A., Wagstaff, J. E., Ng, W. G., & Packman, S. (1992). Neurologic complications in galactosemia. *Pediatric Neurology, 8*(3), 217–20.

Kohlschutter, A., Laabs, R., & Albani, M. (1988). Juvenile neuronal ceroid lipofuscinosis (JNCL): Quantitative description of its clinical variability. *Acta Paediatrica, 77,* 867–872.

Kok, F., Neumann, S., Sarde, C.-O., Zheng, S., Wu, K.-H., Wei, H.-M., Bergin, J., Watkins, P. A., Gould, S., Sack, G., Moser, H., Mandel, J.-L., & Smith, K. D. (1995). Mutational analysis of patients with X-linked adrenoleukodystrophy. *Human Mutation, 6,* 104–115.

Kolodny, E. H., Raghavan, S., & Krivit, W. (1991). Late-onset Krabbe disease (globoid cell leukodystrophy): Clinical and biochemical features of 15 cases. *Developmental Neuroscience, 13*(4–5), 232–239.

Koo, B., Becker, L. E., Chuang, S., Merante, F., Robinson, B. H., MacGregor, D., Tein, I., Ho, V. B., McGreal, D. A., Wherrett, J. R., & Logan, W. J. (1993). Mitochondrial encephalomyopathy, lactic acidosis, stroke-like episodes (MELAS): Clinical, radiological, pathological, and genetic observations. *Annals of Neurology, 34*(1), 25–32.

Korenke, G. C., Fuchs, S., Krasemann, E., Doerr, H. G., Wilichowski, E., Hunneman, D. H., & Hanefeld, F. (1996). Cerebral adrenoleukodystrophy (ALD) in only one of monozygotic twins with an identical ALD genotype. *Annals of Neurology, 40*(2), 254–257.

Kristensen, K., & Lou, H. (1983). Central nervous system dysfunction as early sign of neuronal ceroid lipofuscinosis Batten's disease. *Developmental Medicine and Child Neurology, 25,* 588–590.

Krivit, W., Henslee-Downey, J., Klemperer, M., Cowan, M., Peters, C., Sanders, J., Saunders, F., Weinstein, H., Williams, T., Harris, R., Kirkpatrick, D., Bowen, T., Falk, P., Bayever, E., Bunin, N., Johnson, L.,

Sender, W., de Alacron, P., Shapiro, E., Lockman, L., & Anderson, J. (1995). Bone marrow transplantation for Hurler's syndrome. *Bone Marrow Transplantation, 15*(Suppl.), S182–S185.

Krivit, W., Lockman, L., & Shapiro, E. (1996a). Childhood onset of cerebral adrenoleukodystrophy: Effective treatment by bone marrow transplantation. In J. R. Hobbs & P. G. Riches (Eds.), *Correction of certain genetic diseases by transplantation 1995* (pp. 48–56). London: The Cogent Trust.

Krivit, W., Lockman, L., & Shapiro, E. (1996b). Metachromatic leukodystrophy. In J. R. Hobbs & P. G. Riches (Eds.), *Correction of certain genetic diseases by transplantation 1995* (pp. 41–47). London: The Cogent Trust.

Krivit, W., Lockman, L., Watkins, P. A., Hirsch, J., & Shapiro, E. (1995). The future for treatment by bone marrow transplantation for adrenoleukodystrophy, metachromatic leukodystrophy, globoid cell leukodystrophy and Hurler syndrome. *Journal of Inherited Metabolic Disease, 18*, 398–412.

Krivit, W., & Shapiro, E. (1994). Bone marrow transplant for storage diseases. In S. J. Forman, E. D. Thomas, & K. Blume (Eds.), *Bone marrow transplantation* (pp. 883–891). Oxford: Blackwell Scientific.

Krivit, W., Shapiro, E., Balthazor, M., Lockman, L., Summers, G., Hourse, J., Ogilvie, J., Whitley, C., Belani, K., Braunlin, E., Hirsch, J., Latchaw, R., Peters, C., Dusenbery, K., & Wagner, J. (1996). Hurler syndrome: Outcomes and planning following bone marrow transplantation. In J. R. Hobbs & P. G. Riches (Eds.), *Correction of certain genetic diseases by transplantation 1995* (pp. 25–40). London: The Cogent Trust.

Krivit, W., Shapiro, E., Kennedy, W., Lipton, M., Lockman, L., Smith, S., Summers, C., Wenger, D., Ramsey, N., Kersey, J., Yao, J. K., & Kaye, E. (1990). Effective treatment of late infantile metachromatic leukodystrophy by bone marrow transplantation. *New England Journal of Medicine, 322*, 28–32.

Krivit, W., Shapiro, E., Peters, C., Wagner, J., Cornu, G., Kurtzberg, J., Wenger, D., Kolodny, E., Vanier, M., Loes, D., Dusenbery, K., & Lockman, L. (1998). Hematopoietic stem cell transplantation in globoid cell leukodystrophy. *New England Journal of Medicine, 338*, 1119–1126.

Krivit, W., Sung, J. H., Shapiro, E. G., & Lockman, L. A. (1995). Microglia: The effector cell for reconstitution of the central nervous system following bone marrow transplantation for lysosomal and peroxisomal storage diseases. *Cell Transplantation, 4*, 385–392.

Kruse, B., Barker, P. B., van Zijl, P. C., Duyn, J. H., Moonen, C. T., & Moser, H. W. (1994). Multislice proton magnetic resonance spectroscopic imaging in X-linked adrenoleukodystrophy. *Annals of Neurology, 36*(4), 595–608.

Kuhne, T., Bubl, R., & Baumgartner, R. (1991). Maternal vegan diet causing a serious infantile neurological disorder due to vitamin B12 deficiency. *European Journal of Pediatrics, 150*(3), 205–208.

Kyllerman, M., Skjeldal, O. H., Lundberg, M., Holme, I., Jellum, E., von Dobeln, U., Fossen, A., & Carlsson, G. (1994). Dystonia and dyskinesia in glutaric aciduria type I: Clinical heterogeneity and therapeutic considerations. *Movement Disorders, 9*, 22–30.

Lee, C., Dineen, T. E., Brack, M., Kirsch, J. E., & Runge, V. M. (1993). The mucopolysaccharidoses: Characterization by cranial MR imaging. *American Journal of Neuroradiology, 14*(6), 1285–1292.

Ligtenberg, M. J., Kemp, S., Sarde, C. O., van Geel, B. M., Kleijer, W. J., Barth, P. G., Mandel, J. L., van Oost, B. A., & Bolhuis, P. A. (1995). Spectrum of mutations in the gene encoding the adrenoleukodystrophy protein. *American Journal of Human Genetics, 56*, 44–50.

Lockman, L., Shapiro, E., & Krivit, W. (1993). Studies of eight adrenoleukodystrophy patients at least one year after bone marrow transplantation [Abstract]. *Annals of Neurology, 32*, 447.

Loes, D. J., Hite, S., Moser, H., Stillman, A. E., Shapiro, E., Lockman, L., Latchaw, R. E., & Krivit, W. (1994). Adrenoleukodystrophy: A scoring method for brain MR observations. *American Journal of Neuroradiology, 15*(9), 1761–1766.

Lowry, R. B., Applegarth, D. A., Toone, J. R., MacDonald, E., & Thunem, N. Y. (1990). An update on the frequency of mucopolysaccharide syndromes in British Columbia. *Human Genetics, 85*, 389–390.

Lyon, G., Hagberg, B., Evrard, P., Allaire, C., Pavone, L., & Vanier, M. (1991). Symptomatology of late onset Krabbe's leukodystrophy: The European experience. *Developmental Neuroscience, 13*(4–5), 240–244.

Maestri, N. E., Brusilow, S. W., Clissold, D. B., & Bassett, S. S. (1996). Long-term treatment of girls with ornithine transcarbamylase deficiency. *New England Journal of Medicine, 335*(12), 855–859.

Mandel, H., Braun, J., El-Peleg, O., Christensen, E., & Berant, M. (1991). Glutaric aciduria type I: Brain CT features and a diagnostic pitfall. *Neuroradiology, 33*, 75–78.

Merinero, B., Perez-Cerda, C., Font, L. M., Garcia, M. J., Aparico, M., Lorenzo, G., Martinez Pardo, M., Garzo, C., Martinez-Bermejo, A., Castroviejo, I. P., Christensen, E., & Ugarte, M. (1995). Variable clinical and biochemical presentation of seven Spanish cases with glutaryl-CoA-dehydrogenase deficiency. *Neuropediatrics, 26*, 238–242.

McKinnis, E. J., Sulzbacher, S., Rutledge, J. C., Sanders, J., & Scott, C. R. (1996). Bone marrow transplantation in Hunter syndrome. *Journal of Pediatrics, 129*(1), 145–148.

Moller, H. E., Ullrich, K., Vermathen, P., Schuierer, G., & Koch, H. G. (1995). In vivo study of brain metabolism in galactosemia by 1H and 31P magnetic resonance spectroscopy. *European Journal of Pediatrics, 154*(7, Suppl. 2), S8–S13.

Moser, H., Moser, A. K. S., Bergin, A., Borel, J., Shankroff, J., Stine, O. C., Merette, C., Ott, J., Krivit, W., & Shapiro, E. (1992). Adrenoleukodystrophy: Phenotypic variability and implications for therapy. *Journal of Inherited Metabolic Disease, 15,* 645–664.

Moser, H. W., Kok, F., Neumann, S., Borel, J., Bergin, A., Mostafa, S. D., Panoscha, R., Davoli, C. T., Shankroff, J., & Smith, K. (1994). Adrenoleukodystrophy update: Genetics and effect of Lorenzo's oil therapy in symptomatic patients. *International Pediatrics, 9,* 196–204.

Moser, H. W., Moser, A. B., Naidu, S., & Bergin, A. (1991). Clinical aspects of adrenoleuko-dystrophy and adrenomyeloneuropathy. *Developmental Neuroscience, 13*(4–5), 254–261.

Moser, H. W., Smith, K. D., & Moser, A. (1995). X-linked adrenoleukodystrophy. In C. R. Scriver, A. L. Beaudet, W. S. Sly, & D. Valle (Eds.), *Metabolic and molecular basis of inherited diseases* (7th ed., pp. 2325–2349). New York: McGraw-Hill.

Mosser, J., Douar, A. M., Sarde, C. O., Kioschis, P., Feil, R., Moser, H., Poustka, A. M., Mandel, J. L., & Aubourg, P. (1993). Putative X-linked adrenoleukodystrophy gene shares unexpected homology with ABC transporters. *Nature, 361,* 726–30.

Mosser, J., Lutz, Y., Stoeckel, M. E., Sarde, C. O., Kretz, C., Douar, A. M., Lopez, J., Aubourg, P., & Mandel, J. L. (1994). The gene responsible for adrenoleukodystrophy encodes a peroxisomal membrane protein. *Human Molecular Genetics, 3*(2), 265–271.

Msall, M., Batshaw, M. L., Suss, R., Brusilow, S. W., & Mellits, E. D. (1984). Neurologic outcome in children with inborn errors of urea synthesis. Outcome of urea-cycle enzymopathies. *New England Journal of Medicine, 310*(23), 1500–1505.

Muller, K., Kahn, T., & Wendel, U. (1993). Is demyelination a feature of maple syrup urine disease? *Pediatric Neurology, 9*(5), 375–382.

Nardocci, N., Verga, M. L., Binelli, S., Zorzi, G., Angelini, L., & Bugiani, O. (1995). Neuronal ceroid-lipofuscinosis: A clinical morphological study of 19 patients. *American Journal of Medical Genetics, 57,* 137–141.

Navarro, C., Dominguez, C., Fernandez, J. M., Fachal, C., & Alvarez, M. (1995). Case report: Four-year follow-up of bone marrow transplantation in late juvennile metachromatic leukodystrophy. *Journal of Inherited Metabolic Disease, 18*(2), 157–158.

Navarro, C., Fernandez, J. M., Dominguez, C., Fachal, C., & Alvarez, M. (1996). Late juvenile metachromatic leukodystrophy treated with bone marrow transplantation; a 4-year follow-up study. *Neurology, 46*(1), 254–256.

Nelson, C. D., Waggoner, D. D., Donnell, G. N., Tuerck, J. M., & Buist, N. R. (1991). Verbal dyspraxia in treated galactosemia. *Pediatrics, 88*(2), 346–350.

Nelson, D. (1995). Verbal dyspraxia in children with galactosemia. *European Journal of Pediatrics, 154*(7, Suppl. 2), S6–S7.

Nelson, M. D., Jr., Wolff, J. A., Cross, C. A., Donnell, G. N., & Kaufman, F. R. (1992). Galactosemia: Evaluation with MR imaging. *Radiology, 184*(1), 255–261.

Nidiffer, F. D., & Kelly, T. E. (1983). Developmental and degenerative patterns associated with cognitive, behavioral and motor difficulties in the Sanfilippo syndrome: An epidemiological study. *Journal of Mental Deficiency Research, 27,* 185–203.

Nord, A., van Doorninck, W. J., & Greene, C. (1991). Developmental profile of patients with maple syrup urine disease. *Journal of Inherited Metabolic Disease, 14*(6), 881–889.

Oehlmann, R., Zlotogora, J., Wenger, D. A., & Knowlton, R. G. (1993). Localization of the Krabbe disease gene (GALC) on chromosome 14 by multipoint linkage analysis. *American Journal of Human Genetics, 53*(6), 1250–1255.

Ozand, P. T., Thompson, J. N., Gascon, G. G., Sarvepalli, S. B., Rahbeeni, Z., Nester, M. J., & Brismar, J. (1994). Sanfilippo type D presenting with acquired language disorder but without features of mucopolysaccharidosis. *Journal of Child Neurology, 9*(4), 408–411.

Parsons, V. J., Hughes, D. G., & Wraith, J. E. (1996). Magnetic resonance imaging of the brain, neck and cervical spine in mild Hunter's syndrome (mucopolysaccharidosis type II). *Clinical Radiology, 51*(10), 719–723.

Peters, C., Balthazor, M., Shapiro, E., King, R., Kollman, C., Hegland, J., Henslee-Downey, J., Trigg, M., Cowan, M., Sanders, J., Bunin, N., Weinstein, H., Lenarsky, C., Falk, P., Harris, R., Bowen, T., Williams, T., Grayson, G., Warkentin, P., Sender, L., Cool, V., Crittenden, M., Whitley, C., Packman, S., Kaplan, P., Lockman, L., Anderson, J., Krivit, W., Dusenbery, K., & Wagner, J. (1996). Outcome of unrelated donor bone marrow transplantation in forty children with Hurler syndrome. *Blood, 87,* 4894–4902.

Peters, C., Shapiro, E., Anderson, J., Henslee-Downey, P. J., Klemperer, M., Cowan, M. J., Saunders, E. F., deAlarcon, P. A., Twist, C., Nachman, J. B., Hale, G. A., Harris, R. E., Rozans, M. K., Kurtzberg, J., Grayson, G. H., Williams, T. E., Lenarsky, C., Balthazor, M., Cool, V. A., Crittenden, M., Clarke, J. T. R., Packman, S., Shapira, E., Lockman, L. A., Dusenbery, K., Wagner, J. E., & Krivit, W. (1998). Hurler syndrome: II. Outcome of HLA-genotypically identical sibling and non-genotypically identical related donor bone marrow transplantation in fifty-four children. *Blood, 91*, 2601–2608.

Peters, C., Shapiro, E., & Krivit, W. (1998). Hurler syndrome: Past, present, and future [Editorial]. *Journal of Pediatrics, 133*, 7–9.

Pridjian, G., Humbert, J., Willis, J., & Shapira, E. (1994). Presymptomatic late-infantile metachromatic leukodystrophy treated with bone marrow transplantation. *Journal of Pediatrics, 125*(5, Pt. 1), 755–758.

Pridmore, C. L., Clarke, J. T., & Blaser, S. (1995). Ornithine transcarbamylase deficiency in females: An often overlooked cause of treatable encephalopathy. *Journal of Child Neurology, 10*(5), 369–374.

Rajanayagam, V., Balthazor, M., Shapiro, E., Krivet, W., Lockman, L., & Stillman, A. (1997). Proton MR spectroscopy and neuropsychological testing in adrenoleukodystrophy. *American Journal of Neuroradiology, 18*, 1909–1914.

Rajanayagam, V., Grad, J., Krivit, W., Loes, D. J., Lockman, L., Shapiro, E., Balthazor, M., Aeppli, D., & Stillman, A. E. (1996). Proton MR spectroscopy of childhood adrenoleukodystrophy. *American Journal of Neuroradiology, 17*(6), 1013–1024.

Rapin, I. (1976). Progressive genetic–metabolic diseases of the central nervous system in children. *Pediatric Annals, 5*, 313–349.

Reiss, A. L., Faruque, F., Naidu, S., Abrams, M., Beaty, T., Bryan, R. N., & Moser, H. (1993). Neuroanatomy of Rett syndrome: A volumetric imaging study. *Annals of Neurology, 34*(2), 227–234.

Resnick, J. M., Whitley, C. B., Leonard, A. S., Krivit, W., & Snover, D. C. (1994). Light and electron microscopic features of the liver in mucopolysaccharidosis. *Human Pathology, 25*(3), 276–286.

Rosebush, P. I., MacQueen, G. M., Clark, J. T., Callahan, J. W., Strasberg, P. M., & Mazurek, M. F. (1995). Late-onset Tay–Sachs disease presenting as catatonic schizophrenia: Diagnostic and treatment issues. *Journal of Clinical Psychiatry, 56*, 347–353.

Rourke, B. P. (1987). Syndrome of nonverbal learning disabilities: The final common pathway of white-matter disease/dysfunction. *Clinical Neuropsychologist, 1*, 209–234.

Sansom, D., Krishnan, V. H., Corbett, J., & Kerr, A. (1993). Emotional and behavioural aspects of Rett syndrome. *Developmental Medicine and Child Neurology, 35*(4), 340–345.

Schaap, T., & Bach, G. (1980). Incidence of mucopolysaccharidoses in Israel: Is Hunter disease a 'Jewish disease'? *Human Genetics, 56*, 221–223.

Schachern, P. A., Shea, D. A., & Paparella, M. M. (1984). Mucopolysacchraridosis I-H (Hurler's syndrome) and human temporal bone histopathology. *Annals of Otolaryngology and Laryngology, 93*, 65–69.

Schweitzer, S., Shin, Y., Jakobs, C., & Brodehl, J. (1993). Long-term outcome in 134 patients with galactosaemia. *European Journal of Pediatrics, 152*(1), 36–43.

Scott, H. S., Litjens, T., Hopwood, J. J., & Morris, C. P. (1992). A common mutation for mucopolysaccharidosis type I associated with a severe Hurler syndrome phenotype. *Human Mutation, 1*(2), 103–108.

Scott, H. S., Litjens, T., Nelson, P. V., Brooks, D. A., Hopwood, J. J., & Morris, C. P. (1992). Alpha-ʟ-iduronidase mutations (Q70X and P533R) associated with a severe Hurler phenotype. *Human Mutation, 1*(4), 333–9.

Shani, N., & Valle, D. (1996). A *Saccharomyces cerevisiae* homolog of the human adrenoleukodystrophy transporter is a heterodimer of two half ATP-binding cassette transporters. *Proceedings of the National Academy of Sciences USA, 93*(21), 11901–11906.

Shapiro, E. (1997a). *Neuropsychological features of siblings with ornithine transcarbamylase deficiency.* Unpublished manuscript.

Shapiro, E. (1997b). *Neuropsychological features of five children with Hallerworden–Spatz disease.* Unpublished manuscript.

Shapiro, E., Aubourg, P., Lockman, L., Jambaque, I., Cowan, M., Harris, R., Crittenden, M., Ris, D., Loes, D., Ziegler, R., Peters, C., Moser, M., Cox, C., & Krivit, W. (1997). Adrenoleukodystrophy: Five year follow-up of 12 engrafted cases [Abstract]. *Annals of Neurology, 41.*

Shapiro, E., Balthazor, M., Lockman, L., & Krivit, W. (1994). Bone marrow transplantation in Hurler disease: Positive neuropsychological outcome [Abstract]. *Annals of Neurology, 36*, 491.

Shapiro, E., Balthazor, M., & Rajanayagam, V. (1995). *Magnetic resonance spectroscopy in Hurler syndrome.* Unpublished manuscript.

Shapiro, E., & Klein, K. (1993). Childhood dementia: Neuropsychological assessment and treatment of degenerative childhood diseases. In M. G. Tramontana & S. R. Hooper (Eds.), *Advances in child neuropsychology* (Vol. 3, pp. 119–171). New York: Springer-Verlag.

Shapiro, E., Lipton, M. E., & Krivit, W. (1992). White matter dysfunction and its neuropsychological correlates: A longitudinal study of a case of metachromatic leukodystrophy treated with bone marrow transplant. *Journal of Clinical and Experimental Neuropsychology, 14*(4), 610–624.

Shapiro, E., Lockman, L. A., Knopman, D., & Krivit, W. (1994). Characteristics of the dementia in late-onset metachromatic leukodystrophy. *Neurology, 44*(4), 662–665.

Shapiro, E., Lockman, L., Balthazor, M., & Krivit, W. (1995). Neuropsychological outcomes of several storage diseases with and without bone marrow transplantation. *Journal of Inherited Metabolic Disease, 18,* 413–429.

Shapiro, E., Lockman, L., Balthazor, M., Loes, D., Rajanayagam, V., Ziegler, R., Peters, C., & Krivit, W. (1997). Neuropsychological and neurological function and quality-of-life before and after bone marrow transplantation for adrenoleukodystrophy. In C. G. Steward & J. R. Hobbs (Eds.), *Correction of genetic diseases by transplantation IV* (pp. 52–62). London: The Cogent Trust.

Shapiro, E., Lockman, L., Kennedy, W., Zimmerman, D., Kolodny, E., Raghavan, S., Widershcain, G., Wenger, D. A., Sung, J. H., Summers, C. G., & Krivit, W. (1991). Bone marrow transplantation as treatment for globoid cell leukodystrophy. In R. Desnick (Ed.), *Treatment of genetic diseases* (pp. 223–238). Edinburgh: Churchill Livingstone.

Shapiro, E., McPhee, J., Abbot, A., & Sulzbacher, S. (1994). Minnesota Preschool Affect Rating Scales: Development, reliability, and validity. *Journal of Pediatric Psychology, 19,* 325–345.

Shapiro, E., Salter, J., Balthazor, M., Lockman, L., & Krivit, W. (1995). *Emotional and social behavior in children with Hurler syndrome before and after bone marrow transplantation.* Unpublished manuscript, University of Minnesota.

Shapiro, E., Thrall, M., Peters, C., Ziegler, R., Lockman, L., & Krivit, W. (1999). *Hematopoietic Stem Cell Transplant (HSCT) in Hurler Syndrome: Neuropsychological and health outcome profiles.* Proceedings of the meetings of the COGENT society.

Shevell, M. I., Matiaszuk, N., Ledley, F. D., & Rosenblatt, D. S. (1993). Varying neurological phenotypes among muto and mut– patients with methylmalonylCoA mutase deficiency. *American Journal of Medical Genetics, 45*(5), 619–624.

Shull, R. M., Kakkis, E. D., McEntee, M. F., Kania, S. A., Jonas, A. J., & Neufeld, E. F. (1994). Enzyme replacement in a canine model of Hurler syndrome. *Proceedings of the National Academy of Sciences USA, 91*(26), 12937–12941.

Sørensen, J. B., & Parnas, J. (1979). A clinical study of 44 patients with juvenile amaurotic familial idiocy. *Acta Psychiatrica Scandinavica, 59,* 449–461.

Specola, N., Vanier, M. T., Goutieres, F., Mikol, J., & Aicardi, J. (1990). The juvenile and chronic forms of GM2 gangliosidosis: Clinical and enzymatic heterogeneity. *Neurology, 40,* 145–150.

Streifler, J. Y., Gornish, M., Hadar, H., & Gadoth, N. (1993). Brain imaging in late-onset GM2 gangliosidosis. *Neurology, 43,* 2055–2058.

Sulzbacher, S., McKinnis, E. J. R., Sanders, J., & Scott, R. (1994). Marrow transplantation for genetic storage diseases: A hope for success with metachromatic leukodystrophy, but not with Hunter syndrome [Abstract]. In *Transplantation in children: Current results and controversies.* University of Iowa symposium, Abstract 17. Iowa City: University of Iowa.

Suzuki, K., Suzuki, Y., & Suzuki, K. (1995). Galactosylceramide lipidosis: Globoid-cell leukodystrophy (Krabbe disease). In C. R. Scriver, A. L. Beaudet, W. S. Sly, & D. Valle (Eds.), *The metabolic and molecular bases of inherited disease* (7th ed., pp. 2671–2692). New York: McGraw-Hill.

Swaiman, K. F. (1991). Hallervorden–Spatz syndrome and brain iron metabolism. *Archives of Neurology, 48*(12), 1285–1293.

Swift, A. V., Dyken, P. R., & DuRant, R. H. (1984). Psychological follow-up in childhood dementia: A longitudinal study of subacute sclerosing panencephalitis. *Journal of Pediatric Psychology, 9,* 469–483.

Taccone, A., Schiaffino, M. C., Cerone, R., Fondelli, M. P., & Romano, C. (1992). Computed tomography in maple syrup urine disease. *European Journal of Radiology, 14*(3), 207–212.

Taccone, A., Tortori Donati, P., Marzoli, A., Dell'Acqua, A., Gatti, R., & Leone, D. (1993). Mucopolysaccharidosis: thickening of dura mater at the craniocervical junction and other CT/MRI findings. *Pediatric Radiology, 23*(5), 349–352.

Tandon, V., Williamson, J. B., Cowie, R. A., & Wraith, J. E. (1996). Spinal problems in mucopolysaccharidosis I (Hurler syndrome). *Journal of Bone and Joint Surgery—British Volume, 78*(6), 938–944.

Tsika, A., Ball, W. S., Vigneron, D. B., Dunn, R. S., Nelson, S. J., & Kirks, D. R. (1993). Childhood adrenoleukodystrophy: Assessment with proton MR spectroscopy. *Radiology, 189,* 467–480.

van de Kamp, J. P., Niermeijer, M. F., von Figura, K., & Giesberts, M. A. (1981). Genetic heterogeneity and clinical veriability in the Sanfilippo syndrome types A, B, and C. *Clinical Genetics, 20,* 152–160.

van der Meer, S. B., Poggi, F., Spada, M., Bonnefont, J. P., Ogier, H., Hubert, P., Depondt, E., Rapoport, D., Rabier, D., Charpentier, C., Parvy, P., Bardet, J., Kamoun, P., & Saudubray, J. M. (1994). Clinical outcome of long-term management of patients with vitamin B12–unresponsive methylmalonic acidemia. *Journal of Pediatrics, 125*(6, Pt. 1), 903–908.

van Heest, A., House, J., Krivit, W., & Walker, K. (1998). Surgical treatment of carpal tunnel syndrome and trigger digits in children with mucopolysaccharide storage disorders. *Journal of Hand Surgery, 23*(2), 236–243.

van Schrojenstein-de Valk, H. M., & van de Kamp, J. J. (1987). Follow-up on seven adult patients with mild Sanfilippo B-disease. *American Journal of Medical Genetics, 28*(1), 125–129.

Vellodi, A., Young, E., New, M., Pot-Mees, C., & Hugh-Jones, K. (1992). Bone marrow transplantation for Sanfilippo disease type B. *Journal of Inherited Metabolic Disease, 15*(6), 911–918.

Vellodi, A., Young, E. P., Cooper, A., Wraith, J. E., Winchester, B., Meaney, C., Ramaswami, U., & Will, A. (1997). Bone marrow transplantation for mucopolysaccharidosis type I: Experience of two British centres. *Archives of Disease in Childhood, 76*(2), 92–99.

Watkins, P. A., Gould, S. J., Smith, M. A., Braiterman, L. T., Wei, H. M., Kok, F., Moser, A. B., Moser, H. W., & Smith, K. D. (1995). Altered expression of ALDP in X-linked adrenoleukodystrophy. *American Journal of Human Genetics, 57*(2), 292–301.

Whitley, C. B., Belani, K. G., Chang, P. N., Summers, C. G., Blazar, B. R., Tsai, M. Y., Latchaw, R. E., Ramsay, N. K., & Kersey, J. H. (1993). Long-term outcome of Hurler syndrome following bone marrow transplantation. *American Journal of Medical Genetics, 46*(2), 209–218.

Whitley, C. B., McIvor, R. S., Aronovich, E. L., Berry, S. A., Blazar, B. R., Burger, S. R., Kersey, J. H., King, R. A., Faras, A. J., Latchaw, R. E., McCullough, J., Pan, D., Ramsay, N. K., & Stroncek, D. F. (1996). Retroviral-mediated transfer of the iduronate-2-sulfatase gene into lymphocytes for treatment of mild Hunter syndrome (mucopolysaccharidosis type II). *Human Gene Therapy, 7,* 537–549.

Wraith, J. E., Danks, D. M., & Rogers, J. G. (1987). Mild Sanfilippo syndrome: A further cause of hyperactivity and behavioural disturbance. *Medical Journal of Australia, 147*(9), 450–451.

Young, I. D., & Harper, P. S. (1983). The natural history of the severe form of Hunter's syndrome: A study based on 52 cases. *Developmental Medicine and Child Neurology, 25,* 481–489.

9

ENVIRONMENTAL NEUROTOXICANTS AND PSYCHOLOGICAL DEVELOPMENT

KIM N. DIETRICH

In comparison to other areas of pediatric neuropsychology, prenatal and postnatal exposure to environmental chemicals is a very recent area of scientific inquiry and concern (e.g., Dietrich & Bellinger, 1994; Jacobson, Jacobson, Fein, Schwartz, & Dowler, 1984; Pearson & Dietrich, 1985). Nevertheless, it is virtually certain that human embryos, fetuses, infants, and children have been exposed to anthropogenic sources of pollution for centuries (Markham, 1994), and they have definitely been exposed to toxic concentrations of environmental contaminants since the advent of industrial culture. Clinical commentaries on the adverse effects of environmental chemicals on child development can be found in the medical literature of the 19th and early 20th centuries (Gibson, Love, Hardline, Bencroft, & Turner, 1892; Oliver, 1911; Warkany, 1966).

Exposure to environmental toxicants and drugs has historically posed numerous risks to fetal and child health and development, including mortality, disabling or disfiguring congenital defects, and cancer (Shephard, 1994). However, the nonfatal but disabling impact of environmental pollution on the immature central nervous system (CNS) has been the area of greatest public health concern and the most intensive study in the environmental health sciences (Rees, Francis, & Kimmel, 1990; Needleman & Bellinger, 1994). This is also an area within the domains of environmental health and developmental psychology that has engendered considerable controversy and, regrettably, a significant amount of misunderstanding and scorn (e.g., Scarr, 1985, 1991; Palca, 1992).

ENVIRONMENTAL NEUROTOXICITY AND THE DEVELOPING ORGANISM

It is now widely recognized that the human placenta does not serve as an impervious barrier to developmentally toxic substances, and, furthermore, that the embryonic/fetal CNS is particularly sensitive to a number of xenobiotics. Table 9.1 lists some of the human

TABLE 9.1. Known or Suspected Human Developmental Neurotoxicants

Cocaine	Methadone
Diphenylhydantoin (anticonvulsant)	Methylmercury
Ethanol	Organochlorines
Heroin	Retinoic acid
Lead	X-irradiation
Marijuana	

developmental neurotoxicants that have been proven through rigorous study to be associated with neonatal mortality or neurobehavioral morbidity. In addition to structural defects, exposure to these drugs, chemicals, or forces *in utero* has been associated with deficits on various measures of behavioral and intellectual functioning.

Chemically mediated interference with early organogenesis during the first 2 to 8 weeks of postconceptual life typically results in malformations so severe that many of these conceptuses are spontaneously aborted. Although the probability of major malformation diminishes with the conclusion of the embryonic stage, the risks for suboptimal development continue well beyond this period. The CNS, like other organ systems, is refractory to the induction of major malformations during the period of advanced organogenesis and maturation, but it remains at risk for more subtle developmental deviations throughout the fetal period (Dobbing, 1981). Parturition does not mark the end of neurodevelopmental vulnerability, however, because processes such as cell proliferation and growth—especially cortical cellular migration, myelination, dendritic arborization, and synaptogenesis—continue for a considerable period of time after birth. Indeed, the human brain does not attain its mature form until approximately 21 years after conception (Rodier, 1994).

ENVIRONMENTAL EXPOSURES

It is estimated that 70,000 chemicals are in commercial use. However, very few have been extensively evaluated for their developmentally toxic potential. Excluding pharmaceutical agents, fewer than 10% of chemicals currently in commerce have been subjected to neurotoxicity testing (Landrigan, Graham, & Thomas, 1994), and even fewer have been targeted for developmental neurotoxicity testing (Rees et al., 1990). Thus, while the number of toxicants that could be candidates for discussion is quite large, this chapter focuses primarily on elemental and organic mercury (Hg) , the organochlorines (polychlorinated biphenyls [PCBs] and related compounds) and inorganic lead (Pb). These substances have been disseminated widely in the environment, and their developmental toxicity has been investigated in both humans and animals with a high degree of methodological rigor (Burbacher, Rodier, & Weiss, 1990; Davis, Otto, Weil, & Grant, 1990; Tilson, Jacobson, & Rogan, 1990). Although hundreds of exogenous agents have been shown to produce morphological and functional developmental defects in animals, the only environmental chemicals that are currently considered to be documented human teratogens are methylmercury (MeHg) and the organochlorines, as they alone are so recognized in the authoritative *Catalog of Teratogenic Agents* (Shephard, 1994).

ENVIRONMENTAL NEUROTOXICOLOGY
AND PEDIATRIC NEUROPSYCHOLOGY

Epidemiological studies of environmental chemical influences on child development sel-dom appear in the pages of the major neuropsychological journals. Indeed, there has been a tendency among some in the psychological sciences to dismiss environmental chemical exposures as a potential threat to the normal neuropsychological development of children (e.g., Scarr, 1985). On the other hand, the relatively few researchers working in the area of human developmental neurotoxicology have been rather slow to bring a neuropsycho-logical perspective to their studies. Rather than employing measures that might help to elucidate brain–behavior relationships, they have often relied primarily on global measures of sensory–motor development and cognition—such as the Bayley Scales of Infant Devel-opment (Bayley, 1969, 1993) or various IQ tests (e.g., McCarthy, 1972; Wechsler, 1974, 1989)—to study dose–effect/dose–response relationships (Dietrich & Bellinger, 1994). Reliance on these global measures is mostly attributable to the fact that public health of-ficials are more likely to base environmental regulatory and health policy decisions on IQ deficits rather than diminished scores on neuropsychological measures, whose results mean less to nonspecialists (Bellinger, 1995). Governmental officials, lawyers, legislators, and econometricians can more readily assess the benefits and costs of reducing pollution in terms of IQ measures than in terms of the number of errors on tests of visual–motor integration, the time required to complete a task assessing manual dexterity, the number of errors and false alarms on a continuous-performance test, or the efficiency of short-term memory (e.g., see Schwartz, 1994a).

CLINICAL AND SUBCLINICAL NEUROTOXICITY

Developmental exposure to environmental toxicants can result in both *clinical* and so-called *subclinical* neurotoxicity. Thus, for example, pediatric blood Pb concentrations greater than 80 µg/dL have been associated with gross alterations in behavior, seizures, coma, and death (McKhann, 1926; Perlstein & Attala, 1966), while concentrations below 25 µg/dL have been linked to more subtle deficits in measures of intellectual attainment, such as scores on IQ tests (Bellinger & Dietrich, 1994). At high doses, Hg in its organic form is associ-ated with clinical neurological disease in children; if untreated, this proceeds from paraes-thesia to speech disturbances, ataxia, blindness, and ultimately death (Takeuchi, Eto, & Eto, 1979). However, as with Pb, lower-dose exposure to MeHg has been linked to delays in motor development and lower scores on measures of development and IQ (Marsh et al., 1987; Cox et al., 1989; Kjellstrom, Kennedy, & Wallis, 1989; McKeown-Eyssen, Reudy, & Neims, 1983; Myers et al., 1995).

The age at which a patient is exposed to an environmental agent is a critically impor-tant factor in the determination of mortality, or, among survivors, the severity of develop-mental morbidity and the potential for recovery. For some environmental neurotoxicants such as MeHg, the fetal CNS is exquisitely sensitive to exposure. Widespread developmental damage to cortical and subcortical structures can occur, as well as a cortical degenerative syndrome following birth consisting of neuromotor signs similar to those observed in ce-rebral palsy, but always accompanied by mental retardation (Harada, 1977; Takeuchi, 1968). The damage is likely to be less widespread when exposure occurs later in childhood or beyond. Figure 9.1 compares the distribution of cerebral lesions among adult, infant, and fetal brains exposed to MeHg (Takeuchi, 1968). Whereas MeHg is a selective neuro-

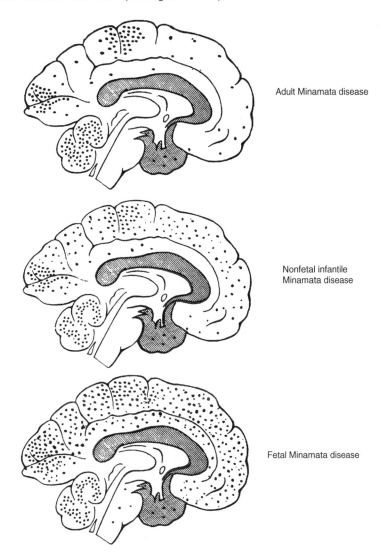

Adult Minamata disease

Nonfetal infantile
Minamata disease

Fetal Minamata disease

FIGURE 9.1. A comparison of the distribution of lesions in the brain of adult (I), nonfetal infant (II), and fetal (III) victims of Minamata disease. From Takeuchi (1968). Copyright 1968 by Kumamoto University, Study Group of Minamata Disease. Reprinted by permission of the author and the National Institute for Minamata Disease.

toxicant in the adult, involving only discrete areas of the mature brain such as the cerebellum and parietal and occipital lobes, damage to infant and especially fetal brains is much more widespread. Thus fetal MeHg poisoning is associated with a vast reduction of brain size, wide distribution of lesions, extensive hypoplastic changes of cytoarchitecture and neuronal malfunction (Reuhl & Chang, 1979; Takeuchi, 1968).

One of the issues developmental neurotoxicologists typically ponder is whether or not an environmental toxicant under study has a characteristic behavioral signature. Pediatric neuropsychologists would also be interested in this question, since brain–behavior relationships and accurate diagnoses are of utmost concern. Unfortunately, attempts to define specific neurobehavioral syndromes have been hampered by the aforementioned reliance on global measures of neurobehavioral development. It is also quite possible that the particular neurobehavioral manifestations of exposure may depend on other factors, such as age, nutrition, quality of caregiving, and other sociohereditary variables. For this reason, reviews of studies measuring the CNS effects of environmental toxicant exposure must take into account biological and sociohereditary background factors before passing judgment on the consistency of positive or negative findings (Bellinger, 1995). Although prenatal and postnatal exposure to Hg is reported to have some fairly specific neurobehavioral manifestations, studies of Pb have not revealed a similarly consistent pattern of neurobehavioral signs. For the organochlorines, there are presently too few studies of high quality to permit a specific neurobehavioral syndrome to be conclusively defined.

INORGANIC AND ORGANIC MERCURY

Background

Hg is an element that has fascinated humankind over several millennia for its "mysterious" fluid characteristics at ambient temperatures, its imagined curative qualities, and its real iatrogenic properties (Clarkson, 1990). Hg has been used for more than 3,000 years in religious ceremonies, medical practices, and diverse forms of commerce. Its modern uses are wide-ranging, from its application as an antifungal agent in the manufacture of paper products to electronics.

Environmental Hg exists in three forms: elemental Hg, inorganic Hg salts, and organic Hg. These forms of Hg differ in their bioavailability and neurotoxicity, with elemental and especially organic mercurials (e.g., MeHg) being the most bioavailable and toxic to the developing CNS (Agency for Toxic Substances and Disease Registry [ATSDR], 1992, 1994).

The methylation process is the key to understanding why MeHg is so feared as a health risk. Sediments in both fresh and marine waters, through the action of microorganisms, convert inorganic Hg to the methylated form of organic Hg (MeHg). Upon release, MeHg begins to ascend the aquatic food chain, attaining its highest concentrations in larger, predatory species of fish (e.g., snapper, pike, swordfish, tuna, and shark). Shellfish also accumulate high concentrations of MeHg in contaminated waters. Thus MeHg accumulates in the kinds of marine life that humans usually harvest and consume. Many experts are now especially concerned about human exposure to MeHg from the consumption of marine life, as the acidification of lakes by "acid rain" is believed to increase the level of MeHg in the edible tissues of fish (Clarkson, 1990). As we shall see, contamination of the human diet by MeHg resulted in two of the most infamous epidemics of environmentally related neurological disease.

Health Consequences

As a scientific discipline, the area of human developmental neurotoxicology owes a great deal to the study of Hg. The health misfortunes resulting from several mass epidemics of Hg poisoning have taught at least two important lessons to developmental neurotoxicologists. First, a substantial amount of interindividual variability can be expected in the response of fetuses and children to equal doses of an environmental contaminant. These differences in response may be due to genetic, nutritional, maternal metabolic, or any other of a multitude of premorbid and comorbid factors. Second, fetuses and children are almost always highly sensitive to environmental contaminants, frequently expressing signs and symptoms of toxicity at doses that fail to produce any outward indications of neurological disease in adults.

The study of Hg, especially MeHg, has proven to be an excellent experimental model for research on the developmental neurotoxicity of heavy metals. As a result, more is understood about how Hg can perturb CNS development and function than about any other environmental contaminant.

In the United States and Europe, Hg poisoning during infancy and childhood has been associated historically with exposure to inorganic mercurials in prescription and over-the-counter medicines. Calomel (mercurous chloride) was frequently prescribed by physicians during the first half of this century to treat a wide variety of childhood disorders, including teething pain, constipation, diarrhea, helminthism, colic, and almost any febrile infirmity of unknown cause (Warkany, 1966). Some infants and children who were administered these preparations developed a complex of cutaneous, neurological, and psychiatric symptoms that physicians have referred to as *acrodynia* ("painful extremities") or *pink disease*. Now a rare syndrome, acrodynia is characterized by the protean clinical signs and symptoms of irritability, paresthesias, insomnia, depression, anorexia, excessive sweating, leg cramps, painful pink to red fingers, hands and feet, and peeling skin. In the most severe cases of acrodynia, there is oral involvement (excessive salivation, severe irritation of the gums, and tooth loss). It is still unknown why only infants and children are affected by elemental Hg in this way. Another curious aspect of this environmental disease is that it affects only a small percentage of children who are exposed to the metal, thus suggesting an as-yet-unknown genetic factor in determining individual susceptibility. Even so, it was estimated that between 1939 and 1948 a total of 585 children under 2 years of age died of acrodynia in England and Wales alone (Warkany, 1966). Although Hg was identified as the probable iatrogenic agent in these medications as early as 1920 (Bilderback, 1920, cited in Warkany, 1966), it was more than 30 years later before mercurial compounds were eliminated from the shelves of pharmacies, groceries, and other dispensaries.

The identification of medicinal preparations as a cause of acrodynia in young children represents a fascinating chapter in human developmental neurotoxicology. Josef Warkany, one of the founders of modern teratology and a key figure in solving this medical puzzle, has written a vivid "postmortem" of this disease of infancy and early childhood (Warkany, 1966). Unfortunately, acrodynia is not yet a disease for the history books alone. Although elemental Hg intoxication in children is rare, there are sufficient sources of the metal in the environment and household products to result in occasional toxicity. One contemporary source of exposure today is discarded flasks of Hg discovered by young children near industrial dumping sites or abandoned factories. Children are naturally attracted to the appearance and unique properties of liquid elemental Hg. Other sources of potential exposure include interior latex paint containing Hg as a fungicide and bactericide, broken fluorescent light bulbs, thermometers, folk medicines, and Hg contamination of the home attributable to the hobbies or occupations of parents (Agocs et al., 1990; McNeil, Oliver, Issler, & Wrong, 1984; *Mortality and Morbidity Weekly Report*, 1991; Tunneson, McMahon, & Baser, 1987). Silver dental amalgams, which can contain up to 50% elemental Hg by weight, can also be a source of low-dose exposure. The mechanical action of chewing on a filling releases trace quantities of Hg vapor, which are partially absorbed. It should be noted, however, that this typically represents a very small percentage of a child's total Hg exposure. A National Institutes of Health expert panel has concluded that the Hg in silver amalgam restorations poses no health risks of medical significance (ATSDR, 1992).

Inorganic Mercury

There are no large-scale pediatric studies of the neurobehavioral effects of exposure to inorganic Hg. The neuropsychological effects of inorganic Hg exposure have usually been studied in adults exposed in the workplace. Although the tests used to assess the neurobehavioral effects of Hg exposure in the workplace vary from study to study, a general pattern of psychomotor disturbances, intellectual deterioration, and emotional lability has been observed (e.g., see Hanninen, 1982).

Medically confirmed cases of inorganic Hg poisoning in childhood are now quite rare. Only case studies provide detailed descriptions of neuropsychological sequelae. One representative example is by Yeates and Mortensen (1994), who reported on the health outcome of Hg vapor poisoning in two young adolescents. The two children became ill following a move into an apartment where a flask of elemental Hg had been spilled and the area had been improperly abated of the toxic metal. Both of the children were given neuropsychological examinations following hospitalization and during chelation therapy with dimercaptosuccinic acid (succimer). The children were examined again 1 year later. Both patients displayed substantial deficits in visual-perceptual and constructional skills, nonverbal memory, and abstract reasoning. These deficits were more severe than expected, given their estimated premorbid functioning. Some improvement in emotionality, attention, and cognitive speed was noted 1 year later, but deficits in the aforementioned areas persisted. The parents of the children appeared to be unaffected by exposure, despite having similarly elevated levels of Hg in their 24-hour urine specimens. The authors speculated that the deficits in nonverbal skills and abstraction identified in their subjects may have been due to damage to cortical white matter pathways, since Hg is known to cause demyelination in the peripheral nervous system. This interpretation is in concordance with what is known about the sensitivity of the developing brain to Hg, since the myelination of neural fibers continues for many years after birth (Rodier, 1994).

Most pediatric neuropsychologists will never encounter a case of pink disease in their practice, and controlled research is not practical, given the small number of cases that are available for study. Nevertheless, an understanding of the signs and symptoms of this rare environmentally induced disease may prove unexpectedly useful to the clinician. A letter to the editor of the *British Medical Journal* from a Manchester physician reinforces this point:

> Sir—It is now many years since pink disease has been a common disorder, and one wonders whether the importance of Hg as a toxic agent in infants is appreciated by younger doctors who may not have seen the condition in the past. I have written this letter because in the last few weeks I have seen two cases of what I had thought was an almost extinct disease . . . (Feldman, 1966, p. 165)

Organic Mercury

The form of Hg most toxic to the developing CNS is MeHg (Clarkson, Hursh, Sager, & Syverson, 1988). Ingested MeHg is almost completely absorbed by humans. It also crosses the placenta with ease, with human neonatal blood concentrations exceeding maternal levels by 50% to 100%. In humans, fecal excretion accounts for most of the elimination process; thus one reason for MeHg's potency as a toxicant to the fetus is the inability to eliminate the metal *in utero*. Furthermore, animal data have shown that fetal brain concentrations of MeHg are more than twice as high as those in the maternal brain, attributable in part to the immaturity of the fetal blood–brain barrier (Null, Gartside, & Wei, 1973).

The first published report of MeHg poisoning in humans was by Hunter and Russell (1954). They described the health problems of four men who were poisoned by inhaling MeHg compounds in a London factory where fungicides were being applied to seeds being prepared and packaged for agriculture. This classic description of the sequential neurological manifestations of the disease later helped to identify MeHg as the causative agent in several mass poisonings. The Hunter–Russell Syndrome, as it came to be called, begins with paraesthesia, deterioration in fine motor coordination, and restriction of the visual fields, and proceeds to gross ataxia, dementia, and death. On autopsy, Hunter and Russell found marked destruction of neurons. The cerebrum was grossly atrophied in both hemispheres.

Minamata Disease

Although the clinical series reported by Hunter and Russell was of great significance, the full extent of our understanding of the developmental toxicity of MeHg in fetuses and children is largely attributable to two widely known and well-documented environmental disasters, where the poison found its way into the diets of thousands of people. These episodes occurred in Minamata, Japan, in the 1950s, and in southern Iraq in the early 1970s.

The Chisso corporation, located near the shores of Minamata Bay in southern Japan, had been using Hg oxide as a catalyst in the production of acetaldehyde and vinyl chloride. Hg oxide was converted to MeHg in the company's acetylene reaction tanks. As a result, massive amounts of MeHg were discharged as part of the factory's effluent into Minamata Bay. The compound rapidly bioaccumulated up the marine food chain, reaching ever-higher concentrations in animal tissues—starting with plankton and other microorganisms, and ending with the large pisciverous fish and carnivorous marine mollusks that were harvested by local fishermen for human consumption.

The adverse ecobiological effects of Chisso's method of disposal of industrial waste were first observed in animals. Marine birds were reported to be falling from the sky; sluggish or dead marine animals were collected near the shoreline by children; and bizarre behaviors were observed in cats, pigs, and other domestic animals that fed on the marine offal. Then, in 1956, what the community had come to refer to as the "strange disease" took on the proportions of an epidemic. In April of that year, a 5-year-old girl was admitted to the pediatrics ward of Chisso's Minamata Corporate Hospital for observation, due to a progressive neurological disease of unknown etiology that had left her ataxic, verbally incoherent, and delirious. Fetuses and children were more severely affected than adults (e.g., see Figure 9.1). Neurological signs and symptoms similar to cerebral palsy were noted; these were accompanied by severe sensory deficits in vision and hearing, as well as by intellectual retardation, emotional disturbances, and untimely death. Exposed infants were sometimes grossly neurologically normal at birth, but would progressively deteriorate over the first 2 years of life. Adults who consumed significant quantities of the poisoned seafood from Minamata Bay were affected as well. Among the most common neurological and neurobehavioral symptoms were disturbances in superficial and deep cutaneous sensation, constriction of the visual field, dysarthria, hearing impairment, tremor, and mental deterioration. The suffering of Minamata Bay area residents, and their struggle for official recognition of their plight, support for medical treatment, and reasonable remuneration, have been poignantly presented in an extraordinary photographic essay by Eugene and Aileen Smith (Smith & Smith, 1975). The Smiths' volume also contains a brilliantly detailed medical report on the natural and social history of the disease by Masazumi Harada. Other accounts of this tragic episode have been published in the English medical literature (e.g., Tsuchiya, 1992).

The Iraqi Episode

The other major MeHg poisoning epidemic occurred in Iraq in the winter of 1971–1972. MeHg had been used for years as an inexpensive and effective fungicide for seed grain. Unfortunately, owing to a drought that winter, some of the seed grain was used to make bread that subsequently contained high concentrations of MeHg. More than 6,000 cases of severe poisoning were reported, 10% of which resulted in death (Clarkson, 1992). As in Minamata, numerous fetuses also fell victim to congenital MeHg cerebral syndrome. Major symptoms included hypertonicity, blindness, deafness, and mental retardation.

Professor Thomas Clarkson and his group at the University of Rochester, in close collaboration with colleagues in Iraq, have studied the neurodevelopmental sequelae of intrauterine MeHg exposure in great detail (Marsh et al., 1987). The Rochester group developed a unique method for recapitulating prenatal MeHg exposure by examining the concentration of the metal in maternal scalp hair. Scalp hair grows at a known rate during pregnancy (approximately 1.1 cm/month), so the history of embryonic/fetal exposure can be reconstructed by sectioning strands of maternal hair for elemental analyses. A high correlation between the concentration of MeHg in maternal hair during pregnancy and infants' brains has been recently reported (Cernichiari et al., 1995).

A finding often cited from the Iraqi study is that fetal toxicity to MeHg occurred at levels of exposure far below those associated with signs and symptoms in adults. Figure 9.2 illustrates the level of prenatal exposure associated with minor symptoms in adults (paresthesia) and with more serious signs of psychomotor retardation in children (e.g., failure to walk independently by 18 months of age). As illustrated in this graphic summary of a linear–plateau or "hockey-stick" regression analysis, the level of prenatal exposure (as assessed by the estimated concentration of Hg in maternal hair during pregnancy) associated with significant developmental morbidity in infants is 10 times lower than the level associated with the mildest neurological symptoms in adults. This is frequently presented as one of the best examples in the human neurotoxicology literature of fetal toxicity in the virtual absence of maternal toxicity (Clarkson, Nordberg, & Sager, 1985). However, recent reanalyses of the Iraqi data have shown that the deviance profile for the point estimate (threshold) for fetal effects is so extreme as to call into serious question the reference value of 10 parts per million of MeHg in maternal hair (Crump et al., 1995). The threshold value reported by the Rochester group appears to be highly dependent on a relatively small number of developmentally abnormal cases at the lower end of the dose–response curve. Nevertheless, these data have been the driving force behind the regulation of MeHg in the United States and elsewhere for many years (World Health Organization, 1990).

The uncertainty of estimates of adverse neurobehavioral health effects could be due to the insensitivity of the measures (e.g., maternal questionnaires, neurological examinations) used to determine developmental delay. The Iraqi battery did not include measures that would reflect less severe delays in the achievement of motor developmental milestones

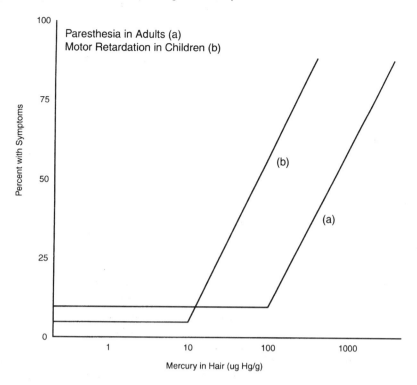

FIGURE 9.2. Dose–response relationships as determined by "hockey-stick" regression analyses for adult (a) and prenatal (b) exposures to methylmercury. From Clarkson et al. (1981). Copyright 1981 by Plenum Publishing Corporation. Reprinted by permission.

or more subtle manifestations of neurological dysfunction. However, it should be acknowledged that investigators of the Japanese and Iraqi MeHg poisoning episodes were responding to environmental health emergencies. They did not originally set out to collect neurodevelopmental data for the purposes of establishing a solid basis for risk assessment. Consequently, researchers and public health officials perceived an urgent need for more carefully designed prospective studies of lower-level exposures in populations at risk for MeHg exposure via diet (principally seafood).

In studies of so-called "asymptomatic" exposures to MeHg, more subtle dose-related deficits in psychomotor functions have been identified. Thus, for example, McKeown-Eyssen et al. (1983) examined 234 Cree children from four Native communities in northern Quebec. These communities subsist on fish from lakes known to support elevated MeHg levels in fish. An interesting sexual dimorphism was observed, with male infants in particular presenting with dose-related deficits in sensory–motor behaviors as assessed by the Bayley Scales of Infant Development. Kjellstrom et al. (1989) found that at the age of 4 years, New Zealand children with mothers that had higher maternal hair MeHg concentrations had lower scores on the Denver Developmental Screening Test; at 6 years, they had significantly lower scores on the Wechsler Intelligence Scale for Children—Revised (WISC-R) and the Test of Language Development. Maternal hair Hg levels accounted for about 3% of the variance in IQ.

Two particularly ambitious prospective studies of the developmental effects of lower-level MeHg exposure *in utero* have recently commenced in the Faroe and Seychelle Islands.

These studies represent a new generation of neurotoxicological investigation in the area of MeHg research. Both studies are superbly designed, with large sample sizes (700–1,000 births), use of individually administered and well-validated psychometric measures, and the direct measurement of perinatal and postnatal covariates and potential confounders (e.g., the Home Observation for Measurement of the Environment [Caldwell, 1979]; measures of maternal IQ). The Seychellois study (Davidson et al., 1995; Myers, Marsh, et al., 1995; Myers, Davidson, et al., 1995; Davidson et al., 1998) has reported results of analyses of the main cohort to approximately 5½ years of age. No significant associations between scores on standardized measures of mental and motor development (Bayley Scales of Infant Development [Bayley, 1969]; Fagan Test of Infant Intelligence [Fagan & Shephard, 1987]; McCarthy Scales of Children's Abilities [McCarthy, 1972] and other tests) and MeHg exposure have been reported thus far for the main study.

Early results of the Faroese study have shown an unexpected positive association between cord blood MeHg concentrations and birthweight (Grandjean et al., 1992; Grandjean, Weihe, & White, 1995). The authors attribute the finding to the benefits of *n*-3 polyunsaturated fatty acids in a high-seafood diet. Selenium may also play a protective role against MeHg neurotoxicity. Infant hair MeHg concentrations at 12 months were also positively associated with the attainment of motor developmental milestones. The authors attributed this unexpected correlation to the benefits of breast feeding, which in itself can lead to higher MeHg intake by an infant.

However, later results of neuropsychological testing of the Faroese children presented a very different picture (Dahl et al., 1996). Using a computerized assessment battery (the Neurobehavioral Evaluation System; Letz, 1990), the investigators measured motor speed (finger tapping), hand–eye coordination, and attention (a continuous-performance task adapted for young children). Higher cord blood and maternal hair MeHg concentrations were associated with poorer performance on all tests following adjustment for covariates, including acquaintance with computers and visual acuity. At 7 years of age, 917 of the Faroese children underwent detailed neurobehavioral evaluations. MeHg-related neuropsychological deficits were found in the domains of language, attention, and memory, and to a lesser degree in visual–spatial and motor functions (Grandjean et al., 1997). The negative results obtained so far in the Seychellois cohort should be interpreted with caution, given the effects on performance observed in later life in the New Zealand and Faroese cohorts. Let us hope that every effort will be made to continue follow-up of the Seychellois cohort into the school-age years.

Biological Mechanisms

Among the heavy metals, a unique aspect of MeHg poisoning is that the mechanism of action in the developing CNS is relatively well established. Developmentally, inhibition of cell division and maturation is one of the presumed mechanisms by which this compound expresses its toxic effects. A major molecular mechanism underlying this process is interference with microtubular assembly. One of the biological targets of MeHg appears to be the protein tubulin. The high affinity of Hg to sulfhydryl groups makes it an extremely potent spindle fiber poison. Methylmercury depolymerizes microtubules, which play an integral role in neuronal and neuroglial cell duplication, migration, and nutrition. The results are fewer neurons (microcephaly) and misalignment of the cytoarchitecture and ectopic neurons (Clarkson, 1991).

ORGANOCHLORINES: POLYCHLORINATED BIPHENYLS AND RELATED COMPOUNDS

Background

PCBs are a family of 209 synthetic hydrocarbons (congeners) that were once used in a wide variety of industrial products and processes, including insulating oil, microscope immersion oil, hydraulic fluids, plasticizers, electrical capacitors, transformers, and even carbonless copy paper. Although PCBs were banned in the United States in the 1970s and somewhat later internationally, careless disposal practices have left PCB residues in air, water, soil, and sediment around the world, and such residues can be detected in biological tissues sampled from most residents of industrial countries (Jensen, 1989). These organochlorine compounds are fat-soluble and have long half-lives in humans. They also cross the placenta and, owing to their lipophilic nature, can be present in high concentrations in human breast milk. Indeed, lactation is the single circumstance in which substantial quantities of PCBs are excreted over a relatively brief period of time (Masuda et al., 1978). Thus infants who are breast-feeding are sometimes regarded as most at risk for developmentally neurotoxic exposures.

PCBs were first identified as human teratogens in 1968 when, in Japan, large quantities of PCBs and their even more toxic thermal degradation by-products (e.g., polychlorinated dibenzofurans) were accidentally mixed with cooking oil during the decolorization process (Kuratsune, 1989). This resulted in an outbreak of severe cystic acne among the residents of Kyusho. It was estimated that more than 1,500 adults were affected. A similar episode occurred in Taiwan in 1979, in which approximately 2,000 individuals were exposed and developed clinical symptoms. The ensuing infirmities following these exposures were referred to as *Yusho* and *Yu-cheng* ("oil disease") in Japan and Taiwan, respectively.

Many of the neonates exposed *in utero* in both episodes were born with low birthweights, dark pigmentation of the skin and nails, early eruption of teeth, swollen eyelids and gums, and an acneform rash called *chloracne*. In some cases, intrauterine exposure resulted in neonatal fatalities (Hsu et al., 1985). Developmentally, survivors of intrauterine poisoning typically lagged behind their unexposed peers in sensory–motor and cognitive abilities (Harada, 1976; Rogan et al., 1988). Survivors of the Yu-cheng episode have been carefully followed over the last two decades. Persistent deficits in cognitive development and an increased incidence of behavioral disorders have been noted in older children exposed prenatally (Chen, Guo, Hsu, & Rogan, 1992; Chen, Yu, Rogan, Gladen, & Hsu, 1994). However, the degree of observed deficits was smaller than one might expect, given the relatively high levels of transplacental PCBs and related contaminants to which these children were exposed *in utero*. For example, preschool and elementary school children exposed prenatally had IQ scores only about 5 points (0.33 standard deviations) lower than those of matched controls. Furthermore, no relationship was found between PCB-related dysmorphology at birth and severity of neurobehavioral deficits (Chen et al., 1992, 1994).

Although most residents of industrialized countries are exposed to low levels of PCBs, no outbreaks of clinical symptomatic disease have been noted in persons who have not been occupationally exposed. Most of the concern is presently focused on fetal exposure and the possibility of embryonic/fetal CNS developmental effects at low doses (Environmental Protection Agency, 1993).

Neuropsychological Consequences of Low-Level Exposure

Relative to the number of studies of developmental exposures to other environmental chemicals, such as Hg and Pb, the data on the effects of low-level exposure to PCBs in fetuses and children are meager. Indeed, only three neuroepidemiological studies of high quality have been conducted thus far—one on the southeastern shores of Lake Michigan (Jacobson & Jacobson, 1994), another in North Carolina (Rogan et al., 1986), and a third in upstate New York (Stewart et al., in press). One of the principal dietary sources of exposure to PCBs in the United States is the consumption of sports fish caught in the shallower shoreline waters of contaminated lakes, as well as consumption of some ocean fish and mollusca. In the late 1970s, Greta Fein, Joseph and Sandra Jacobson, and their colleagues at Wayne State University recruited a cohort of neonates born to women who had consumed variable quantities of contaminated sports fish harvested from the southeastern shores of Lake Michigan. The final sample included approximately 300 mothers and children who were recruited to overrepresent families who consumed relatively large quantities of Lake Michigan sports fish (Fein, Jacobson, Jacobson, Schwartz, & Dowler, 1984). Walter Rogan and his group at the National Institute of Environmental Health Sciences recruited a random sample of 900 children in North Carolina born to mothers who were exposed to only background levels of PCBs—that is, levels of PCBs to which individuals in the southeastern United States would typically be exposed by virtue of their residence in a modern industrialized country (Rogan et al., 1986). Both studies used similar methods in the assessment of intrauterine dose, neuropsychological assessment, and examination of potential confounding variables.

The Michigan and North Carolina studies initiated neurobehavioral assessments almost immediately after birth with the Neonatal Behavioral Assessment Scale (Brazelton, 1984). Newborns of Michigan mothers who had consumed the highest quantities of contaminated fish exhibited weaker reflexes and were less responsive to visual and auditory stimulation (Jacobson et al., 1984). Although cord serum PCB levels were unrelated to newborn neurological status, this may have been due in part to limitations in the chemical analytic procedures available at that stage of the study (Jacobson & Jacobson, 1994). Because cord blood is relatively lean, PCBs were undetectable in a significant portion (66%) of the samples, according to the chemical analytic technology then available.

Similar findings were reported for neonates born to North Carolina women (Rogan et al., 1986): Nonoptimal neurobehavioral signs, such as weak reflexes and delayed or absent orientation to presented stimuli, were directly related to chemical estimates of perinatal PCB exposure. In this case, the assessment of dose was based on an omnibus measure of organochlorine dose, derived from two samples of prenatal maternal blood and several samples of breast milk collected while each infant was being nursed. Nevertheless, analytic problems also plagued the North Carolina study; for example, 80% of the cord serum PCB concentrations were below the level of detection with the methods available at that time. Despite such limitations, it is worth noting that the much more highly exposed and symptomatic *Yusho* infants were also reported to be less responsive to stimulation and hypotonic (Harada, 1976).

In further follow-up studies of the North Carolina cohort, higher prenatal exposure to PCBs was associated with poorer performance on the Bayley (1969) Psychomotor Development Index at 12, 18, and 24 months (Gladen et al., 1988). No measures of prenatal PCB exposure were significantly associated with the Bayley Mental Development Index. No neurobehavioral effects related to intrauterine exposure to PCBs were observed on the standard scores derived from the Bayley Scales in the Jacobsons' Michigan sample, although cord serum PCB concentrations were significantly associated with deficits on a cluster of Bayley items assessing fine motor coordination (Jacobson & Jacobson, 1994).

In addition to the Bayley scales, the Michigan sample was examined with the Fagan Test of Infant Intelligence (Fagan & Shephard, 1987). This instrument assesses an infant's ability to discriminate a novel visual stimulus when it is paired with another visual stimulus that was previously presented during a "familiarization" period. If the infant gazes for a longer period of time at the novel stimulus, the inference is that the familiar stimulus has been cognitively encoded, retained, and discriminated. Both cord serum PCB levels and maternal consumption of contaminated fish were associated in a dose-dependent fashion with poorer visual recognition memory scores on the Fagan test at 7 months (Jacobson, Fein, Jacobson, Schwartz, & Dowler, 1985).

One of the most striking aspects of the Michigan studies is the specificity of the reported neurobehavioral effects. For example, when these children were evaluated at 4 years of age with the McCarthy Scales of Children's Abilities (McCarthy, 1972), the strongest associations between measures of perinatal PCB exposure, such as cord serum and breast milk concentrations, and neuropsychological performance were found for the McCarthy Memory subscale (Jacobson, Jacobson, & Humphrey, 1990). As was previously observed on the Fagan Test of Infant Intelligence, the ability to encode and retain information appeared to be especially affected by intrauterine exposure to PCBs. Paradoxically, however, the duration of postnatal exposure to PCBs in breast milk was not inversely related to 4-year cognitive performance. One explanation for this finding is that mothers who breast-fed for longer periods of time provided a postnatal environment that was more conducive to mental development in their offspring, thus compensating for any adverse developmental effects of postnatal exposure to PCBs via breast milk. It seems likely that the inverse association between the concentration of PCBs in maternal breast milk and cognitive performance reflected prenatal as opposed to postnatal exposure, since the concentration of PCBs in breast milk shortly after birth would be highly correlated with prenatal maternal body burden of the chemical and its transplacental transfer to the fetus. Furthermore, the fact that the effects associated with maternal milk levels paralleled those associated with cord serum PCB concentrations provides substantial support for this interpretation (Jacobson & Jacobson, 1994).

Given that the effects of prenatal exposure to PCBs seem to be specific to neuropsychological factors related to information retention and retrieval, the effect of PCBs on information-processing efficiency was further evaluated in the Michigan sample with supplementary measures of memory, reaction time, visual discrimination, and sustained attention (Jacobson, Jacobson, Padgett, Brumitt, & Billings, 1992). As was found for the McCarthy scales, cord serum and breast milk PCB concentrations were significantly associated in a dose-dependent fashion with information-processing efficiency as assessed by the measures of memory, stimulus discrimination, and reaction time, but unrelated to the amount of contaminated milk consumed. Again, the effect of maternal milk PCB concentration presumably reflected greater prenatal exposure rather than postnatal breast-feeding exposure.

The study conducted in North Carolina of fetuses exposed to background levels of PCBs did not report a relationship between any measure of intrauterine exposure and neurocognitive skills of children following school entry (as assessed by the McCarthy Scales) or academic achievement (as determined by the examination of school records, such as report cards) (Gladen & Rogan, 1991). The Michigan cohort was also examined at school age (11 years) with a battery of IQ and achievement tests (Jacobson & Jacobson, 1996). For this analysis, a composite measure of prenatal PCB exposure was derived from cord blood and maternal blood and breast milk samples. Postnatal PCB exposure was assessed in blood samples collected at 4 and 11 years of age. Blood Pb and hair Hg concentrations were also obtained at these ages. The blood samples obtained from children were also analyzed for polybrominated biphenyls and for seven organochlorine pesticides, including dichlorodiphenyl trichloroethane (DDT). Following covariate adjustment, higher levels of PCB exposure were related to deficits in Full Scale Wechsler IQ, and subtests measuring mnemonic and attentional performance were observed. The greatest deficits (–6.2 IQ points on average) were reserved for the 30 children in the highest-exposure quintile (>1.25 mg/ml fat basis). The most highly exposed children were approximately three times more likely to present with IQ scores associated with learning problems (<84), and they were twice as likely to be more than 2 years behind age-based norms for reading mastery (as assessed by the Wookcock Reading Mastery Test—Revised). Among the other environmental contaminants examined, only Pb and Hg were significantly related to any of the outcomes assessed.

The reason for the discrepancy between these two epidemiological studies is not clear. Both studies found effects of PCBs during infancy, but these effects persisted only in the Michigan study. Furthermore, the neurobehavioral deficits in the Michigan study were cognitive, while only psychomotor effects were found in North Carolina. Exposures in the two samples appeared to overlap, but differences in the analytic procedures used to determine the concentration of PCBs in sampled tissues complicate attempts to compare and contrast the absolute levels of prenatal exposures in the two studies. Furthermore, whereas the Michigan study examined perinatal exposure to PCBs directly in cord serum, the North Carolina study had to construct a measure of perinatal dose from several highly intercorrelated measures of fetal exposure, including concentrations in maternal serum and breast milk. It should be emphasized, however, that both the Michigan and North Carolina studies were using the best analytic methods available at the time the tissues were analyzed. Many of the previous problems associated with PCB analysis have been since resolved (Mullin et al., 1984). It is also conceivable that the neurobehavioral data collected in the Michigan study were of somewhat better quality, owing to the fact that all assessments were individually administered by a relatively small number of highly trained psychometricians, whose proficiency and reliability were well established prior to data collection and closely monitored throughout the study.

It is important to note that a more recent study that employed advanced environmental chemical analytical techniques has replicated many of the Michigan findings (Stewart, Reihman, Darvill, & Lonky, 1998). The Oswego study of Great Lakes fish eaters found a number of significant dose–effect relationships between measures of prenatal exposure to highly chlorinated PCB homologs in fish and measures of newborn, infant, and preschool neurologic status, memory, and other measures of cognitive performance.

Both the human and animal literature suggest that the effects of organochlorines on the CNS are potentially complex, and this may also help to explain some of the perceived inconsistencies in the literature. The degree of chlorination is one critical factor that could not be investigated in the early studies due to chemical analytical limitations. The more highly chlorinated congeners (PCBs with 7 or more chlorine atoms per biphenyl nucleus) are believed to be most persistent and toxic. These particular PCB congeners may be more prevalent in fish (Stewart et al., in press). Furthermore, the variable effects observed across studies may also be due to the action of metabolites of various PCB congeners, the interactions among different congeners, or some combination of these factors (Kodavanti & Tilson, 1997).

Biological Mechanisms

There is now considerable scientific evidence that PCBs and related compounds exercise many of their developmentally toxic effects through changes in hormonal function, either by altering the circulating concentrations of hormones or by affecting receptor numbers or affinity in target cells. Thus, for example, some of the developmental neurotoxicity of PCBs may be associated with the antiestrogenic characteristics of dioxin-like PCB congeners, which in turn can affect neurochemistry (e.g., dopaminergic functions) during development (Korach, Sarver, Chae, McLachlan, & McKinney, 1987; Environmental Protection Agency, 1993). PCBs and related compounds are also structurally similar to the thyroid hormones. Thyroid hormones are essential for normal CNS development; they increase the rate of neuronal proliferation and help initiate the process of neuronal maturation and differentiation (Hambaugh, Mendoza, Burkhart, & Weil, 1971). It has been posited that PCBs and related compounds, even at low doses, could alter neurological development through their action on thyroid hormone availability during critical periods of brain development (Porterfield, 1994). Such alterations could express themselves later in subtle deficits in neuropsychological functions (Jacobson & Jacobson, 1994).

INORGANIC LEAD

Background

Pb is the environmental contaminant pediatric psychologists are most likely to encounter in their practice. A pediatric neuropsychologist's attention to Pb as a causal factor in neurobehavioral problems is particularly critical when a practice includes infants and children living in older substandard housing. Owing to its usefulness for a wide variety of industrial applications, such as paint pigments and smoothers, stabilizers, batteries, plumbing, agricultural chemicals, and antiknock compounds, Pb is a ubiquitous environmental contaminant.

For pregnant women, the major sources of exposure are occupational, since the levels of Pb in the atmosphere and diet have decreased substantially due to regulatory actions by the Environmental Protection Agency and the Food and Drug Administration (Annest et al., 1983; Bolger, Carrington, Capar, & Adams, 1991). For children living in older housing with Pb paint, a serious hazard continues to exist, despite the fact that the concentration of Pb in the blood of children and adults has declined dramatically at the national level since the 1980s (Pirkle et al., 1994).

No developmental neurotoxicant has received as much attention over so long a period of time as has Pb. As early as the mid-19th century, the adverse effects of Pb on the health of workers were described by Tanquerel des Planches (1839/1848). The distinctive problem of Pb poisoning in children was not widely appreciated until much later. Thus the disease as it occurs in children was first described by J. L. Gibson and colleagues among children living in Brisbane, Australia (Gibson et al., 1892). Some years later, Gibson identified chalking and flaking Pb-based paint in homes as the environmental source of the problem (Gibson, 1904). This led to the initial appreciation of the hazards of childhood Pb exposure in the United States (Thomas & Blackfan, 1914). However, during the first part of this century it was widely believed that children surviving the acute stage of the disease would inevitably be uncompromised in later life (McKhann, 1932).

It was not until 1943 that Randolph Byers, chief of pediatric neurology at the Boston Children's Hospital, followed up on 20 children who had recovered from Pb encephalopathy and found that 19 of the 20 children had learning or behavior disorders (Byers & Lord, 1943). Thus Byers was the first to advance the modern neurotoxicological hypothesis that Pb's effects are not simply due to the necrosis of brain cells, but also are attributable to interference with the normal development of a child's CNS.

Neuropsychological Consequences of High-Dose Exposure

Frank Pb encephalopathy is now rare, although cases, and even Pb-related fatalities, still occasionally occur in the United States and elsewhere (Selbst, Henretig, & Pearce, 1985; Centers for Disease Control, 1991a). Lead encephalopathy becomes a clinical possibility when blood Pb levels exceed 80–100 µg/dl in children. A blood Pb concentration in excess of 70 µg/dl is a medical emergency requiring immediate treatment. Autopsy studies of nonsurvivors have shown severe cerebral edema attributable to injury to the capillaries, as well as a direct effect on neurons, including neuronal death in areas where neuronal cells are concentrated (such as the gray matter and basal ganglia). In this syndrome there is a progression from lethargy, anorexia, and irritability to loss of mental developmental milestones, anemia, ataxia, gasping respirations, reduced consciousness, seizures, coma, and sometimes death.

Neuropsychological Consequences of Low-Dose Exposure

A comprehensive review of the literature on low-dose Pb exposure is well beyond the scope of this chapter. For the details of studies conducted in this area, the reader should consult recent environmental health criteria documents published by the Centers for Disease Control (1991b) and the World Health Organization (1995).

The modern era of research on pediatric low-dose Pb exposure began with a study by Herbert Needleman of school children in Chelsea and Somerville, Massachusetts (Needleman et al., 1979). This study addressed many of the methodological problems of past investigations by assessment of historical or cumulative exposure to Pb (through measurement of Pb in teeth), assessment of potential confounding factors, and the use of multivariate statistical procedures. The authors reported a covariate-adjusted difference in child IQ of approximately 4.5 points between groups "high" and "low" in tooth Pb. Teacher ratings of children's behavior in the classroom also suggested more behavioral problems and academic difficulties in children with higher concentrations of Pb in their shed teeth. Most of the cross-sectional studies of Pb and child development that followed the Needleman et al. (1979) report were attempts to replicate these findings. The question of low-level Pb effects raised by the Chelsea and Somerville studies also spawned a number of prospective studies of lead and child development in the United States, Europe, and Australia (Bellinger & Dietrich, 1994). The Needleman et al. results ultimately provoked a bitter debate, which pitted the interests of children's health against the economic interests of the lead industry and their spokespersons in the academies (e.g., see Needleman, 1992).

Low-Level Prenatal Exposure to Lead

Some of the first prospective studies of Pb and child development reported an inverse relationship between low-level prenatal Pb exposure and measures of fetal growth (Dietrich et al., 1987; McMichael, Vimpani, Robertson, Baghurst, & Clark, 1986). Initial findings indicated that low-level fetal Pb exposure (as represented by maternal or cord blood Pb concentrations in the range of 1 to 25 µg/dl) was associated with delays in mental and motor development in infants 2 years of age and under, as assessed by the Bayley Scales of Infant Development (Bellinger, Leviton, Waternaux, Needleman, & Rabinowitz, 1987; Dietrich et al., 1987; Wigg et al., 1988). Subsequent follow-up of these cohorts revealed that deficits were transient or only captured by measures of early sensory–motor abilities. The single exception to these findings came from the prospective investigation conducted in the Pb-smelting region around Kosovska Mitrovica (a city in Kosovo, a now much better-known part of the former Yugoslavia), where a highly significant inverse association between prenatal maternal blood Pb concentrations and mental development was observed at 4 years of age (Wasserman et al., 1994). However, it should be noted that the women in this study with the highest exposures had blood Pb concentrations in the range associated with higher-level occupational, as opposed to lower-level general community, exposures. Thus most of the data coming from the prospective studies suggest that the developmental effects of low-level prenatal Pb exposure are subtle and transient (Bellinger, 1994).

An interesting but unexpected repercussion of these findings was the attempt by some industries to revive turn-of-the-century fetal protection policies designed to exclude women from the workplace. In particular, the employment of women in the manufacture of Pb acid batteries was contested. The U.S. Supreme Court ultimately ruled that such policies violated federal law (see Bertin, 1994).

Low-Level Postnatal Exposure to Lead

According to contemporary definitions, "low-level postnatal exposure" refers to exposures to environmental Pb that result in blood concentrations between 1 and 30 µg/dl. The vast majority of these studies have relied on standardized measures of psychometric intelligence, as opposed to neuropsychological batteries designed to assess specific abilities or learning processes. From the results of this vast psychometric literature, two conclusions may be reached. First, studies with adequate power and with multivariate adjustment for confounding factors have revealed an unequivocal relationship between low-level Pb exposure and decreased IQ (Bellinger & Dietrich, 1994; Needleman & Gatsonis, 1990; Pocock, Smith, & Baghurst, 1994; Schwartz, 1994b; World Health Organization, 1995). Second, the effect observed at the lowest levels of Pb exposure is small. Thus, for example, meta-analytic studies estimate that an increase in mean lifetime blood Pb concentration from 10 to 20 µg/dl is associated with a decrease in Full Scale IQ of approximately 2 points (95% confidence interval, -0.3 to -3.6 points; $p \leq .01$) (World Health Organization, 1995). The effect estimate for Pb depends to some degree on the period of exposure being considered. For example, Figure 9.3 presents the results of a meta-analysis of four prospective studies that followed subjects into the elementary years of education. The combined evidence supports an inverse association between early exposure to Pb (birth to 3 years) and Full Scale IQ on the order of -2.6 points (confidence interval, -1.2 to -4.0 points; $p < .001$) for an increase in blood Pb from 10 to 20 µg/dl. A meta-analysis of the larger cross-sectional studies conducted since 1980 produced similar estimates.

However, it is important to bear in mind that these analyses do not address the intellectual consequences of blood Pb concentrations above this highly restricted range (i.e., 20–70 µg/dl). This question is of critical public health as well as clinical significance, as children living in Pb-contaminated housing are at considerable risk for blood Pb elevations in excess of 20–30 µg/dl. For example, in one study (Dietrich, Berger, Succop, Hammond, & Bornschein, 1993), first-graders with average lifetime blood Pb concentra-

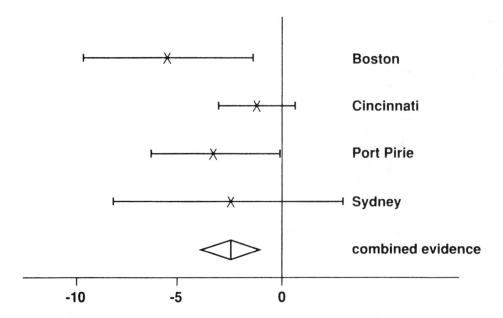

FIGURE 9.3. Estimated mean change in IQ for an increase in blood Pb concentration from 10 to 20 µg/dL. From World Health Organization (1995). Copyright 1995 by the World Health Organization. Reprinted by permission.

tions of greater than 20 µg/dl had Performance IQs that were on average 7–9 points lower than those of children whose blood lead concentrations remained under 10 µg/dl. Children with higher blood Pb concentrations also displayed statistically and clinically significant deficits in fine motor coordination when assessed in kindergarten (Dietrich, Berger, & Succop, 1993).

Neuropsychological Evaluations

Attempts to elucidate the neuropsychological bases for Pb-associated deficits in IQ have been limited by the reliance on global measures of cognitive development. The data that exist are limited, but performance on measures of motor speed, executive regulatory functions, visual–spatial skills, and visual–motor integration appears to be poorer in particular (Baghurst et al., 1992, 1995; Dietrich, Berger, & Succop, 1993; Dietrich, Succop, Berger, & Keith, 1992; Stiles & Bellinger, 1993; Winneke, Brockhaus, Ewers, Kramer, & Neuf, 1990). In the Port Pirie, Australia cohort study, postnatal blood Pb concentrations were most consistently associated with lower scores on measures of visual–spatial abilities, such as the Block Design subtest of the WISC-R and the Developmental Test of Visual–Motor Integration (Beery, 1982). The Cincinnati prospective study reported that postnatal blood Pb concentrations were inversely associated with the Simultaneous Processing subscale of the Kaufman Assessment Battery for Children (Kaufman & Kaufman, 1983) administered at 4 and 5 years of age. Furthermore, the Fine Motor Composite of the Bruininks–Oseretsky Test of Motor Proficiency (Bruininks, 1978) was significantly lower in children with elevated neonatal and postnatal blood Pb levels. In the European multicenter cross-sectional study on Pb and child development, the most consistent associations were found for a measure of visual–motor integration (error scores on the Goettinger Formreproduktiontest) and a measure of serial choice reaction performance (the Vienna Reaction Device). In a study of the relationships between low-level Pb exposure and neuropsychological functions, the most consistent finding was an increase in the percentage of perseverative errors on the Wisconsin Card Sorting Test among 10-year-old children with higher recent or concurrent blood Pb concentrations (Stiles & Bellinger, 1993). Bellinger (1995) has made a strong case that the observed effects of Pb in any given study may be a function not only of toxicant dose, but of contextual factors that may act to buffer or exacerbate the effects of Pb-related neuronal developmental insult.

Behavioral Effects

A relatively neglected area of research is the impact of lower-level Pb exposure on behavior. Among the survivors of Pb encephalopathy, Byers and Lord (1943) reported a high prevalence of behavior problems in school. In his memoirs, Byers noted that some children treated for Pb poisoning were referred back to him by parents and teachers for "violent aggressive behavioral difficulties, such as attacking teachers with knives or scissors" (quoted in Needleman, Riess, Tobin, Biesecker, & Greenhouse, 1996). Some case–control studies have reported higher tooth Pb concentrations among children with diagnoses of hyperactivity or attention deficit disorder (e.g., Gittelman & Eskanazi, 1983). Low levels of Pb in blood and/or teeth have also been associated with teacher ratings of hyperactive behavior or attentional problems (Fergusson, Fergusson, Horwood, & Kinzett, 1988; Fergusson, Horwood, & Lynskey, 1993; Silva, Hughes, Williams, & Faed, 1988; Thomson et al., 1989; Yule, Urbanowicz, Lansdown, & Millar, 1984). In the seminal study by Needleman et al. (1979), children with higher concentrations of Pb in dentine were more likely to be rated unfavorably by teachers on the dimensions of distractibility, persistence in work, organizational ability, dependence, impulsivity, daydreaming, frustration tolerance, and ability to follow simple or complex directions. Bellinger, Leviton, Allred, and Rabinowitz (1994) observed a significant relationship between tooth Pb concentrations and total Behavior Problem scores on the Teacher's Report Form of the Achenbach Child Behavior Checklist (Achenbach & Edelbrock, 1986).

There are no published studies on the relationship between early Pb exposure and the development of antisocial behavior in adolescence. In the only study of its kind thus far, Needleman et al. (1996) examined the relationship between bone Pb concentrations as assessed by K-line X-ray fluorescence spectroscopy (another measure of lifetime cumulative exposure) and the delinquent behavioral tendencies of children in the Pittsburgh Youth Study at 7 and 11 years of age. At 11 years of age, both teachers and parents reported a significant Pb-related association with the Delinquency and Aggressive clusters of the Child Behavior Checklist (Achenbach, 1983). Indeed, higher bone Pb concentration was associated with an increased risk of exceeding the clinical score on the Attention, Aggression, and Delinquency subscales at 11 years of age. The authors concluded that Pb exposure is associated with an increased risk for aggressive, antisocial, and delinquent behaviors. These findings are intriguing, but the issue needs to be studied further in other cohorts.

Early Exposure and Neurobehavioral Status in Adolescence and Early Adulthood

Only a very meager amount of data are available in regard to longer-term effects of early Pb exposure on neurobehavioral status. Needleman, Schell, Bellinger, Leviton, and Allred (1990) conducted a long-term follow-up investigation of their cohorts in Chelsea and

Somerville, Massachusetts; Needleman et al. (1979) had initially examined this sample in the first and second grades. For several important measures, the authors reported a statistically significant association between early Pb exposure and adverse outcomes when these children were assessed at 17–18 years of age. Compared to subjects with tooth Pb concentrations less than 10 µg/g, subjects with concentrations in excess of 20 µg/g had a covariate-adjusted odds ratio for failure to graduate from high school of 7.4 (95% confidence interval, 1.4–40.8). Reading disabilities were also significantly more likely in children with higher tooth Pb concentrations. Other outcomes significantly associated with tooth Pb concentrations were lower class rank, increased absence from school, poorer grammatical reasoning and vocabulary scores, slower finger tapping, poorer eye–hand coordination, and longer reaction times in response to auditory and visual stimuli.

Methodological Controversies

It has been stated that the least controversial thing one can say about pediatric Pb research is that it has been attended by controversy and acrimony (Bellinger, 1995). The principal difficulties with studying the effects of lead on child development are the measurement and "control" of cofactors that might potentially confound the relationship. The risk of undue Pb exposure is not randomly distributed in the population. An elevated blood Pb level is often a marker of social disadvantage. Children from the poorest families, living in substandard housing, are most often the victims of Pb poisoning. Undernutrition and poor caretaking may also contribute to the problem (Dietrich et al., 1985; Dietrich, 1991). Thus, in many cases, Pb exposure is correlated with adverse social and other biomedical factors that contribute to suboptimal neurobehavioral development. Not surprisingly, this has brought biostatistical and experimental design issues to the forefront of the debate. Although a complete treatment of the methodological controversies in this area is beyond the scope of this chapter, the reader may wish to refer to some excellent recent commentaries (e.g., Bellinger, 1995).

Biological Mechanisms

Although Pb has been shown to have a number of adverse physiological effects on the CNS, including changes in capillary integrity, synaptogenesis, myelination, and catecholamine metabolism, no single mechanism capable of integrating these various effects has yet been advanced. Silbergeld (1992) has commented that there are probably two broad but interrelated categories of mechanisms, including neurodevelopmental (cell development, migration, and synaptogenesis) and neuropharmacological (cell-to-cell biochemical interactions and neurotransmitter metabolism).

Recent studies suggest that Pb may disrupt the process whereby synaptic connections are established in the developing CNS (Goldstein, 1992). Marcovac and Goldstein (1988) found that Pb activated phosphokinase C at extremely low concentrations. They argue that this may be part of a fundamental mechanism for the neurodevelopmental toxicity of Pb. Because an essential event in brain development is the pruning of neural cellular aggregations (i.e., programmed cell death), the increase in neuronal responsivity promoted by an increase in phosphokinase C activity could alter the higher-order cerebral architecture of the brain.

In rodent studies, Pb has been shown to disrupt desialylation of the neural cell adhesion molecule, a morphoregulator that plays key roles in fiber outgrowth, neural migration, and synaptogenesis (Cookman, King, & Regan, 1987). Low-level Pb exposure has also been shown to induce precocious development of rat glial cells, thus potentially disrupting their trophic, supportive, and nutritional roles in the CNS (Cookman, Hemmens, Keane, King, & Regan, 1988).

As a neuropharmacological agent, Pb affects several calcium-dependent aspects of neurotransmission and signal transduction. Effects such as these could alter the developmental processes by which neuronal connections are established (Pounds & Rosen, 1988).

Pb Poisoning: A Treatable Environmental Disease of Childhood

A unique aspect of lead poisoning relative to other environmentally mediated diseases of childhood is that it is commonly treated with various chelating drugs that help the body to excrete the toxicant. Elemental Hg poisoning is also treated with chelating agents, but these treatments are uncommon, given the relatively low incidence of the disease.

The current standard of care calls for pharmacological intervention when blood Pb concentrations exceed 44 µg/dl. In the past, these interventions have usually meant hospital treatment with parenteral administration of calcium disodium ethylenediaminetetraacetic acid (EDTA). At higher blood Pb concentrations, treatment with EDTA may be accompanied by intramuscular injection of dimercaprol (British antilewisite, or BAL). Today, pharmacotherapy is increasingly conducted on an outpatient basis with a newly approved, orally administered drug—dimercaptosuccinic acid (succimer), a congener of BAL. In addition to drug treatment, it is absolutely essential to identify the sources of Pb exposure and to eliminate any further contact with them.

A major gap in our knowledge is the lack of information with regard to whether such treatments improve the developmental prognosis of exposed infants and children. Ruff, Bijur, Markowitz, Ma, and Rosen (1993) examined behavioral changes in children with blood Pb concentrations between 25 and 55 µg/dl who were treated either pharmacologically (if eligible) or through iron supplementation. The residences of all subjects were inspected for Pb, and abatement proceeded if deemed necessary. Long-term (6-month) declines in blood Pb concentrations were significantly related to Bayley or Stanford–Binet cognitive scores following covariate adjustment. The facts that the study involved a limited sample and that treatments were combined or unsystematic make the findings somewhat difficult to interpret. Nevertheless, the results of this investigation suggest that there may be developmental advantages to pharmacological treatment at lower levels of exposure.

A multiple-center, randomized clinical trial is currently underway under the auspices of the National Institute of Environmental Health Sciences to determine the developmental and behavioral benefits of oral chelation with succimer in preschool children with blood Pb concentrations in the range of 20–44 µg/dl (Rogan, 1998).

CONCLUSION

As in many areas of epidemiological research, clinicians, investigators, and other observers of the literature on environmental chemical influences on child development have reached disparate conclusions. Unfortunately, these conclusions are often based on assumptions that lie in the "transcientific domain," where the interests of an investigator's sponsors become an obstacle to good science (Needleman, 1992). Very few credible clinicians or scientists would argue today that exposure to moderate to high doses of Hg, organochlorines, or Pb *in utero* is inconsequential in terms of CNS development. Given the continued vulnerability of the human CNS to developmentally perturbing influences after birth, most scientists agree that limiting the exposure of infants and toddlers to these neurotoxicants is equally important.

Not all nonpharmaceutical chemical exposures suffered by fetuses are accidental or involuntary. For example, the recent increase in women of reproductive age who abuse readily available chemical solvents such as toluene has attracted the attention of clinicians and researchers, who have described a syndrome in surviving newborns that bears a striking similarity to fetal alcohol syndrome (Pearson, Hoyme, Seaver, & Rimsza, 1994; Arnold, Kirby, Langendoerfer, & Wilkins-Haug, 1994).

Pediatric neuropsychologists would do well to keep informed of new developments in this emerging field. Very few of the environmental chemical pollutants to which fetuses and children are daily exposed have been characterized in terms of their developmental impact. A working knowledge of this area will not only enhance the clinical and scientific acumen of the pediatric neuropsychologist, but may eventually help to identify as yet undiscovered environmental risks to normal CNS development. Clinicians, after all, were the first to identify some of the best-known environmental and pharmaceutical chemical risks to CNS development (Byers & Lord, 1943; Hanson & Smith, 1975; Harada, 1976; Jones, Smith, Streissguth, & Myrianthopoulos, 1974; Lammer et al., 1985).

REFERENCES

Achenbach, T. M., & Edelbrock, C. (1983). *Manual for the Child Behavior Checklist and revised Child Behavior Profile.* Burlington: University of Vermont, Department of Psychiatry.

Achenbach, T. M., & Edelbrock, C. (1986). *Manual for the Teacher's Report Form and Teacher Version of the Child Behavior Profile.* Burlington: University of Vermont, Department of Psychiatry.

Agency for Toxic Substances and Disease Registry (ATSDR). (1992). Hg toxicity. *American Family Physician, 46,* 1731–1741.

Agency for Toxic Substances and Disease Registry (ATSDR). (1994). *Toxicological profile for Hg: Update.* Atlanta, GA: U.S. Department of Health and Human Services.

Agocs, M. M., Etzel, R. A., Parrish, R. G., Paschal, D. C., Campagna, P. R., Cohen, D. S., Kilbourne, E. M., & Hesse J. L. (1990). Hg exposure from interior latex paint. *New England Journal of Medicine, 323,* 1096–1101.

Annest, J. L., Pirkle, J. L., Makuc, D., Neese, J. W., Bayse, D. D., & Kovar, M. G. (1983). Chronological trends in blood lead levels between 1976 and 1980. *New England Journal of Medicine, 308,* 1373–1377.

Arnold, G. L., Kirby, R. S., Langendoerfer, S., & Wilkins-Haug, L. (1994). Toluene embryopathy: Clinical delineation and developmental follow-up. *Pediatrics, 93,* 216–220.

Baghurst, P. A., McMichael, A. J., Tong, S., Wigg, N. R., Vimpani, G. V., & Robertson, E. F. (1995). Exposure to environmental lead and visual–motor integration at age 7 years: The Port Pirie Cohort Study. *Epidemiology, 6,* 104–109.

Baghurst, P. A., McMichael, A. J., Wigg, N. R., Vimpani, G. V., Robertson, E. F., Roberts, R. J., & Too, S. L. (1992). Environmental exposure to lead and children's intelligence at the age of seven years. *New England Journal of Medicine, 327,* 1279–1284.

Bayley, N. (1969). *Manual for the Bayley Scales of Infant Development.* New York: Psychological Corporation.

Bayley, N. (1993). *Bayley scales of infant development* (2nd ed.). San Antonio, TX: Psychological Corporation.

Bellinger, D. (1994). Teratogen update: Lead. *Teratology, 50,* 367–373.

Bellinger, D. (1995). Interpreting the literature on lead and child development: The neglected role of the "experimental system." *Neurotoxicology and Teratology, 17,* 201–212.

Bellinger, D., & Dietrich, K. N. (1994). Low level lead exposure and cognitive function in children. *Pediatric Annals, 23,* 600–605.

Bellinger, D., Leviton, A., Allred, E., & Rabinowitz, M. (1994). Pre- and postnatal lead exposure and behavior problems in school-age children. *Environmental Research, 66,* 12–30.

Bellinger, D., Leviton, A., Waternaux, C., Needleman, H., & Rabinowitz, M. (1987). Longitudinal analyses of prenatal and postnatal lead exposure and early cognitive development. *New England Journal of Medicine, 316,* 1037–1043.

Beery, K. E. (1982). *Revised administration, scoring, and teaching manual for the Developmental Test of Visual–Motor Integration.* Cleveland, OH: Modern Curriculum Press.

Bertin, J. E. (1994). Reproductive hazards in the workplace: lessons learned from the *UAW v. Johnson Controls.* In H. L. Needleman & D. Bellinger (Eds.), *Prenatal exposure to toxicants: Developmental consequences* (pp. 297–316). Baltimore: Johns Hopkins University Press.

Bolger, P. M., Carrington, C. D., Capar, S. G., & Adams, M. A. (1991). Reductions in dietary lead exposure in the United States. *Chemical Speciation and Bioavailability, 3,* 31–36.

Brazelton, T. B. (1984). *Neonatal Behavioral Assessment Scale* (Clinics in Developmental Medicine No. 88). Philadelphia: J. B. Lippincott.

Bruininks, R. H. (1978). *Bruininks–Oseretsky Test of Motor Proficiency.* Circle Pines, MN: American Guidance Service.

Burbacher, T. M., Rodier, P. M., & Weiss, B. (1990). Methylmercury developmental neurotoxicity: A comparison of effects in humans and animals. *Neurotoxicology and Teratology, 12,* 191–202.

Byers, R. K., & Lord, E. E. (1943). Late effects of lead poisoning on mental development. *American Journal of Diseases of Children, 66,* 471–494.

Caldwell, B., & Bradley, R. (1979). *Home Observation for Measurement of the Environment (HOME).* Unpublished manual, University of Arkansas, Little Rock, AR.

Centers for Disease Control. (1991a). Fatal pediatric poisoning from leaded paint—Wisconsin, 1990. *Journal of the American Medical Association, 265,* 2050–2051.

Centers for Disease Control. (1991b, October). *Preventing lead poisoning in young children: A statement by the Centers for Disease Control.* Atlanta, GA: Author.

Cernichiari, E., Brewer, R., Myers, G. J., Marsh, D. O., Lapham, L. W., Cox, C., Shamlaye, C. F., Berlin, M., Davidson, P. W., & Clarkson, T. W. (1995). Monitoring methylmercury during pregnancy: Maternal hair predicts fetal brain exposure. *Neurotoxicology, 16,* 705–709.

Chen, Y. C. J., Guo, Y. L., Hsu, C. C., & Rogan, W. J. (1992). Cognitive development of Yu-cheng ("oil disease") children prenatally exposed to heat-degraded PCBs. *Journal of the American Medical Association, 268,* 3213–3218.

Chen, Y. C. J., Yu, M. L. M., Rogan, W. J., Gladen, B. C., & Hsu, C. C. (1994). A 6-year follow-up of behavior and activity disorders in the Taiwan Yu-cheng children. *American Journal of Public Health, 84,* 415–421.

Clarkson, T. W. (1990). Hg—an element of mystery. *New England Journal of Medicine, 323,* 1137–1139.

Clarkson, T. W. (1991). Methylmercury. *Fundamental and Applied Toxicology, 16,* 20–21.

Clarkson, T. W., Cox, C., Marsh, D. O., Myers, G. J., Al-Tikriti, S. K., Amin-Zaki, L., & Dabbagh, A. R. (1981). Dose-response relationships for adult and prenatal exposures to methylmercury. In G. G. Berg & H. D. Maillie (Eds.), *Measurement of risk* (pp. 111–130). New York: Plenum Press.

Clarkson, T. W., Hursh, J. B., Sager, P. R., & Syverson, T. L. M. (1988). Hg. In T. W. Clarkson, L. Friberg, G. F. Nordberg, & P. R. Sager (Eds.), *Biological monitoring of toxic metals* (pp. 199–246). New York: Plenum Press.

Clarkson, T. W., Nordberg, G. F., & Sager, P. R. (1985). Reproductive and developmental toxicity of metals. *Scandinavian Journal of Work and Environmental Health, 11,* 145–154.

Cookman, G. R., Hemmens, S. E., Keane, G. J., King, W. B., & Regan, C. M. (1988). Chronic low level lead exposure precociously induces rat glial development in vitro and in vivo. *Neuroscience Letters, 86,* 33–37.

Cookman, G. R., King, W. B., & Regan, C. M. (1987). Chronic low level lead exposure impairs embryonic to adult conversion of the neural cell adhesion molecule. *Journal of Neurochemistry, 49,* 399–403.

Cox, C., Clarkson, T. W., Marsh, D. O., Amin-Zaki, L., Tikriti, S., & Myers, G. J. (1989). Dose–response analysis of infants prenatally exposed to methylmercury: An application of a single compartment model to single strand hair analysis. *Environmental Research, 49,* 318–332.

Crump, K., Viren, J., Silvers, A., Clewell, H., Gearhart, J., & Shipp, A. (1995). Reanalysis of dose-response data from the Iraqi methylmercury poisoning episode. *Risk Analysis, 15,* 523–532.

Dahl, R., White, R. F., Weihe, P., Sorensen, N., Letz, R., Hudnell, H. K., & Otto, D. A. (1996). Feasibility and validity of three computer-assisted neurobehavioral tests in 7-year old children. *Neurotoxicology and Teratology, 18,* 413–419.

Davidson, P. W., Myers, G. J., Cox, C., Axtell, C. Shamlaye, M. B., Sloane-Reeves, J. Cernichiari, E., Needham, L., Choi, A., Yining, W., Berlin, M., & Clarkson, T. W. (1998). Effects of prenatal and postnatal methylmercury exposure from fish consumption on neurodevelopment. *Journal of the American Medical Association, 280,* 701–707.

Davidson, P. W., Myers, G. J., Cox, C., Shamlaye, C. F., Marsh, D. O., Tanner, M. A., Berlin, M., Sloane-Reeves, J., Cernichiari, E., Choisy, O., Choi, A., & Clarkson, T. W. (1995). Longitudinal neurodevelopmental study of Seychellois children following *in-utero* exposure to methylmercury from maternal fish ingestion: Outcomes at 19 and 29 months. *Neurotoxicology, 16,* 677–688.

Davis, J. M., Otto, D. A., Weil, D. E., & Grant, L. D. (1990). The comparative developmental neurotoxicity of lead in humans and animals. *Neurotoxicology and Teratology, 12,* 215–229.

des Planches, L. T. (1848). *Lead diseases: A treatise* (S. L. Dana, Trans.). Lowell, MA: Daniel Bixby. (Original work published 1839)

Dietrich, K. N. (1991). Lead toxicity, mineral intake, and child development. *Clinics in Applied Nutrition, 1,* 27–38.

Dietrich, K. N., & Bellinger, D. (1994). The assessment of neurobehavioral development in studies of the effects of prenatal exposure to toxicants. In H. L. Needleman & D. Bellinger (Eds.), *Prenatal exposure to toxicants: Developmental consequences* (pp. 57–85). Baltimore: Johns Hopkins University Press.

Dietrich, K. N., Berger, O. G., & Succop, P. A. (1993). Lead exposure and the motor developmental status of urban six-year-old children in the Cincinnati Prospective Study. *Pediatrics, 91,* 301–307.

Dietrich, K. N., Berger, O. G., Succop, P. A., Hammond, P. B., & Bornschein, R. L. (1993). The developmental consequences of low to moderate prenatal and postnatal lead exposure: Intellectual attainment in the Cincinnati Lead Study cohort following school entry. *Neurotoxicology and Teratology, 15,* 37–44.

Dietrich, K. N., Krafft, K. M., Bornschein, R. L., Hammond, P. B., Berger, O., Succop, P. A., & Bier, M. (1987). Low-level fetal lead exposure effect on neurobehavioral development in early infancy. *Pediatrics, 80,* 721–730.

Dietrich, K. N., Krafft, K. M., Pearson, D. T., Bornschein, R. L., Hammond, P. B., & Harris, L. (1985). Contribution of social and developmental factors to lead exposure during the first year of life. *Pediatrics, 75,* 1114–1118.

Dietrich, K. N., Succop, P. A., Berger, O. G., & Keith, R. (1992). Lead exposure and the central auditory processing abilities and cognitive development of urban children: The Cincinnati Lead Study cohort at age 5 years. *Neurotoxicology and Teratology, 14,* 51–56.

Dobbing, J. (1981). The later development of the brain and its vulnerability. In J. A. Davis & J. Dobbing (Eds.), *Scientific foundations of pediatrics* (pp. 744–759). London: Heinemann.

Environmental Protection Agency. (1993). *Workshop report on developmental neurotoxic effects associated with exposure to PCBs.* Lexington, MA: Eastern Research Group.

Fagan, J. F., & Shephard, P. A. (1987). *The Fagan Test of Infant Intelligence.* Cleveland, OH: Infantest.

Feldman, G. V. (1966). Pink disease [Letter]. *American Journal of Diseases of Children, 112,* 165.

Fergusson, D., Fergusson, J., Horwood, L., & Kinzett, N. (1988). A longitudinal study of dentine lead levels, intelligence, school performance, and behaviour. *Journal of Child Psychology and Psychiatry, 29,* 811–824.

Fergusson, D., Horwood, L., & Lynskey, M. (1993). Early dentine lead levels and subsequent cognitive and behavioural development. *Journal of Child Psychiatry and Psychology, 34,* 215–227.

Fein, G. G., Jacobson, J. L., Jacobson, S. W., Schwartz, P. M., & Dowler, J. K. (1984). Prenatal exposure to polychlorinated biphenyls: Effects on birth size and gestational age. *Journal of Pediatrics, 105,* 315–320.

Gibson, J. L. (1904). A plea for painted railings and painted walls of rooms as the source of lead poisoning amongst Queensland children. *Australian Medical Gazette, 23,* 149–153.

Gibson, J. L., Love, W., Hardine, D., Bencroft, P., & Turner, D. (1892). Note on lead poisoning as observed among children in Brisbane. *Transactions of the 3rd Intercolonial Medical Congress, Sydney* (pp. 76–83).

Gittelman, R., & Eskanazi, B. (1983). Lead and hyperactivity revisited: An investigation of nondisadvantaged children. *Archives of General Psychiatry, 40,* 827–833.

Gladen, B. C., & Rogan, W. J. (1991). Effects of perinatal polychlorinated biphenyls and dichlordiphenyl dichlorethene on later development. *Journal of Pediatrics, 119,* 58–63.

Gladen, B. C., Rogan, W. J., Hardy, P., Thullen, J., Tingelstad, J., & Tulley, M. (1988). Development after exposure to polychlorinated biphenyls and dichlorodiphenyl dichloroethene transplacentally and through human milk. *Journal of Pediatrics, 113,* 991–995.

Goldstein, G. (1992). Developmental neurobiology of lead toxicity. In H. L. Needleman (Ed.), *Human lead exposure* (pp. 125–135). Boca Raton, FL: CRC Press.

Grandjean, P., Weihe, P., Jorgensen, P. J., Clarkson, T. W., Cernichiari, E., & Videro, T. (1992). Impact of maternal seafood diet on fetal exposure to mercury, selenium, and lead. *Archives of Environmental Health, 47,* 185–195.

Grandjean, P., Weihe, P., & White, R. F. (1995). Milestone development in infants exposed to methylmercury from human milk. *Neurotoxicology, 16,* 27–33.

Grandjean, P., Weihe, P., White, R. F., Debes, F., Arki, S., Yokoyama, K., Murata, K., Sorensen, N., Dahl, R., & Jorgensen, P. J. (1997). Cognitive deficit in 7-year-old children with prenatal exposure to methylmercury. *Neurotoxicology and Teratology, 19,* 417–428.

Hambaugh, M., Mendoza, L. A., Burkhart, J. F., & Weil, F. (1971). The thyroid as a time clock in the developing nervous system. In D. C. Pease (Ed.), *Cellular aspects of neuronal growth and differentiation* (pp. 321–328). Berkeley: University of California Press.

Hanninen, H. (1982). Behavioral effects of occupational exposure to Hg and lead. *Acta Neurologica Scandinavica, 66,* 167–175.

Hanson, J. W., & Smith, D. W. (1975). The fetal hydantoin syndrome. *Journal of Pediatrics, 87,* 285–290.

Harada, M. (1976). Intrauterine poisoning: Clinical and epidemiological studies of the problem. *Bulletin of the Institute of Constitutional Medicine of Kumamoto University, 25,* 1–60.

Harada, Y. (1977). Congenital Minamata disease. In T. Tsubaki & K. Irukayama (Eds.), *Methylmercury poisoning in Minamata and Niigata, Japan* (pp. 209–239). New York: Elsevier.

Hsu, S. T., Ma, C. I., Hsu, S. K., Wu, S. S., Hsu, N. H., Yeh, C. C., & Wu, S. B. (1985). Discovery and epidemiology of PCB poisoning in Taiwan: A four year follow-up. *Environmental Health Perspectives, 59,* 5–10.

Hunter, D., & Russell, D. S. (1954). Focal cerebral and cerebellar atrophy in a human subject due to organic Hg compounds. *Journal of Neurology, Neurosurgery and Psychiatry, 17,* 235–241.

Jacobson, J. L., & Jacobson, S. W. (1994). The effects of perinatal exposure to polychlorinated biphenyls and related contaminants. In H. L. Needleman & D. Bellinger (Eds.), *Prenatal exposure to toxicants: Developmental consequences* (pp. 130–147). Baltimore: Johns Hopkins University Press.

Jacobson, J. L., & Jacobson, S. W. (1996). Intellectual impairment in children exposed to polychlorinated biphenyls *in utero. New England Journal of Medicine, 335,* 783–789.

Jacobson, J. L., Jacobson, S. W., Fein, G. G., Schwartz, P. M., & Dowler, J. K. (1984). Prenatal exposure to an environmental toxin: A test of the multiple effects model. *Developmental Psychology, 20,* 523–532.

Jacobson, J. L., Jacobson, S. W., & Humphrey, H. E. B. (1990). Effects of *in utero* exposure to polychlorinated biphenyls on cognitive functioning in young children. *Journal of Pediatrics, 116,* 38–45.

Jacobson, J. L., Jacobson, S. W., Padgett, R. J., Brumitt, G. A., & Billings, R. L. (1992). Effects of prenatal PCB exposure on cognitive processing efficiency and sustained attention. *Developmental Psychology, 28,* 297–306.

Jacobson, S. W., Fein, G. G., Jacobson, J. L., Schwartz, P. M., & Dowler, J. K. (1985). The effect of PCB exposure on visual recognition memory. *Child Development, 56,* 853–860.

Jensen, A. A. (1989). Background levels in humans. In R. D. Kimbrough & A. A. Jensen (Eds.), *Topics in environmental health: Vol. 4. Halogenated biphenyls, napthalenes, dibenzodioxins, and related products* (pp. 385–390). Amsterdam: Elsevier.

Jones, K. L., Smith, D. W., Streissguth, A. P., & Myranthopoulos, N. C. (1974). Outcome of offspring of chronic alcoholic women. *Lancet, i,* 1076–1078.

Kaufman, A. S., & Kaufman, N. L. (1983). *Kaufman Assessment Battery for Children.* Circle Pines, MN: American Guidance Service.

Kjellstrom, T., Kennedy, P., & Wallis, S. (1989). *Physical and mental development of children with prenatal exposure to Hg from fish: Stage 2. Interviews and psychological tests at age 6* (Report No. 3642). Solna: National Swedish Environmental Protection Board.

Kodavanti, P. R. S., & Tilson, H. A. (1997). Comments on "Developmental neurotoxicity of PCBs in humans: What do we know and where do we go from here?" *Neurotoxicology and Teratology, 19,* 1–2.

Korach, K. S., Sarver, P., Chae, K., McLachlan, J. A., & McKinney, J. D. (1987). Estrogen receptor-binding activity of polychlorinated hydroxybiphenyls: Conformationally restricted structural probes. *Molecular Pharmacology, 33,* 120–126.

Kuratsune, M. (1989). Yusho with reference to Yu-cheng. In R. D. Kimbrough & A. A. Jensen (Eds.), *Topics in environmental health: Vol. 4. Halogenated biphenyls, terphenyls, napthalenes, dibenzodioxins, and related products* (pp. 381–400). Amsterdam: Elsevier.

Lammer, E. J., Chen, D. T., Hoar, R. M., Agnish, N. A., Benke, P. J., Braun, J. T., Curry, C. J., Fernhoff, P. M., Grix, A. W., & Lott, I. T. (1985). Retinoic acid embryopathy. *New England Journal of Medicine, 313,* 837–841.

Landrigan, P. J., Graham, D. G., & Thomas, R. D. (1994). Environmental neurotoxic illness: Research for prevention. *Environmental Health Perspectives, 102*(Suppl. 2), 117–120.

Letz, R. (1990). The Neurobehavioral Evaluation System (NES): An international effort. In B. L. Johnson, W. K. Anger, A. Duraw, & C. Xinteras (Eds.), *Advances in neurobehavioral toxicology: Applications in environmental and occupational health* (pp. 189–202). Chelsea, MI: Lewis.

Markham, A. (1994). *A brief history of pollution*. New York: St. Martin's Press.

Markovac, J., & Goldstein, G. (1988). Picomolar concentrations of lead stimulate brain protein kinase C. *Nature, 334,* 71–73.

Marsh, D. O., Clarkson, T. W., Cox, C., Myers, G. J., Amin-Zaki, L., & Al-Tikriti, S. (1987). Fetal methyl-mercury poisoning. *Archives of Neurology, 44,* 1017–1022.

Masuda, Y., Kagawa, R., Kuroki, H., Kuratsune, M., Yoshimura, T., Taki, I., Kasuda, M., Yamashita, F., & Hayashi, M. (1978). Transfer of polychlorinated biphenyls from mothers to fetuses and infants. *Food and Cosmetic Toxicology, 16,* 543–546.

McCarthy, D. (1972). *McCarthy Scales of Children's Abilities*. New York: Psychological Corporation.

McKeown-Eyssen, G. E., Reudy, J., & Neims, A. (1983). Methylmercury exposure in northern Quebec: II. Neurological findings in children. *American Journal of Epidemiology, 118,* 470–479.

McKhann, C. F. (1926). Lead poisoning in children. *American Journal of Diseases of Children, 32,* 386–392.

McKhann, C. F. (1932). Lead poisoning in children: The cerebral manifestations. *Archives of Neurology and Psychiatry, 27,* 294–298.

McMichael, A. J., Vimpani, G. V., Robertson, E. F., Baghurst, P. A., & Clark, P. D. (1986). The Port Pirie cohort study: Blood lead and pregnancy outcome. *Journal of Epidemiology and Community Health, 40,* 18–25.

McNeil, N. I., Oliver, R. E., Issler, H. C., & Wrong, O. M. (1984). Domestic metallic Hg poisoning. *Lancet, i,* 269–271.

Mortality and Morbidity Weekly Report. (1991). Acute chronic poisoning, residential exposures to elemental Hg—Michigan, 1989–1990. *Journal of the American Medical Association, 266,* 196–197.

Mullin, M. D., Pochini, C. M., McCrindle, S., Romkes, M., Safe, S., & Safe, L. (1984). High resolution PCB analysis: The synthesis and chromatographic properties of all 209 PCB congeners. *Environmental Science and Technology, 18,* 468–476.

Myers, G. J., Marsh, D., Davidson, P. W., Shamlaye, C. F., Tanner, M. A., Choi, A., Cernichiari, E., Choisy, O., & Clarkson, T. W. (1995). Main neurodevelopmental study of Seychellois children following *in-utero* exposure to methylmercury from a maternal fish diet: Outcome at six months. *Neurotoxicology, 16,* 653–664.

Myers, G. J., Davidson, P. W., Cox, C., Shamlaye, C. F., Tanner, M. A., Choisy, O. C., Sloane-Reeves, J., Marsh, D. O., Cernichiari, E., Choi, A., Berlin, M., & Clarkson, T. W. (1995). Neurodevelopmental outcomes of Seychellois children sixty-six months after *in utero* exposure to methylmercury from a maternal fish diet: Pilot study. *Neurotoxicology, 16,* 639–652.

Needleman, H. L. (1992). Salem comes to the National Institutes of Health: Notes from inside the crucible of scientific integrity. *Pediatrics, 90,* 977–981.

Needleman, H. L., & Bellinger, D. C. (Eds.). (1994). *Prenatal exposure to toxicants: Developmental consequences.* Baltimore: Johns Hopkins University Press.

Needleman, H. L., & Gatsonis, C. (1990). Low level lead exposure the IQ of children. *Journal of the American Medical Association, 263,* 673–678.

Needleman, H. L., Gunnoe, C., Leviton, A., Reed, R., Peresie, H., Maher, C., & Barrett, P. (1979). Deficits in psychologic and classroom performance of children with elevated dentine lead levels. *New England Journal of Medicine, 300,* 689–695.

Needleman, H. L., Riess, J. A., Tobin, M. J., Biesecker, G. E., & Greenhouse, J. B. (1996). Bone lead levels and delinquent behavior. *Journal of the American Medical Association, 275,* 363–369.

Needleman, H. L., Schell, A., Bellinger, D., Leviton, A., & Allred, E. N. (1990). The long-term effects of low doses of lead in childhood: An 11-year follow-up report. *New England Journal of Medicine, 322,* 83–88.

Null, D. H., Gartside, P. S., & Wei, E. (1973). Methylmercury accumulation in brains of pregnant, non-pregnant and fetal rats. *Life Sciences, 12,* 65–72.

Oliver, T. (1911). Lead poisoning and the race. *British Medical Journal, i,* 1096–1098.

Palca, J. (1992). Lead researcher confronts accuser in public hearing. *Science, 256,* 437–438.

Pearson, D. T., & Dietrich, K. N. (1985). The behavioral toxicology and teratology of childhood: Models, methods and implications for intervention. *Neurotoxicology, 6,* 165–182.

Pearson, M. A., Hoyme, E., Seaver, L. H., & Rimsza, M. A. (1994). Toluene embryopathy: Delineation of the phenotype and comparison with fetal alcohol syndrome. *Pediatrics, 93,* 211–215.

Perlstein, M. A., & Attala, R. (1966). Neurologic sequelae of plumbism in children. *Clinical Pediatrics, 5,* 292–298.

Pirkle, J. L., Brody, G., Gunter, E., Kramer, R., Paschal, D., Flegal, K., & Matte, T. (1994). The decline in blood lead levels in the United States: The National Health and Nutrition Examination Surveys (NHANES). *Journal of the American Medical Association, 272,* 284–291.

Pocock, S. J., Smith, M., & Baghurst, P. (1994). Environmental lead and children's intelligence: A systematic review of the epidemiological evidence. *British Medical Journal, 309,* 1189–1197.

Porterfield, S. P. (1994). Vulnerability of the developing brain to thyroid abnormalities: Environmental insults to the thyroid system. *Environmental Health Perspectives, 102*(Suppl. 2), 125–130.

Pounds, J., & Rosen, J. (1988). Cellular Ca^{2+} homeostasis and Ca^{2+}-mediated cell processes as critical targets for toxicant action: Conceptual and methodological pitfalls. *Toxicology and Applied Pharmacology, 94,* 331–341.

Rees, D. C., Francis, E. Z., & Kimmel, C. A. (1990). Scientific and regulatory issues relevant to assessing risk for developmental neurotoxicity: An overview. *Neurotoxicology and Teratology, 12,* 175–181.

Reuhl, K. R., & Chang, L. W. (1979). Effects of methylmercury on the development of the nervous system: A review. *Neurotoxicology, 1,* 21–55.

Rodier, P. M. (1994). Vulnerable periods and processes during central nervous system development. *Environmental Health Perspectives, 102*(Suppl. 2), 121–124.

Rogan, W. J. (1998). The treatment of lead-exposed children (TLC) clinical trial: Design and recruitment for a study of the effect of oral chelation on growth and development of toddlers. *Pediatric and Perinatal Epidemiology, 12,* 313–333.

Rogan, W. J., Gladen, B. C., Mckinney, J. B., Carreras, N., Hardy, P., Thullen, J., Tingelstad, J., & Tully, M. (1986). Neonatal effects of transplacental exposure to PCBs and DDE. *Journal of Pediatrics, 109,* 335–341.

Rogan, W. J., Gladen, B. C., Hung, K., Koong, S., Shih, L., Taylor, J. S., Wu, Y., Yang, D., Ragan, N. B., & Tully, M. (1988). Congenital poisoning by polychlorinated biphenyls and their contaminants in Taiwan. *Science, 241,* 334–336.

Rogan, W. J., Gladen, B. C., McKinney, J. D., Carreras, N., Hardy, P., Thullen, J., Tingelstad, J., & Tully, M. (1986). Polychlorinated biphenyls (PCBs) and dichlorodiphenyl dichlorethene (DDE) in human milk: Effects of maternal factors and previous lactation. *American Journal of Public Health, 76,* 172–177.

Ruff, H. A., Bijur, P. E., Markowitz, M., Ma, Y. C., & Rosen, J. F. (1993). Declining blood lead levels and cognitive changes in moderately lead-poisoned children. *Journal of the American Medical Association, 269,* 1641–1646.

Scarr, S. (1985). Constructing psychology: Making facts and fables for our times. *American Psychologist, 40,* 499–512.

Scarr, S. (1991, October 30). [Transcript of grand rounds, Massachusetts Mental Health Center].

Schwartz, J. (1994a). Societal benefits of reducing lead exposure. *Environmental Research, 66,* 105–124.

Schwartz, J. (1994b). Low level lead exposure and children's I.Q.: A meta-analysis and search for a threshold. *Environmental Research, 65,* 42–55.

Selbst, S. M., Henretig, F. M., & Pearce, J. (1985). Lead encephalopathy. *Clinical Pediatrics, 24,* 280–285.

Shephard, T. H. (1994). *Catalog of teratogenic agents* (8th ed.). Baltimore: Johns Hopkins University Press.

Silbergeld, E. (1992). Mechanisms of lead neurotoxicity, or looking beyond the lamppost. *FASEB Journal, 6,* 3201–3206.

Silva, P., Hughes, P., Williams, S., & Faed, J. (1988). Blood lead, intelligence, reading attainment and behaviour in eleven year old children in Dunedin, New Zealand. *Journal of Child Psychology and Psychiatry, 29,* 43–52.

Smith, W. E., & Smith, A. W. (1975). *Minamata.* New York: Holt, Rinehart & Winston.

Stewart, P., Reihman, J., Darvill, T., & Lonky, E. (1998, August). *The Oswego Newborn and Infant Development Project: Examining the impact of exposure to environmental contaminants on cognitive and behavioral development in children.* First International Conference on Children's Health and Environment, Amsterdam, Netherlands.

Stewart, P., Daly, H., Darvill, T., Olonky, E., Reihman, J., Pagano, J., & Bush, B. (in press). Assessment of prenatal exposure to PCB's from maternal consumption of Great Lakes fish: An analysis of PCB pattern and concentration. *Environmental Research.*

Stiles, K. M., & Bellinger, D. C. (1993). Neuropsychological correlates of low-level lead exposure in school-age children: A prospective study. *Neurotoxicology and Teratology, 15,* 27–35.

Takeuchi, T. (1968). Pathology of Minamata disease. In *Minamata disease* (pp. 141–228). Minamata, Kumamoto Japan: Kumamoto University, Study Group of Minamata Disease.

Takeuchi, T., Eto, N., & Eto, K. (1979). Neuropathology of childhood cases of methylmercury poisoning (Minamata disease) with prolonged symptoms, with particular reference to the decortication syndrome. *Neurotoxicology, 1,* 1–20.

Thomas, H. M., & Blackfan, K. D. (1914). Recurrent meningitis due to lead in a child of 5 years. *American Journal of Diseases of Children, 8,* 377–380.

Thomson, G., Raab, G., Hepburn, W., Hunter, R., Fulton, M., & Laxen, D. (1989). Blood-lead levels and children's behavior: Results from the Edinburgh lead study. *Journal of Child Psychology and Psychiatry, 30*, 515–528.

Tilson, H. A., Jacobson, J. L., & Rogan, W. J. (1990). Polychlorinated biphenyls and the developing nervous system: Cross-species comparisons. *Neurotoxicology and Teratology, 12*, 239–248.

Tsuchiya, K. (1992). The discovery of the causal agent of Minamata disease. *American Journal of Industrial Medicine, 21*, 275–280.

Tunnessen, W. W., McMahon, K. J., & Baser, M. (1987). Acrodynia exposure to Hg from fluorescent light bulbs. *Pediatrics, 79*, 786–789.

Warkany, J. (1966). Acrodynia—postmortem of a disease. *American Journal of Diseases of Children, 112*, 147–156.

Wasserman, G. A., Graziano, J. H., Factor-Litvak, P., Popovac, D., Morina, N., Musabegovic, A., Vrenezi, N., Capuni-Paracka, S., Lekic, V., Preteni-Redjepi, E., Hadzialjevic, S., Slavkovich, V., Kline, J., Shrout, P., & Stein, Z. (1994). Consequences of lead exposure and iron supplementation on childhood development at age 4 years. *Neurotoxicology and Teratology, 16*, 233–244.

Wechsler, D. (1974). *Wechsler Intelligence Scale for Children—Revised*. New York: Psychological Corporation.

Wechsler, D. (1989). *Wechsler Preschool and Primary Scale of Intelligence—Revised*. San Antonio, TX: Psychological Corporation.

Wigg, N. R., Vimpani, F. V., McMichael, A. J., Baghurst, P. Q., Robertson, S. F., & Roberts, R. J. (1988). Port Pirie cohort study: Childhood blood lead and neuropsychological development at age two years. *Journal of Epidemiology and Community Health, 42*, 213–219.

Winneke, G., Brockhaus, A., Ewers, U., Kramer, U., & Neuf, M. (1990). Results from the European multicenter study on lead neurotoxicity in children: Implications for risk assessment. *Neurotoxicology and Teratology, 12*, 553–559.

World Health Organization, International Programme on Chemical Safety. (1990). *Environmental health criteria 101—methylmercury*. Geneva: Author.

World Health Organization, International Programme on Chemical Safety. (1995). *Environmental health criteria 165—inorganic lead*. Geneva: Author.

Yeates, K. O., & Mortensen, M. E. (1994). Acute and chronic neuropsychological consequences of mercury vapor poisoning in two early adolescents. *Journal of Clinical and Experimental Neuropsychology, 16*, 209–222.

Yule, W., Urbanowicz, M., Lansdown, R., & Millar, I. (1984). Teacher's ratings of children's behaviour in relation to blood lead levels. *British Journal of Developmental Psychology, 2*, 295–305.

PART III

Central Nervous System Dysfunction in Other Medical Disorders

10

PREMATURITY AND LOW BIRTHWEIGHT

ERIN M. PICARD
JEREL E. DEL DOTTO
NAOMI BRESLAU

Although considerable strides have been made toward decreasing the mortality and morbidity rates associated with low birthweight (LBW), its prevalence has remained essentially unchanged. Far from being eradicated, the rates of LBW and its principal determinant—preterm birth—have not improved in the United States since 1970 (Paneth, 1995).

Advances in perinatal medicine have exerted the greatest impact on birthweight-specific mortality rates, thus contributing to an overall decline in infant mortality (Berkowitz & Papiernik, 1993). Evidence suggests that the major factor responsible for the decline in infant mortality throughout the 1970s was the increased survival of high-risk infants—that is, those of LBW and very low birthweight (VLBW). Continued interest in LBW is fueled by the fact that the proportion of these births has remained relatively impervious to interventions. Moreover, LBW has been demonstrated to be a significant determinant of postneonatal mortality and of infant and childhood morbidity.

DEFINITION AND HISTORY

Traditionally, births have been classified as either LBW (≤2,500 g) or normal birthweight (NBW; >2,500 g), to reflect the striking differences in outcome between the two groups (Kleinman, 1992). Increasing survival rates of the smallest LBW infants has led to further refinements of this nomenclature. Consequently, distinctions among LBW, VLBW (≤1,500 g), and extremely low birthweight (ELBW; ≤1,000 g) have been drawn in the recent literature. Evidence to suggest a gradient relationship between LBW and mortality/morbidity rates supports the use of a more precise classification. That is, adverse pregnancy outcomes decrease with increasing birthweights.

A more detailed classification may be created by supplementing birthweight data with information regarding gestational age (GA) and size in relation to GA. Thus it is possible to distinguish preterm (<37 weeks) from postterm (>42 weeks) infants, and to classify birthweights as small for gestational age (below the 10th percentile of birthweight) or large for gestational age (above the 90th percentile; Kleinman, 1992).

Admittedly, the term LBW has been applied to a heterogeneous group of infants of varying degrees of preterm birth or growth retardation. Nevertheless, its use is supported by evidence to suggest that preterm delivery is the principal determinant of LBW in the United States. Furthermore, in contrast to the difficulties inherent in the measurement of GA, birthweight can be measured precisely and routinely (Kleinman, 1992).

Prior to the advent of neonatal intensive care, the survival of infants weighing less than 1,000 g at birth was the exception, not the rule. Although attempts were made to promote the survival of high-risk infants in the era preceding the implementation of neonatal intensive care, these efforts had a negligible effect on survival rates and often had devastating consequences. Such practices may have contributed to the particularly dismal outlook observed among infants weighing less than 1,500 g during this period (Hack, Klein, & Taylor, 1995). Significant changes in survival rates were not realized until technological advances grounded in research and an understanding of the neonate's physiology were implemented. The medical innovations responsible for improved survival rates included phototherapy for jaundice, pharmacological treatment for patent ductus arteriosus, and management of respiratory distress syndrome (RDS) through surfactant replacement and increase in ventilatory assistance (Hack et al., 1995).

Because few infants weighing less than 1,000 g at birth survived in the era preceding the implementation of neonatal intensive care, outcome studies during this earlier period focused on children of birthweights greater than 1,500 g. Now that advances in perinatal medicine have resulted in decreased mortality rates of LBW infants, particularly those weighing less than 1,500 g, VLBW and ELBW infants have been emphasized in the majority of more recently published studies.

Contemporary neonatal practices have resulted in particularly dramatic improvements in the survival of infants with birthweights under 750 g or GAs under 29 weeks. Survival in this subgroup, however, has not been won without cost. The expense involved in treating these infants is exorbitant, and the risk of severe handicap is high. As it would appear that we are fast encroaching upon the limit of biological viability, it is difficult to envision any further lowering of the range of LBW in surviving children. Given the constraints of biological viability, prevention becomes an appropriate target for further improvements in care. Unfortunately, our armamentarium of preventive strategies has proven woefully inadequate in effecting change in the rates of LBW births, due in large part to our limited understanding of the determinants of preterm birth (Paneth, 1995).

Improved survival among increasingly smaller neonates has also raised concerns regarding the developmental morbidity of LBW. Long-term sequelae include neuropsychological deficits, even in children in whom early complications have resolved. Moreover, developmental problems not easily identified during the preschool years may later become apparent.

EPIDEMIOLOGY

Mortality rates associated with LBW decreased from the late 1960s to the early 1980s at a rate of approximately 4% annually (Kempe et al., 1992). All ethnic groups have since shown a leveling off in this downward trend. Despite substantial declines in mortality rates, the frequency of LBW births has not declined appreciably. What little decline there has been has been attributed to a reduction in full-term LBW births (Berkowitz & Papiernik, 1993).

The rates of LBW vary according to both ethnicity and country. In the United States in 1991, the LBW rate was 13.6% among African American infants and 5.8% among European American infants (Paneth, 1995). The high rate of LBW has not been observed among other ethnic minorities in the United States. In fact, there is little difference in the prevalence of LBW among Americans of European, Cuban, Mexican, Native, and Asian descent (Kleinman, 1992).

LBW births account for roughly 6.0–6.9% of all live births. Among developed countries, the United States has an unusually high rate of LBW. This high rate cannot be attributed solely to racial differences, given that the European American population, considered separately, would rank no better than 13th in international comparisons (Paneth, 1995).

LBW arises secondary to preterm birth, intrauterine growth retardation (IUGR), or some combination thereof. Although the causes of preterm birth and IUGR are poorly understood, these conditions are associated with different risk factors, and are therefore believed to represent pathophysiologically distinct processes.

In affluent societies such as the United States, preterm birth is the principal determinant of LBW (Paneth, 1995). The likelihood that preterm birth is the mechanism responsible increases with decreasing birthweights. In developing countries, conversely, LBW is more commonly related to IUGR.

In the absence of adequate information regarding the etiology of preterm birth and IUGR, a considerable body of research has accumulated about risk factors—factors that predispose the fetus to either of these conditions. Multiple factors are associated with LBW, including social and economic conditions, maternal size, maternal health, smoking during pregnancy, lack of prenatal care, geographic locale, ethnicity, toxic exposure during pregnancy, and poor pregnancy history. For the most part, the factors associated with preterm birth are related to reproductive history. By way of contrast, the factors associated with IUGR are predominantly demographic (Kramer, 1987a, 1987b).

MEDICAL COMPLICATIONS

LBW is perhaps best conceptualized as an index of biological risk (Hack et al., 1995). Because it is simply an index of risk, LBW defines a group of children who are heterogeneous with respect to neurodevelopmental outcome. At least some of the variability in outcome, however, is thought to be related to early medical complications associated with prematurity (Landry, Fletcher, Denson, & Chapieski, 1993). The likelihood of medical complications increases with decreasing birthweight. Thus as many as 70% of children weighing less than 1,600 g may experience medical complications (Landry et al., 1993). At most, these complications may permanently disrupt the functioning of the central nervous system; at the very least, they may resolve with no obvious adverse sequelae.

Due to the immaturity of multiple organ systems, the preterm infant is at risk for the development of a number of conditions. The most common medical disorder observed among premature infants is hyaline membrane disease (HMD), also known as RDS (Oh & Stern, 1987). RDS/HMD is the result of immature lung development accompanied by surfactant deficiency. *Surfactant* is a substance that coats the alveoli of the lungs, thereby preventing their collapse. By 37 weeks' gestation, a sufficient amount of this substance is available to produce respiratory stability (Wyly, 1995). In infants with RDS/HMD, breathing becomes labored as the alveoli collapse, resulting in grunting, nasal flaring, and synchrony in breathing. RDS/HMD is diagnosed if two of the following symptoms are evident within the first 6 hours of life: respiration rate persistently above 60 per minute, costal or sternal recession, and expiratory grunting (Vulliamy & Johnston, 1987). The clinical management involves ventilatory support and surfactant replacement, to an extent depending upon GA. From 10% to 20% of premature infants are affected by HMD/RDS, with the incidence rising to 65% among those with birthweights below 1,000 g (Wyly, 1995). According to Oh and Stern (1987), many of the complications associated with prematurity are secondary to RDS/HMD. Three of these complications—patent ductus arteriosus, bronchopulmonary dysplasia (BPD), and extrapulmonary extravasation of air—are described below. Although Oh and Stern (1987) included periventricular hemorrhage (PVH) or intraventricular hemorrhage (IVH) among the possible complications of RDS/HMD, this opinion appears to be controversial.

1. *Patent ductus arteriosus.* Shortly after birth, and partly in response to a rise in oxygen saturation, the ductus arteriorsus (a fetal blood vessel that joins the aorta and pulmonary artery) closes in normal-term neonates (Oh & Stern, 1987). In preterm infants with RDS/HMD, however, it is not uncommon for the ductus to remain patent for several days or weeks, leading to pulmonary edema.

2. *Extrapulmonary extravasation of air.* This process is associated with pulmonary interstitial emphysema, pneumomediastinum, and pneumothorax. These latter conditions are the results of air in the pulmonary interstitial tissues, the anterior mediastinum, and the pleural cavity, respectively (Oh & Stern, 1987).

3. *Bronchopulmonary dysplasia.* A third complication of RDS/HMD is BPD, which is most commonly observed among the least mature infants who require assisted ventilation. BPD may be accompanied by prolonged oxygen dependence and respiratory symptoms that persist up to 6 months of life. The etiology of BPD is due to some combination of alveolar damage from RDS/HMD, exposure to high oxygen concentrations, the use of a respirator, the use of endotracheal intubation, and the prolonged duration of these therapies (Oh & Stern, 1987).

Premature infants are also susceptible to PVH or IVH (Dietch, 1992). PVH/IVH occurs when there is bleeding into the subependymal germinal matrix (Volpe, 1987, 1989, 1992). The germinal matrix becomes less prominent over the final 12 to 16 weeks of gestation, until it is exhausted at term (Volpe, 1987). The vulnerability of the germinal matrix to injury probably plays a pivotal role in the pathogenesis of PVH/IVH (Dietch, 1992). PVH/IVH is characteristic of a premature infant, particularly one of less than 32 weeks' gestation. According to Volpe (1987), PVH/IVH is most likely to occur in a premature infant with RDS severe enough to require mechanical ventilation. In approximately 90% of cases, the onset is within the first 72 hours of life. The severity of PVH/IVH ranges from grade 1, in which there is evidence of hemorrhage in the germinal matrix with little or no intraventicular involvement, to grade 4, in which there is intracerebral involvement or other parenchymal lesions (Volpe, 1987). Neuropathological consequences of PVH/IVH include germinal matrix destruction, periventricular hemorrhagic infarction, and hydrocephalus (Volpe, 1989). Periventricular leukomalacia and pontine neuronal necrosis are associated with neuropathological conditions that are not felt to have a casual relationship to PVH/IVH.

A number of pre- and perinatal factors may lead to alterations in brain growth and development. Damage may be mediated by inadequate oxygenation, in the case of respiratory problems, or it may be the result of direct injury caused by PVH/IVH (Landry et al.,

1993). Sequelae associated with such alterations may range from frank neurological disorders to more subtle deficits, such as impairments in neuropsychological functioning. Adverse outcomes nevertheless are associated with more severe medical complaints, such as higher grades of PVH/IVH or the presence of BPD.

NEUROPATHOLOGY

The brain of the preterm infant is susceptible to damage of diverse origins involving pathophysiologically distinct processes. Although the effects of LBW are generally presumed to be mediated by pre- or perinatal brain injury, it is only recently, with the introduction of cranial ultrasound, that investigators have been able to study relationships between brain lesions and outcome.

According to Forfar et al. (1994), three distinct pathologies of the preterm brain are now recognized: (1) PVH or IVH, with or without posthemorrhagic hydrocephalus; (2) infarctive periventricular leukomalacia; and (3) noninfarctive perinatal telencephalic leukoencephalopathy. The corresponding abnormalities detected by cranial ultrasonography may be classified as uncomplicated IVH/PVH, ventricular dilatation, posthemorrhagic hydrocephalus, and cerebral atrophy (Roth et al., 1993). Each of the three pathologies is presumed to have a different perinatal etiology. Infarctive periventricular leukomalacia is probably ischemic in nature, and is best prevented by supporting myocardial function (Forfar et al., 1994). Conversely, noninfarctive perinatal telencephalic leukoencephalopathy has been linked to toxic and nutritional factors.

Lesser degrees of hypoxic–ischemic injury leading to localized periventricular leukomalacia or to diffuse gliosis may go unrecognized by ultrasound imaging (Stewart et al., 1989). Moreover, subtle forms of injury, such as alterations of dendritic arborization and synaptogenesis, may not be detectable. Lesions such as these may account for neurocognitive impairment.

In relating ultrasound findings to neurodevelopmental outcome, investigators have found that ventricular dilatation, hydrocephalus, and cerebral atrophy are the conditions that carry the poorest prognosis. Uncomplicated PVH, conversely, confers no significant adverse effect on outcome (Roth et al., 1993).

A spectrum of neurological abnormalities may be found among LBW children, the most common of which is cerebral palsy. Rates of neurosensory/neuromotor abnormalities among LBW, VLBW, and ELBW children are approximately 6–8%, 14–17%, and 20%, respectively (Forfar et al., 1994). According to Forfar et al. (1994), many of these impairments are manifestations or correlates of cerebral palsy, including abnormal posture and mobility, epilepsy, deafness, and visual problems.

DEVELOPMENTAL OUTCOMES

As early as the 1940s, LBW children were described as having varying degrees of neurocognitive impairment during infancy and early childhood (Benton, 1940; Knobloch, Rider, Harper, & Pasamanick, 1956; Lilienfeld & Pasamanick, 1955; Lilienfeld, Pasamanick, & Rogers, 1955; Pasamanick & Knobloch, 1961; Pasamanick & Lilienfeld, 1955; Pasamanick, Rogers, & Lilienfeld, 1956). A review of the literature on cohorts of children born during the 1950s and 1960s, prior to the introduction of neonatal intensive care, suggests that LBW infants of this era also demonstrated poorer development relative to their NBW peers (Benton, 1940). Although the early studies in this area differ from contemporary investigations in methodology, evidence for neuropsychological sequelae of LBW is long-standing. There is less consensus, however, with regard to the nature and extent of these sequelae.

Investigations of school-age children since the late 1980s have consistently revealed that LBW groups score lower in IQ than NBW controls (Breslau et al., 1994; Hack et al., 1992; Klein, Hack, & Breslau, 1989; Levy-Shiff, Einat, Mogilner, Lerman, & Kriker, 1994; Lloyd, Wheldall, & Perks, 1988; Marlow, Roberts, & Cooke, 1989; McCormick, Brooks-Gunn, Workkman-Daniels, Turner, & Peckham, 1992; Rickards et al., 1993; Saigal, Szatmari, Rosenbaum, Campbell, & King, 1991; Teplin, Burchinal, Johson-Martin, Humphry, & Kraybill, 1991). At school age, VLBW children have also been found to perform more poorly than their NBW peers on measures of diverse neuropsychological abilities and academic achievement (Breslau et al., 1988; Hack et al., 1991, 1992, 1994; Hunt, Cooper, & Tooley, 1988; Klein et al., 1989; Marlow et al., 1989; McCormick et al., 1992; Rickards et al., 1993; Saigal et al., 1991; Teplin et al., 1991). Although some researchers have found that neurobehavioral sequelae of LBW are restricted to the visual–motor domain (Klein et al., 1989; Rickards et al., 1993), others have presented evidence to suggest deficits spanning verbal and nonverbal domains (Breslau, 1995; Breslau, Chilcoat, Del Dotto, Andreski, & Brown, 1996; Hack et al., 1992; Hoy, Bill, & Sykes, 1988; Saigal et al., 1991; Teplin et al., 1991). The lack of uniformity in LBW sequelae is hardly surprising, given the diversity of methods used and the wide age ranges of children included in these studies. Long-term studies beginning in early childhood and extending through adolescence may help to clarify the nature of LBW outcomes in different age groups and the manner in which sequelae change over time.

EVIDENCE FOR A BIRTHWEIGHT-RELATED GRADIENT IN SEQUELAE

The bulk of research conducted over the past 20 years has been devoted to determining the long-term developmental outcome of VLBW children, although this group represents only 15% of LBW births. The study of LBW infants weighing more than 1,500 g has been all but neglected. Children with birthweights of 1,500–2,500 g rarely require neonatal intensive care and are much less likely than lower-birthweight children to suffer adverse neurodevelopmental consequences. However, this higher-birthweight group does in fact suffer adverse sequelae when compared to their NBW peers. Consequently, the much larger subset of LBW children with birthweights at the higher end of the LBW range clearly merit consideration. Some studies, for example, have documented a gradient relationship between birthweight and IQ, with mean differences in IQ ranging from as little as 3.8 points for LBW children at the upper end of the LBW spectrum to as much as 15.2 points for LBW children at the lower end of this continuum (Hack & Breslau, 1986). In two studies (Breslau et al., 1994; McCormick et al., 1992), the gradient relationship between IQ and birthweight was discovered to extend to children with birthweights greater than 1,500 g. In other studies, evidence has accrued to suggest that the gradient effect of birthweight applies to measures of neuropsychological functioning in addition to IQ (Hack, Taylor, Klein, & Eiben, 1993; Taylor, Klein, & Hack, 1994).

Little is known, however, about outcomes in relatively recent cohorts of LBW children with birthweights above 1,500 g. To test the hypothesis that children with less extreme LBW are nevertheless at some risk for adverse outcomes, we tested children 6–7 years of age with birthweights up to 2,500 g (Breslau et al., 1994). The study evaluated large groups of LBW and NBW children, randomly selected from the 1983–1985 newborn lists of two major hospitals in Michigan, one serving an urban population and the other a suburban population. Because our purpose was to evaluate the long-term sequelae of LBW in children who had survived infancy without severe handicaps, children with identifiable neurological abnormalities in whom cognitive deficits might be most apparent were excluded. The mean IQ of LBW children was lower than that of NBW children by one-third of a standard deviation, even after population site, maternal IQ, maternal education, and race were controlled for. Furthermore, a gradient relationship with IQ was detected, with the largest deficit observed in children born weighing under 1,500 g, an intermediate deficit in children born weighing 1,501–2,000 g, and the least pronounced deficit in children born weighing 2,001–2,500 g. The results suggested that the linear relationship between birthweight and IQ continues well beyond the conventional LBW cutoff. The difference between LBW and NBW children, and the gradient relationship between birthweight and cognitive outcome, applied equally for Wechsler Verbal IQ and Performance IQ (Breslau et al., 1994).

To illustrate methods of neuropsychological research on LBW children, and to clarify the nature of the cognitive sequelae observed in these children, the procedures and findings of our own work in this area are described in further detail below. The fact that our sample represented the entire range of LBW provided an opportunity to test for graded relationships between birthweight and measures of abilities, as well as to evaluate the status of heavier LBW children (i.e., those with birthweights of 1,500–2,500 g). Administration of a comprehensive neuropsychological battery also allowed us to investigate whether LBW is associated with selective cognitive deficits (e.g., in visual–motor skills), or rather with a more generalized lowering of abilities.

Sample and Data

As described more fully in Breslau et al. (1994), random samples of LBW and NBW newborns were drawn from each hospital, for each year from 1983 through 1985. Children with identifiable neurological impairment, ascertained at time of recruitment, were excluded. The participation rate was 75%, yielding a total of 823 children (473 LBW and 350 NBW children), with approximately equal numbers of LBW and NBW in the urban and suburban subsamples.

The neuropsychological battery included the Wechsler Intelligence Scale for Children—Revised (Wechsler, 1974) and tests designed to measure aspects of language development, spatial skills, fine motor coordination, tactile perception, attention, and memory. The conceptual rationale for the battery has been described in detail elsewhere (Rourke & Del Dotto, 1994). Briefly, tests of general and specific abilities were selected to provide measures sensitive to deficits believed to be associated with LBW, and at the same time predictive of academic difficulties and diagnosable learning disorders. Specific measures included in the test battery are listed in Table 10.1. All assessments were conducted in the age range of 6 to 7 years, and testing was performed by evaluators unaware of the children's LBW status. Maternal IQ was measured by the Two-Subtest Short Form of the Wechsler Adult Intelligence Scale—Revised (Silverstein, 1983), also administered by trained psychometricians. Additional information on demographic and family characteristics was gathered from interviews conducted by trained staff members.

TABLE 10.1. Neuropsychological Test Battery

Domain	Skills	Instruments	References
Language—syntax	Expressive	CELF-R[a]: Formulated Sentences	Semel et al. (1987)
	Receptive	CELF-R: Sentence Structure	
Language—semantic	Word knowledge	WISC-R[b]: Vocabulary	Wechsler (1974)
	Verbal reasoning	WISC-R: Similarities	
Language—phonological	Expressive	Verbal Fluency	Petrauskas & Rourke (1979)
	Receptive	Auditory Analysis Test	Rosner & Simon (1970)
Spatial	Visual–motor	Developmental Test of Visual–Motor Integration	Beery (1989)
	Visual-perceptual	Judgment of Line Orientation Test	Benton (1983)
Fine motor coordination	Dexterity and sequencing	Grooved Pegboard Test (combined)	Gardner & Broman (1979)
Tactile perception	Localization	Finger Agnosia	Reitan & Davison (1974)
	Recognition	Fingertip-Writing Recognition	Reitan & Davison (1974)
Attention	Focused attention	Underlining Test	Rourke & Petrauskas (1977)
	Vigilance	Continuous-Performance Test	Rosvold et al. (1956)
Memory	Nonverbal	Nonverbal Selective Reminding Test	Fletcher (1985)

From Breslau et al. (1994). Copyright 1994 by N. Breslau. Reprinted by permission.
[a]CELF-R, Clinical Evaluation of Language Functioning—Revised.
[b]WISC-R, Wechsler Intelligence Scale for Children—Revised.

Analysis

The hypothesis that LBW is associated with lower performance across neurocognitive domains was tested in a series of multiple-regression analyses that included the following covariates: geographic subsample (urban and suburban), maternal education (less than high school, high school, part college, college), maternal IQ (measured as a continuous variable), and race (African American and European American). These analyses were preceded by a repeated-measures two-way analysis of variance (ANOVA) to test for a statistical interaction between geographic subsample and birthweight group, in order to determine whether the effect of LBW varied between the two subsamples. The repeated-measures ANOVA also tested the interaction between birthweight group and the 14 tests in the battery. A significant interaction between birthweight status and the series of tests would suggest that the effect of LBW varied across neurocognitive domains and might be observed only in selected areas.

The hypothesis concerning the gradient relationships of cognitive abilities across levels of LBW was tested by multiple-regression analysis, in which LBW was defined by a set of three dichotomous variables representing conventional birthweight categories (VLBW, ≤1,500 g; intermediate LBW, 1,501–2,000 g; and high LBW, 2,001–2,500 g); NBW was used as a reference category, and the set of covariates was included. Tests of linear and higher-order effects were applied.

The initial analyses constitute an example of a sample contrasted-groups design. Though commonly used, this design is valid only if the groups being compared are relatively homogeneous. When the groups being contrasted are heterogeneous, group means may be misleading and may obscure important within-groups features. Recent research with learning-disabled populations has convincingly shown that in pediatric populations, homogeneity tends to be the exception rather than the rule (Fletcher et al., 1994). Thus, in the next stage of our investigation, we attempted to identify subtypes within our sample via cluster analysis.

Results

Characteristics of the Urban and Suburban Samples

The urban and suburban samples differed markedly in racial composition, maternal education, and single-parent status. Differences on these indices between the LBW and NBW groups within sites were small. The LBW and NBW subsets in the urban site were similar to their suburban counterparts with respect to the proportions with low Apgar scores, history of neonatal intensive care, and maternal history of substance use.

Comparisons of LBW and NBW Children

An ANOVA of the test battery detected significant main effects of LBW and population site, but no significant interactions involving LBW and site. The results further indicated that the effect of LBW and the effect of site varied across tests. On all 14 tests, ANOVAs revealed that LBW children scored more poorly than their NBW counterparts, with suburban children scoring significantly higher than urban children on all tests. There were no significant interactions noted between LBW status and site.

When the adjusted differences between LBW and NBW groups were analyzed, the urban and suburban samples were combined, and population site was included in the list of covariates. A series of multiple-regression analyses was than carried out to compare LBW and NBW children from the combined sample, with population site, race, maternal education, and IQ as covariates. Adjusted differences between LBW and NBW children were evaluated on the combined sample. Significant differences were found for 9 of the 14 tests, including tests of language (receptive syntax, verbal reasoning, and receptive phonological awareness), spatial ability, fine motor coordination, tactile perception, and focused attention. These results indicate that although the effect of LBW differed across the 14 tests, the differences were in magnitude. On most tests (9 of 14), differences remained significant when adjusted for potential confounders. Further ANOVAs with the 9 tests showed no significant interaction between LBW and tests.

Comparisons of LBW and NBW Children with Normal IQs

We also investigated comparisons of LBW and NBW children with IQs of 80 and above, since 80 is the IQ cutoff commonly used in the definition of learning disorders. Significant differences were detected on tests of syntactic and phonological receptive language, verbal reasoning, spatial skills, tactile perception, and focused attention. According to these results, the observed deficits associated with LBW were not confined to the subset with subnormal IQs: On principal cognitive domains (both verbal and nonverbal), LBW children scored significantly lower than NBW children, even when population site and other determinants of children's cognitive development were controlled for.

Performance Gradient by Level of LBW

A series of multiple-regression analyses was used to estimate the relationship of neurocognitive status with LBW. As noted earlier, LBW was classified into three levels—VLBW (≤1,500 g), intermediate LBW (1,501 to 2,000 g), and high LBW (2,001 to 2,500 g)—with NBW (≥2,500 g) as a reference. The model included population site, maternal IQ, maternal education, and race as covariates. Linear tests for trend were statistically significant for all tests. No significant higher-order effects were detected. Pairwise tests revealed that each of the three LBW groups scored significantly lower than the NBW groups on verbal reasoning, receptive syntax, receptive phonological awareness, spatial tests, tactile perception, and focused attention.

Cluster Analysis

The scores on the nine variables derived from the multiple-regression analysis were subjected to a number of cluster-analytic procedures. These analyses generated a five-cluster solution. To determine the characteristics of the five clusters, mean scores on each of the neuropsychological measures were calculated for each subtype. These results are presented in Figure 10.1. The mean profile of the first subtype (*n* = 87) suggested low-average performance on most language and visual–spatial measures, with average performances on tasks of tactile, fine motor, and attentional processes. The mean profile of the second subtype (*n* = 64) revealed normal to high-normal functioning on all of the neuropsychological measures. The third subtype (*n* = 29) demonstrated average performances on nearly all of the neuropsychological measures, with the exception of a conspicuously poor performance on a measure of speeded eye–hand coordination. The mean profile of the fourth subtype (*n* = 35) also revealed generally average performances on most neurocognitive tasks, with the exception of a mildly impaired score on a measure of tactile symbol recognition. The final subtype (*n* = 29) was characterized by roughly average performances on measures of tactile symbol recognition and focused attention; low-average to borderline-impaired performances on measures of receptive language, spatial thinking, and fine finger dexterity; and a markedly impaired performance on a measure of tactile finger localization.

The five clusters were also subdivided according to site and race. The relative frequency distributions of blacks and whites were comparable within clusters 1 and 5, and approximately equal proportions of urban and suburban children were assigned to each of these clusters. There was a tendency for a greater proportion of whites to be found in clusters 2 (69% vs. 31% for blacks) and 4 (75% vs. 25% for blacks), and a tendency for a greater proportion of suburban children to be found in each of these clusters (61% and 74%, respectively). However, cluster 3 was characterized by a greater proportion of urban children.

Summary

The results of this study can be summarized as follows:

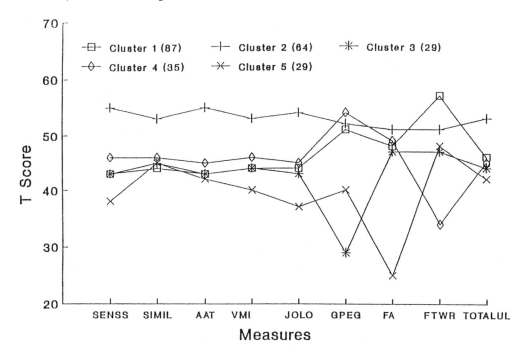

FIGURE 10.1. Cluster profiles for LBW subjects. SENSS, Sentence Structure; SIMIL, Similarities; AAT, Auditory Analysis Test; VMI, Developmental Test of Visual–Motor Integration Test; JOLO, Judgment of Line Orientation Test; GPEG, Grooved Pegboard Test; FA, Finger Agnosia; FTWR, Fingertip-Writing Recognition; TOTALUL, Underlining Test.

1. LBW children at 6 years of age scored significantly lower than NBW children on 9 of 14 neuropsychological tests measuring language, spatial, fine motor, tactile, and attention skills, even when population site, maternal IQ, education, and race were controlled for. The group differences did not vary significantly in urban versus suburban samples.

2. The associations between LBW and the array of neurocognitive abilities held when the analysis was repeated for the subset with IQs of 80 or below.

3. Level of LBW, defined according to conventional cutoffs, showed graded relationships with IQ and with most other outcome measures. Nonetheless, even children with moderate or high LBW (i.e., 1,501–2,000 g and 2,001–2,500 g, respectively) performed more poorly in testing than did NBW children.

4. Cluster analysis revealed that the LBW children exhibited distinct subtypes of neuropsychological impairments, which are strikingly similar to those identified in previous multivariate studies of learning disability subtypes (Rourke, 1985, 1991; Rourke & Del Dotto, 1994). Broadly speaking, these included learning disabilities characterized primarily by disorders of auditory/linguistic functioning, disorders of nonverbal functioning, and output disorders in multiple modalities.

The inclusion of the full range of LBW in the study exposed a gradient relationship with neurocognitive performance across levels of LBW. This issue has rarely been addressed in recent research, which has focused on the extreme low end of the LBW distribution. While VLBW children performed more poorly than heavier LBW children, even children at the intermediate and high LBW levels performed significantly worse than NBW chil--

dren. Moreover, even within the relatively narrowly defined birthweight levels, performance varied by birthweight. The conventional cutoff of 1,500 g (VLBW) used to classify children at high risk for adverse sequelae does not appear to signify a discrete boundary with respect to neurocognitive outcome: Below the 1,500-g cutoff, as well as above it, higher birthweight signaled better performance at 6 years of age. In addition, the conventional LBW cutoff of 2,500 g appears to be an arbitrary boundary with respect to key neurocognitive outcomes, as performance continues to improve in NBW children (i.e., those with birthweights over 3,500 g). Unfortunately, the small number of children with birthweights over 3,500 g in our study limits our ability to identify the optimal birthweight region with respect to cognitive performance at the beginning of schooling.

The findings reported above parallel previous analyses of the relationship between LBW and IQ (Breslau et al., 1994). In both sets of analyses, associations between LBW and cognitive abilities were observed in two socioeconomically disparate populations. Although the urban and suburban children varied markedly on indices of social disadvantage, there was no evidence that the effect of LBW varied between sites. In addition, a gradient relationship with birthweight that extended well beyond 3,000 g was observed in this previous study for general cognitive development (as measured by IQ) and for specific developmental skills (such as language development, visual–motor integration, and attention). The exclusion of LBW children with frank neurological abnormality, such as cerebral palsy or severe sensory impairment, probably resulted in an underestimation of the total spectrum of cognitive deficits associated with premature birth. In addition to lower cognitive abilities across key domains observed in our sample of children who survived infancy relatively intact, subsets of LBW children excluded from our sample might have shown marked deficits in selected cognitive areas.

CONCLUSIONS AND FUTURE RESEARCH DIRECTIONS

It was not so long ago that infants weighing less than 1,500 g at birth were not considered viable. Improved perinatal practices over the past several decades have led to greater survival rates among LBW neonates; currently, infants of less than 500 g and 23 weeks' gestation are surviving. A sharp decrease in morbidity rates among LBW survivors accompanied the advent of neonatal intensive care. Survival rates continued to improve throughout the 1970s and 1980s, but there was little further change in the rates of cerebral palsy and neurodevelopmental handicap (Hack et al., 1995). The result has been a net increase in the prevalence of handicapping conditions. Due to increased survival rates, we are now confronted with the impact of a philosophy of "survival at any cost" on long-term developmental outcome.

Several studies of LBW children have consistently indicated poorer performance in VLBW as compared with NBW children across a wide range of neurocognitive domains. Our own research in this area extends these findings to the entire LBW range, up to 2,500 g. Although several studies have suggested that LBW is associated specifically with visual–motor deficits, there is evidence that the association also applies to indices of language development, fine motor and tactile abilities, and attention—a finding consistent with studies that have reported generalized deficits. The language skills on which LBW and NBW children differed in our own research (even when those with IQs of 80 or less were excluded) were receptive syntax, verbal reasoning, and receptive phonological awareness. The clinical significance of deficits in receptive phonological ability for learning disabilities is well documented (Fletcher et al., 1994). An explanation for the stronger LBW effects on some of the language tests than on others is not readily available. Follow-up of the children as they mature is likely to shed light on the developmental implications of these early findings.

The biological bases for the observed deficits associated with LBW may include intrauterine brain damage, perinatal complications, chronic neonatal disease, and brain growth failure in infancy (Hack et al., 1986). The prevalence of these complications is highest in VLBW children, in whom neurocognitive deficits are most pronounced. The biological bases for the observed gradient relationships and the lower performance of VLBW children relative to NBW children are unclear. The presence of sequelae in this subgroup of LBW children suggests the possibility of suboptimal development either *in utero* or postnatally as an additional mechanism, apart from detectable brain damage. Long-term follow-up assessments of these and other samples of VLBW children will shed light on the persistence of these deficits and their implications for learning and social adaptation.

Due to the rapid pace of medical innovations in the past several decades, the characteristics of survivors of LBW vary by year of birth. Arguably, LBW survivors born in the era predating neonatal intensive care (circa 1960) represented a group of hardy and mature infants compared to their peers of the 1970s and 1980s, who have been the beneficiaries of advances in perinatal medicine. The findings of early research are not likely to be comparable to those of contemporary investigations. The fact that outcomes may differ in studies conducted in different eras does not imply that the early research is devoid of scientific value, but it does underscore the importance of taking sample characteristics into account in interpreting findings. Additional methodological issues to consider in evaluating studies of LBW outcomes include survival rates in the sample, numbers and characteristics of refusers and dropouts, the nature of the control group, follow-up duration, corrections for preterm birth, the sensitivity and comprehensiveness of assessment procedures, and criteria for inclusion–exclusion of participants (Hack et al., 1995).

REFERENCES

Benton, A. L. (1940). Mental development of prematurely born children. *American Journal of Orthopsychiatry*, 10, 719–746.

Benton, A. L. (1983). Judgment of Line Orientation Test. In A. L. Benton, K. Hamsher, N. R. Varney, & O. Spreen (Eds.), *Contributions to neuropsychological assessment* (pp. 44– 54). New York: Oxford University Press.

Beery, K. E. (1989). *Developmental Test of Visual–Motor Integration: Administration, scoring, teaching manual.* Cleveland, OH: Modern Curriculum Press.

Berkowitz, G. S., & Papiernik, E. (1993). Epidemiology of preterm birth. *Epidemiologic Reviews*, 15(2), 414– 443.

Breslau, N. (1995). Psychiatric sequelae of low birth weight. *Epidemiologic Reviews*, 17, 96–106.

Breslau, N., Chilcoat, H., Del Dotto, J. E., Andreski, P., & Brown, G. (1996). Low birthweight and neurocognitive status at six years of age. *Biological Psychiatry*, 40, 389–397.

Breslau, N., Del Dotto, J. E., Brown, G. G., Kumar, S., Ezhuthachan, S., Hufnagle, K. G., & Petersen, E. L. (1994). A gradient relationship between low birth weight and IQ at age 6 years. *Archives of Pediatric and Adolescent Medicine*, 148, 377–383.

Breslau, N., Klein, N., & Allen, L. (1988). Very low birth weight: Behavioral sequelae at nine years of age. *Journal of the American Academy of Child and Adolescent Psychiatry*, 27(5), 605–612.

Dietch, J. S. (1992). Periventricular–intraventricular hemorrhage in the very low birth weight infant. *Neonatal Network*, 12(1), 7–16.

Fletcher, J. M. (1985). Memory for verbal and nonverbal stimuli in learning disability subtypes: Analysis by selective reminding. *Journal of Experimental Child Psychology*, 40, 244–259.

Fletcher, J. M., Shaywitz, S. E., Shankweiler, D. P., Katz, L., Liberman, I. Y., Stuebing, K. K., Francis, D. J., Fowler, A. E., & Shaywitz, B. A. (1994). Cognitive profiles of reading disability: Comparisons of discrepancy and low achievement definitions. *Journal of Educational Psychology*, 86(1), 6–23.

Forfar, J. O., Hume, R., McPhail, F. M., Maxwell, S. M., Wilkinson, E. M., Lin, J. P., & Brown, J. K. (1994). Low birth weight: A 10-year outcome study of the continuum of reproductive casualty. *Developmental Medicine and Child Neurology, 36,* 1037–1048.

Gardner, R. A., & Broman, M. (1979). *Purdue Pegboard normative data.* Lafayette, IN: Lafayette Instrument.

Hack, M., & Breslau, N. (1986). Very low birth weight infants: Effects of brain growth during infancy on intelligence quotient at 3 years of age. *Pediatrics, 77,* 196–202.

Hack, M., Breslau, N., Weissman, B., Aram, D., Klein, N., & Borowoski, E. (1991). Effect of very low birth weight and subnormal head size on cognitive abilities at school age. *New England Journal of Medicine, 323*(4), 231–237.

Hack, M., Breslau, N., Aram, D., Weissman, B., Klein, N., & Borawski-Clark, E. (1992). The effect of very low birth weight and social risk on neurocognitive abilities at school age. *Journal of Developmental and Behavioral Pediatrics, 13,* 412–420.

Hack, M., Klein, N. K., & Taylor, H. G. (1995). Long term developmental outcomes of low birth weight infants. *The Future of Children, 5*(1), 176–196.

Hack, M., Taylor, H. G., Klein, N., & Eiben, R. (1993). Outcome of <750 gm birth weight children at school age. *New England Journal of Medicine, 331,* 753–759.

Hack, M., Taylor, H. G., Klein, N., Eiben, R., Schatschneider, C., & Mercuri-Minich, N. (1994). School-age outcomes in children with birth weights under 750 g. *New England Journal of Medicine, 331*(12), 753–759.

Hoy, E. A., Bill, J. M., & Sykes, D. H. (1988). Very low birth weight: A long term developmental impairment? *International Journal of Behavioral Development, 11,* 37–67.

Hunt, J. V., Cooper, B. A. B., & Tooley, W. H. (1988). Very low birth weight infants at 8 and 11 years of age: Role of neonatal illness and family status. *Pediatrics, 81,* 596–603.

Kempe, A., Wise, P. H., Barkan, S. E., Sappenfield, W. M., Sachs, B., Gortmaker, S. L., Sobol, A. M., First, L. R., Pursley, D., Rinehart, H., Kotelchuck, M., Cole, S., Gunter, N., & Stockbauer, J. W. (1992). Clinical determinants of the racial disparity in very low birth weight. *New England Journal of Medicine, 327*(14), 969–973.

Klein, N. K., Hack, M., & Breslau, N. (1989). Children who were very low birth weight: Development and academic achievement at nine years of age. *Journal of Developmental and Behavioral Pediatrics, 10,* 32–37.

Kleinman, J. C. (1992). The epidemiology of low birth weight. In S. L. Friedman & M. D. Sigman (Eds.), *Annual advances in applied developmental psychology: The psychological development of low birth weight children* Vol. 6 (pp. 21–36). Norwood, NJ: Ablex.

Knobloch, H., Rider, R. V., Harper, P. A., & Pasamanick, K. B. (1956). The neuropsychiatric sequelae of prematurity. *Journal of the American Medical Association, 161,* 581–585.

Kramer, M. S. (1987a). Determinants of low birth weight: Methodological assessment and meta-analysis. *Bulletin of the World Health Organization, 65*(5), 663–737.

Kramer, M. S. (1987b). Intrauterine growth and gestational duration. *Pediatrics, 80*(4), 502–511.

Landry, S. H., Fletcher, J. M., Denson, S. E., & Chapieski, M. L. (1993). Longitudinal outcome for low birth weight infants: Effects of intraventricular hemorrhage and bronchopulmonary dysplasia. *Journal of Clinical and Experimental Neuropsychology, 15*(2), 205–218.

Levy-Shiff, R., Einat, G., Mogilner, M. B., Lerman, M., & Kriker, R. (1994). Biological and environmental correlates of developmental outcome of prematurely born infants in early adolescence. *Journal of Pediatric Psychology, 19,* 63–78.

Lilienfeld, A. M., & Pasamanick, B. (1955). The association of maternal and fetal factors with the development of cerebral palsy and epilepsy. *American Journal of Obstetrics and Gynecology, 70,* 93–101.

Lilienfeld, A. M., Pasamanick, B., & Rogers, M. (1955). Relationship between pregnancy experiences and the development of certain neuropsychiatric disorders in childhood. *American Journal of Public Health, 45,* 637–643.

Lloyd, B. W., Wheldall, K., & Perks, D. (1988). Controlled study of intelligence and school performance of very low-birth weight children from a defined geographic area. *Developmental Medicine and Child Neurology, 30,* 36–42.

Marlow, N., Roberts, B. L., & Cooke, R. W. I. (1989). Motor skills in extremely low birthweight children at the age of 6 years. *Archives of Diseases in Childhood, 64,* 839–847.

McCormick, M. C., Brooks-Gunn, J., Workkman-Daniels, K., Turner, J., & Peckham, G. J. (1992). The health and developmental status of very low-birth-weight children at school age. *Journal of the American Medical Association, 167,* 2204–2208.

Oh, W., & Stern, L. (1987). Respiratory diseases of the newborn. In L. Stern & P. Vert (Eds.), *Neonatal medicine* (pp. 389–402). Cambridge, MA: Masson.

Paneth, N. S. (1995). The problem of low birth weight. *The Future of Children, 5*(1), 19–34.

Pasamanick, B., & Knobloch, H. (1961). Epidemiologic studies on the complications of pregnancy and the birth process. In G. Caplan (Ed.), *Prevention of mental disorders in children* (pp. 133–168). New York: Basic Books.

Pasamanick, B., & Lilienfeld, A. M. (1955). Association of maternal and fetal factors with development of mental deficiency: Abnormalities in the prenatal and perinatal periods. *Journal of the American Medical Association, 159*, 155–160.

Pasamanick, B., Rogers, M. E., & Lilienfeld, A. M. (1956). Pregnancy experience and the development of behavior disorders in children. *American Journal of Psychiatry, 112*, 613–618.

Petrauskas, R. J., & Rourke, B. P. (1979). Identification of subtypes of retarded readers: A neuropsychological multivariate approach. *Journal of Clinical Neuropsychology, 1*, 17–37.

Reitan, R. M., & Davison, L. A. (1974). *Clinical neuropsychology: Current status and applications.* New York: Wiley.

Rickards, A. L., Kitchen, W. H., Doyle, L. W., Ford, G. W., Kelly, E. A., & Callanan, C. (1993). Cognition, school performance, and behavior in very low birth weight and normal birth weight children at 8 years of age: A longitudinal study. *Journal of Developmental and Behavioral Pediatrics, 14*, 363–368.

Rosner, J., & Simon, D. P. (1970). *Auditory Analysis Test: An initial report.* Pittsburgh, PA: University of Pittsburgh, Learning Research and Development Center.

Roth, S. C., Baudin, J., McCormick, D. C., Edwards, A. D., Townsend, J., Stewart, A. L., & Reynolds, E. O. R. (1993). Relation between ultrasound appearance of the brain of very preterm infants and neuro-developmental impairment at eight years. *Developmental Medicine and Child Neurology, 35*, 755–768.

Rosvald, H. E., Mirsky, A. F., Sarason, I., Bransom, E. D., & Beck, I. H. (1956). A continuous performance test of brain damage. *Journal of Consulting Psychology, 20*, 343–349.

Rourke, B. P. (Ed.). (1985). *Neuropsychology of learning disabilities: Essentials of subtype analysis.* New York: Guilford Press.

Rourke, B. P. (Ed.). (1991). *Neuropsychological validation of learning disability subtypes.* New York: Guilford Press.

Rourke, B. P., & Del Dotto, J. E. (1994). Learning disabilities: A neuropsychological perspective. In M. C. Roberts & C. E. Walker (Eds.), *Handbook of clinical child psychology* (pp. 511–536). New York: Wiley.

Rourke, B. P., & Petrauskas, R. J. (1977). *Underlining Test—Revised.* Windsor, Ontario, Canada: University of Windsor, Department of Psychology.

Saigal, S., Szatmari, P., Rosenbaum, P., Campbell, D., & King, S. (1991). Cognitive abilities and school performance of extremely low birth weight children and matched term control children at age 8 years: A regional study. *Journal of Pediatrics, 118*, 751–760.

Semel, E., Wiig, E. H., & Secord, W. (1987). *Clinical Evaluation of Language Fundamentals—Revised.* New York: Psychological Corporation.

Silverstein, A. B. (1983). *Two- and four-subtest short forms of the Wechsler Adult Intelligence Scale—Revised.* New York: Psychological Corporation.

Stewart, A. L., del Costello, A. M., Hamilton, P. A., Baudin, J., Townsend, J., Bradford, B. C., & Reynolds, E. O. R. (1989). Relationship between neurodevelopmental status of very preterm infants at one and four years. *Developmental Medicine and Child Neurology, 31*, 756–765.

Taylor, H. G., Klein, N., & Hack, M. (1994). Academic functioning in <750 gm birth weight children who have normal cognitive abilities: Evidence for specific learning disabilities. *Pediatric Research, 35*, 289A.

Teplin, S. W., Burchinal, M., Johnson-Martin, N., Humphry, R. A., & Kraybill, E. N. (1991). Neurodevelopmental, health, and growth status at age 6 years of children with birth weights less than 1001 grams. *Journal of Pediatrics, 118*, 768–777.

Volpe, J. J. (1987) *Neurology of the newborn.* Philadelphia: W. B. Saunders.

Volpe, J. J. (1989). Intraventricular hemorrhage in the premature infant: Current concepts, Part I. *Annals of Neurology, 25*(1), 3–11.

Volpe, J. J. (1992). Brain injury in the premature infant: Current concepts of pathogenesis and prevention. *Biology of the Neonate, 62*, 231–242.

Vulliamy, D. C., & Johnson, P. G. B. (1987). *The newborn child* (6th ed.). Edinburgh: Churchill Livingstone.

Wechsler, D. (1974). *Wechsler Intelligence Scale for Children—Revised.* New York: Psychological Corporation.

Wyly, M. W. (1995). *Premature infants and their families: Developmental interventions.* San Diego: Singular.

11

TURNER SYNDROME

DANIEL B. BERCH
BRUCE G. BENDER

HISTORICAL OVERVIEW

In 1938, Henry Turner first formally identified a syndrome consisting of sexual infantilism, short stature, primary amenorrhea, webbed neck, and cubitus valgus (wide carrying angle at the elbow). Wilkins and Fleischmann (1944) subsequently demonstrated that ovarian dysgenesis was another cardinal feature of what later came to be known as Turner syndrome (TS). Numerous other physical malformations and clinical manifestations have since been detected in individuals with TS, albeit with a relatively wide variation in frequency. These include a shield chest, low hairline, various skeletal abnormalities, lymphedema at birth, coarctation of the aorta, recurrent otitis media, hearing loss, and renal abnormalities (see Table 11.1 for a more complete listing of the clinical findings). It is of historical interest to note that as early as 1768, Morgagni provided a clinical description of a small woman based on an autopsy that included no identifiable gonadal tissue, along with several other anatomical features corresponding to the physical stigmata that now characterize TS (Tesch & Rosenfeld, 1995). However, it was not until 1959 that the sex chromosome constitution of individuals with TS was determined to be abnormal. Ford, Jones, Polani, De Almedia, and Briggs (1959) demonstrated that a woman presenting with classic clinical features had a 45,X karyotype, or complete monosomy of the second X chromosome. Figure 11.1 (top) shows the karyotype of one such TS female.

Historically, the study of TS individuals has been of interest to researchers in a variety of disciplines, including clinical genetics, behavioral genetics, pediatric endocrinology, pediatric psychology, and developmental psychology. However, the study of children with this type of sex chromosome abnormality has received comparatively little emphasis within the domain of pediatric neuropsychology. One of the reasons for this may be that in some cases the condition does not become evident until late adolescence or early adulthood, when ascertainment is frequently made on the basis of primary or secondary amenorrhea. Second, although it has been known for some time that various cognitive deficits are associated with TS, the underlying neuropathology of these impairments has been much less clear than it has been for many of the central nervous system disorders and systemic illnesses

TABLE 11.1. Clinical Findings in TS

Type	Characteristics
Classical	Short stature Short webbed neck Broad chest Cubitus valgus Gonadal dysgenesis
Growth	Decreased mean birthweight Lack of pubertal growth spurt
Skeletal	Scoliosis Madelung wrist deformity Genu valgum Exostosis medial tibial condyle Short metacarpals, metatarsals
Craniofacial	Craniosynostosis Narrow palate Micrognathia Strabismus Malrotation of ears Inner ear defects
Cardiovascular	Aortic coarctation Bicuspid aortic valve Mitral valve prolapse Septal defect Partial anomalous venous return
Renal	Horseshoe or pelvic kidney Unilateral aplasia or hypoplasia Unilateral double ureter
Lymphatic	Intestinal lymphangiectases Congential lymphedema hands, feet
Hair and skin	Low posterior hairline Increased pigmented nevi Hypoplastic nails Dermatoglyphic variations

Note. Adapted from White (1994). Copyright 1994 by Lawrence Erlbaum Associates. Adapted by permission.

represented in this volume. As Fletcher (1994) recently pointed out, until the 1980s attempts to study "brain–behavior" relationships in developmental disorders such as TS, Williams syndrome, and autism "would generally have been met with firm skepticism—if not outright cynicism—because of the absence of known brain lesions as a basis for the syndrome" (p. 299). Consequently, Fletcher (1994) argued that much of the research concerning children with syndromes such as TS may more appropriately be regarded as the study of "behavior–brain" relationships, with the behavioral features motivating the search for neurobiological correlates. Third, due to the relatively low incidence of this syndrome, along with the lack of severe intellectual, psychopathological, or neuromotor difficulties (albeit subtle ones), most pediatric neuropsychologists are unlikely to encounter many children with this condition. Nonetheless, an awareness of recent advances in the study of the neurocognitive and psychosocial factors associated with TS has important implications not only for improving the diagnosis and remediation of the behavioral sequelae of this

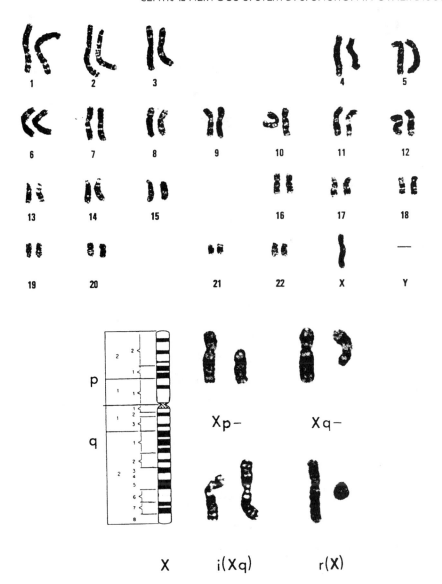

FIGURE 11.1. Top: The complete karyotype of a 45,X TS female. Bottom: Four types of structural abnormalities of the X chromosome found in other TS females, including Xp– (X short-arm deletion), Xq– (X long-arm deletion), i(Xq) (isochromosome for the X long arm), and r(X) (ring X chromosome). In each case, the normal X from the same cell is on the left. From White (1994). Copyright 1994 by Lawrence Erlbaum Associates. Reprinted by permission.

sex chromosome abnormality, but also for advancing theoretical conceptions of the biological mechanisms underlying neuropsychological development in general.

EPIDEMIOLOGY AND PATHOPHYSIOLOGY

The incidence of TS is estimated at 1 in 2,000 to 1 in 5,000 live female births. Fewer than 2% of 45,X conceptions survive to term. Moreover, approximately 10% of all spontaneously aborted fetuses have a 45,X karyotype. It has been estimated that approximately 50% of all females with TS have a pure 45,X karyotype (Hall, Sybert, Williamson, Fisher, & Reed, 1982). An X chromosome monosomy can result from meiotic nondisjunction during either spermatogenesis or oogenesis, or from an error in mitosis after conception (Ross, 1990). TS is not associated either with increased maternal or paternal age (Mathur et al., 1991) or with birth order. Several studies have demonstrated that in more than 70% of 45,X live births and aborted fetuses, it is the paternal sex chromosome that is absent (see Mathur et al., 1991).

In addition to the 45,X karyotype, there are a considerable number of cytogenetic variants associated with TS (see bottom portion of Figure 11.1). These include various kinds of structural abnormalities, such as partial X monosomy (e.g., deletions of the short or long arm of the X chromosome), isochromosome (duplication of the long arm of the second X chromosome), and mosaicism (i.e., two or more cell populations existing simultaneously in the same person, most typically a karyotype involving a combination of cells missing the second X chromosome and those with a normal complement of 46). Whereas earlier reports suggested that TS females with mosaicism may not be as severely affected as nonmosaic 45,X individuals, others have argued that for a number of reasons, it is particularly difficult to assess relationships between specific karyotypic variations and phenotypic clinical features (Sybert, 1990). White (1994) has suggested that the most accurate associations between karyotype and phenotype should emerge from studies comparing 45,X individuals with nonmosaic females who have a structural abnormality of the second X chromosome.

NEUROPATHOLOGY

The lack of sex chromatin material can influence the development of structural aspects of the brain in various ways, including both direct and indirect means (Rovet, 1990). A review of early electroencephalographic studies of TS women revealed that although anywhere from 25% to 75% might exhibit aberrant wave patterns, no consistent abnormalities were apparent (Nielsen, Nyborg, & Dahl, 1977). Neuropathological evidence based on autopsies has been relatively sparse, with assorted case reports yielding evidence of very different types of cerebral anomalies (Brun & Skold, 1968; Reske-Nielsen, Christensen, & Nielsen, 1982). In addition, as Reiss et al. (1993) have noted, wide age variations along with diverse clinical aberrations in these individuals (e.g., cerebrovascular disease or epilepsy) greatly limit the generalizability of the results. At the very least, the autopsy data do not definitively implicate an innate, localized brain abnormality in TS females (Rovet, 1990).

Abnormalities in brain structure and function have also been investigated via neuroimaging techniques. Two case reports of mentally retarded adolescents provided evidence from computed tomography of agenesis of the corpus callosum (Araki et al., 1987; Kimura, Nakajima, & Yoshino, 1990). A positron emission tomography study of five TS individuals with different karyotypes indicated reduced glucose metabolism in both the occipital and parietal cortex, bilaterally (Clark, Konoff, & Hayden, 1990). In a preliminary analysis of magnetic resonance imaging (MRI) data gathered from 8 TS girls and 13 controls, Ross, Reiss, Freund, Roeltgen, and Cutler (1993) provided evidence of increased bilateral ventricular volume for the TS girls, on average, along with greater variance in these indices for the TS girls than for the controls. The authors concluded that these results suggest a generalized process influencing brain development, along with contributions from other genetic, endocrine, or environmental factors. In a recent MRI study of monozygotic twins discordant for TS, Reiss et al. (1993) reported a number of interesting anatomical differences between an 11-year-old TS girl and her unaffected twin. In comparison with her sister, the TS girl had overall increased cerebrospinal fluid (CSF) volumes (25%), as well as a corresponding decrease in volume of gray matter. According to the authors, these results suggest a mild, generalized hypoplasia during neural development. The largest regional differences in CSF and gray matter were in right prefrontal, right posterior parieto-occipital, and left parietoperisylvian cortical areas. Finally, there were differences in the posterior fossa, with a 50% enlargement of the fourth ventricle and cisterna magna, but a reduction (10–15%) in the size of the cerebellar vermis, pons, and medulla.

Examining the MRI scans of 18 TS adults (9 with a 45,X karyotype and 9 with mosaicism) and 19 healthy controls, Murphy et al. (1993) found evidence for bilateral abnormalities that were greater on the right side than on the left. Specifically, as compared with controls, 45,X women exhibited smaller bilateral volumes of cerebral hemispheric and parieto-occipital brain matter, as well as hippocampus, lenticular, and thalamic nuclei, even after corrections for differences in head size. However, these investigators did not detect any difference in the volumes of the lateral ventricles—a finding that conflicts with that of Ross et al. (1993). The mosaic TS subjects yielded values that fell between those of 45,X women and controls for right-hemisphere volume (brain matter plus CSF) and left-hemisphere brain matter, as well as for lenticular, caudate, and thalamic nuclei.

Finally, Reiss, Mazzocco, Greenlaw, Freund, and Ross (1995) have more recently demonstrated somewhat lower proportions of gray and white tissue in the right inferior parietal–occipital region in girls who have TS than in unaffected controls.

In sum, the evidence thus far suggests that monosomy of the X chromosome influences the developing brain in a manner that yields bilateral abnormalities of the cerebral hemispheres, but perhaps to a greater extent on the right side. Although evidence is accruing that indicates reduced total gray matter volume, conclusions regarding more localized structural alterations must await confirmation of the intriguing findings that have just begun to emerge with the use of modern neuroimaging techniques. Furthermore, some efforts have been initiated with the objective of providing more direct links between measures of cognitive function and their presumed neuroanatomical substrates (see Rovet & Buchanan, 1999, for a more thorough treatment of a cognitive neuroscience approach to the study of Turner syndrome).

NEUROPSYCHOLOGICAL SEQUELAE

Neurocognitive Impairments

That TS is associated with neuropsychological impairment has been recognized for over 30 years. The nature of that association, however, has not been well understood, and though a large volume of information from a variety of studies has clarified this picture, some misunderstandings persist.

Early reports indicated that mental retardation was a feature of TS (Grumbach, Van Wyck, & Wilkins, 1955; Haddad & Wilkins, 1959; Polani, 1961). Although numerous debates ensued as to whether mental retardation is increased in TS, the fact that most TS females are not mentally retarded has been well established. However, the initial apparent association between TS and mental retardation created a stereotype of the condition that is not easily dispelled. For example, as late as 1986, one of us used a major introductory psychology text in which a brief mention was made that TS, like Down syndrome, results in mental retardation. This error was pointed out by an undergraduate female with TS who eventually received an A for the course.

As more TS patients became available for observation and study, investigators began to detect a more specific effect of this syndrome on development of cognitive skills. Initial observations suggested a visual–spatial deficit, as evidenced by a large discrepancy between the Verbal and Performance IQs on the Wechsler scales, with the former score falling within the normal range and the latter score much below the average range (Cohen, 1962; Shaffer, 1962). Figure 11.2 shows a typical profile of subtest scores on the Wechsler scales. Labeling the spatial deficit as "space-form blindness," Money (1963) overdramatized the nature of this impairment, bolstering an emergent stereotype that the neurocognitive deficit in TS was severe and homogeneous. Indeed, numerous related deficiencies were subsequently associated with TS, including impaired left–right orientation (Waber, 1979), mental rotation (Berch & Kirkendall, 1986 [see Figure 11.3 for a sample stimulus pair used in this

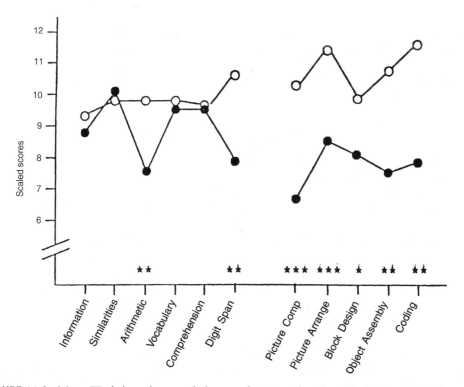

FIGURE 11.2. Mean Wechsler subtest scaled scores for 23 TS females (filled circles) and 23 control females (open circles) with mean chronological ages of 15.4 years and 15.2 years, respectively (asterisks indicate varying levels of significance). From Rovet (1990). Copyright 1990 by AAAS and Westview Press. Reprinted by permission.

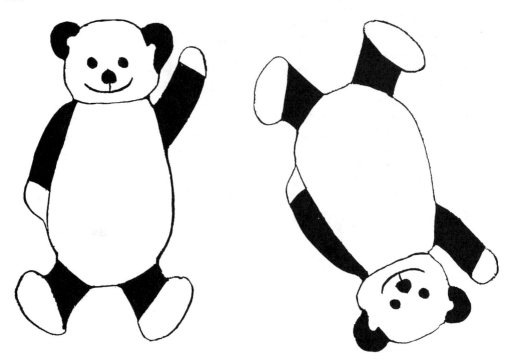

FIGURE 11.3. Sample stimulus pair from a mental rotation task in which a child is asked to decide as quickly as possible, without making errors, whether the bear on the right would have the same (or a different) arm raised as the bear on the left if it were standing upright. From Marmor (1977). Copyright 1977 by the American Psychological Association. Reprinted by permission.

study]; Rovet & Netley, 1980, 1982), visual–perceptual and visual–conceptual skills (Temple & Carney, 1995), drawing (Silbert, Wolff, & Lilienthal, 1977), arithmetic (Garron, 1977), and handwriting (Pennington, Bender, Puck, Salbenblatt, & Robinson, 1982). Garron (1977) argued that when standardized IQ tests are administered, TS patients demonstrate reduced Performance but not Verbal IQs, in support of the view of Money and Alexander (1966) that verbal skills in TS are average to above average. Such findings led to speculations about impaired right-hemisphere functioning (Alexander & Money, 1966; Silbert, Wolff, & Lilienthal, 1977), specifically in the right parietal lobe (Money, 1973).

Subsequent studies have shown that the neuropsychological deficits in children with TS are not limited to the well-documented impairment in spatial thinking, and that these children do exhibit a slightly increased rate of mental retardation. Although most females with TS are not mentally retarded, there is evidence of a mild decrease in Verbal as well as Full Scale IQ. Rovet (1990) reviewed 13 studies reporting IQ scores for a total of 226 individuals with TS and 142 female control subjects. Wechsler Performance IQ scores for TS females were dramatically lower than those of controls (15.1 points), but these individuals also obtained lower scores on Verbal IQ (3.5 points) and Full Scale IQ (9.1 points). Given a normal distribution of IQs in this population, these findings indicate that rates of IQ scores of less than 70 are somewhat higher in women with TS (10.2%) than in the general population (2.3%). It should also be noted that Van Dyke, Wiktor, Roberson, and Weiss (1991) reported that TS women with the cytogenetic variant known as a small X ring chromosome are at increased risk for mental retardation. These women are also more growth-retarded than other individuals with TS and have relatively smaller head circumference.

A number of studies have identified language difficulties in females with TS, and, even more specifically, deficits of verbal memory. Bender, Puck, Salbenblatt, and Robinson (1984) conducted an evaluation of language skills in nine TS and nine chromosomally normal girls as part of the only study in the United States that has incorporated an unselected sample of TS girls, identified not because of clinical presentation but through the chromosome screening of 40,000 consecutive newborns in Denver, Colorado between 1964 and 1974. The school-age TS group was found to have significantly reduced scores in the areas of auditory short-term memory and verbal fluency. Similar TS-related verbal difficulties have been reported by others (Pennington et al., 1985; Rovet & Netley, 1982; Waber, 1976, 1979).

Finally, there is some evidence of poorer performance in girls with TS on tasks that assess executive function skills, putatively subserved by the frontal lobes, although these deficits may be somewhat task specific (Temple, Carney, & Mullarkey, 1996). For example, Temple et al. (1996) demonstrated impaired performance on the Stroop and verbal fluency tasks, but not on the Wisconsin Card Sorting Test or the Tower of London.

Hemispheric Asymmetries

Several investigators have shown that TS women may have neuropsychological impairment suggestive of bilateral brain involvement. In one study, a comprehensive neuropsychological battery was administered to 11 TS patients (13 to 23 years of age). In contrast to normal female controls matched for age and Wechsler Verbal IQ, the TS women demonstrated impaired motor coordination, visual memory, word fluency, and right–left discrimination (Waber, 1979). A similar study of 10 TS adults identified moderately impaired auditory processing, memory, attention, language fluency, and concept development (Pennington et al., 1985). The authors of both studies concluded that, contrary to previously held beliefs, the neuropsychological test performance of persons with TS was not consistent with right-hemisphere brain impairment, but rather with more broad-based dysfunction implicating both hemispheres. When Pennington et al. (1985) contrasted the performance of their TS participants with that of other patient groups assessed with the same neuropsychological battery, the TS group's performance was comparable to that of neurological patients with diffuse bilateral damage, as opposed to that of patients with right-hemisphere damage.

Other data relevant to the issue of hemispheric asymmetries come from studies of atypical cerebral lateralization in persons with TS. After reviewing five studies that made use of the dichotic listening procedure, Rovet (1990) concluded that TS females consistently show weaker left-hemisphere involvement in verbal information processing, sometimes accompanied by increased right-hemisphere involvement. She also reported some of her own data indicating that adolescents and young adults with TS show greater than normal levels of left-hemisphere involvement for the processing of nonverbal information. Consistent with the suggestion of weaker left-hemisphere involvement in verbal processing, Portellano-Perez, Bouthelier, and Asensio-Monge (1996) reported greater activation of right- than left-hemisphere beta rhythms in TS girls (8 to 14 years old) during silent reading and in an arithmetic computation task. However, the TS girls in this study also showed a similar pattern of greater right-hemisphere activation in a puzzle-solving task, whereas controls exhibited the opposite pattern.

Electrophysiological Recording

Evidence emerging from the use of other technologies has begun to enhance our understanding of brain–cognition relationships in TS individuals. For example, Johnson and his colleagues used the event-related potential (ERP) paradigm to assess the magnitude and timing of information-processing operations in "untreated" TS children and adolescents (i.e., subjects were tested prior to receiving hormone replacement therapy). These authors contend that by quantifying the amplitudes and latencies of different ERP components, one can disentangle the relative contributions of various processing stages (e.g., sensory and motor components) to general cognitive impairments (Johnson, Rohrbaugh, & Ross, 1993; Johnson & Ross, 1994). Using an auditory discrimination task referred to as the "oddball" paradigm, Johnson et al. (1993) found that the ERPs in the younger TS girls did not differ from those of their controls. In contrast, amplitudes of ERPs were larger in the postpubertal TS subjects than in their age-matched controls. The specific finding of a frontal negative wave of longer duration in the postpubertal females was interpreted as being consistent with a maturational deficit. Reaction times were slower in both pre- and postpubertal TS subjects than in their controls, leading to the conclusion that these results are consistent with a congenital deficit. The ERP data suggested that the slow reaction times are entirely attributable to deficits in the response-processing stages of selection, preparation, and execution, rather than to impairments in earlier stages of sensory or cognitive processing.

Using a left–right discrimination task (hand identification) with the same sample of females with TS, Johnson and Ross (1994) subsequently reported that both ERP and reaction time data indicated considerable cognitive and motor deficits at both pre- and postpubertal age levels. According to the authors, the fact that the same types of deficits were observed at all ages is suggestive of a congenital deficit. The validity of this conclusion rests on the assumption that congenital lesions produce developmental trajectories that fall below, yet parallel, rates of change in normal individuals (Ris, 1995). Ris (1995) has criticized this premise, arguing that substantial evidence from the developmental neuropsychology literature is incompatible with such an assumption and suggests that growth trajectories for neurologically affected and unaffected groups diverge over time.

BIOLOGICAL MECHANISMS

Attempting to understand biological links between abnormal karyotype and abnormal neuropsychological phenotype, many investigators have made the common error of assuming that two co-occurring events are causally related. In this case, the recognition that sex hormones may play a role in determining sex-related differences in cognitive performance (Williams, Barnet, & Meck, 1990), and that TS patients have abnormally low sex hormone levels, has frequently led investigators to hypothesize that sex hormone abnormalities underlie neuropsychological impairment in TS. The theory of hormone mediation of TS deficits enjoys wide appeal, having been proposed more than 30 years ago (Shaffer, 1962) and continuing to appear in current discussions (Temple & Carney, 1993). It is acknowledged that there is no pre- to postpuberty change in ability profiles that differentiates females with TS from chromosomally normal girls; therefore, the most popularly held belief is that the absence of normal exposure to prenatal endogenous sex hormones sets the stage for incomplete brain development and a subsequent lifetime of neuropsychological impairment. That this theory of the influence of prenatal hormones on cognitive development has minimal scientific support has not diluted its popularity. Unfortunately, after years of such theorizing, no solid evidence of hormone-mediated impairment in TS has emerged to date. However, some progress is being made in this area (Ross & Zinn, 1999). Moreover, as both Collaer and Hines (1995) and Buchanan, Pavlovic, and Rovet (1998) have pointed out, the TS population affords a distinctive opportunity for separating the effects of hormonal and chromosomal factors on cognitive skills, because of almost the complete absence of endogenous estrogen production coupled with the postponement of estrogen therapy until middle to late adolescence. Speculating along these lines, Buchanan et al. (1998) have hypothesized that the chromosomal anomaly in TS may contribute to perceptual impairments independently of deficits in selective attention and orientation, which may reflect an acquired abnormality.

Most psychological studies of TS have considered this condition in isolation. When TS is examined in the broader context of other sex chromosome abnormalities, the hormone mediation theory becomes less plausible. Of the other three sex chromosome abnormalities involving a single chromosome aneuploidy (47,XXX, 47,XXY, and 47,XYY), sex hormone deficiencies are present only among 47,XXY men. However, all these conditions are associated with intellectual deficits and learning disabilities (Bender, Linden, & Robinson, 1993). Furthermore, whereas the cognitive deficiencies of 47,XXX women are even greater than those associated with TS, 47,XXX women have normal levels of sex hormones. Although 47,XXX women do not exhibit the specific deficits seen in TS women, the fact that all four of these sex chromosome abnormalities involve cognitive deficiencies strongly suggests that there is a common causal mechanism independent of sex hormones.

Another neurodevelopmental theory has been proffered to explain the impact of sex chromosomes upon the developing central nervous system. Specifically, some evidence indicates that the absence of an X chromosome shortens the cell cycle, thus accelerating the rate of cell division and subsequently altering the rate of brain growth (Barlow, 1973; Polani, 1977). Netley (1977) hypothesized that normal critical periods during which the brain's hemispheres develop their specialized information-processing capacities are disrupted in the case of TS, leading to atypical lateralization and cognitive impairment. Although the finding that chromosomally normal children with delayed growth have cognitive deficits bolsters this theory slightly, there remains little additional supportive evidence.

PSYCHOSOCIAL ADAPTATION

Several studies have described an increased incidence of depression, anorexia nervosa, and schizophrenia in TS women (Darby, Garfinkel, Vale, Kirwan, & Brown, 1981; Halmi & DeBault, 1974; Raft, Spencer, & Toomey, 1976; Sabbath, Morris, Menzer-Benaron, & Sturgis, 1961). These findings may have been subject to a selection bias, however, since these studies were based on convenient samples of clinical patients. Results from four larger and possibly less biased studies indicate that psychopathology is present in a relatively low proportion of these women. Eleven percent of TS patients (5 of 45) in Denmark (Nielsen et al., 1977), 8% of TS patients (4 of 49) in Finland (Taipale, 1979), 13% of TS patients (9 of 68) in the United States (Money & Mittenthal, 1970), and 0% of TS patients (0 of 103) in a second Danish study (Nielsen & Sillesen, 1981) met criteria for clinical disorders.

Although obvious psychopathology may be relatively uncommon, difficulties of psychological adaptation and the existence of distinct personality styles in TS females have been identified. TS females are frequently described as immature and socially reluctant. Based on interviews with 86 TS women, Nielsen and Sillesen (1981) found that the majority of individuals in their sample were normally adjusted, but that one-third of the group had behavioral difficulties including insecurity, shyness, and excessive sensitivity. Shaffer (1962) administered the Minnesota Multiphasic Personality Inventory (MMPI) to 13 TS adolescents and adults. The results of the MMPI suggested that the group had low energy, a nonreactive personality style, and somewhat overcooperative behavior. This theme of unassertive and overcompliant behavior was echoed in a subsequent study of 73 TS patients by Money and Mittenthal (1970). McCauley (1990), providing a slightly more positive portrayal of this pattern of personality and adaptation, reviewed nine TS studies and concluded that many of these women with TS possess an unambiguous female gender identification, strong heterosexual orientation, and an inclination to follow traditional, somewhat stereotyped patterns of female behavior and goals.

The behavioral difficulties associated with TS vary with developmental level. In a study of two age groupings of TS patients (9–14 years and 17–29 years), younger subjects demonstrated immaturity and muted affect, whereas the older subjects, who also had received hormone treatments, were viewed as more mature but with diminished heterosexual activity and a lessened capacity to understand the nuances of social interaction (Rothchild & Owens, 1972). Sonis et al. (1983) identified increased activity level and difficulty with concentration in 6- to 11-year-old TS girls, whereas they observed anxious, depressed, and socially withdrawn behavior in 12- to 16-year-old girls. Others have also reported an increase in distractibility and hyperactivity in TS girls under 11 years of age (Rovet, 1986; Rovet & Ireland, 1994; Swillen et al., 1993).

By adolescence, low self-esteem and social withdrawal are common correlates of TS (McCauley, Ross, Kushner, & Cutler, 1995). In a study of 17 TS girls and 16 short-stature female controls, McCauley, Ito, and Kay (1986) conducted psychological evaluations consisting of a clinical interview and self-report questionnaires. The TS girls, 17 years of age or younger, were found to be more socially immature and to have fewer friends than short-stature controls. Increased anxiety (Rovet, 1986), difficulty with social interactions, and immature sexual development (Rothchild & Owens, 1972) have also been described in TS adolescents.

Attempts have been made to establish a causal relationship between the spatial deficits and social immaturity found in TS patients. According to Rourke (1989), neurologically based nonverbal learning disabilities can interfere with an individual's ability to perceive and understand subtle social cues. As a result, the nuances of facial expressions and gestures are not always appreciated, and appropriate responses to the behavioral signals that govern social relationships are not forthcoming (Semrud-Clikeman & Hynd, 1990). Applying this theoretical model to TS, McCauley, Kay, Ito, and Treder (1987) evaluated 17 TS and 17 short-stature control girls with a series of questionnaires and the Affective Discrimination Task. In the latter, subjects were presented with a series of videotaped facial expressions, each of which must be judged as to whether the facial expression indicates approach or avoidance. The TS group was significantly less accurate in interpreting the facial expressions. The ability to interpret facial expressions was also correlated with parents' ratings of social skills.

The finding of decreased ability to read social cues is interesting and may help explain some of the difficulty experienced by TS girls in psychosocial adaptation. The documented difficulty these girls have with verbal fluency, noted earlier (e.g., Waber, 1979), may also contribute to problems in socialization. Still, neither of these cognitive deficits is likely to account for more than a small portion of the difficulties TS females have in social adaptation. Short stature, physical stigmata, and the knowledge of one's own infertility are powerful factors that may well interfere with positive self-esteem and social confidence. Results from interviews of 22 middle-aged TS women indicated that they had usually isolated themselves from peers as a result of feeling "different." Ovarian failure and infertility were described by these women as issues that represented major psychological hurdles, frequently resulting in depression (Sylven, Magnusson, Hagenfeldt, & von Schoultz, 1993). In a study involving mailed-in questionnaires rather than personal interviews of 20 TS women, 50% expressed social insecurity, low self-confidence, and depression (Delooz, van de Berghe, Swillen, Kleczkowska & Fryns, 1993). The majority of women in both of the latter studies were married and gainfully employed outside the home.

Although they generally demonstrate a primary heterosexual orientation (Money & Mittenthal, 1970), TS women tend to date later than peers (Senzer et al., 1973), have lower sexual drive (Garron & Vander Stoep, 1969), have sex later and less often (Nielsen et al., 1977), and struggle with painful intercourse related to vaginal constriction and sore membranes (Sylven et al., 1993). As compared with chromosomally normal females, TS women are less likely to have a significant heterosexual relationship or to get married (Hampson, Hampson, & Money, 1955; Nielsen et al., 1977).

An intriguing finding regarding a possible genetic origin for social adjustment difficulties in TS females was recently reported by Skuse et al. (1997). These investigators demonstrated that in subjects 11 to 25 years of age, a much lower proportion of the TS females whose single X chromosome was of paternal origin exhibited clinically significant social difficulties (28.6%) as compared with the proportion of TS females demonstrating such problems whose X chromosome was of maternal origin (72.4%). As the former group also showed higher scores on a measure of social cognition along with superior verbal and executive function skills, which are thought to mediate social interactions, the researchers concluded that their results demonstrate an imprinted X-linked locus for social cognitive skills.

In summary, psychopathology is relatively rare among TS girls and women. Diminished concentration and hyperactivity are relatively common among TS girls, whereas TS adolescents report being self-conscious, anxious, depressed, and socially isolated. Although many TS women marry and succeed educationally and vocationally (Orten & Orten, 1992), social immaturity, anxiety, depression, and low self-confidence are found more frequently in this group than among their chromosomally normal peers (Bender, Harmon, Linden, Bucher-Bartelson, & Robinson, 1999).

Given that most TS children are neither mentally retarded nor psychologically maladjusted, how might we best characterize the range of their more subtle neurocognitive deficits and psychosocial dysfunctions? Citing evidence of decreased math and memory scores and increased reports of impulsivity and social isolation in TS girls, Williams and colleagues (Williams, 1994; Williams, Richman, & Yarbrough, 1991, 1992) have argued that this pattern of difficulties is very similar to that found in children with nonverbal learning disabilities. One study of 13 TS children included groups of 13 female and 14 male controls with nonverbal learning disabilities (Williams et al., 1992). All three groups performed similarly on tests of verbal memory, sequential memory, sustained attention, and comprehension. Although the absence of tests of other cognitive abilities limits the generalizability of these findings, the investigators concluded that TS and nonverbal learning disabilities are quite similar. The above-normal rates of arithmetic deficits, hyperactivity, and social isolation among girls and women with TS are consistent with this view.

METHODOLOGICAL ISSUES

Various methodological issues have emerged with the publication of a large number of psychological studies of TS in the past two decades. Some investigators working in this field have been well aware of the limitations of their own research, frequently raising these issues when attempting to interpret their results. Previous reviews of the psychological literature have also highlighted some of the more prominent difficulties associated with this research area (Bender, Linden, & Robinson, 1994; Berch, 1990; McCauley, 1990; Rovet, 1990). In this section, we discuss the major methodological problems that arise in neuropsychological research with TS populations, along with some suggestions for improved research designs. The most common methodological weaknesses include sampling bias, small sample sizes, heterogeneity of karyotypes, failure to consider physical anomalies, inappropriate comparison groups, and misapplication of statistical procedures.

Ascertainment and Sampling Bias

As Smith (1990) has noted, the methods for ascertainment of potential participants are extremely important in carrying out research in both genetics and psychology. Rovet and Ireland (1994) suggest that a sampling bias may occur when children with problems are referred for psychological evaluation by their pediatricians, pediatric endocrinologists, or clinical geneticists. In addition, these authors argue that samples of children recruited directly from endocrine clinics may be biased, because parents whose children have preexisting behavioral problems may be more amenable to participating in a psychological study.

Consistent with this viewpoint, it is typically believed that the use of selected samples of individuals with any type of sex chromosome aneuploidy is likely to yield a negative bias for cognitive status, primarily for the reasons discussed above. However, this account cannot explain the finding that the mean Wechsler Full Scale IQ score for unselected TS females in the Bender et al. (1984) prospective study, which is the only study of unselected TS subjects in the United States, is about 10 points lower than that reported by Rovet (1990). The latter investigation pooled data from 226 selected TS females across 13 studies. There has been an increasing awareness of the condition worldwide over the past decade, following the impact of contact groups (e.g., the U.S. and Canadian Turner's Syndrome Societies, operating at local, state or province, and national levels). There has also been access to a wider range of TS girls participating in growth hormone therapy trials. As a result of the increasing recognition of TS, the samples in the studies surveyed by Rovet may actually have consisted of TS females representing the higher end of the distribution; that is, a positive bias may have been present. It is possible that TS adults who are willing to participate in these studies are those who are better educated and adjusted, and who are also interested in the purposes of such projects. Likewise, parents who permit their TS children and adolescents to participate in psychological studies are almost by definition more interested in learning about their children's strengths as well as their impairments—a characteristic that may correlate with higher overall family functioning.

One possible source of evidence in support of this hypothesis comes from a study by Rovet (1993) of psychoeducational characteristics of 67 TS children averaging 12.2 years of age (range = 6 to 16 years). She argued that because the TS children were referred for psychological evaluation to Toronto's Hospital for Sick Children as part of their initial diagnostic workup, there was probably no ascertainment bias. However, the mean IQ score of this sample was 90—midway between the mean reported for the unselected sample of Bender et al. (1984) and the mean computed by Rovet (1990) for selected TS samples. Furthermore, Rovet's (1993) TS children scored significantly lower in IQ than a comparison group of sixth-grade children, although she concluded that this difference was due to significantly poorer performance on certain subtests rather than to globally reduced intelligence.

In a study by Orten and Orten (1992), 750 members of the U.S. Turner Syndrome Society were contacted with questions about educational achievement, occupational status, and personal happiness. Responses from the 411 TS subjects who completed the questionnaire led the authors to conclude that educational and vocational achievement in TS is similar to that of the genetically normal population. Given the very real possibility that higher-achieving women might have responded more willingly to such a questionnaire, the findings would have been positively biased and their generalizability suspect.

Small Sample Sizes

Many studies have been limited by small sample sizes. Examination of the 16 studies of intellectual characteristics compiled by Rovet (1990; see her Table 3.1) reveals a median sample size of 12. As Rovet (1990) noted, the use of small samples increases the probability of a type II error (i.e., not finding an effect when there in fact is one). Another problem arising in studies with small sample sizes is that in order to recruit enough subjects, investigators frequently have had to include TS individuals varying widely in age. In 12 of the 16 studies reviewed by Rovet (1990) (the others did not report age ranges, or consisted of case studies), the median age range was 12.5 years. In at least two-thirds of these studies, the ages ranged from preadolescence to young adulthood. Reiss et al. (1993) argued that the inclusion of both pre- and postpubertal females in the same study potentially complicates the interpretation of findings, because of hormonal and genetic factors that may increase the variance within the TS sample.

One possible solution to the problem of small sample sizes is a multicenter collaborative study. Studies of this type have recently become more feasible, primarily as a result of attempts at a national level to conduct large clinical trials of growth hormone therapy. The report by Rovet and Ireland (1994), which summarizes psychosocial characteristics of TS children, is the product of such an approach. Their subjects were recruited from a target group of 130 TS children (aged 7 to 13 years) participating in the Canadian TS Humatrope trial. This project was conducted at 13 pediatric endocrine clinics in major Canadian cities. According to Rovet and Ireland (1994), this approach circumvents most of the types of sampling biases described earlier, and can also yield large samples of children falling within relatively restricted age ranges. These researchers argue that although this strategy may not totally eliminate sampling bias, the reasons for participating in a growth hormone study are not likely to be correlated with the types of variables investigated in psychological research. However, Rovet and Ireland (1994) also state that psychological studies of TS children recruited from growth hormone trials may yield a negative bias. This is because children with less severe phenotypic characteristics are probably not included in such trials, since a diagnosis of TS may not be made until later in development, due to delayed sexual maturation, infertility, or early menopause.

Heterogeneous Samples

The vast majority of TS samples have consisted of females with a variety of different karyotypes, including mosaicism. McCauley (1990) has argued that this karyotypic heterogeneity increases phenotypic heterogeneity and precludes a more fine-grained analysis of karyotypic subgroups, especially in light of the small sample sizes that typically characterize TS research. Even with a comparatively large sample size, this problem is not easily ameliorated. For example, in their study of 112 girls, Rovet and Ireland (1994) reported that there were 8 or fewer children in six of the karyotype subgroups. This made it difficult to draw firm conclusions with regard to relationships between psychosocial functioning and karyotype.

Role of Physical Anomalies

McCauley (1990) has also argued that in contrast to other types of sex chromosome aneuploidies, the physical anomalies associated with TS can complicate the interpretation of impairments in psychosocial functioning. In other words, short stature along with other phenotypic stigmata may directly influence how others treat TS females, which in turn can influence the development of various dimensions of self-esteem (Bender et al., 1994). For example, recent research (Young-Hyman, 1990) suggests that children with short stature due to constitutional growth delay are not pervasively low in self-esteem or socially withdrawn, but that these children are at risk for the development of various psychosocial difficulties, including displeasure with their body image and physical adequacy. Without appropriate comparison groups, a researcher cannot therefore confidently attribute dysfunctional behaviors to the sex chromosome abnormality per se.

Another approach to studying the impact of physical anomalies is to examine relationships between the degree of physical abnormality and the severity of behavioral dysfunction, as long as a sample is large enough to permit a meaningful correlational analysis. Rovet and Ireland (1994), for example, found a significant within-group, positive relationship between height and social competence, but no relationship between height and behavior problems. In contrast, McCauley et al. (1995) reported that the level of social competence within their sample of 93 TS girls was unrelated to height. One final complication that can ensue from the easily identifiable physical anomalies of many persons with TS is that a psychologist cannot evaluate the participants in person without being aware which subjects have TS (McCauley, 1990).

Comparison Groups

One of the most challenging aspects of designing methodologically sound psychological studies of TS females is arriving at a judicious choice of a comparison group. The modal approach has been to match controls to persons with TS based on a single characteristic, such as chronological age or Verbal IQ. Less frequently, investigators have employed a multivariate matching procedure (see Berch, 1990, for detailed descriptions of various types of matching techniques). As Rovet (1990) has summarized, TS researchers have matched for chronological age, Wechsler Full Scale IQ, Wechsler Verbal IQ, socioeconomic status, race and/or ethnicity, and physical stature. Others have used female siblings as controls. Berch (1990) has suggested that the nature of the hypothesis being tested should dictate the choice of matching procedures, and that appropriate matching can illuminate biological mechanisms underlying neuropsychological dysfunction. A study by Pennington et al. (1985) represents one such application of this approach. These investigators incorporated various groups of controls with brain damage (either diffuse or lateralized) to assess similarities and differences in patterns of neuropsychological impairment between TS females and patients with defined lesions. Another example of this approach is a study by Mazzocco (1998) that made use of a control group of girls with fragile X syndrome who had IQ scores within the normal range. This group was included in order to delineate more precisely the specificity of the mathematics profiles of TS girls, given that girls with fragile X syndrome also generally exhibit poor mathematical skills.

As Reiss et al. (1993) have argued, interpretation of findings from studies employing matched-pairs designs is typically complicated by potential genetic and hormonal heterogeneity in the TS sample. Matching for short stature, for example, cannot control either for autosomal genetic influences or for the family environment. Even the use of female siblings does not control for the majority of autosomal genetic factors.

A more optimal way to control for the influence of factors that could otherwise confound the interpretations of performance differences between TS females and standard comparison groups is the use of twins, with one member of the pair being the individual with TS and the other her unaffected sister. Although this type of occurrence is extremely rare, Rovet (1990) has summarized the results of data from three such sets of twins. In each case, a discrepancy between the Wechsler Verbal and Performance IQ scores was found. Unfortunately, zygosity data were not available, clouding the interpretation of these results. More recently, however, Reiss et al. (1993) reported the results of a study of 11-year-old monozygotic twins discordant for TS, with no evidence of chromosomal mosaicism. Generally, the neurocognitive and psychosocial assessments yielded mild impairments exclusive to the TS twin; however, both girls were extremely unrepresentative in terms of their global cognitive status, with Wechsler Full Scale IQs of 135 and 145 for the TS twin and her sister, respectively. Furthermore, as the authors point out, other factors associated with twinning could complicate the interpretation of results from such studies, including risks due to unfavorable conditions *in utero*, and differences in cytoplasmic inheritance or the occurrence of postzygotic mutations that could differentially influence brain development in monozygotic twins.

Statistical Matters

An unfortunately common practice in research on small samples of individuals with TS involves carrying out numerous statistical tests to compare the performance levels of TS and control subjects on a variety of neurocognitive and psychosocial measures. Unless one controls for the level of experimentwise error rate through the use of techniques such as the Bonferroni adjustment, type I error may occur (i.e., finding effects that are more likely to be attributable to chance). In an analysis of small-sample research, Bates and Appelbaum (1994) discuss how to protect against multiple significance tests, using techniques that go beyond the classical methods for type I error control. Furthermore, they provide a list of other "homilies" for small-sample research, one of which is relevant to conducting research with TS samples. Specifically, with small samples of individuals from special populations, critical assumptions underlying the use of standard parametric techniques (e.g., the *t* test) are frequently violated. To handle such problems, Bates and Appelbaum suggest the use of other statistical methods, such as randomization tests. Although such tests are computationally intensive because of the need to create an empirically based randomization distribution, these authors argue that with the innovation of an "approximate" randomization test (Edgington, 1987) and the advent of high-speed personal computers, use of this kind of methodology has recently become much more feasible.

FUTURE DIRECTIONS

As we look toward future directions in neuropsychological research with TS children and adolescents, it is useful to review recent suggestions from other investigators and to determine the extent to which these recommendations have been followed. A survey of major articles and book chapters suggests a need for (1) increased sample sizes, (2) multicenter collaborative efforts, (3) better controls, (4) more attempts to investigate the contribution of environmental risk factors such as family dysfunction, (5) additional efforts to explore associations between cytogenetic variants and behavioral phenotypes, (6) computerized testing, (7) neuroimaging and ERP techniques, (8) theoretically driven study of cognitive deficits, and (9) application of causal modeling approaches for purposes of data analysis and interpretation.

Although some headway has been made with regard to many of these recommendations, much remains to be done. For example, causal modeling and path-analytic techniques represent potentially useful approaches for examining putative causal relationships among cytogenetic, hormonal, neuroanatomical, and neuropsychological variables in the study of sex chromosome abnormalities (Berch, 1990). Nevertheless, to our knowledge, these tools have not yet been applied to the study of TS. This may be attributable in large part to the complexities involved in the use and interpretation of these techniques. However, readable introductory texts on causal modeling are now available (e.g., Loehlin, 1987), and most advanced statistical packages for personal computers contain relatively easy-to-follow procedures for testing various types of path-analytic models.

Another issue that has received rather limited attention is the role of environmental risk factors. In the only such study to date, Bender, Linden, and Robinson (1987) explored the relationship between the quality of the family environment and the phenotypic expression of sex chromosome abnormalities. They found that TS girls from dysfunctional families were more impaired in psychosocial adjustment, school adaptation, and neuromotor development than TS girls from good-functioning families. Differences between TS girls and chromosomally normal control children were apparent only when analysis was restricted to children from dysfunctional family environments. As Rovet (1993) has argued, these results highlight the importance of studying the effects of environmental risk factors on the biological and psychological development of TS children. We agree that further investigation of these issues is necessary in order to achieve a more complete account of the neurocognitive and psychosocial sequelae of a 45,X karyotype.

Fletcher (1994) has suggested that it might be especially illuminating if researchers were to compare cognitive functioning in relationship to biological variables within subgroups of TS children. Consistent with this recommendation, Murphy et al. (1994) investigated what they referred to as an "X chromosome dosage effect" by comparing the neurocognitive performance of two subgroups of TS adult females (45,X individuals and mosaics), and also by examining associations between neuropsychological measures and percentage of lymphocytes having a 45,X karyotype in the mosaic TS subjects. In the latter analysis, the percentage of lymphocytes was strongly correlated with visual–spatial ability ($r = -.76$); specifically, the greater the percentage of lymphocytes, the slower the speed of mental rotation of various letter stimuli. This is a most intriguing finding that bears replication and extension.

A common theme in research on neuropsychological outcomes of pediatric conditions is the need for a theoretically driven foundation for the measures one chooses to employ. For example, in discussing neuropsychological research with TS children, Fletcher (1994) has noted that "the bulk of the research on the behavioral phenotype consists of clinical studies of IQ scores and other more traditional measures" (p. 305). Fletcher additionally argues, "Contemporary models of cognition have not been applied to children with Turner syndrome" (p. 305). The recent application by Rovet, Szekely, and Hockenberry (1994) of a cognitive model of mathematical processing (McCloskey, Caramazza, & Basili, 1985) to arithmetic error patterns exhibited by children with TS constitutes an important step in this direction. Using this model, these investigators demonstrated that mathematical difficulties in TS children are attributable to inadequate procedural skills (such as carrying out basic arithmetic calculations) rather than to poorer conceptualization ability.

Consistent with both the approach and results of Rovet et al. (1994), Mazzocco (1998) recently reported that TS girls make more operation errors (e.g., subtracting instead of adding) and more alignment errors than girls with fragile X syndrome, who also experience difficulties with mathematics. Concomitantly, by administering a series of tasks based on the McCloskey et al. model (1985), Temple and Marriott (1998) also found impaired calculation skills in TS females. These girls exhibited more multiplication and division errors than their unaffected controls and also retrieved addition facts at a slower rate. The latter finding apparently does not reflect a general slowness of responding in TS girls, given that their oral reading rate is no slower than that of controls (Temple & Carney, 1996).

Another potentially useful direction for future research might be to draw upon the conceptual frameworks that have proven helpful in studying other populations with neuropsychological disorders. Models of working memory, such as that of Baddeley and Hitch (1974), provide excellent examples of a potentially productive theoretical approach to the study of neuropsychological deficits (Becker, 1994). Berch (Berch, 1996; Berch & Hartmann, 1992) has already drawn upon this conception as a framework for interpreting cognitive deficits associated with TS. Specifically, he has suggested that the impaired Backward Digit Span performance of TS children, adolescents, and adults could be reflective of a reduced working memory capacity, and that this deficit may underlie the weaknesses exhibited by TS females across a wide spectrum of cognitive tasks. Evidence in support of this hypothesis has recently been reported by Buchanan et al. (1998).

Finally, it is important to realize that the future study of TS in particular and sex chromosome aneuploidy in general is likely to have significant implications for the larger domain of pediatric neuropsychology. In this regard, Pennington and Smith (1988) noted that "the study of genetically influenced learning disabilities may provide for developmental neuropsychology what the study of acquired lesions has provided for adult neuropsychology" (p. 822). Smith (1990) subsequently proposed that the study of variations in sex chromosome abnormalities illustrates the range of influences of genetic factors on cognition and behavior. We concur that these consequences include subtle variations in functioning within the normal range.

EPILOGUE

In recent years, it has become almost routine to end a discourse on the topic of TS with a caveat concerning the tendency to make inappropriate generalizations based on either average or modal behavioral outcomes reported in the literature. In other words, a call for the recognition of the extreme variability of phenotypic features exhibited by TS individuals is usually in order. This heterogeneity became particularly evident to both of us upon attending an international contact group meeting of several hundred TS females, ranging from infants to the elderly. At the very least, one comes away from such an event with a true appreciation of the sizable range of physical, neuropsychological, psychiatric, psychosocial, educational, socioeconomic, and vocational characteristics in this population. These personal encounters, together with published case reports, reveal that individuals with TS run the gamut from mentally retarded to intellectually gifted, from clumsy to well coordinated, from ill to healthy, from obese to anorectic, from socially inept to socially adept, from affectively flat to ebullient, from well to poorly educated, from laborers to highly specialized professionals, from low in visual–spatial ability to artistically talented (e.g., a graphic artist, a sculptor), and from inordinately weak in arithmetic to highly skilled in advanced mathematics (e.g., an astrophysicist). Thus, when forming a conception of the prototypical female with TS, pediatric neuropsychologists and other medical and professional personnel should bear in mind that various as-yet-unknown biological and environmental factors may attenuate or potentiate the influence of a missing X chromosome on developing physical and behavioral phenotypes.

ACKNOWLEDGMENTS

Preparation of this chapter was supported in part by Grant No. MCJ-399156-07-0 from the Maternal and Child Health Bureau, Health Resources and Services Administration, Public Health Service, U.S. Department of Health and Human Services (DHHS), and by Award No. 09DD0328/03 from the Administration on Developmental Disabilities, Administration for Children and Families, DHHS. The opinions expressed in this chapter do not necessarily represent the views of the U.S. Department of Education.

REFERENCES

Alexander, D., & Money, J. (1966). Turner's syndrome and Gerstmann's syndrome: Neuropsychologic comparisons. *Neuropsychologia, 4*, 165–273.

Araki, K., Matsumoto, K., Shiraishi, T., Ogura, H., Kurashige, T., & Kitamura, I. (1987). Turner's syndrome with agenesis of the corpus callosum, Hashimoto's thyroiditis and horseshoe kidney. *Acta Paediatrica Japonica, 29*, 622–626.

Baddeley, A. D., & Hitch, G. J. (1974). Working memory. In G. H. Bower (Ed.), *The psychology of learning and motivation* (Vol. 8, pp. 47–90). San Diego, CA: Academic Press.

Barlow, D. (1973). The influence of inactive chromosomes on human development. *Humangenetik, 17*, 105–136.

Bates, E., & Appelbaum, M. (1994). Methods of studying small samples: Issues and examples. In S. H. Broman & J. Grafman (Eds.), *Atypical cognitive deficits in developmental disorders: Implications for brain function* (pp. 245–280). Hillsdale, NJ: Erlbaum.

Becker, J. T. (1994). Introduction to the special section: Working memory and neuropsychology—Interdependence of clinical and experimental research. *Neuropsychology, 8*, 483–484.

Bender, B. G., Harmon, R. J., Linden, M. G., Bucher-Bartelson, B., & Robinson, A. (1999). Psychosocial competence of unselected young adults with sex chromosome abnormalities. *Neuropsychiatric Genetics, 88*, 200–206.

Bender, B. G., Linden, M., & Robinson, A. (1987). Environment and developmental risk in children with sex chromosome abnormalities. *Journal of the American Academy of Child Psychiatry, 26*, 499–503.

Bender, B. G., Linden, M. G., & Robinson, A. (1993). Neuropsychological impairment in 42 adolescents with sex chromosome abnormalities. *American Journal of Medical Genetics (Neuropsychiatric Genetics), 48*, 169–173.

Bender, B. G., Linden, M. G., & Robinson, A. (1994). Neurocognitive and psychosocial phenotypes associated with Turner syndrome. In S. H. Broman & J. Grafman (Eds.), *Atypical cognitive deficits in developmental disorders: Implications for brain function* (pp. 197–216). Hillsdale, NJ: Erlbaum.

Bender, B. G., Puck, M., Salbenblatt, J., & Robinson, A. (1984). Cognitive development of unselected girls with complete and partial X monosomy. *Pediatrics, 73*, 175–182.

Berch, D. B. (1990). Methodological issues in SCA research. In D. B. Berch & B. G. Bender (Eds.), *Sex chromosome abnormalities and human behavior: Psychological studies* (pp. 185–222). Boulder, CO: AAAS/Westview Press.

Berch, D. B. (1996). Memory. In J. F. Rovet (Ed.), *Turner syndrome across the lifespan* (pp. 140–145). Toronto: Klein Graphics.

Berch, D. B., & Hartmann, L. A. (1992, October). Digit span, processing efficiency, and IQ in Turner syndrome. In B. G. Bender & R. J. Harmon (Cochairs), *Psychological development of children, adolescents, and adults with sex chromosome abnormalities.* Symposium presented at the meeting of the American Academy of Child and Adolescent Psychiatry, Washington, DC.

Berch, D. B., & Kirkendall, K. L. (1986, May). Spatial information processing in 45,X children. In A. Robinson (Chair), *Cognitive and psychosocial dysfunctions associated with sex chromosome abnormalities.* Symposium presented at the meeting of the American Association for the Advancement of Science, Philadelphia.

Brun, A., & Skold, G. (1968). CNS malformations in Turner's syndrome: An integral part of the syndrome? *Acta Neuropathologica, 10*, 159–161.

Buchanan, L., Pavlovic, J., & Rovet, J. (1998). A re-examination of the visuospatial deficit in Turner syndrome: Contributions of working memory. *Developmental Neuropsychology, 14*, 341–367.

Clark, C., Klonoff, H., & Hayden, M. (1990). Regional cerebral glucose metabolism in Turner syndrome. *Canadian Journal of Neurosciences, 17*, 140–144.

Cohen, H. (1962). Psychological test findings in adolescents having ovarian dysgenesis. *Psychosomatic Medicine, 24*, 249–256.

Collaer, M. L., & Hines, M. (1995). Human behavioral sex differences: A role for gonadal hormones during early development? *Psychological Bulletin, 118*, 55–107.

Darby, P. L., Garfinkel, P. E., Vale, J. M., Kirwan, P. J., & Brown, G. M. (1981). Anorexia nervosa and Turner syndrome: Cause or coincidence? *Psychological Medicine, 11*, 141–145.

Delooz, J., Van den Berghe, H., Swillen, A., Kleczkowska, A., & Fryns, J. P. (1993). Turner syndrome patients as adults: A study of their cognitive profile, psychosocial functioning and psychopathological findings. *Genetic Counseling, 4*, 169–179.

Edgington, E. S. (1987). *Randomization tests* (2nd ed.). New York: Marcel Dekker.

Fletcher, J. M. (1994). Afterword: Behavior–brain relationships in children. In S. H. Broman & J. Grafman (Eds.), *Atypical cognitive deficits in developmental disorders: Implications for brain function* (pp. 297–326). Hillsdale, NJ: Erlbaum.

Ford, C. E., Jones, K. W., Polani, P. E., De Almedia, J. C., & Briggs, J. H. (1959). A sex-chromosome anomaly in a case of gonadal dysgenesis (Turner's syndrome). *Lancet, i*, 711.

Garron, D. C. (1977). Intelligence among persons with Turner's syndrome. *Behavior Genetics, 7*, 105–127.

Garron, D. C., & Vander Stoep, L. R. (1969). Personality and intelligence in Turner's syndrome. *Archives of General Psychiatry, 21*, 339–346.

Grumbach, M. M., Van Wyck, J. J., & Wilkins, L. (1955). Chromosomal sex in gonadal dysgenesis relationship to male pseudohermaphroditism and theories of human sex differentiation. *Journal of Clinical Endocrinology, 15*, 1161–1193.

Haddad, H. M., & Wilkins, L. (1959). Congenital abnormalities associated with gonadal aplasia: Review of 55 cases. *Pediatrics, 23*, 885–902.

Hall, J. G., Sybert, V. P., Williamson, R. A., Fisher, N. L., & Reed, S. D. (1982). Turner's syndrome. *Western Journal of Medicine, 137*, 32–44.

Halmi, K. A., & DeBault, L. E. (1974). Gonosomal aneuploidy in anorexia nervosa. *American Journal of Human Genetics, 26*, 195–198.

Hampson, J. L., Hampson, J. C., & Money, J. (1955). The syndrome of gonadal agenesis (ovarian agenesis) and male chromosome pattern in girls and women: Psychologic studies. *Bulletin of Johns Hopkins Hospital, 97*, 207–226.

Johnson, R., Jr., Rohrbaugh, J. W., & Ross, J. L. (1993). Altered brain development in Turner's syndrome: An event-related potential study. *Neurology, 43*, 801–808.

Johnson, R., Jr., & Ross, J. L. (1994). Event-related potential indications of altered brain development in Turner syndrome. In S. H. Broman & J. Grafman (Eds.), *Atypical cognitive deficits in developmental disorders: Implications for brain function* (pp. 217–242). Hillsdale, NJ: Erlbaum.

Kimura, M., Nakajima, M., & Yoshino, K. (1990). Ullrich–Turner syndrome with agenesis of the corpus callosum. *American Journal of Medical Genetics, 37,* 227–228.

Loehlin, J. C. (1987). *Latent variable models: An introduction to factor, path, and structural analysis.* Hillsdale, NJ: Erlbaum.

Marmor, G. S. (1977). Mental rotation and number conservation: Are they related? *Developmental Psychology, 13,* 320–325.

Mathur, A., Stekol, L., Schatz, D., MacLaren, N. K., Scott, M. L., & Lippe, B. (1991). The parental origin of the single X chromosome in Turner syndrome: Lack of correlation with parental age or clinical phenotype. *American Journal of Human Genetics, 48,* 682–686.

Mazzocco, M. M. M. (1998). A process approach to describing mathematics difficulties in girls with Turner syndrome. *Pediatrics, 108*(Suppl.), 492–496.

McCauley, E. (1990). Psychosocial and emotional aspects of Turner syndrome. In D. B. Berch & B. G. Bender (Eds.), *Sex chromosome abnormalities and human behavior: Psychological studies* (pp. 78–99). Boulder, CO: AAAS/Westview Press.

McCauley, E., Ito, J., & Kay, T. (1986). Psychosocial functioning in girls with Turner syndrome and short stature. *Journal of the American Academy of Child Psychiatry, 25,* 105–112.

McCauley, E., Kay, T., Ito, J., & Treder, R. (1987). The Turner syndrome: Cognitive deficits, affective discrimination and behavior problems. *Child Development, 58,* 464–473.

McCauley, E., Ross, J. L., Kushner, H., & Cutler, G., Jr. (1995). Self-esteem and behavior in girls with Turner syndrome. *Journal of Developmental and Behavioral Pediatrics, 16,* 82–88.

McCloskey, M., Caramazza, A., & Basili, A. (1985). Cognitive mechanisms in number processing and calculation: Evidence from dyscalculia. *Brain and Cognition, 4,* 171–196.

Money, J. (1963). Cytogenetic and psychosexual incongruities with a note on space-form blindness. *American Journal of Psychiatry, 119,* 820–827.

Money, J. (1973). Turner's syndrome and parietal lobe functions. *Cortex, 9,* 385–393.

Money, J., & Alexander, D. (1966). Turner's syndrome: Further demonstration of the presence of specific cognitional deficiencies. *Journal of Medical Genetics, 3,* 47–48.

Money, J., & Mittenthal, S. (1970). Lack of personality pathology in Turner syndrome: Relations to cytogenetics, hormones and physique. *Behavior Genetics, 1,* 43–56.

Murphy, D. G. M., Allen, G., Haxby, J. V., Largay, K. A., Daly, E., White, B. J., Powell, C. M., & Schapiro, M. B. (1994). The effects of sex steroids, and the X chromosome, on female brain function: A study of the neuropsychology of adult Turner syndrome. *Neuropsychologia, 32,* 1309–1323.

Murphy, D. G. M., DeCarli, C., Daly, E., Haxby, J. V., Allen, G., White, B. J., McIntosh, A. R., Powell, C. M., Horwitz, B., Rapoport, S. I., & Schapiro, M. B. (1993). X-chromosome effects on female brain: A magnetic resonance imaging study of Turner's syndrome. *Lancet, 342,* 1197–1200.

Netley, C. (1977). Dichotic listening of callosal agenesis and Turner's syndrome. In S. J. Segalowitz & F. A. Gruber (Eds.), *Language development and neurological theory* (pp. 133–143). New York: Academic Press.

Nielsen, J., Nyborg, H., & Dahl, G. (1977). Turner's syndrome: A psychiatric–psychological study of 45 women with Turner's syndrome, compared with their sisters and women with normal karyotypes, growth retardation, and primary amenorrhea. *Acta Jutlandica, 45*(Medicine Series 21).

Nielsen, J., & Sillesen, I. (1981). Turner's syndrome in 115 Danish girls born between 1955 and 1966. *Acta Jutlandica, 54*(Medicine Series 22).

Orten, J. D., & Orten, J. L. (1992). Achievement among women with Turner's syndrome. *Journal of Contemporary Human Services, 73,* 424–431.

Pennington, B. F., Bender, B., Puck, M., Salbenblatt, J., & Robinson, A. (1982). Learning disabilities in children with sex chromosome anomalies. *Child Development, 53,* 1182–1192.

Pennington, B. F., Heaton, R. K., Karzmark, P., Pendleton, M. G., Lehman, R., & Shucard, D. W. (1985). The neuropsychological phenotype in Turner syndrome. *Cortex, 21,* 391–404.

Pennington, B. F., & Smith, S. D. (1988). Genetic influences on learning disabilities: An update. *Journal of Consulting and Clinical Psychology, 56,* 817–823.

Polani, P. E. (1961). Turner's syndrome and allied conditions. *British Medical Bulletin, 17,* 200–205.

Polani, P. E. (1977). Abnormal sex chromosomes, behaviour and mental disorder. In J. Tanner (Ed.), *Developments in psychiatric research* (pp. 89–128). London: Hoddler & Stoughton.

Portellano-Perez, J. A., Bouthelier, R. G., & Asensio-Monge, I. (1996). New neurophysiological and neuropsychological contributions on Turner syndrome. In J. F. Rovet (Ed.), *Turner syndrome across the lifespan* (pp. 52–57). Toronto: Klein Graphics.

Raft, D., Spencer, R. F., & Toomey, T. C. (1976). Ambiguity of gender identity and fantasies and aspects of normality and pathology in hypopituitary dwarfism and Turner's syndrome: Three cases. *Journal of Sex Research, 12,* 161–172.

Reiss, A. L., Freund, L., Plotnick, L., Baumgardner, T., Green, K., Sozer, A. C., Reader, M., Boehm, C., & Denckla, M. B. (1993). The effects of X monosomy on brain development: Monozygotic twins discordant for Turner's syndrome. *Annals of Neurology, 34,* 95–107.

Reiss, A. L., Mazzocco, M. M. M., Greenlaw, R., Freund, L., & Ross, J. L. (1995). Neurodevelopmental effects of X monosomy: A volumetric imaging study. *Annals of Neurology, 38,* 731–738.

Reske-Nielsen, E., Christensen, A. L., & Nielsen, J. (1982). A neuropathological and neuropsychological study of Turner's syndrome. *Cortex, 18,* 181–190.

Ris, M. D. (1995). Developmental neuropsychology at its best. *Contemporary Psychology, 40,* 366–367.

Ross, J. L. (1990). Disorders of the sex chromosomes: Medical overview. In C. S. Holmes (Ed.), *Psychoneuroendocrinology: Brain, behavior, and hormonal interactions* (pp. 127–137). New York: Springer-Verlag.

Ross, J. L., Reiss, A. L., Freund, L., Roeltgen, D., & Cutler, G. B., Jr. (1993). Neurocognitive function and brain imaging in Turner syndrome—preliminary results. *Hormone Research, 39*(Suppl. 2), 65–69.

Ross, J. L., & Zinn, A. (1999). Turner syndrome: Potential hormonal and genetic influences on the neurocognitive profile. In H. Tager-Flusberg (Ed.), *Neurodevelopmental disorders* (pp. 251–268). Cambridge, MA: MIT Press.

Rothchild, E., & Owens, R. P. (1972). Adolescent girls who lack functioning ovaries. *Journal of the American Academy of Child Psychiatry, 11,* 88–113.

Rourke, B. P. (1989). *Nonverbal learning disabilities: The syndrome and the model.* New York: Guilford Press.

Rovet, J. (1986, May). Processing deficits in 45,X females. In A. Robinson (Chair), *Cognitive and psychosocial dysfunctions associated with sex chromosome abnormalities.* Symposium presented at the meeting of the American Association for the Advancement of Science, Philadelphia.

Rovet, J. F. (1990). The cognitive and neuropsychological characteristics of females with Turner syndrome. In D. B. Berch & B. G. Bender (Eds.), *Sex chromosome abnormalities and human behavior: Psychological studies* (pp. 38–77). Boulder, CO: AAAS/Westview Press.

Rovet, J. F. (1993). The psychoeducational characteristics of children with Turner syndrome. *Journal of Learning Disabilities, 26,* 333–341.

Rovet, J., & Buchanan, L. (1999). Turner syndrome: A cognitive neuroscience approach. In H. Tager-Flusberg (Ed.), *Neurodevelopmental disorders* (pp. 223–249). Cambridge, MA: MIT Press.

Rovet, J., & Ireland, L. (1994). Behavioral phenotype in children with Turner syndrome. *Journal of Pediatric Psychology, 19,* 779–790.

Rovet, J., & Netley, C. (1980). The mental rotation task performance of Turner syndrome subjects. *Behavior Genetics, 10,* 437–443.

Rovet, J., & Netley, C. (1982). Processing deficits in Turner's syndrome. *Developmental Psychology, 18,* 77–94.

Rovet, J., Szeleky, C., & Hockenberry, M. (1994). Specific arithmetic calculation deficits in children with Turner syndrome. *Journal of Clinical and Experimental Neuropsychology, 16,* 820–839.

Sabbath, J. C., Morris, T. A., Menzer-Benaron, D., & Sturgis, S. H. (1961). Psychiatric observation in the adolescent girls lacking ovarian function. *Psychosomatic Medicine, 23,* 224–231.

Semrud-Clikeman, M., & Hynd, G. W. (1990). Right hemispheric dysfunction in nonverbal learning disabilities: Social, academic, and adaptive functioning in adults and children. *Psychological Bulletin, 107,* 196–209.

Senzer, N., Aceto, T., Cohen, M. M., Ehrhardt, A. A., Abbassi, V., & Capraro, V. J. (1973). Isochromosome X. *American Journal of Diseases of Children, 126,* 312–316.

Shaffer, J. W. (1962). A specific cognitive deficit observed in gonadal aplasia (Turner's syndrome). *Journal of Clinical Psychology, 18,* 403–406.

Silbert, A., Wolff, P. H., & Lilienthal, J. (1977). Spatial and temporal processing in patients with Turner's syndrome. *Behavior Genetics, 7,* 11–21.

Skuse, D. H., James, R. S., Bishop, D. V. M., Coppin, B., Dalton, P., Aamodt-Leeper, G., Bacarese-Hamilton, M., Creswell, C., McGurk, R., & Jacobs, P. A. (1997). Evidence from Turner's syndrome of an imprinted x-linked locus affecting cognitive function. *Nature, 387,* 705–708.

Smith, S. D. (1990). The contribution of studies on sex chromosome aneuploidies to the understanding of genetic influences on behavior. In D. B. Berch & B. G. Bender (Eds.), *Sex chromosome abnormalities and human behavior: Psychological studies* (pp. 223–233). Boulder, CO: AAAS/Westview Press.

Sonis, W. A., Levine-Ross, J., Blue, J., Cutler, G. B., Loriaux, P. L., & Klein, R. P. (1983, October). *Hyperactivity of Turner's syndrome.* Paper presented at the meeting of the American Academy of Child Psychiatry, San Francisco.

Swillen, A., Fryns, J. P., Kleczkowska, A., Massa, G., Vaderschueren-Lodeweyckx, M., & van den Berghe, H. (1993). Intelligence, behaviour, and psychosocial development in Turner syndrome. *Genetic Counseling, 4,* 7–18.

Sybert, V. P. (1990). Mosaicisms in Turner syndrome. *Growth Genetics and Hormones, 6,* 4–8.

Sylven, L., Magnusson, C., Hagenfeldt, K., & von Schoultz, B. (1993). Life with Turner's syndrome—a psychosocial report from 22 middle-aged women. *Acta Endocrinologica, 129,* 188–194.

Taipale, V. (1979). *Adolescence in Turner's syndrome.* Helsinki: Children's Hospital, University of Helsinki.

Temple, C. M., & Carney, R. A. (1993). Intellectual functioning of children with Turner syndrome: A comparison of behavioural phenotypes. *Developmental Medicine and Child Neurology, 35,* 691–698.

Temple, C. M., & Carney, R. A. (1995). Patterns of spatial functioning in Turner's Syndrome. *Cortex, 31,* 109–118.

Temple, C. M., & Carney, R. A. (1996). Reading skills in children with Turner's Syndrome: An analysis of hyperlexia. *Cortex, 32,* 335–345.

Temple, C. M., Carney, R. A., & Mullarkey, S. (1996). Frontal lobe function and executive skills in children with Turner's syndrome. *Developmental Neuropsychology, 12,* 343–363.

Temple, C. M., & Marriott, A. J. (1998). Arithmetical ability and disability in Turner's syndrome: A cognitive neuropsychological analysis. *Developmental Neuropsychology, 14,* 47–67.

Tesch, L. G., & Rosenfeld, R. C. (1995). Morgagni, Ullrich, and Turner: The discovery of gonadal dysgenesis. *Endocrinologist, 5,* 327–328.

Turner, H. H. (1938). A syndrome of infantilism, congenital webbed neck, and cubitus valgus. *Endocrinology, 23,* 566–574.

Van Dyke, D. L., Wiktor, A., Roberson, J. R., & Weiss, L. (1991). Mental retardation in Turner syndrome. *Journal of Pediatrics, 118,* 415–417.

Waber, D. P. (1976). Sex differences in cognition: A function of maturation rate? *Science, 192,* 572–574.

Waber, D. P. (1979). Neuropsychological aspects of Turner syndrome. *Developmental Medicine and Child Neurology, 21,* 58–70.

White, B. J. (1994). The Turner syndrome: Origin, cytogenetic variants, and factors influencing the phenotype. In S. H. Broman & J. Grafman (Eds.), *Atypical cognitive deficits in developmental disorders: Implications for brain function* (pp. 183–195). Hillsdale, NJ: Erlbaum.

Wilkins, L., & Fleischmann, W. (1944). Ovarian agenesis: Pathology, associated clinical symptoms, and the bearing on theories of sexual differentiation. *Journal of Clinical Endocrinology, 4,* 357–375.

Williams, C. L., Barnett, A. M., & Meck, W. H. (1990). Organizational effects of early gonadal secretions on sexual differentiation in spatial memory. *Behavioral Neuroscience, 104,* 84–97.

Williams, J. K. (1994). Behavioral characteristics of children with Turner syndrome and children with learning disabilities. *Western Journal of Nursing Research, 16,* 26–29.

Williams, J. K., Richman, L. C., & Yarbrough, D. B. (1991). A comparison of memory and attention in Turner syndrome and learning disability. *Journal of Pediatric Psychology, 5,* 585–593.

Williams, J. K., Richman, L. C., & Yarbrough, D. B. (1992). Comparison of visual–spatial performance strategy training children with Turner syndrome and learning disabilities. *Journal of Learning Disabilities, 25,* 658–664.

Young-Hyman, D. L. (1990). Psychosocial functioning and social competence in growth hormone deficient, constitutionally delayed and familial short-stature children and adolescents. In C. S. Holmes (Ed.), *Psychoneuroendocrinology: Brain, behavior, and hormonal interactions* (pp. 40–55). New York: Springer-Verlag.

12

PHENYLKETONURIA

MARILYN WELSH
BRUCE PENNINGTON

The study of phenylpyruvic amentia [PKU] may throw light on the whole problem of mental deficiency. (Jervis, 1939, quoted in Knox, 1972, p. 266)

The future study of phenylketonuria [is] an endeavor which has the potential of furnishing insight into the nature and mechanism of development of the intellectual functions. (Knox, 1972, p. 266)

Variation in performance among PKU children suggests that the disorder may be an ideal one in which to study risk and protective mechanisms in the development of EF [executive function] impairment. (Welsh, Pennington, Ozonoff, Rouse, & McCabe, 1990, p. 1709)

These three quotes from researchers studying the phenomenon of phenylketonuria (PKU) across the decades illustrate how the implications of this research have changed with advances in identification, treatment, and both the cognitive and neuropsychological assessment of individuals with this disorder.

When Jervis (1939) suggested that the study of PKU may illuminate our understanding of "mental deficiency," he was reflecting the "state of the art" in the 1930s—a time when individuals with PKU went unidentified for years and essentially untreated, the consequences of which were severe mental retardation and behavioral disturbance. Thus the scientific community viewed PKU as a genetic disorder that provided new and useful information regarding the nature of global mental deficiency.

The comment by Knox (1972) represents the advances in our understanding of PKU that occurred with the advent of reliable identification and generally effective treatment of the disease. His statement that the study of PKU would furnish "insight into the nature and mechanism of development of the intellectual functions" indicates a more specific focus on how assessment of children identified and treated at various ages might reveal important findings relevant to both the normal and abnormal course of intellectual development. Clearly, the issue was no longer global mental deficiency, but the more

275

focal effects of the biochemical (and presumably neurological) changes noticed with PKU on intellectual functioning.

As our knowledge about the unique pathophysiology of PKU increased, and as our assessment tools became more sophisticated, it became possible to test more specific neuropsychological models of PKU. The Welsh et al. (1990) quote summarizes the interest of current researchers on targeted neuropsychological sequelae, the selection of which is based on accumulating knowledge regarding neurochemical perturbations of PKU and their effects on neurological functions (e.g., Pueschel, 1996).

The objective of this chapter is to examine a wide range of evidence that bears on the question of whether PKU—in particular, early-treated PKU—results in a relatively specific neuropsychological phenotype. As noted throughout the chapter, PKU is a disorder in which the links among gene, enzyme, biochemistry/neurochemistry, brain functioning, and behavior are clearer than in most other neurodevelopmental disorders. For example, we know that the genetic mutation inactivates the enzyme responsible for converting or hydroxylating phenylalanine (Phe) into tyrosine. This relative lack of tyrosine should have adverse effects on neurochemical metabolism, and in particular on metabolism of catecholamines such as dopamine (DA). There is evidence, for example, for an inverse association between Phe and DA in treated PKU individuals (Krause et al., 1985). Given that the prefrontal cortex is highly sensitive to reductions in DA (Chiodo, Bannon, Grace, Roth, & Bunney, 1984), neuropsychological sequelae reflective of a prefrontal dysfunction have been suggested (Chamove & Molinaro, 1978). The major questions to be addressed in this chapter are these: First, to what extent are there relatively specific neurochemical and neurophysiological effects of PKU that result in specific neuropsychological sequelae? And, second, can a case be made that this disorder should be considered a "natural model" of prefrontal cortical dysfunction (Diamond et al., 1993; Diamond, Prevor, Callender, & Druin, 1997; Welsh et al., 1990)?

In what follows, we review several issues regarding PKU, including (1) history of identification and treatment, (2) epidemiology and developmental course, (3) genetics and neuropathology, and (4) neuropsychological sequelae. We conclude with a scientific critique and a discussion of directions for future research. At relevant points throughout this review, the specificity hypothesis of prefrontal cortical dysfunction is examined in light of the empirical evidence available to date.

HISTORICAL OVERVIEW

The following historical review of the discovery, identification, and treatment of PKU is based on that of Knox (1972). In 1934, Folling described 10 patients, clustered in several families, who excreted phenylpyruvic acid in their urine and were mentally retarded. Following this, Jervis (1939, cited in Knox, 1972) and colleagues suggested that the condition was inherited through a single autosomal recessive gene and resulted in a abnormal buildup of Phe in the tissues of these patients. Jervis (1947, 1953; both references cited in Knox, 1972) also identified the metabolic error as one in which the ability to hydroxylate Phe to tyrosine is disrupted; phenylalanine hydroxylase (PAH) is inactive in the liver, and Phe is converted instead into phenylpyruvic acid. Given this understanding of the metabolic deficit, an effective preventive treatment was devised in which the dietary levels of Phe were restricted (Armstrong & Tyler, 1955, and Bickle, Gerrard, & Hickmans, 1954; both references cited in Knox, 1972). A Phe tolerance test was developed to identify heterozygous carriers of PKU (Hsia, Driscoll, Troll, & Knox, 1956, cited in Knox, 1972). The tolerance test was soon followed by an effective neonatal screening procedure that detected elevated plasma Phe and thus identified newborns who were homozygous for the disorder (Guthrie & Susi, 1963, cited in Knox, 1972). As of 1980, more than 40 million newborns have been screened for PKU in the years since Folling's discovery (Scriver & Clow, 1980), averting severe mental retardation and psychiatric disturbance in individuals who would have otherwise been institutionalized.

EPIDEMIOLOGY AND DEVELOPMENTAL COURSE

Epidemiology

The incidence of PKU varies by ethnic group and hence across populations. In the U.S. population, PKU has been reported in 1 in 14,000 newborns (Standbury, Wyngaarden, & Fredrickson, 1983). An incidence of 1 in 18,000 was reported in a survey of frequency in British Columbia, Canada (Tischler & Lowry, 1978). If random mating is assumed, these incidence rates translate into carrier frequencies of 1.5% and 1.7%, respectively (the odds of two heterozygotes' mating is the carrier frequency squared; hence one-fourth of their children will be homozygous recessive).

Prior to the widespread availability of newborn screening programs, the primary data for calculating the incidence of PKU consisted of its frequency among institutionalized mentally retarded individuals (Knox, 1972). These epidemiological studies indicated that the disease incidence was approximately 1 in 20,000 among mixed populations in northern European countries (which translates into a carrier frequency of 1.4%). Most individuals with PKU were found in institutions, where they made up about 1% of persons with mental retardation. In one of the first comprehensive surveys of the institutionalized population, Jervis (1954, cited in Knox, 1972) included 48,536 mentally retarded patients from 12 countries. He found a total of 312 PKU patients, or an average incidence of 0.64% of the worldwide institutionalized retarded population. The incidence in single institutions varied across geographical locations, ranging from 0% in French-speaking Canada to 2.7% in England. Jervis noted that PKU was most common in northern European and Scandinavian countries and in genetically related populations. In an earlier study, Jervis (1937, cited in Knox, 1972) found that of all groups represented in a U.S. sample of individuals with mental retardation, PKU was least common among Jews and African Americans.

Jervis's comprehensive epidemiological survey of PKU failed to identify a sex difference in incidence. The characteristics of the untreated disease in males and females are not different, but there appears to be a higher death rate among affected males (Lang, 1955, and Partington, 1961; both references cited in Knox, 1972). More males than females have been identified as having elevated Phe levels by neonatal screening; however, a percentage of these males are eventually not diagnosed with PKU, resulting in relatively equal rates of diagnosis during infancy.

Developmental Course

The natural history of the disease involves changes in manifestation across development in both untreated and early-treated cases of PKU. The developmental course of the disease in untreated individuals was studied extensively after discovery of PKU and development of techniques to diagnose this disease in institutionalized individuals. Knox (1972) pointed out that there are no consistent neonatal abnormalities associated with PKU in the first month or two of life, but that there are striking delays in developmental milestones during the next few years. Paine (1957) studied 106 untreated PKU individuals with mental retardation who had been identified in institutions by means of urine tests for phenylpyruvic acid. He found significant delays in the developmental milestones of these patients, such as sitting unsupported, walking, and talking. For example, the mean age for producing single words was between 3 and 4 years of age, compared to developmental standards of 13 to 18 months for this skill (Bloom, 1993).

Paine (1957) found a history of seizure activity in 26% of the patients, and this appeared to be related to the degree of mental retardation. In contrast, abnormal electroencephalograms (EEGs) were found in 79% of the sample, and the incidence of this abnormality was *not* associated with degree of retardation. Microcephaly was more apparent in the severely retarded group (IQ under 25). The patients with microcephaly and low IQ demonstrated stereotypes that are also observed in other severely retarded groups and in persons with autism:

> The [hand] postures are variable and difficult to describe. They include rhythmic pill-rolling movements of the hands, irregular tic-like motions, aimless to and from movements of the fingers and frequently habitual fiddling of the fingers close before the eyes. The patients may also twist of dangle pieces of string or other objects in front of the eyes. All of this activity is often accompanied by a rhythmic rocking back and forth which may continue for hours. (Paine, 1957, pp. 296–297)

The degree to which these abnormal behaviors are the consequences of very low intelligence in general versus PKU in particular is unclear, as the two conditions are confounded in untreated individuals. However, the striking resemblance of these symptoms to those found in association with autism is consistent with the frontal lobe/DA deficiency hypothesis model that has been proposed to account for *both* PKU and autism, as discussed further in later sections of this chapter.

Knox (1972) suggested that the most striking clinical characteristic of untreated PKU is "the transformation of an apparently normal baby into a severely defective one during the first year or so of life" (p. 269). Combining cross-sectional data from many studies of intellectual development in untreated individuals, Knox (1972) concluded that intelligence declines sharply and linearly over the first 10 months of life, with slower declines until about 3 years, and no further intellectual loss thereafter. At the point of this plateau, the average IQ of individuals reported in these studies was 40.2 (*SD* = 3.2). Overall, the behavior of untreated individuals was described in this early literature as "unpleasant." More specifically, these children were observed to be restless, anxious, jerky, fearful, hyperactive, irritable, and destructive, with uncontrollable temper tantrums, night terrors, and noisy psychotic episodes in a small minority of patients (Wright & Tarjan, 1957).

The developmental course of the physiological and behavioral disturbances in early-treated PKU individuals is far less clear. It has been only about 3 decades since the initiation of widespread neonatal screening and dietary therapy. Moreover, important parameters of the dietary regimen (e.g., age at initiation, early termination vs. maintenance of diet, strictness of diet) have changed over the years as knowledge regarding the disease and its sequelae has advanced. Comparison of early-treated individuals of different ages is subject to the same interpretive problems that beset cross-sectional studies of the consequences of preterm birth, in which the age of subjects is confounded with changes in medical knowledge, technology, and treatment. Therefore, the natural history of PKU in early-treated individuals remains largely unknown. As discussed later (see

"Scientific Critique and Future Directions"), a better understanding of natural history will require greater attention to developmental processes in both neurological functioning and behavior.

GENETICS AND NEUROPATHOLOGY

Genetics

Scriver and Clow (1980) suggest that PKU is a classic example of a genetic disorder because it adheres to the three historic principles of human and medical genetics proposed by Vogel and Motulsky (1979). First, PKU is inherited as an autosomal recessive trait, in accordance with Mendel's law of segregation. Second, as an "inborn error of metabolism," it reflects Garrod's (1902) principle of gene action: Genetic factors specify chemical and enzymatic reactions that ultimately relate to clinical abnormality. Third, the disease of PKU is manifested only when the mutant allele is expressed in an "obligatory environment containing an abundance of the essential amino acid L-phenylalanine" (Scriver & Clow, 1980, p. 1337). Thus PKU is a classic example of a "nature–nurture" interaction, in which both the expression and treatment of the disease are dependent on the genetic predisposition and the individual's immediate environment (i.e., the amount of Phe exposure).

In classical PKU, PAH enzymatic activity is absent; either the enzyme is not synthesized at all, or its structure is fundamentally altered (Ciaranello, Wong, & Rubenstein, 1990). One year after the discovery of this enzyme, the work of Penrose (1935) revealed that PKU is a genetic disorder transmitted as an autosomal recessive trait. Fifty years later, gene-cloning studies identified a single gene for PAH (Woo, Lidsky, Guther, Chandra, & Robson, 1983). Studies of classical PKU patients and their extended families with restriction fragment polymorphism analysis have shown the locus of the human PAH gene to be on chromosome 12 (Woo et al., 1985). Interestingly, Woo (1991) reports that classical PKU is not caused by deletion of the entire PAH gene. Instead, there may be distinct mutations of the gene involving at least two types of base substitutions (Ciaranello et al., 1990), and the exact mutation may vary across PKU individuals.

Neurochemistry

The major biochemical abnormality characteristic of PKU involves the inability of PAH to oxidize Phe into tyrosine in the liver. The effect that this genetic mutation has on the synthesis and function of neurotransmitters in the brain is of central importance to the neuropsychological consequences of this disease. As far back as the 1950s, it was documented that the synthesis of serotonin, DA, and norepinephrine was impaired in untreated PKU, as measured by decreased plasma or urine concentrations of the neurotransmitters or their metabolites (Armstrong & Robinson, 1954, cited in Knox, 1972; Paere, Sandler, & Stacey, 1957; Weil-Malherbe, 1955). McKean (1972) demonstrated that the levels of these three biogenic amines were lower in the autopsied brains of untreated PKU individuals than in the brains of control patients, showing that the impairment in synthesis occurred in the brain rather than peripherally. Moreover, McKean found decreased cerebrospinal fluid levels of the DA metabolite homovanillic acid in PKU patients. Because concentrations of both homovanillic acid and 5-hydroxyindoleacetic acid (the serotonin metabolite) are significantly increased by lowering Phe levels through dietary means (McKean, 1972; Butler, O'Flynn, Seifert, & Howell, 1981), Guttler and Lou (1986) concluded that high levels of

Phe disrupt the biosynthesis of serotonin and DA in the central nervous system (CNS), and that this effect is reversible through a Phe-restricted diet.

There are at least three mechanisms by which PKU is thought to interfere with the synthesis of biogenic amines, and these processes are particularly clear in the case of the catecholamine DA. First, the genetic mutation inactivates PAH, the enzyme necessary to convert Phe to tyrosine. Tyrosine is an essential precursor amino acid for the synthesis of DA. Peterson, Shah, Raghupathy, and Rhoads (1983) found that the availability of tyrosine for catecholamine synthesis is reduced twofold in PKU, and that this is solely the consequence of a reduction in CNS tyrosine.

A second mechanism involves the metabolites resulting from high Phe concentrations, which inhibit the enzymes necessary for critical chemical reactions, such as tyrosine hydroxylase (catabolizes tyrosine to L-dopa) and DA decarboxylase (catabolizes L-dopa to DA). The first enzyme is involved in the rate-limiting step in the synthesis of DA (Curtius, Baerlocher, & Vollmin, 1972). Phe metabolites have a similar effect in the synthesis of serotonin. In this case, metabolites can inhibit the activity of 5-hydroxytryptophan decarboxylase, resulting in a decrease in serotonin synthesis (Sandler, 1982).

Third, Aragon and colleagues (Aragon, Gimenez, Major, Marivizon, & Valdivieso, 1981; Aragon, Gimenez, & Valdivieso, 1982) have demonstrated that Phe and tyrosine share a common transport system at presynaptic terminals. Given limited capacity for transport, the high CNS levels of Phe characteristic of PKU would competitively inhibit the uptake of tyrosine via this system. Again, because tyrosine is necessary for the rate-limiting step in DA synthesis, CNS DA levels would be significantly reduced (Peterson et al., 1983).

How does this neurochemical evidence bear on the specificity hypothesis of PKU? Suggestions of depleted DA are consistent with a prefrontal dysfunction model because of the heightened sensitivity of the dopaminergic neurons in the prefrontal cortex to small reductions in DA (Chiodo et al., 1984; Thierry et al., 1977; Bannon, Bunney, & Roth, 1981; Tam, Elsworth, Bradberry, & Roth, 1991). This sensitivity is thought to be due to the relative lack of synthesis-modulating autoreceptors present on dopaminergic neurons in the prefrontal cortex, as compared to other brain regions (Bannon, Michaud, & Roth, 1981; Bannon, Reinhard, Bunney, & Roth, 1982; Chiodo et al., 1984).

A potential problem with the specificity hypothesis is that mechanisms responsible for disruption of the DA system will also interfere with synthesis of other neurochemicals. For example, DA is converted to norepinephrine by DA-beta-decarboxylase; therefore, depleted DA should result in reduced concentrations of norepinephrine. Moreover, Phe metabolites inhibit the action of enzymes necessary for the synthesis of DA *and* serotonin; metabolites of both neurochemicals are reduced in PKU individuals. The fact that the neurochemical perturbations in early-treated PKU are *not* specific to DA alone casts some doubt on the specificity hypothesis. It is nevertheless possible that the changes in DA concentrations are more severe than other neurochemicals, or that prefrontal cortical function is more sensitive to DA reductions than other brain systems are sensitive to reductions in norepinephrine and serotonin. Further research is needed to examine these possibilities.

Neurological Damage

Evidence of structural damage to the brain has been gleaned from three sources: autopsies of the brains of untreated PKU individuals; *in vivo* imaging (computed tomography [CT], magnetic resonance imaging [MRI]) of the brains of treated and untreated PKU patients; and examination of the brains of animals with experimentally induced hyper-phenylalaninemia.

Knox (1972) reviewed earlier studies in which the brains of 25 untreated PKU individuals were examined on autopsy (Crome & Pare, 1960; Knox, 1960; both references cited in Knox, 1972). A typical finding was that these individuals had abnormally small brains of about two-thirds the normal weight. An additional finding was that of defective myelination, sometimes with secondary fibrillary gliosis (Poser & Van Bogaert, 1959). Knox (1972) pointed out that the defective myelination appears to be a consequence of abnormal myelin *formation*, rather than of demyelination, and that it was unclear whether or how high Phe concentrations disrupted the complex myelination process. A later autopsy study of a 27-year-old man with both PKU and autism indicated a reduced density in dendritic spines of pyramidal neurons in the cortex; similar abnormalities were noted in the cortex of a man diagnosed with autism alone (Williams, Hauser, Purpura, DeLong, & Swisher, 1980).

Recent reviews of MRI studies of treated PKU patients suggest that as Phe level concentrations increase, the water content of brain white matter increases and produces visible neuroradiological changes (Smith, 1994; Ullrich et al., 1994). Consistent with early morphological analyzes of autopsied brains, MRI findings also reveal abnormalities in myelination. These anomalies are most often present in posterior/periventricular white matter—brain regions characterized by late myelination in humans (Bick et al., 1993; McCombe et al., 1992; Ullrich et al., 1994). The MRI data from more severely affected PKU patients indicate defective myelination in the frontal and subcortical white matter, involving the corpus callosum and the association fibers (Bick et al., 1993).

Interestingly, these MRI changes are not correlated with an individual's history of treatment, such as age at dietary initiation, mean Phe levels during treatment, or quality of dietary control prior to diet termination or relaxation (Bick et al., 1993; Pearson, Gean-Marton, Levy, & Davis, 1990; Walter, Tyfield, Holton, & Johnson, 1993; Lou et al., 1992). The transient abnormalities in white matter water content visible on an MRI scan are instead related to concurrent hyperphenylalaninemia (Cleary et al., 1994; Thompson et al., 1993). Moreover, these MRI changes can be reversed if Phe level is decreased (Walter, Cleary, Wraith, & Jenkins, 1994). It is also important to note that MRI changes in treated PKU thus far have been found to be uncorrelated with neurological symptoms (e.g., spasticity, fine motor deficits, or intellectual impairment), electrophysiological data, or neuropsychological performance (Bick et al., 1993; Cleary et al., 1994; Ludolph, Ullrich, Nedjat, Masur, & Bick, 1992; Pearson et al., 1990; Thompson et al., 1990, 1993; Weglage, Pietsch, Funders, Koch, & Ullrich, 1995).

Consistent with the human data reviewed above, Huether, Kaus, and Neuhoff (1982) found that induced hyperphenylalaninemia in rats disrupted myelination in the spinal cord and cortex. Myelin formation in the cortex appeared to be delayed for up to 20 postnatal days, but thereafter the rate of myelination was not significantly different from that observed in control animals. Hogan and Coleman (1981) found that experimental hyperphenylalaninemia in one sample of rats adversely affected dendritic branching of the pyramidal cells in the motor cortex, and in another sample caused smaller dendritic trees of the Purkinje cells in the cerebellum.

Evidence of neuroanatomical damage does *not* provide unequivocal support for the specificity hypothesis of prefrontal dysfunction in PKU. The one consistent result across different research paradigms (autopsy, MRI, animal models) is the existence of defective myelination. Pietz, Meyding-Lamade, and Schmidt (1996) report MRI findings of abnormalities in the parieto-occipital periventricular white matter; these abnormalities extended to the frontal cortex only in the more severe cases of PKU. Another common observation from the autopsy and animal studies is reduced dendritic branching of pyramidal neurons. Given that the pyramidal tract of neurons begins in the motor cortex within the frontal lobe, and that this system is thought to have executive control over voluntary movements (Spreen, Risser, & Edgell, 1985), the reduced dendritic branching is somewhat consistent with the prefrontal dysfunction model of PKU.

Functional Neurological Changes

In addition to morphological analysis of the brain, one can explore the neurological consequences of PKU by examining the changes in brain functions that are characteristic of the disease. In general, past research has focused on the measurement of brain electrical activity in untreated and treated PKU samples. The choice of brain electrical recordings may have been dictated by the fact that untreated individuals were often severely mentally retarded and sometimes psychotic, and that most early-treated individuals were children, given the relative recency of early identification and treatment. As the early-treated PKU population enters adulthood, more "active" and sometimes invasive methodologies, such as positron emission tomography (PET) and regional cerebral blood flow, may be applied to study the functional correlates of this condition.

The EEG records synaptic potentials from large numbers of neurons simultaneously, and in that sense can be considered a rather "crude summation of the electrical activity of cerebral neurons" (Rolle-Daya, Pueschel, & Lombroso, 1975, p. 899). Nevertheless, abnormal EEGs in individuals with PKU may be markers of a neurological insult caused by the genetic mutation and its resultant biochemical consequences. Rolle-Daya et al. (1975) found that the majority of PKU subjects treated after 6 months of age (late-treated) had abnormal EEGs, most of which involved paroxysmal discharges (spiking). In contrast, early-treated individuals (prior to 6 months) generally showed normal EEGs. The EEG patterns were not related to age of diet initiation after 6 months, nor were they associated with dietary control. Some studies have documented a correlation between Phe level and background abnormalities of EEG rhythms (Donker, Reits, Van Sprang, Storm van Leewen, & Wadman, 1979; Storm van Leewen, Donker, & Van Sprang, 1975) and EEG epileptiform patterns (Degiorgio, Antonozzi, Del Castello, & Loizzo, 1982) in early-treated patients. Two studies reported that the most common EEG anomalies observed in their treated PKU subjects were focal paroxysmal discharges, primarily in the frontal region (Blaskovics, Engel, Podosin, Azen, & Friedman, 1981; Gross, Berlow, Schuett, Ruggero, & Fariello, 1981).

An alternative to the EEG for studying brain electrical activity is the event-related potential (ERP). The ERP measures synchronous firing of a population of neurons from a specific brain region or regions in response to an external stimulus (visual, auditory, or somatosensory) or in association with a designated movement (Bashore, 1993). ERP data consist of information with regard to the amplitude and latency of various positive- and negative-going peaks or components that are assumed to reflect different elements of stimulus and response processing. Although few studies of ERPs in individuals with early-treated PKU have been conducted, Pueschel, Fogelson-Doyle, Kammerer, and Matsumiya (1983) measured visual, auditory, and somatosensory evoked potentials (EPs) while young children were on diets and again after diet termination. EPs are a class of ERPs that are elicited under passive conditions; that is, a subject simply sits and receives stimulation, with no assigned processing or decision-making requirements. Thus EPs are presumed to reflect the activation of primary sensory pathways, rather than the engagement of higher-order cognitive processes. The only abnormality observed by Pueschel et al. was in later components of the somatosensory EP. This abnormal EP was related to lower IQs, perceptual–motor problems, and poor dietary control in these subjects. Similarly, abnormalities in the visual EP have been found in treated PKU patients under poor dietary control (McCombe et al., 1992). In contrast to these results, Creel and Buehler (1982) found that the visual EPs of mentally retarded PKU subjects who were not treated early were surprisingly normal.

Research exploring brain functioning has *not* provided data consistent with any specific neuropsychological phenotype. Two studies that found focal paroxysmal discharges in the frontal lobe support the prefrontal dysfunction model; however, the evidence of abnormal somatosensory and visual EPs is inconsistent with this hypothesis. Data relevant to specificity hypotheses are most likely to emerge from cognitive psychophysiological paradigms in which the ERP is linked to specific stages of information processing, as opposed to the traditional EEG and EP methodologies.

NEUROPSYCHOLOGICAL STUDIES OF EARLY-TREATED PHENYLKETONURIA

The previous review of the genetic, biochemical, neuroanatomical, and neurophysiological effects of PKU as we currently understand them leads us to behavioral manifestations— the final step in Garrod's sequence of gene action. The past 60 years of research on PKU have identified the genetic mutation and many of the concomitant biochemical changes. Whereas there is clear evidence for disrupted neurochemical synthesis, the resultant effects on the structure and function of the brain remain unclear. Application of the newer neuro-imaging technologies to the study of PKU is likely to lead to isolation of specific neurological consequences of the disorder. A careful examination of the behavioral sequelae should provide evidence that converges with information on anomalies of brain structure and function.

In what follows, the phrase *neuropsychological consequences* is interpreted broadly to include the early studies of intelligence and intellectual development, investigations of general behavior and psychopathology, and more focused analyzes of cognitive processes and neuropsychological models in the early-treated PKU population.

Intelligence and Intellectual Development

Studying the impact of treated PKU on intellectual functioning and development was motivated less by hypotheses about the effects of PKU on brain functions per se than by a pragmatic concern. Since intellectual deterioration was one of the most striking symptoms in untreated PKU, it was of the utmost interest to evaluate whether the recently developed Phe-restricted dietary therapy would avert mental retardation (and, if so, to what degree). That is, the preservation of intellectual function became the primary yardstick by which the effectiveness of the treatment was measured. Since specific diet-related factors (e.g., dietary control, age at initiation, and age at termination) varied across individuals, the effects of these factors on IQ could be explored.

Waisbren, Schnell, and Levy (1980) reviewed 19 studies conducted between 1962 and 1979 that examined the effects of diet termination on IQ. Whereas 9 studies demonstrated significant losses in IQ after diet termination, the remaining 10 revealed no loss in intellectual function. These studies differed in important parameters of the diet, including age at initiation and age at termination. Across the 19 studies, age at diet termination, which ranged from 2 years to 9 years, did not appear to be associated with IQ changes following diet termination (loss vs. no loss). As Waisbren et al. (1980) pointed out, however, five methodological problems common to these studies made it difficult to draw any general conclusions. These problems included (1) use of multiple examiners, (2) single test observations, (3) use of different intelligence tests, (4) lack of control groups, and (5) different methods of assessing statistical significance.

The PKU Collaborative Study (Williamson, Dobson, & Koch, 1977) addressed many of the methodological concerns noted by Waisbren et al. (1980). In this study, Phe levels were monitored in children from infancy through 4 years of age, culminating in Stanford–Binet IQ assessment. The primary purpose of this multicenter project was to assess the effectiveness of dietary therapy for children with PKU. Dobson, Williamson, Azen, and Koch (1977), who reported the earliest results from the Collaborative Study, found that the children exhibiting lower Phe levels after 6 months of age scored higher on the IQ test at age 4. However, higher IQ at this age was also associated with *higher* Phe levels from birth to 6 months of age. The latter, somewhat counterintuitive result is consistent with findings reported by Fuller and Shuman (1971) in which low Phe (less than 5 mg/dl) of long duration was related to lower developmental quotients in PKU toddlers. An explanation for this finding is that maintaining Phe concentrations at a very low level through dietary restrictions and supplements may limit the developing brain's access to important nutrients and proteins.

In assessing children from the Collaborative Study at 6 years of age, Williamson, Koch, Azen, and Chang (1981) found that the mean IQ of the sample was 98 (clearly within the normal range), and that the best predictors of intelligence were maternal IQ, age at diet initiation, and quality of dietary control. That is, the later in development the low-Phe diet was initiated and the poorer the quality of dietary control, the more likely it was that the IQ score would be lower than normal (i.e., Full Scale IQ of 103, the mean of the non-PKU sibling group).

To further assess the effects of diet, children participating in the Collaborative Study were randomly assigned to continue or discontinue dietary therapy at age 6, and Koch, Azen, Friedman, and Williamson (1982) compared the performances of these two groups at ages 6 and 8. The two diet groups, continuers and discontinuers, did not significantly differ in IQ at either assessment; in fact, IQ remained stable through age 8 in both groups. Phe levels increased over time in both groups, but more dramatically in discontinuers. However, the two groups did not differ in terms of the effects of these increases on IQ or achievement scores.

The 8-year-olds' IQ and achievement data were later analyzed with regard to how the PKU subjects performed in comparison to unaffected sibling controls (Koch, Azen, Friedman, & Williamson, 1984). Discrepancies between PKU subjects and siblings in IQ and achievement (favoring siblings) were positively correlated with lifetime Phe level, maximum diagnostic Phe in infancy, and Phe levels at 6 and 8 years of age. Discrepancies were observed only in the group of discontinuers. Thus, although the discontinuers were performing in the "normal range" as reported by Koch et al. (1982), they were not performing as well as would be predicted from their siblings' scores.

In the follow-up assessment at age 10, Holtzman, Kronmal, van Doorninck, Azen, and Koch (1986) found that the best predictor of IQ, achievement, and behavior problems at age 10 was the age at which dietary control was lost. The poorest outcomes were observed in children who lost dietary control (based on elevated Phe levels) prior to age 6 years; these children were also the most discrepant from their parents in intelligence.

Two studies of intellectual outcomes in individuals with PKU not affiliated with the PKU Collaborative Study were conducted by Berry, O'Grady, Perlmutter, and Bofinger (1979) and by Waisbren, Mahon, Schnell, and Levy (1987). Berry et al. (1979) examined the IQ and achievement scores of an early-treated PKU sample ranging widely in age (4–35 years). Consistent with the Williamson et al. (1981) findings from the Collaborative Study, these investigators found that the average IQ of their subjects was 98 and that the PKU subjects' IQ scores and arithmetic achievement were lower than those of unaffected siblings. Moreover, there was a negative relationship between Phe level measured after 1 year of age and current IQ. Waisbren et al. (1987) also studied an early-treated PKU sample that ranged widely in age (3–24 years). Two-thirds of the sample had terminated the PKU diet at age 5, and one-third was currently on the diet. The overall mean IQ for the PKU group was again 98, with about a 10-point difference in favor of the on-diet sub-group. The best predictors of current Full Scale IQ were age and Phe level while on the diet. Lower intelligence scores were associated with greater age and with Phe levels above 16 mg/dl. The best predictors of IQ change over a 5-year period were dietary status (on or off diet) and Phe level while on diet.

In general, studies of intelligence provide evidence of the effectiveness of the dietary treatment when initiated very early in development. Early-treated PKU children exhibit intellectual levels well within the normal range (low to high 90s). However, it is also clear that their intellectual functioning does not achieve the levels predicted from their parents' and siblings' intelligence, and that IQ declines with age during the school years in some children. Declining mental abilities appear to be related to elevations in Phe caused by poor or absent dietary control. Little is known, however, about the neuropsychological changes that mediate these declining abilities, and in particular about whether specific or general cognitive dysfunctions are contributory.

Behavior and Psychopathology

The rationale for evaluation of intellectual outcomes of PKU also motivated early studies of general behavior and symptoms of psychopathology in early-treated individuals. Given that untreated PKU patients frequently exhibited severe behavioral disturbances, it was important to explore the degree to which these symptoms were averted or ameliorated by a Phe-restricted diet.

With regard to general behavioral characteristics, Schor (1983) found that parents of 3- to 7-year-old early-treated children rated them as more rhythmic, more intense, and less persistent than their unaffected siblings. Median Phe level was inversely related to persistence ratings. In a similar study of 8- to 12-year-old early-treated PKU children, Schor (1984) found that parents rated the children as lower in persistence and higher in distractibility compared to published age norms. In a sample of 41 early- and later-treated patients who had discontinued dietary therapy during childhood, Michals, Dominik, Schuett, Brown, and Matalon (1985) identified 22 patients with symptoms of hyperactivity, attention deficits, and irritability.

Stevenson et al. (1979) compared a sample of 99 early-treated PKU children to a teacher-selected sample of 197 age-matched unaffected controls on the Rutter Scales of Behavioral Deviance. Each teacher of a PKU subject selected two control subjects from the PKU child's class of the same sex and a similar age. The control group was thus not randomly selected, nor was it matched to the PKU group on IQ. The results revealed an interesting sex difference in rates of behavioral deviance. The PKU boys exhibited higher levels of neurotic deviance than controls, even after the group difference in IQ was controlled for. In contrast, only PKU girls with low IQ (under 70) showed greater behavioral deviance than control subjects. Although the authors suggested several possible explanations for the existence of behavioral deviance in the PKU population, none of these explanations is relevant to the gender difference found.

Fisch, Sines, and Chang (1981) also found that early-treated male PKU subjects exhibited more evidence of psychopathology than their unaffected parents and siblings, particularly poor impulse control, intrapsychic tension, and disturbed interpersonal relations. Comparisons involving early-treated PKU females to family members failed to reveal similar differences. Fisch et al. (1981) noted that in this study and in the larger PKU Collaborative Study, female PKU subjects had higher IQs than male PKU subjects. In addition, Thompson (1957) found that male relatives of PKU patients had a higher incidence of mental disorders than did female relatives. Although these findings are intriguing, the genetic and biochemical mechanisms responsible for these sex differences in the sequelae of PKU are not well understood.

In a later study, Realmuto et al. (1986) investigated attention problems in a sample of early-treated PKU subjects ranging in age from 9 to 20 years. After an experimental elevation of Phe level ("Phe load"), the researchers failed to find the predicted decrement in sustained attention and inhibition. However, they did note that 6 of their 13 subjects met the diagnostic criteria for attention deficit disorder (as defined by the *Diagnostic and Statistical Manual of Mental Disorders*, third edition), either currently or at some point in the past. In a direct comparison between early-treated PKU children and children diagnosed with attention-deficit/hyperactivity disorder (ADHD), Kalverboer et al. (1994) found that the PKU children exhibited more problems in task orientation than controls, but that these problems were less marked than in the ADHD children.

To summarize, problems with attention, impulse control, distractibility, persistence, and hyperactivity have been found in early-treated individuals with PKU. These symptoms are consistent with a diagnosis of ADHD; in fact, some proportion of early-treated PKU individuals receive such a diagnosis. Historically, there has also been a link between PKU and autism. Autism has been found frequently in samples of untreated or late-treated PKU children (Friedman, 1969). Conversely, undiagnosed cases of PKU are occasionally identified within groups of children diagnosed with autism (Lowe, Tanaka, Seashore, Young, & Cohen, 1980). Of particular note, Friedman (1969) found that manipulating Phe levels through dietary treatment in PKU children with both mental retardation and autism had an effect on the severity of autistic symptoms, but not on intelligence. Given evidence of abnormalities in DA and prefrontal function in ADHD, and possibly in autism as well, these findings are congruent with a prefrontal dysfunction/DA depletion neuropsychological model of PKU. Moreover, the findings of Stevenson et al. (1979) and Fisch et al. (1981) converge to indicate a tendency toward neuroticism in early-treated PKU children, which may include symptoms of anxiety and depression. Although not yet tested directly, it is possible that these symptoms could relate to serotonin depletion.

It is important to note here that children with early-treated PKU do not present with a consistent clinical profile; indeed, some of these children do not have clinically significant problems. Just as in children with other genetic disorders, there are wide individual differences within this group, reflecting both environmental and other genetic influences that vary across individuals (e.g., Shiwach & Sheikha, 1998). However, a few generalizations may be drawn from the research reviewed in this chapter. Basically, research exploring psychopathological and neuropsychological sequelae of PKU suggest that, on average, an early-treated child will present with the symptoms of mild ADHD; that is, there will be evidence of hyperactivity, impulsivity, and less task persistence. Thus completing self-directed academic tasks, especially those that require more planning and organization (e.g., book reports, research projects), may be problematic. These children would be more likely to have problems with mathematics than they would have with reading. There are also indications that an early-treated PKU child may present with increased irritability; however, whether this should be considered a primary or secondary characteristic of the disorder is unclear.

Specific Cognitive and Neuropsychological Processes

As newborn identification and dietary treatment were well underway by the mid-1970s, studies of the sequelae of PKU turned from assessments of general intelligence (which appeared to be "normal") to explorations of more specific cognitive processes. The processes investigated in these studies have been traditional cognitive domains, such as visual–spatial skills, perceptual–motor functions, language, and short- and long-term memory.

More recently, interest has focused on specific neuropsychological models, in an effort to gain insight into the particular neurological systems that are affected by the disease. The most prominent of these neuropsychological models proposes a prefrontal cortical dysfunction as the underlying neuropathological correlate of PKU, and problems in executive functioning (EF) as the primary neuropsychological manifestation of the disorder (Welsh & Pennington, 1988). EF, which involves cognitive processes that subserve goal-directed, future-oriented activities, transcends the traditional cognitive domains listed above. Among the processes that have been grouped under the rubric of EF are planning, working memory, organized search, flexibility, and inhibition. Earlier research findings with regard to PKU-related deficits in the more traditional cognitive domains can be reinterpreted within this EF framework in examining support for the prefrontal dysfunction model of PKU.

Several cognitive studies of children with early-treated PKU conducted in the 1970s and 1980s suggested deficits in visual–spatial problem solving. Studies of school-age and older individuals, for example, found problems in "visual analysis and synthesis" on tasks such as the Bender–Gestalt (Davis, McIntyre, Murray, & Mims, 1986; Fischler et al., 1987; Mims, McIntyre, & Murray, 1981, 1983), the Matching Familiar Figures Test (Davis et al., 1986), and the Embedded Figures Test (Davis et al., 1986). It is unclear, however, whether these deficits were due to problems with spatial cognition or to other deficient cognitive processes. For instance, Mims et al. (1983) observed that their PKU subjects had particular difficulty translating the perception of the figure to be copied on the Bender–Gestalt into an accurate mental representation. The ability to generate and manipulate mental representations is consistent with the concept of working memory (Case, 1992). Similarly, the Matching Familiar Figures Test and Embedded Figures Test require such EF processes as organized search, hypothesis testing, inhibition, and flexibility, in addition to visual–spatial analysis. Brunner, Berch, and Berry (1987) developed a test of complex spatial analysis in which parts of a figure had to be mentally manipulated in order to determine whether it matched another figure—possibly tapping working memory processes. The authors found that their PKU group was significantly impaired on this task as compared to a control group. Although they suggested that this deficit could be due to metacognitive or "executive" strategies, the group difference did not remain significant after IQ was covaried.

Impairments in the domain of perceptual–motor skills, or psychomotor functions, have also been identified. Because the Bender–Gestalt requires both perception and fine motor coordination, difficulties of individuals with PKU on this task have also been attributed to perceptual–motor deficits (Fischler et al., 1987; Koff, Boyle, & Pueschel, 1977; Mims et al., 1983). Mims et al. (1983) tested children with PKU and matched controls on four experimental conditions of a grapheme copying task, similar to the Bender–Gestalt. These conditions were designed to tease apart the perceptual, conceptual, and motor demands of the traditional Bender–Gestalt test. Based on the results, the authors concluded that the poor Bender–Gestalt performance of early-treated PKU children could not be accounted for by specific motor incoordination.

Two studies identified perceptual–motor deficits on the Tactual Performance Test of the Halstead–Reitan neuropsychological battery (Brunner, Jordan, & Berry, 1983; Pennington, van Doorninck, McCabe, & McCabe, 1985). This test requires a blindfolded subject to fit objects of various geometric shapes into the appropriate spaces on a board. It is well established that a wide range of brain lesions can disrupt performance on this task. In addition to spatial cognition, the Tactual Performance Test requires mental flexibility and novel problem solving. Efficient performance on this task is also guided by a mental representation of the tactile information provided.

The psychomotor hyperexcitability, poor concentration, and a lack of persistence observed by Cabalska et al. (1977) in early-treated PKU children 8 to 10 years of age constitutes further anecdotal evidence for EF deficits. Such problems with concentration and persistence—also observed in Schor's (1983, 1984) samples, discussed earlier—could certainly contribute to deficits seen in perceptual–motor tests and the visual–spatial tasks discussed above. Similarly, Brunner et al. (1987) note that impulsive responding was a factor in the impaired visual–spatial problem-solving abilities of their PKU subjects.

Language is another traditional domain of cognition that has been explored in early-treated PKU subjects, although less extensively than visual–spatial skills. The limited research data available indicate that as a group, early-treated PKU children do not exhibit speech and language deficits (Melnick, Michals, & Matalon, 1981; O'Grady, Berry, & Sutherland, 1971; Ozanne, Krimmer, & Murdoch, 1990). However, Ozanne, Murdoch, and Krimmer (1990, cited in Ozanne et al., 1990) did find a small subset of individuals with poor dietary control that displayed language impairment. These researchers concluded that language and speech difficulties may be part of the clinical profile of an older PKU child with a history of elevated Phe levels.

Even when evidence of specific language problems is reported in the literature, these deficits can be interpreted within the EF framework. For example, although O'Grady et al. (1971) failed to detect a deficit in overall psycholinguistic ability in their early-treated PKU group, their findings did reveal a significant impairment in spontaneous verbal expression. The latter skill is closely associated with verbal fluency, a language function that is frequently deficient in patients with frontal damage (Kolb & Whishaw, 1990).

Studies of the cognitive skills of early-treated PKU children conducted in the 1970s and 1980s thus suggest a pattern of cognitive function characterized by intact speech and language skills, but impaired visual–spatial and perceptual–motor abilities. These conclusions are based on a relatively small set of studies, many of which used the same task (e.g., Bender–Gestalt) and in which inferences about both spatial and perceptual–motor deficits were drawn from performance on a limited range of tasks. Nevertheless, a closer examination of the impairments revealed in these studies suggest that one problem exhibited by early-treated PKU subjects is the ability to generate and manipulate a mental representation of spatial information. Given that the ability to use mental representations to guide problem solving, while inhibiting maladaptive responses, is a primary feature of EF (Diamond, Werker, & LaLonde, 1994; Welsh & Pennington, 1988), deficits in the latter area may be responsible for many of the performance problems observed in these earlier studies.

Prefrontal Cortex Dysfunction Model

The cognitive research reviewed in the preceding section indicates some reduction in IQ and greater deficits on nonverbal tasks than on verbal tasks. The prefrontal cortex dysfunction hypothesis has the potential to account for this profile in terms of both underlying cognitive processes and brain mechanisms.

Several lines of evidence support the hypothesis of prefrontal cortex dysfunction in early-treated PKU. First, as previously discussed, the biochemical alterations resulting from the genetic mutation cause a disruption in catecholamine biosynthesis. One of these catecholamines, DA, is essential for prefrontal cortical functioning. Chamove and Molinaro (1978) artificially elevated Phe levels in rhesus monkeys and observed behaviors that were similar to those displayed by monkeys with frontal lesions. In a later animal model of PKU, Diamond, Ciaramitaro, Donner, Djali, and Robinson (1994) disrupted PAH in order to raise Phe levels in rats. As a consequence, DA metabolism was selectively reduced in the prefrontal cortex, and behavior on a task mediated by this brain region was impaired. More indirect evidence for prefrontal cortex dysfunction in PKU is the similarity in neuropathology and behavior between this disorder and two other conditions thought to involve frontal dysfunction and low DA: ADHD and autism. The fact that early-treated PKU children have difficulties in visual–spatial and perceptual–motor problem solving, which frequently demand "frontal skills" such as planning, working memory, and inhibition, is a further source of indirect support for the prefrontal hypothesis. In what follows, neuropsychological research that addresses this hypothesis more directly is reviewed.

Three studies evaluated the performance of older children and adults with early-treated PKU on traditional neuropsychological assessment batteries. Two studies that used the Halstead–Reitan batteries, along with additional tests, found evidence of visual–spatial, perceptual–motor, and reasoning deficits (Brunner et al., 1983; Pennington et al., 1985). Pennington et al. (1985) also reported an impairment on a test associated with frontal lobe function in adults, the Wisconsin Card Sorting Test. Perseverative responding on this test by early-treated PKU individuals studied in adulthood was replicated by Ris, Williams, Hunt, Berry, and Leslie (1994).

Faust, Libon, and Pueschel (1986–1987) administered the Luria–Nebraska battery to early-treated individuals aged 7 to 19 and discovered impairments in visual–spatial functions and reasoning, as well as "reduced channel capacity." Memory and language functions were intact. The authors defined reduced channel capacity as "abnormal limits in the amount of information that can be held in mind at one time and manipulated" (p. 174). Unfortunately, Faust et al. (1986–1987) did not identify the specific tests thought to tap channel capacity. The authors suggested that the visual–spatial deficits stemmed from difficulties in "the formation of internal spatial images and/or the performance of internal spatial operations" (p. 173). The descriptions of specific spatial deficits and reduced channel capacity are congruent with most definitions of a working memory deficit. Although Faust et al. (1986–1987) also reported that performance on "frontal lobe tasks" was normal, they did not identify the particular tasks used to measure functioning in this area.

A small set of studies has tested the prefrontal cortex dysfunction model directly by administering EF tasks to early-treated PKU children of various ages. We (Welsh et al., 1990) administered EF tasks measuring planning, organized search, and fluency to 4- and 5-year-old children who were currently on the PKU diet. Although the PKU group performed more poorly than an age- and IQ- matched control group on the EF tasks, the two groups performed comparably on a test of recognition memory. Moreover, EF performance was negatively correlated with concurrent Phe level.

Diamond et al. (1993) conducted a 2-year longitudinal study of early-treated infants and preschoolers with PKU. The results of the study revealed that the PKU subjects were selectively impaired on the "prefrontal cortex tasks," and that performance on these tasks covaried inversely with individual changes in Phe level over time. In a 4-year follow-up of these children, Diamond et al. (1997) found that early-treated children with Phe levels that were three to five times higher than the normal level were selectively impaired on tasks requiring working memory and inhibitory control. These deficits were seen across an age range of 6 months to 7 years.

Finally, Mazzocco et al. (1994) tested the prefrontal cortex dysfunction model by administering tests of EF and other cognitive abilities to early-treated PKU children aged 6 to 13 years. Despite the fact that some of the EF tasks were the same as those used in the Welsh et al. (1990) study, Mazzocco et al. found no group differences on any of the EF tasks. Testing also failed to document PKU-related impairment on the Developmental Test of Visual–Motor Integration, a test of perceptual–motor function. The lack of group difference on this test is surprising, given the preponderance of studies demonstrating perceptual–motor impairments. In addition, performance on this measure was not correlated with Phe level at the time of testing. Unexpectedly, the EF tasks discriminated children on the basis of geographical status (urban vs. rural), instead of on the basis of genetic status (PKU vs. control). Although it was suggested that geographical status might have been a confound in the Welsh et al. (1990) study, further analysis of the latter data set failed to support this possibility.

Findings from these recent neuropsychological studies provide evidence for EF impairments in planning, inhibition, visual search, and flexible set shifting; as such, they are consistent with a prefrontal cortex dysfunction model of early-treated PKU. The variety of tasks used and the wide age range of the samples tested make it difficult to be sure that similar "prefrontal skills" are being measured across studies. For example, evidence of EF impairment is based on tasks as diverse as the Wisconsin Card Sorting Test (Pennington et al., 1985; Ris et al., 1995), the Tower of Hanoi (Welsh et al., 1990), and a modified Stroop task (Diamond et al., 1993). Nevertheless, one common element in these tasks is the need to generate and manipulate a mental representation, as well as to inhibit inappropriate responding. Results from neuropsychological testing, together with the neurochemical evidence of DA depletion, thus appear to justify continued research based on the prefrontal dysfunction model of PKU (Griffiths, Tarrini, & Robinson, 1997; Smith, Klim, Mallozzi, & Hanley, 1996).

Other Neuropsychological Evidence

Several additional studies have investigated sequelae of PKU using a variety of individual neuropsychological measures, speeded information-processing tasks, and measures of attention. Clarke, Gates, Hogan, Barret, and MacDonald (1987) explored the effects of increased and decreased Phe levels on the neuropsychological performance of early-treated PKU children aged 11 to 18 years. They did not find effects of elevated Phe on two EF tasks (verbal fluency or the Stroop inhibition measure); the only task affected by elevated Phe was choice reaction time. It is important to note that the PKU subjects had been off diet for 2 to 11 years at the time of testing, and that the IQ performance reflected this fact (mean IQ = 78; range = 62–90). It is thus possible that the years on an unrestricted diet contributed to permanent neurological damage and cognitive impairment, and that a temporary decrease in Phe level could not reverse this effect.

In a somewhat similar study, Schmidt et al. (1994) investigated the impact on sustained attention of manipulating concurrent Phe level in early-treated PKU adults (mean age = 20.5 years). Unlike the sample tested in the Clarke et al. (1987) study, these adults had maintained the Phe-restricted diet well into adolescence and scored in the normal range of intelligence (mean IQ = 108, range = 89–132). Schmidt et al. found that the high-Phe condition was related to impaired sustained attention and slower reaction times. Lowering Phe improved performance, but not to the level of the unaffected control subjects. These results, like those of Clarke et al. (1987), suggest some degree of permanent impairment of performance in the PKU subjects. Schmidt et al., however, found that test performance *could* be changed by manipulating concurrent Phe levels. One can speculate that the many years on a relatively well-controlled diet averted structural brain damage to a large degree and contributed to the "reversibility" of the deficit. Consistent with this possibility, Stemerdink et al. (1994) found that PKU children and adolescents treated early and continuously, who had relatively low Phe levels and normal IQ, showed no deficits on information-processing tasks relative to unaffected controls.

Another program of research has explored the possibility that the disruption in DA biosynthesis during postnatal brain development might have a greater impact on left-hemisphere function, and that this impact might differ in males and females with early-treated PKU. Craft, Gourovitch, Dowton, Swanson, and Bonforte (1992) found that male, but not female, early-treated PKU subjects exhibited a right-visual-field defect in the ability to disengage attention, suggestive of dysfunction in the left parietal lobe. This defect was related to concurrent Phe level for male subjects only.

In a follow-up study, Gourovitch, Craft, Dowton, Ambrose, and Spartan (1994) assessed interhemispheric transfer time in children with early-treated PKU. In light of the accumulating evidence of deficient myelination, it was hypothesized that the corpus callosum might be compromised in PKU. A manual reaction time paradigm was administered to children with early-treated PKU, children diagnosed with ADHD, and unaffected control children. The authors found that the early-treated PKU group showed slowed interhemispheric transfer from the left to the right hemisphere, compared to the other two groups. The transfer time from left to right hemisphere was related to Phe level at birth, but not to concurrent Phe level.

Although the two studies by Craft and colleagues both suggest a possible left-hemisphere dysfunction, some inconsistencies are also apparent. First, whereas Craft et al. (1992) found evidence of left-hemisphere dysfunction in PKU males only, Gourovitch et al. (1994) found slowed interhemispheric transfer from left to right in a group composed of both male and female subjects. Second, the left-hemisphere dysfunction suggested by the Craft et al. (1992) data was related to concurrent Phe level, whereas the slowed interhemispheric transfer observed by Gourovitch et al. (1994) was related to Phe level at the time of birth. The reasons for these inconsistencies are as yet unclear.

A further problem with the left-hemisphere dysfunction model is its difficulty in accounting for deficits in visual–spatial and perceptual–motor functions in persons with early-treated PKU. These particular functions would presumably be mediated by the *right* parietal lobe. One would also expect that the hypothesized left-hemisphere dysfunction would be associated with greater language impairments than are observed in this population. Recent MRI studies report white matter abnormalities in the posterior structures, but do not suggest a unilateral distribution. MRI findings indicating defective myelination of the fibers of the corpus callosum are nevertheless consistent to some degree with the Gourovitch et al. (1994) data.

SCIENTIFIC CRITIQUE AND FUTURE DIRECTIONS

Prior to the discovery of an effective dietary therapy, PKU served as a model of global deterioration of the brain, behavior and intelligence. Over 60 years after the initial discovery of PKU, routine identification and early dietary treatment of affected individuals have allowed scientists to investigate the more subtle sequelae of the disorder. The growing sophistication in behavioral assessment and neuroimaging techniques has provided the tools necessary to begin to link behavioral sequelae to specific neurological systems. Today's neuropsychological researchers confront two major issues regarding the outcomes of early-treated PKU: (1) To what degree do neuropsychological sequelae change with development? and (2) What neuropsychological model provides the most appropriate description of the behavioral and neurological consequences of the disorder?

Developmental Issues

Now that routine identification and treatment of PKU have existed in industrialized countries for over two decades, a large pool of early-treated individuals is available for research on possible age-related differences in the sequelae of this disorder. The studies of the behavioral and neuropsychological sequelae of early-treated PKU reviewed above have included samples ranging widely in age. Unfortunately, however, these studies have failed to examine the potential influences of age-related factors.

With the exception of the PKU Collaborative Study and more recent neuropsychological investigations (e.g., Diamond et al., 1993; Welsh et al., 1990), past research samples have also failed to focus on individuals within restricted age bands. For example, Ozanne et al. (1990) explored speech and language skills in early-treated PKU subjects from 7 months to 16 years of age, and Gourovitch et al. (1994) examined interhemispheric transfer time in subjects ranging in age from 6 to 16 years. As a result of these recruitment practices, chronological age has been confounded with various treatment variables. An older PKU child, for example, may have been treated at a later age, experienced less stringent dietary control, or terminated the PKU diet at an earlier age than a younger child. Confounds of this type prevent us from being able to address important issues, such as possible age differences in the effects of dietary control.

This lack of appreciation for developmental factors is particularly troublesome when pre- and postpubertal subjects are combined in a single sample (e.g., Brunner et al., 1983, 1987; Clarke et al., 1987; Faust et al., 1986–1987; Gourovitch et al., 1994; Mazzocco et al., 1994; Ozanne et al., 1990; Pennington et al., 1985; Stemerdink et al., 1994). Much of the ingested and endogenous Phe is utilized for protein synthesis during growth. As the rate of growth declines during adolescence, the amount of Phe available for metabolism increases (Levy & Waisbren, 1994). Consequently, even with a consistently controlled diet, blood concentrations of Phe should be higher in adolescents than in younger children. The fact that the PKU diet is usually less well controlled in adolescence leads to even greater age differences in Phe levels. Do these elevated Phe levels in adolescence have the same neuro-psychological consequences as they do in younger children? How do brain development and other physiological changes (e.g., myelin turnover, hormones) after puberty interact with rising Phe levels to affect neuropsychological functioning?

The relevance of these issues to understanding of the sequelae of PKU underscores the importance of recruiting subject samples that are more homogeneous with respect to this variable, and of then assessing the effects of treatment variables with the age factor effectively held constant. Conversely, one can conduct longitudinal studies in which early treatment variables are held constant and age varies within individuals across follow-up. The PKU Collaborative Study provided important longitudinal data on the effects of early diet initiation and age of diet termination on intellectual function. To date, only one longitudinal study of more specific neuropsychological sequelae has been reported (Diamond et al., 1993). Future studies that take into account chronological age, as well as the various treatment parameters, will begin to address the critical question of whether the impairments associated with PKU should be viewed within a developmental lag or deficit model.

Testing Neuropsychological Models

A second challenge that confronts researchers investigating PKU is to identify an appropriate neuropsychological model of the disorder—one that accurately portrays both the nature of the behavioral consequences and the associated neuropathology. In the past, neuropsychological research has been more exploratory than hypothesis-driven. Despite the frequent failure to test specific neuropsychological models, this research has yielded findings implicating prefrontal, left-hemisphere, or attentional systems in the brain. As data accrue from various levels of analysis (genetic, neurochemical, neuroanatomical), researchers need to begin to refine hypothetical neuropsychological models and to test these models by utilizing specific neurocognitive paradigms and methodologies. These are four potentially useful approaches in this regard.

One methodological technique that has paid dividends in other neuropsychological research involves selection of comparison groups to test specific hypotheses about brain dysfunction. For example, if one proposes a prefrontal cortex dysfunction model of PKU, an appropriate clinical comparison group would be one with known or presumed dysfunction in the posterior cortex. Administration of tests of prefrontal functions (e.g., EF) and of posterior cortical functions (e.g., linguistic skills) would then permit the researchers to examine potential double dissociations. Such a dissociation would be evident, for example, if the PKU group performed poorly on the EF tasks and normally on the linguistic tasks, while the clinical comparison group showed the opposite profile.

To our knowledge, no published study of PKU has employed this double-dissociation paradigm. A study by Pennington et al. (1985) employed aspects of this technique by comparing PKU subjects to comparison groups with left-hemisphere, right-hemisphere, or bilateral dysfunction. Although there were similarities in neuropsychological performance between the PKU and right-hemisphere dysfunction groups, the PKU group was distinct from all three groups in terms of a pattern of deficits suggestive of a frontal lobe dysfunction.

A second but related approach would be to select comparison groups consisting of subjects known or presumed to suffer brain dysfunction similar to that proposed to occur in PKU. For example, if one subscribes to a prefrontal dysfunction model of this disorder, an appropriate comparison group would consist of subjects with documented frontal damage or putative frontal dysfunction due to DA depletion, such as ADHD or high-functioning autism. No published study has compared PKU subjects to patients with documented frontal lobe insults, although two behavioral studies to date have compared PKU subjects to individuals diagnosed with ADHD. Kalverboer et al. (1994) found some behavioral similarities between children with PKU and those with ADHD. Gourovitch et al. (1994), however, found differences in interhemispheric transfer time in comparing these two groups of children. Clearly, one would not expect to find the neuropsychological profile of children with PKU to be a *duplicate* of that found in children with frontal damage or ADHD. However, a pattern of findings demonstrating substantial similarities in these profiles, as well as dissimilarities in the profiles of subjects with PKU versus those with suspected posterior cortex damage, would provide convincing support for the proposed prefrontal dysfunction model.

A third approach to hypothesis testing is to manipulate Phe concentrations via random assignment of early-treated PKU individuals to groups receiving high or low levels of Phe. In this manner, the causal effects of Phe level on behavior could be assessed via a true experimental design. Conducting such manipulation studies with samples that are relatively homogeneous with respect to age would allow researchers to assess the impact of DA reductions on brain function and behavior at various points in development. This approach would also yield valuable information regarding the development of brain–behavior relations more generally.

A final approach is to continue tracing the path from genome to neurochemistry to neuropathology to behavior. The fact that increasing numbers of early-treated individuals are entering adulthood may permit the use of more advanced neuroimaging techniques, such as PET. These methods are likely to provide the type of neurophysiological data that are critical to a more rigorous test of the prefrontal cortex dysfunction model, as well as other neuropsychological hypotheses. Similarly, various cognitive psychophysiological paradigms (e.g., measures of heart rate, the P300 components of the ERP, and the lateralized readiness potential) could be employed to test specific information-processing deficits characteristic of PKU (van der Molen & Molenaar, 1994).

CONCLUSIONS

One overall conclusion to be drawn from the present review is that there appears to be relative consistency in findings *within* levels of analysis, but that data from different levels do not yet fit together into a coherent neuropsychological model. There is consensus among molecular geneticists, for example, that the mutation is in the PAH gene on chromosome 12, with the particular nature of this mutation varying across PKU individuals. The neurochemical data indicate that the synthesis of DA, norepinephrine, and serotonin is negatively affected by the disorder, but that DA is most directly affected by the inactive PAH gene. Neuropathological findings from autopsies, MRI, and animal models consistently reveal abnormalities in myelination or in the water content of the myelin. The brain regions affected in this manner vary across studies. Finally, there is some convergence of data from behavioral, cognitive, and neuropsychological studies indicating specific impairments in EF in children with early-treated PKU. These impairments relate specifically to the generation and manipulation of mentally represented spatial information and the ability to inhibit maladaptive responses.

Although PKU provides us with a unique opportunity to trace the path from gene to brain to behavior, the links between these relatively large bodies of knowledge are still tenuous. The emerging neuropsychological "story" does not yet unequivocally support the prefrontal dysfunction hypothesis. The existing data also fail to support alternative proposals with regard to either specific or general neuropsychological dysfunction. Subtle differences in the nature of the genetic mutation may be related to the regional distribution of white matter abnormalities. Similarly, individual differences in the genetic mutation or in white matter abnormalities may account for variability in the clinical manifestations of the disorder. Discovery of associations among these levels of analysis will require continued empirical efforts to specify the nature of PKU-related anomalies of gene, brain, and behavior.

REFERENCES

Aragon, M. C., Giminez, C., & Valdivieso, F. (1982). Inhibition by L-phenylalanine of tyrosine transport by synaptosomal plasma membrane vesicles: Implications in the pathogenesis of phenylketonuria. *Journal of Neurochemistry, 39,* 1185–1187.

Aragon, M. C., Giminez, C., Major, F., Jr., Marivizon, J. G., & Valdivieso, F. (1981). Tyrosine transport by membrane vesicles isolated from rat brain. *Journal of Biochemistry and Biophysics, 646,* 465–470.

Bannon, M. J., Bunney, E. B., & Roth, R. H. (1981). Mesocortical dopamine neurons: Rapid transmitter turnover compared to other brain catecholamine systems. *Brain Research, 218,* 376–382.

Bannon, M. J., Michaud, R. L., & Roth, R. H. (1981). Mesocortical dopamine neurons: Lack of autoreceptors modulating dopamine synthesis. *Molecular Pharmacology, 19,* 270–275.

Bannon, M. J., Reinhard, J. F., Jr., Bunney, E. B., & Roth, R. H. (1982). Unique response to antipsychotic drugs is due to absence of terminal autoreceptors in mesocortical dopamine neurons. *Nature, 296,* 444–446.

Bashore, T. R. (1993). Differential effects of aging on the neurocognitive functions subserving speed at mental processing. In J. Cerella (Ed.), *Adult information processing: Limits on loss* (pp. 37–76). New York: Academic Press.

Berry, H. K., O'Grady, D. J., Perlmutter, L. J., & Bofinger, M. K. (1979). Intellectual development and academic achievement of children treated early for phenylketonuria. *Developmental Medicine and Child Neurology, 21,* 311–320.

Bick, U., Ullrich, K., Stober, U., Moller, H., Schuierer, G., Ludolph, A. C., Oberwitter, C., Weglage, J., & Wendel, U. (1993). White matter abnormalities in patients with treated hyperphenylalaninemia: Magnetic resonance relaxometry and proton spectoscopy findings. *European Journal of Pediatrics, 152,* 1012–1020.

Bickel, H., Gerrard, J., & Hickmans, E. M. (1954). Influence of phenylalanine intake on the chemistry and behavior of a phenylketonuric child. *Acta Paediatrica, 43,* 64.

Blaskovics, M., Engel, R., Podosin, R. L., Azen, C. G., & Friedman, E. G. (1981). EEG pattern in phenylketonuria under early initiated dietary treatment. *American Journal of Diseases of Children, 135,* 802.

Bloom, L. (1993). *The transition from infancy to language: Acquiring the power of expression.* New York: Cambridge University Press.

Brunner, R. L., Berch, D. B., & Berry, H. (1987). Phenylketonuria and complex spatial visualization: An analysis of information processing. *Developmental Medicine and Child Neurology, 29,* 460–468.

Brunner, R. L., Jordan, M. K., & Berry, H. K. (1983). Early treated PKU: Neuropsychologic consequences. *Journal of Pediatrics, 102,* 831–835.

Butler, I. J., O'Flynn, M. E., Seifert, W. E., & Howell, R. R. (1981). Neurotransmitter defects and treatment of disorders of hyperphenylalaninemia. *Journal of Pediatrics, 98,* 729–733.

Cabalska, B., Durzynska, N., Borzymownsky, J., Zorska, K., Kaslacz-Folga, A., & Bozkowa, K. (1977). Termination of dietary treatment in phenylketonuria. *European Journal of Pediatrics, 126,* 253–262.

Case, R. (1992). The role of the frontal lobes in the regulation of cognitive development. *Brain and Cognition, 20,* 51–73.

Chamove, A. S., & Molinaro, T. J. (1978). Monkey retarded learning analysis. *Journal of Mental Deficiency Research, 22,* 223.

Chiodo, L. A., Bannon, M. J., Grace, A. A., Roth, R. H., & Bunney, B. S. (1984). Evidence for the absence of impulse-regulating somatodendritic and synthesis-modulating nerve terminal autoreceptors of subpopulations of mesocortical dopamine neurons. *Neuroscience, 12,* 1–16.

Ciaranello, R. D., Wong, D. L., & Rubenstein, J. L. R. (1990). Application of basic neuroscience to child psychiatry. In S. I. Deutsch, A. Weizman, & R. Weizman (Eds.), *Molecular neurobiology and disorders of brain development* (pp. 9–32). New York: Plenum Press.

Clarke, J. T. R., Gates, R. D., Hogan, S. E., Barret, M., & MacDonald, G. W. (1987). Neuropsychological studies on adolescents with phenylketonuria returned to phenylalanine restricted diets. *American Journal of Mental Retardation, 92,* 255–262.

Cleary, M. A., Walter, J. H., Wraith, J. E., Jenkins, J. P. R., Alani, S. M., Tyler, K., & Whittle, D. (1994). Magnetic resonance imaging of the brain in phenylketonuria: Relationship to intelligence, neuropsychological abnormalities, and biochemical control. *Lancet, 344,* 87–90.

Craft, S., Gourvitch, M. L., Dowton, S. B., Swanson, J. M., & Bonforte. (1992). Lateralized deficits in visual attention in males with developmental dopamine depletion. *Neuropsychologia, 30,* 341–351.

Creel, D., & Buehler, B. A. (1982). Pattern evoked potentials in phenylketonuria. *Electroencephalography and Clinical Neurophysiology, 53,* 220–223.

Curtius, H. C., Baerlocher, K., & Vollmin, J. A. (1972). Pathogenesis of phenylketonuria: Inhibition of dopa and catecholamine synthesis in patients with phenylketonuria. *Clinical Chimica Acta, 42,* 235–239.

Davis, D. D., McIntyre, C. W., Murray, M. E., & Mims, S. S. (1986). Cognitive styles in children with dietary treated phenylketonuria. *Educational and Psychological Research, 6,* 9–15.

Degiorgio, G. F., Antonozzi, I., Del Castello, P. G., & Loizzo, A. (1982). EEG as a possible prognostic tool in phenylketonuria. *Electroencephalography and Clinical Neurophysiology, 55,* 60–68.

Diamond, A., Ciaramitaro, V., Donner, E., Djali, S., & Robinson, M. (1994). An animal model of early-treated PKU. *Journal of Neuroscience, 14,* 3072–3082.

Diamond, A., Hurwitz, W., Lee, E. Y., Bockes, T., Grover, W., & Minarcik, C. (1993). *Cognitive deficits on frontal cortex tasks in children with early-treated PKU: Results of two years of longitudinal study.* Paper presented at the biennial meeting of the Society for Research in Child Development, Los Angeles.

Diamond, A., Prevor, M. B., Callender, G., & Druin, D. P. (1997). Prefrontal cortex cognitive deficits in children treated early and continuously for PKU. *Monographs of the Society for Research in Child Development, 62*(4, Serial No. 252).

Diamond, A., Werker, J. F., & LaLonde, C. (1994). Toward understanding commonalities in the development of object search, categorization, and speech perception. In G. Dawson & K. W. Fischer (Eds.), *Human behavior and the developing brain* (pp. 380–426). New York: Guilford Press.

Dobson, J. C., Williamson, M. L., Azen, C., & Koch, R. (1977). Intellectual assessment of 111 four-year-old children with phenylketonuria. *Pediatrics, 60,* 822–827.

Donker, D. N. J., Reits, D., Van Sprang, F. J., Storm van Leewen, W. S., & Wadman, S. K. (1979). Computer analysis of the EEG as an aid in the evaluation of dietetic treatment in phenylketonuria. *Electroencephalography and Clinical Neurophysiology, 46,* 205–213.

Faust, D., Libon, D., & Pueschel, S. (1986–1987). Neuropsychological functioning in treated phenylketonuria. *International Journal of Psychiatry in Medicine, 16,* 169–177.

Fisch, R. O., Sines, L. K., & Chang, P. (1981). Personality characteristics of nonretarded phenylketonurics and their family members. *Journal of Clinical Psychiatry, 42,* 106–113.

Fischler, K., Azen, C. G., Henderson, R., Friedman, E. G., & Koch, R. (1987). Psychoeducational findings among children treated for phenylketonuria. *American Journal of Mental Deficiency, 92,* 65–73.

Friedman, E. (1969). The "autistic syndrome" and phenylketonuria. *Schizophrenia, 1,* 249–261.

Fuller, R., & Shuman, J. (1971). Treated phenylketonuria: Intelligence and blood phenylalanine levels. *American Journal of Mental Deficiency, 75,* 539–545.

Garrod, A. E. (1902). The incidence of alkaptonuria: A study in chemical individuality. *Lancet, ii,* 1616–1620.

Gourovitch, M. L., Craft, S., Dowton, S. B., Ambrose, P., & Spartan. (1994). Interhemispheric transfer in children with early-treated phenylketonuria. *Journal of Clinical and Experimental Neuropsychology, 16,* 393–404.

Griffiths, P., Tarrini, M., & Robinson, P. (1997). Executive function and psychosocial adjustment in children with early treated phenylketonuria: Correlation with historical and concurrent phenylalanine levels. *Journal of Intellectual Disability Research, 41,* 317–323.

Gross, T., Berlow, S., Schuett, V. E., Ruggero, G., & Fariello, M. D. (1981). EEG in phenylketonuria: Attempt to establish clinical importance of EEG changes. *Archives of Neurology, 38,* 122–126.

Guttler, F., & Lou, H. (1986). Dietary problems of phenylketonuria: Effect on CNS transmitters and their possible role in behavior and neuropsychological function. *Journal of Inherited Metabolic Disease, 9,* 169–172.

Hogan, R. N., & Coleman, P. D. (1981). Experimental hyperphenylalaninemia: Dendritic alterations in cerebellum of rat. *Experimental Neurology, 74,* 218–244.

Holtzman, N. A., Kronmal, R. A., van Doorninck, W., Azen, C., & Koch, R. (1986). Effect of age at loss of dietary control on intellectual performance and behavior of children with phenylketonuria. *New England Journal of Medicine, 314,* 593–598.

Huether, G., Kaus, R., & Neuhoff, V. (1982). Brain development in experimental hyperphenylalaninemia: Myelination. *Neuropediatrics*, *13*, 177–182.

Kalverboer, A. F., van der Schot, L. W. A., Hendrikx, M. M. H., Huisman, J., Slijper, F. M. E., & Stemerdink, B. A. (1994). Social behaviour and task orientation in early-treated PKU. *Acta Paediatrica*, (Suppl. 407), 104–105.

Knox, W. E. (1972). Phenylketonuria. In J. B. Stanbury, J. B. Wyngaarden, & D. S. Fredrickson (Eds.), *The metabolic basis of inherited disease* (pp. 266–295). New York: McGraw-Hill.

Koch, R., Azen, C., Friedman, E. G., & Williamson, M. L. (1982). Preliminary report on the effects of diet discontinuation in PKU. *Journal of Pediatrics*, *100*, 870.

Koch, R., Azen, C., Friedman, E. G., & Williamson, M. L. (1984). Paired comparisons between early treated PKU children and their matched sibling controls on intelligence and school achievement test results at eight years of age. *Journal of Inherited Metabolic Disease*, *7*, 86–90.

Koff, E., Boyle, P., & Pueschel, S. M. (1977). Perceptual–motor functioning in children with phenylketonuria. *American Journal of Disease in Childhood*, *131*, 1084–1087.

Kolb, B., & Whishaw, I. Q. (1990). *Fundamentals of human neuropsychology* (2nd ed.). New York: Freeman.

Krause, W. L., Halminski, M., McDonald, L., Dembure, P., Salvo, R., Friedes, D., & Elsas, L. J. (1985). Biochemical and neuropsychological effects of elevated plasma phenylalanine in patients with treated phenylketonuria: A model for the study of phenylalanine and brain function in man. *Journal of Clinical Investigation*, *75*, 40–48.

Levy, H. L., & Waisbren, S. E. (1994). PKU in adolescents: Rationale and psychosocial factors in diet continuation. *Acta Paediatrica*, (Suppl. 407), 92–97.

Lou, H. C., Toft, P. B., Andreson, J., Nikkelsen, I., Olsen, B., & Guttler, F. (1992). An occipito-temporal syndrome in adolescents with optimally controlled hyperphenylalaninemia. *Journal of Inherited Metabolic Disease*, *15*, 687–695.

Lowe, T. L., Tanaka, K., Seashore, M. R., Young, J. G., & Cohen, D. J. (1980). Detection of phenylketonuria in autistic and psychotic children. *Journal of the American Medical Association*, *243*, 126–128.

Ludolph, A. C., Ullrich, K., Nedjat, S., Masur, H., & Bick, U. (1991). Neurological outcome in 22 treated adolescents with hyperphenylalaninaemia. *Acta Neurologica Scandinavica*, *85*, 243–248.

Mazzocco, M. M., Nord, A. M., Van Doorninck, W. J., Greene, C. L., Kovar, C. G., & Pennington, B. F. (1994). Cognitive development among children with early-treated phenylketonuria. *Developmental Neuropsychology*, *10*, 133–151.

McCombe, P. A., McLaughlin, D. B., Chalk, J. B., Brown, N. N., McGill, J. J., & Pender, M. P. (1992). Spasticity and white matter abnormalities in adult phenylketonuria. *Journal of Neurology, Neurosurgery and Psychiatry*, *55*, 359–361.

McKean, C. M. (1972). The effects of high phenylalanine concentrations on serotonin and catecholamine metabolism in the human brain. *Brain Research*, *47*, 469–476.

Melnick, C. R., Michals, K. K., & Matalon, R. (1981). Linguistic development of children with phenylketonuria and normal intelligence. *Journal of Pediatrics*, *98*, 269–272.

Michals, K., Dominik, M., Schuett, M. S., Brown, E., & Matalon, R. (1985). Return to diet therapy in patients with phenylketonuria. *Journal of Pediatrics*, *106*, 933–936.

Mims, S. K. S., McIntyre, C. W., & Murray, M. E. (1981). Evidence of visual–motor problems in children with dietary treated phenylketonuria. *Educational and Psychological Research*, *1*, 223–230.

Mims, S. K. S., McIntyre, C. W., & Murray, M. E. (1983). An analysis of visual motor problems in children with dietary treated phenylketonuria. *Educational and Psychological Research*, *3*, 111–121.

O'Grady, D. J., Berry, H. K., & Sutherland, B. S. (1971). Cognitive development in early treated phenylketonuria. *American Journal of Diseases of Children*, *121*, 20–23.

Ozanne, A. E., Krimmer, H., & Murdoch, B. E. (1990). Speech and language skills in children with early treated phenylketonuria. *American Journal on Mental Retardation*, *94*, 625–632.

Paere, C. M. B., Sandler, M., & Stacy, R. S. (1957). 5-Hydroxytryptamine deficiency in phenylketonuria. *Lancet*, *i*, 551.

Paine, R. S. (1957). The variability in manifestations of untreated patients with phenylketonuria (phenylpyruvic aciduria). *Pediatrics*, *20*, 290–331.

Pearson, K. D., Gean-Marton, A. D., Levy, H. L., & Davis, K. R. (1990). Phenylketonuria: MR-imaging of the brain with clinical correlation. *Radiology*, *177*, 437–440.

Pennington, B. F., van Doorninck, W. J., McCabe, L. L., & McCabe, E. R. B. (1985). Neuropsychological deficits in early-treated phenylketonurics. *American Journal of Mental Deficiency*, *89*, 467–474.

Penrose, L. S. (1935). Inheritance of phenylpyruvic amentia (phenylketonuria). *Lancet*, *229*, 192–194.

Peterson, N. A., Shah, S. N., Raghupathy, E., & Rhoads, D. E. (1983). Presynaptic tyrosine availability in the phenylketonuric brain: A hypothetical evaluation. *Brain Research*, 272, 189–193.

Pietz, J., Meyding-Lamade, U. K., & Schmidt, H. (1996). Magnetic resonance imaging of the brain in adolescents with phenylketonuria and in one case of 6-pyruvoyl tetrahydropteridine synthase deficiency. *European Journal of Pediatrics*, 155(Suppl. 1), S69–S73.

Poser, C. M., & Van Bogaert, L. (1959). Neuropathologic observations in phenylketonuria. *Brain*, 82, 1–9.

Pueschel, S. M. (1996). Central nervous system effects in individuals with phenylketonuria. *Developmental Brain Dysfunction*, 90, 165–179.

Pueschel, S. M., Fogelson-Doyle, L., Kammerer, B., & Matsumiya, Y. (1983). Neurophysiological, psychological, and nutritional investigations during discontinuation of the phenalanine-restricted diet in children with classic phenylketonuria. *Journal of Mental Deficiency Research*, 27, 61–67.

Realmuto, G. M., Garfinkel, B. D., Tuchman, M., Tsai, M. Y., Chang, P.-N., Fisch, R. O., & Shapiro, S. (1986). Psychiatric diagnosis and behavioral characteristics of phenylketonuric children. *Journal of Nervous and Mental Disease*, 174, 536–540.

Ris, M. D., Williams, S. E., Hunt, M. M., Berry, H. K., & Leslie, N. (1994). Early-treated phenylketonuria: Adult neuropsychologic outcome. *Journal of Pediatrics*, 124, 388–392.

Rolle-Daya, H., Pueschel, S. M., & Lombroso, C. T. (1975). Electroencephalographic findings in children with phenylketonuria. *American Journal of Diseases of Children*, 129, 869–900.

Sandler, M. (1982). Inborn errors and disturbances of central neurotransmission (with special reference to phenylketonuria). *Journal of Inherited Metabolic Disease*, 5(Suppl. 2), 65–70.

Schmidt, E., Rupp, A., Burgard, P., Pietz, J., Weglage, J., & Sonneville, L. (1994). Sustained attention in adult phenylketonuria: The influence of the concurrent phenylalanine-blood-level. *Journal of Experimental Neuropsychology*, 16, 681–688.

Schor, D. P. (1983). PKU and temperament: Rating children three through seven years old in PKU families. *Clinical Pediatrics*, 22, 807–811.

Schor, D. P. (1984, October). *PKU and temperament in 8–12 year old children*. Paper presented at the annual meeting of the American Academy for Cerebral Palsy and Developmental Medicine, Washington, D.C.

Scriver, C. R., & Clow, C. L. (1980). Phenylketonuria: Epitome of human biochemical genetics. Part I. *New England Journal of Medicine*, 303, 1336–1400.

Shiwach, R. S., & Sheikha, S. (1998). Delusional disorder in a boy with phenylketonuria and amine metabolites in the cerebrospinal fluid after treatment with neuroleptics. *Journal of Adolescent Health*, 22, 244–246.

Smith, I. (1994). Treatment of phenylalanine hydroxylase deficiency. *Acta Paediatrica*, (Suppl. 407), 60–65.

Smith M., Klim, P., Mallozzi, E., & Hanley, W. B. (1996). A test of the frontal-specificity hypothesis in the cognitive performance of adults with phenylketonuria. *Developmental Neuropsychology*, 12, 327–341.

Spreen, O., Risser, A. T., & Edgell, D. (1985). *Human developmental neuropsychology*. New York: Oxford University Press.

Standbury, J. B., Wyngaarden, J. B., & Fredrickson, D. S. (Eds.). (1983). *The metabolic basis of inherited disease* (2nd ed.). New York: McGraw-Hill.

Stemerdink, B. A., van der Molen, M. W., Kalverboer, A. F., van der Meere, J. J., Hendrikx, M. M. H., Huisman, J., van der Schot, L. W. A., & Slijper, F. M. E. (1994). Information processing deficits in children with early and continuously treated phenylketonuria. *Acta Paediatrica* (Suppl. 407), 106–107.

Stevenson, J. E., Hawcroft, J., Lobascher, M., Smith, I., Wolff, O. H., & Graham, P. J. (1979). Behavioral deviance in children with early treated phenylketonuria. *Archives of Disease in Childhood*, 54, 14–18.

Storm van Leewen, W., Donker, D. N. J., & Van Sprang, F. J. (1975). The electroencephalogram in inborn errors of metabolism. In M. A. B. Brazier (Ed.), *Growth and development of the brain* (pp. 275–286). New York: Raven Press.

Tam, S.-Y., Elsworth, J. D., Bradberry, C. W., & Roth, R. H. (1991). Mesocortical dopamine neurons: High basal firing frequency predicts tyrosine dependence of dopamine synthesis. *Journal of Neural Transmission*, 81, 97–110.

Thierry, A. M., Tassin, J. P., Blanc, A., Stinus, L., Scatton, B., & Glowinsky, J. (1977). Discovery of the mesocortical dopaminergic system: Some pharmacological and functional characteristics. *Advances in Biomedical Psychopharmacology*, 16, 5–12.

Thompson, A. J., Smith, I., Brenton, D., Youl, B. D., Rylance, G., Davidson, D. C., Kendall, B., & Lee, A. J. (1990). Neurological deterioration in young adults with phenylketonuria. *Lancet*, 336, 602–605.

Thompson, A. J., Tillotson, S., Smith, I., Kendall, B., Moore, S. G., & Brenton, D. P. (1993). Brain MRI changes in phenylketonuria. *Brain*, 116, 811–821.

Thompson, J. H. (1957). Relatives of phenylketonuric patients. *Journal of Mental Deficiency Research*, 1, 67–68.

Tischler, B., & Lowry, R. B. (1978). Phenylketonuria in British Columbia, Canada. *Monographs of Human Genetics, 9,* 102.

Ullrich, K., Moller, H., Weglage, J., Schuierer, G., Bick, U., Ludolph, A., Hahn-Ullrich, H., Funders, B., & Koch, H. G. (1994). White matter abnormalities in phenylketonuria: Results of magnetic resonance measurements. *Acta Paedriatrica,* (Suppl. 407), 78–82.

van der Molen, M. W., & Molenaar, P. C. M. (1994). Cognitive psychophysiology: A window to cognitive development and brain maturation In G. Dawson & K. W. Fischer (Eds.), *Human behavior and the developing brain* (pp. 456–490). New York: Guilford Press.

Vogel, F., & Motulsky, A. G. (1979). *Human genetics: Problems and approaches.* New York: Springer-Verlag.

Waisbren, S. E., Mahon, B. E., Schnell, R. R., & Levy, H. L. (1987). Predictors of intelligence quotient changes in persons treated for phenylketonuria early in life. *Pediatrics, 79,* 351–355.

Waisbren, S. E., Schnell, R. R., & Levy, H. L. (1980). Diet termination in children with phenylketonuria: A review of psychological assessments used to determine outcome. *Journal of Inherited Metabolic Disease, 3,* 149–153.

Walter, J. H., Cleary, M. A., Wraith, J. E., & Jenkins, J. P. R. (1994). Reversal of abnormal resonance imaging in phenylketonuria [Abstract]. In *Symposium on phenylketonuria: Past, present, future, 1994, May 23–25, Elsingore, Denmark* (p. 63).

Walter, J. H., Tyfield, L. A., Holton, J. B., & Johnson, C. (1993). Biochemical control, genetic analysis and magnetic resonance imaging in patients with phenylketonuria. *European Journal of Pediatrics, 152,* 822–827.

Weglage, J., Pietsch, M., Funders, B., Koch, H. G., & Ullrich, K. (1995). Neurological findings in early-treated phenylketonuria. *Acta Paediatrica, 84,* 411–415.

Weil-Malherbe, H. (1955). The concentration of adrenaline in human plasma and its relation to mental activity. *Journal of Mental Sciences, 101,* 733.

Welsh, M. C., & Pennington, B. F. (1988). Assessing frontal lobe function in children: Views from developmental psychology. *Developmental Neuropsychology, 4,* 199–230.

Welsh, M. C., Pennington, B. F., Oznoff, S., Rouse, B., & McCabe, E. R. B. (1990). Neuropsychology of early-treated phenylketonuria: Specific executive function deficits. *Child Development, 61,* 1697–1713.

Williams, R. S., Hauser, S. L., Purpura, D. P., DeLong, F. R., & Swisher, C. N. (1980). Autism and mental retardation: Neuropathological studies performed in four retarded persons with autistic behavior. *Archives of Neurology, 37,* 749–753.

Williamson, M. L., Dobson, J. C., & Koch, R. (1977). Collaborative study of children treated for phenylketonuria: Study design. *Pediatrics, 60,* 815–821.

Williamson, M. L., Koch, R., Azen, C., & Chang, C. (1981). Correlations of intelligence test results in treated phenylketonuric children. *Pediatrics, 68,* 161–167.

Woo, S. L. C. (1991). Genes, brain, and behavior. In P. R. McHugh & V. A. McKusick (Eds.), *Molecular genetic analysis of phenylketonuria and mental retardation* (pp. 193–203). New York: Raven Press.

Woo, S. L. C., Lidsky, A. S., Guttler, F., Chandra, T., & Robson, K. J. H. (1983). Cloned human phenylanine hydroxylase gene allows prenatal diagnosis and carrier detection of classical phenylketonuria. *Nature, 306,* 151–155.

Woo, S. L. C., Guttler, F., Ledley, F. D., Lidsky, A. S., Kwok, S. C., DiLella, A. G., & Robson, K. J. (1985). The human phenylalanine hydroxylase gene. *Progress in Clinical and Biological Research, 177,* 123–135.

Wright, S. W., & Tarjan, G. (1957). Phenylketonuria. *American Journal of Diseases of Children, 93,* 405.

13

ACUTE LYMPHOBLASTIC LEUKEMIA

DEBORAH P. WABER
PHYLLIS J. MULLENIX

Acute lymphoblastic leukemia (ALL) is the most common malignancy of childhood, with approximately 2,000 new cases diagnosed in the United States each year. Its treatment is a remarkable success story. As recently as the late 1960s, this disease was virtually always fatal. The major breakthrough in the treatment of ALL, achieved in the early 1970s, was the addition to the therapeutic regimen of central nervous system (CNS) prophylaxis—usually cranial radiation therapy (CRT) (Pui, 1997). By effectively preventing recurrence of the disease in the CNS, which had been the most common site of relapse after hematological remission was achieved, CRT greatly enhanced the likelihood of long-term disease-free survival. Building on the success of CNS treatment, leukemia treatment programs have achieved long-term survival rates that can exceed 70% in many institutions. The efficacy of therapy depends on several factors, including the combination of therapeutic agents used to treat the disease, intensity of the treatment protocol, and risk for relapse of the disease. Because so many children are now successfully treated, the quality of life for long-term survivors is a key consideration from the moment of diagnosis.

It has long been recognized that the intensive therapies used in treatment of ALL carry an unavoidable burden of toxicity to the CNS—a burden that may be greatest for the youngest, most vulnerable children. Adverse sequelae include endocrine abnormalities and associated growth problems (Katz & Morad, 1993); second malignancies (brain tumors) (Neglia et al., 1991); and, most frequently, learning problems (Cousens, Waters, Said, & Stevens, 1988). Because of the latter phenomenon, neuropsychology has been an important contributor to the development and evaluation of ALL treatment programs.

In addition to their clinical role in serving individual patients, neuropsychologists evaluate the risks and benefits associated with treatment protocols. The ultimate goal of protocol development is to maximize treatment efficacy while minimizing toxicity. The contribution of neuropsychologists to this endeavor is to define and describe neurobehavioral toxicity. The primary question asked of a neuropsychologist is how parameters of a treatment protocol are related to neurobehavioral outcome. As oncologists evaluate risks and benefits associated with treatment protocols, they need to know how outcomes are affected by variations in the intensity and components of treatment. Are the observed sequelae an acceptable risk, given the benefit? How do alternative modalities of treatment differ in terms of toxic burden? Can characteristic cognitive or behavioral sequelae that emerge during a child's development be associated with treatment?

Many years of follow-up are required to answer these questions. Such extended follow-up periods are needed because of the long-term evolution of actual neurotoxic effects, as well as the possibility that some sequelae may emerge only later in response to developmentally relevant challenges (e.g., the increased complexity of information processing and abstract reasoning demanded of older children). An additional complication for researchers is that experimental designs are generally limited by the exigencies of treatment. Treatment protocols are generally designed to focus to a greater extent on the effectiveness of treatment in controlling the disease than on risks for toxicity. Thus control or comparison groups that might be desirable from a methodological standpoint for evaluation of toxicity are often unavailable, or the utility of such groups can be limited by unavoidable confounding variables such as leukemic risk or associated therapies. As a result, neuropsychological research findings may be difficult to interpret or outdated by changes in therapeutic regimens.

The major aim of the present chapter is to highlight the central issues involved in this area of research, largely through description of our own experience evaluating neurobehavioral sequelae associated with a succession of investigational protocols from the Dana–Farber Cancer Institute/Children's Hospital (DF/CH) Consortium ALL program. The working model that has guided this research is also described. Other major collaborative groups, including the Pediatric Oncology Group, the Children's Cancer Group, and St. Jude's Children's Research Hospital, employ somewhat different treatment protocols. Nevertheless, protocols have evolved in a similar manner in all programs; that is, they are increasingly tailored to leukemic risk groups and include attempts to decrease treatment intensity whenever that option is viewed as safe.

NATURAL HISTORY/TREATMENT

As indicated above, ALL is the most common pediatric malignancy, accounting for three-quarters of all leukemias in children and one-quarter of all malignancies (Pui, 1997). Even so, it occurs infrequently. The prevalence in the United States is 3.4 cases per 100,000 children under the age of 15 years (Ries, Miller, & Hankey, 1994). ALL is most typically diagnosed in preschool-age children; the peak incidence occurs between 3 and 4 years of age (Gurney, Severson, Davis, & Robison, 1995). Thus the disease strikes many children during a developmental period when the CNS is presumably highly vulnerable to insult.

Because ALL can progress rapidly, treatment must be swift and intensive. Early attempts at treatment in the 1940s and 1950s included antineoplastic drugs, but treatment generally failed because of relapse in the CNS. The introduction of CNS therapies in the 1960s greatly enhanced the efficacy of treatment, leading to cure in a large number of patients. Advances since the 1970s have come from risk-directed therapies, which permitted refinement of treatments based on clinical signs that connoted good or poor prognosis (Pui, 1997). In general, risk group assignment is based on age and leukocyte count, with a recent consensus by the National Cancer Institute and the Cancer Therapy Evaluation Program that children aged 1 to 9 with a leukocyte count less than 50×10^9/liter fulfill minimal criteria for standard-risk (SR) ALL, and all others are classified as high-risk (HR) (Smith, Arthur, & Camitta, 1996).

Therapeutic protocols entail an initial, highly intensive period of treatment called *remission induction*, when the disease is brought into remission by intensive drug therapy (typically lasting about 1 month). Remission induction is followed by the *intensification phase* of treatment, at the outset of which CNS treatment occurs. This may include combined CRT (typically 1,800 cGy delivered in 10 fractions) and a drug delivered directly into the spinal canal (intrathecal), or, in many institutions, drug therapy only. The intensification period continues for several months and is followed by *maintenance therapy*, which usually lasts about 2 years. These entail drug therapies only, often with periodic intrathecal therapy.

As indicated above, the first successful ALL protocols were uniform for most patients. Contemporary protocols, however, are more individualized, involving careful assignment of children to leukemic risk groups. Children classified as HR receive more intensive therapies. Multiagent therapeutic combinations are the rule, providing opportunities for agent interactions in terms of toxicity, and many of the effective antileukemic agents (e.g., CRT, methotrexate [MTX], prednisone) have known neurotoxic risks.

CNS treatment, which in the past has generally included CRT, has been particularly controversial because of concerns about the neurotoxicity of radiation in the developing brain. Radiation is especially toxic to cells that are migrating or multiplying (Hicks & D'Amato, 1966; Altman, Anderson, & Wright, 1968) and can be selectively toxic to white matter even in mature animals (Mildenberger, Beach, McGeer, & Ludgate, 1990). Radiation given in combination with MTX can be even more neurotoxic (Bleyer, 1988).

For SR patients, most protocols now treat the CNS without CRT, achieving comparable efficacy with intrathecal and systemic drug combinations. HR patients, however, can require CRT to protect the CNS adequately against relapse or even to protect against hematological remission (Nachman et al., 1994). Some studies suggest that the risk for CNS toxicity can be decreased for SR patients by treating the CNS without radiation (Jankovic et al., 1994). The intensive drug therapy required and the neurotoxic potential of these agents, however, raise questions about the extent to which cognition can be thus spared. Indeed, in some studies, comparable neuropsychological sequelae have been documented among children treated with and without CRT (Brown et al., 1992; Kaufman, Moore, Espy, & Hutter, 1994; Mulhern, Fairclough, & Ochs, 1991).

Children can also experience acute neurotoxicity associated with certain treatment agents. On rare and unpredictable occasions, drugs can precipitate catastrophic events, such as acute encephalopathies. More common are the mood changes and temper tantrums that are routinely associated with corticosteroid therapy during maintenance therapy (Drigan, Spirito, & Gelber, 1992). Parents anecdotally report that children lose previously achieved skills while on maintenance therapy (e.g., preschoolers may forget their letters). For older children, acute effects of cancer therapy are further compounded by frequent school absences, necessitated either by the illness or by the need to protect children with compromised immune systems from exposure to the usual childhood illnesses (e.g., chickenpox). The resulting gaps in schooling are thought to have potential long-range consequences as well (Peckham, Meadows, Bartel, & Marrero, 1988).

It is the longer-term neurobehavioral effects of leukemia therapies, however, that are of greatest concern. As survival rates improved during the early 1980s and survivors began to enter school in large numbers, there were frequent clinical reports of school difficulties. It soon became apparent that these were not transient effects associated with the emotional turmoil of a life-threatening illness or of school absence, but long-term, neurologically based consequences of treatment (Eiser, 1978). There is now a substantial literature indicating that the rate of learning disabilities is increased in this population (e.g., Gamis & Nesbit, 1991; Roman & Sperduto, 1995). As oncologists have succeeded in safely reducing doses of some of the most intensive therapies (e.g., reducing CRT dose from 2,400 cGy to 1,800 cGy or less), there is a clear and welcome trend toward less severe neurobehavioral outcomes as well. The alarming consequences observed subsequent to treatment on early-generation protocols (including significantly diminished IQ and pervasive learning problems) are now relatively rare, and sequelae of present-day leukemia treatment, even where radiation is involved, are more subtle. Data from the DF/CH program, which are described in detail later in this chapter, illustrate this trend.

READING THE RESEARCH LITERATURE: FUNDAMENTAL CONSIDERATIONS

Because ALL is such a rare disease, systematic research is typically undertaken in the context of multicenter collaborative groups that in combination can treat large enough numbers of patients to evaluate clinical trials. These include the Children's Cancer Group, Pediatric Oncology Group, and the DF/CH Consortium in the United States, as well as collaborative groups in Europe. The resulting studies therefore represent the efforts of many participating institutions throughout the world. Several comprehensive literature reviews have detailed the methodological issues and broad conclusions of these research studies on late neuropsychological sequelae in ALL (Butler & Copeland, 1993; Cousens et al., 1988; Fletcher & Copeland, 1988; Gamis & Nesbit, 1991; Madan-Swain & Brown, 1991).

An important consideration in evaluating this literture is that recruitment is often selective; therefore, the outcomes reported in a research investigation may not be entirely representative of the population of children diagnosed with ALL. Most studies, probably correctly, report data based on patients who have been in continuous complete remission since diagnosis. Patients who have relapsed, suffered unusual and sometimes catastrophic toxicities, or experienced other unusual adverse events are excluded from these studies. Moreover, the event-free survival rates associated with the relevant protocol are not reported, and in some instances the treatment protocol itself is not adequately described. The toxicity of a particular treatment must be assessed within the broader context of both its documented efficacy in enhancing disease survival and its effects relative to other disease-related sequelae.

An additional consideration in evaluating research in this area is the unit of analysis used to study treatment effects. The most common approach is the one in which the patient serves as the unit of analysis. Most researchers exclude children who have experienced adverse events that may compromise CNS development (e.g., relapse, encephalopathy). Including these children would complicate interpretation of findings with regard to the effects of specific components of treatment on disease outcomes. Thus the standard practice is to study only children who have been in continuous complete remission since diagnosis. Although methodologically sound, this strategy provides a biased view of risks and benefits of treatment, since only the "successes" are studied (e.g., the effective risk of relapse is zero).

A complementary approach is to treat the protocol as the unit of analysis. Since most ALL patients are treated on investigational protocols, this alternative approach entails evaluation of all children on a given treatment protocol, regardless of their medical history. To illustrate the advantage of this approach, children who are treated with a protocol that provides for less intensive initial treatment, and who remain in continuous complete remission, would show only minimal CNS sequelae. Yet children from that protocol could in theory be vulnerable to an increased rate of relapse, requiring intensive retreatment or bone marrow transplantation. The level of morbidity for the entire group receiving that protocol could then be higher than that observed with a protocol involving more intense initial treatment (and therefore somewhat higher levels of impairment for the subset of children in continuous complete remission).

The essential point is that late neuropsychological effects must be evaluated in the broadest possible context. The fact that one treatment is more or less toxic than another is ultimately irrelevant if there are substantial differences in efficacy. Disease control must be the preeminent goal. Seemingly minor modifications of protocols (to mitigate toxicity) could be associated with loss of efficacy. Treatment failure for only a few children, with only a modest statistical decrease in efficacy, is an unacceptable price to pay for a modest or uncertain decrease in the overall prevalence or severity of learning problems.

A proper evaluation of treatment toxicity thus requires an appreciation of the efficacy of the treatment protocol. Specifically, how does the efficacy of one protocol compare with that of other protocols for children with the same leukemia risk characteristics? Past research failed to use standard criteria for defining risk groups, making it difficult to make these comparisons. The new uniform guidelines for definition of risk groups (National Cancer Institute/Cancer Therapy Evaluation Program guidelines), referred to above, can facilitate future efforts in this regard (Smith et al., 1996).

NEUROPSYCHOLOGICAL SEQUELAE OF ALL: DANA–FARBER CANCER INSTITUTE/CHILDREN'S HOSPITAL CONSORTIUM PROTOCOLS

Background

Our research program has been guided by a model of treatment effects that we have refined in the process of evaluating children enrolled in a series of treatment protocols. In brief, our clinical model posits the following: (1) Treatment of ALL affects two distinct sets of cognitive processes; (2) each of these cognitive processes is specifically vulnerable to different components of treatment (i.e., agents); and (3) males and females are differentially sensitive to some of these agents. The evolution of the model is outlined below in relation to each of the clinical protocols evaluated. The protocol number indicates the year in which that protocol was initiated (e.g., children were placed onto Protocol 81-01 beginning in 1981).

A companion animal model (Mullenix et al., 1990, 1994) has permitted experimental testing of hypotheses in a context free of the constraints of clinical investigation. The animal model provides for experimental manipulations of three agents with known neurotoxic effects—MTX, CRT, and glucocorticoid—in developing rats, with behavioral outcomes quantified in terms of the structure of spontaneous behavior. By allowing for these manipulations, the animal work has informed interpretation of the clinical data, corroborating some clinical observations (e.g., sex differences) and predicting others (e.g., steroid effects).

Another feature of our program is that we have relied on a succinct, simple, and reliable battery of psychological tests that has proved highly sensitive to variations in treatment protocols and has permitted us to gain a broader perspective on the outcomes of any given protocol. In our initial study (Waber, Urion, et al., 1990), we used a fairly extensive neuropsychological battery. From our experience with that battery, we were able to identify a relatively limited set of measures that would provide information pertinent to specifying patient and treatment effects. Because the DF/CH Consortium ALL Program includes 10 institutions in North America (3 of which serve primarily non-English-speaking patients), the battery needed to be brief (for convenience), reliable (for use by multiple testers of varying degrees of expertise), and applicable in different languages (English, French, Spanish). It also needed to be sensitive to the strengths and weaknesses likely to be demonstrated by these patients, and to provide estimates of skills of adaptive significance for children (e.g., intelligence, school achievement). Although the battery could be supplemented by more detailed measures of cognitive functions at some sites to provide insight into features of cognitive processing in these children (Kleinman & Waber, 1994; Waber et al., 1994), for purposes of protocol evaluation and model building, the basic psychometric battery was the focus.

This basic battery includes subtests from the Wechsler Intelligence Scales for Children (WISC) needed to estimate Full Scale IQ (Vocabulary, Block Design), long-term memory and knowledge base (Information), reasoning in the concrete domain (Picture Arrangement), and immediate and working memory for rote material (Digit Span). It also includes standardized measures of basic areas of academic achievement (Woodcock–Johnson Word Identification, Reading Comprehension, and Calculation; Wide Range Achievement Test—Spelling), as well as the Rey–Osterrieth Complex Figure Test (Copy and Immediate Recall).

An important feature of our studies is careful screening for preexisting risk by asking parents to complete a developmental history. In each of our studies, we have identified a small but significant number of children who had preexisting risk for learning disability as indicated by either neurological history (e.g., premature birth, meningitis) or developmental history (e.g., delayed motor or language milestones); a few even had a learning disability that was identified prior to diagnosis of the ALL. Because the number of children in these studies is typically not very large, inclusion of even a small number of these children could distort findings.

The design of the studies follows from the investigational protocols on which the patients were treated. The designs allowed for three kinds of analyses: comparing children's performance to normative expectations; determining the relationship of patient variables (sex, age) to performance; and comparing children randomized or assigned to different treatment groups, to ascertain the effects of components of treatment or dose levels. Controls were not included. We learned from experience that comparison to clinical controls can introduce an "apples and oranges" problem (Waber, Urion, et al., 1990), and that the use of healthy controls can introduce bias by virtue of the variables selected for matching. Another option—using pretreatment data as a baseline—was rejected because so many children, especially those at greatest risk, are quite young at diagnosis (when measurement is less reliable or not possible), and because identified children are already quite ill and their families are emotionally upset.

Table 13.1 outlines the primary features of each of the three studies undertaken by our research group, each of which involved a different type of treatment protocol. Tables 13.2 to 13.4 (see below) summarize major findings from each of the three studies and depict schematically the implications of the findings for the model. Because sex differences figure prominently in these results, implications of the model for males and females are shown separately. The "Global" cognitive process, as referred to in the later tables, is

TABLE 13.1. Relevant Features of Treatment Protocols for Three Studies

	Radiation dose (cGy)	MTX dose (induction)	Steroid (prednisone) dose
Study I: Protocols 73-01, 77-01, 80-01	2,400	None	120 mg/m²
Study II: Protocol 81-01	SR: 1,800 HR: 2,800	Randomized HD MTX	SR: 40 mg/m² HR: 120 mg/m²
Study III: Protocol 87-01	SR f: No CRT HR: 1,800	Randomized HD MTX	SR: 40 mg/m² HR: 120 mg/m²

manifested empirically in terms of IQ scores, and the "Specific" process is defined in terms of scores on tests of academic achievement and verbal memory. Although we do not yet have a clear understanding of the core nature of the specific process, it is referred to in the model as "verbal memory/coding."

Study I: DF/CH Protocols 73-01, 77-01, 80-01

The earliest successful ALL treatment protocols, of the mid- to late 1970s, took a "one size fits all" approach to therapy. The standard CNS prophylactic regimen was 2,400 cGy of CRT given in combination with intrathecal MTX. Systemic drugs included in the DF/CH protocols included prednisone, doxorubicin, vincristine, MTX, and asparaginase. Our initial study of the effects of treatment for ALL examined outcomes among 51 children treated on these protocols whose median elapsed time from diagnosis was 8 years (Waber, Urion, et al., 1990). Because children were not assigned to different intensities of treatment based on risk group, as is the current practice, these early protocols provided a particularly good opportunity to document the age and sex differences in patient vulnerability to the adverse effects of treatment. Since protocols with different treatment intensities are now used with different ALL risk groups, the effects of child variables can be more difficult to discern in the context of treatment variables.

The most striking feature of our initial studies was the dramatic and unexpected vulnerability of female patients to late effects, especially given the fact that most studies of learning-disabled children report a preponderance of males. Whereas all children exhibited specific difficulties involving academic skills and symbolic processing, females showed a generalized depression of cognitive functioning, manifested in lower IQ scores, that was related to age at diagnosis. A Cognitive Impairment Index, ranging from 0 to 4, was devised from IQ and achievement scores. We found that 15% of females but no males were rated as most severely affected; conversely, 46% of males but only 11% of females were rated as without measurable deficits. Young females appeared to be most vulnerable to the insult associated with treatment. Males showed no such age effect.

On the basis of these findings, we hypothesized

> that there is a generalizable factor, common to all pediatric cancer victims, or at least all children treated with systemic and/or CNS anti-cancer therapy. This factor operates along with a second, developmentally determined factor, and the latter can operate only in a nervous system at the critical stage of ontogenesis (the timing, or existence of which, may be endocrine-related). This vulnerability is evident only among females treated at younger ages, and results

in neuropsychological deficit that is most consistent with a subcortical locus (Waber, Gioia, et al., 1990). This suggests that the insult occurs primarily in myelinating tracts rather than in neurons or in already myelinated tracts (Rourke, 1987). (Waber, Urion, et al., 1990, p. 245)

In an extension of the study cited above (Waber, Gioia, et al., 1990), we concluded that treatment affects global cognitive abilities in females, including organizational skills as well as alertness/arousal. The most salient differences between males and females emerged for sensitivity to organizational structure on the Rey–Osterrieth Complex Figure and performance on a measure of alerted reaction time. Moreover, variance in these measures accounted for variance in performance on measures of academic skill, especially arithmetic and reading comprehension. In contrast, academic skills dependent on verbal coding and phonology—that is, single-word recognition and spelling—were depressed in both sexes. The differential outcomes by sex in this study provided an initial clue as to how the two fundamental processes could be cleaved.

The dual-cognitive-process model, displayed in its initial, simplest form in Table 13.2, posits that two cognitive processes are affected by ALL treatment. As described earlier, we refer to one of these processes as Global and the other as Specific. Females exhibit greater vulnerability with respect to the Global process only (putatively related to damage to white matter), whereas both sexes are vulnerable to treatment-related deficits in the Specific process. Although the Global and Specific processes are conceptualized as distinct, it is important to recognize that as a phenomenological matter they are functionally integrated. Impairment in the Global process, for example, may compromise performance on a measure of the Specific process, such as academic achievement. Because Study I involved assessment of the effects of a treatment protocol that was uniform for all children, the results of this study did not provide data relevant to the effects of particular treatment agents. Studies of subsequent protocols, however, did provide information in this regard.

Study II: DF/CH Protocol 81-01

Protocol 81-01 was the first DF/CH investigational ALL protocol to stratify children by risk group. SR patients were assigned to receive 1,800 cGy of CRT, and HR patients were assigned to 2,800 cGy of CRT. Comparison of these two groups thus allowed us to evaluate the impact of radiation dose on outcome. The two groups, however, also differed in terms of the systemic dose of certain drugs. Specifically, the HR group received higher cumulative doxorubicin and asparaginase doses and higher prednisone doses than did the

TABLE 13.2. Findings and Questions Posed by Study I

Cognitive function	Finding	Sex affected	Agent
Global: IQ	Females scored lower than males	Females	?
Specific: Verbal memory/ coding	Males and females scored below expectations	Both	?

SR group. In addition, many of the children on this protocol were randomized to receive intravenous methotrexate (IV MTX) during remission induction, either as a single conventional (low) dose (CD) of 40 mg/m^2 or as a single high dose (HD) of 33 g/m^2 or 4 g/m^2. Children not participating in this randomization were assigned to CD MTX.

Fifty-one patients received neuropsychological evaluation a median of 6 years after treatment (Waber, Tarbell, Kahn, Gelber, & Sallan, 1992). Children ranged from 6 to 16 years of age at testing. The findings of this study were consistent with the dual-cognitive-process model. First, as was the case for the earlier study (Waber, Urion, et al., 1990), females exhibited greater global vulnerability to toxicity associated with treatment than did males, as documented by lower IQ scores. Surprisingly, however, the results failed to document a relationship between radiation dose and IQ. Instead, females randomized to receive HD MTX were far more likely to exhibit low IQ (<90), regardless of risk group (i.e., CRT dose). MTX dose was not related to outcomes in boys. For both sexes, however, children in the HR group exhibited poorer scores on measures of verbal memory (WISC Digit Span) and academic achievement than did children in the SR group.

These findings suggested further modification of the model. Global cognitive impairment (IQ) was again seen in females only. Contrary to expectation, however, this impairment was associated with MTX dose, rather than with radiation dose! Even though the HD MTX was administered systemically and not intrathecally (i.e., directly to the CNS), late cognitive effects apparently ensued. Although the basis for the possible damage to white matter was not clear, we commented that

> white-matter changes in long-term survivors are observed most prominently in children whose treatment included CRT, and such changes can be effected in animals treated only with CRT. Because all children in this study received CRT, the possibility exists that MTX administered during the induction phase of treatment had a potentiating effect, increasing subsequent vulnerability to CRT. (Waber et al., 1992, p. 815)

Since all the children treated on this protocol received radiation, we could not tell from these findings whether the observed effect was due solely to the HD MTX or whether the adverse outcome associated with MTX depended on subsequent CRT.

In contrast, both sexes had deficits in discrete academic skills (e.g., reading, spelling, arithmetic), and these appeared to be associated with the higher dose of CRT received by the HR group. Certain drugs, however, were also given in higher doses to the HR children. Prednisone is of particular interest because of its known CNS effects:

> There is substantial evidence that glucocorticoids can induce injury to hippocampal neurons or impair the ability of these neurons to survive insults. In addition, prednisone therapy has been associated with verbal memory changes in pediatric asthma patients. Whether the treatment effects observed in this study are attributable to the higher dose of CRT, to corticosteroids, or to some synergy of treatment agents remains open to question. (Waber et al., 1992, p. 815)

To summarize, evaluation of Protocol 81-01 substantiated in a new cohort the prior finding of greater female vulnerability to a Global deficit following ALL therapy (see Table 13.3). A Global deficit of this type is consistent with damage to white matter. The results of this study further indicated that these treatment effects are associated with MTX dose, even when the drug is given systemically. Furthermore, these consequences are apparently related to a single HD of this drug. The study could not resolve, however, whether the relevant toxic agent is MTX alone or MTX interacting synergistically with CRT.

TABLE 13.3. Findings and Questions Posed by Study II

Cognitive function	Finding	Sex affected	Agent
Global: IQ	Females who received HD MTX scored lower than other females and males	Females	HD MTX ± (?) CRT
Specific: Verbal memory/ coding	Males and females scored below expectations	Both	CRT? Steroid?

As indicated above, the absence of an association between CRT dose and IQ was surprising. Although we could not categorically rule out an effect (given the modest numbers of children sampled), there was adequate statistical power to detect a large effect, and none was observed. Nevertheless, a deficit in the Specific cognitive process, as manifested in academic skills (symbolic processing), was related to risk group and thus to CRT dose in this protocol. Whether the responsible agent was indeed CRT or some other agent also associated with risk group (e.g., glucocorticoid) could not be ascertained due to confounds inherent in the treatment protocol. Because of the known neurobehavioral impact of glucocorticoids, particularly on the hippocampus, we proposed that the observed effect could be related to CRT, to prednisone, or even to both.

Study III: DF/CH Protocol 87-01

As Table 13.1 indicates, Protocol 87-01 was the most elaborate of the protocols to date. Here again, children were assigned to treatment on the basis of risk group. SR children did not receive CRT, whereas HR children received 1,800 cGy of CRT. Children on this protocol were again randomized to a single intravenous HD of MTX or the CD. This protocol therefore provided an opportunity to refine the model further. For the first time, outcomes in children who had received CRT could be compared to those of children who had not. Moreover, we were able to attempt to replicate our earlier finding concerning HD MTX, and to determine whether these adverse effects are dependent on subsequent CRT treatment.

For this study (Waber et al., 1995), 66 children were evaluated at a median of 4 years after diagnosis. The test battery was comparable to that which had been used in the previous studies, including subtests from the WISC-R, measures of academic achievement, and a measure of visual–spatial organizational skill (Rey–Osterrieth Complex Figure). Since the time elapsed between diagnosis and assessment was briefer than had been the case in our previous studies, some of the children who had been treated at the youngest ages were not yet old enough for the evaluation (minimum age = 7 years). Younger children are likely to be most vulnerable to treatment effects, and the underrepresentation of this group of patients bears on our interpretation of the findings.

With the exception of one subgroup of patients, the results of this study failed to reveal an impact of 1,800 cGy of CRT on cognitive outcomes. The exception was that females treated with HD MTX who subsequently received CRT had lower IQ scores than the rest of the sample. A second finding was that scores on rote verbal memory (Digit Span) and spelling were decreased relative to other abilities for the entire group, regardless of treatment (a profile that we had observed in previous studies).

These findings not only reinforce the working model, but also permit additional elaboration. Female vulnerability to treatment was once again documented, and was related specifically to a high dose of systemic MTX. The adverse impact of MTX, however, was synergistic; that is, the effect emerged clearly only in those girls who received HD MTX followed by CRT. Significantly, neither HD MTX without CRT nor CRT with CD MTX was associated with diminished IQ. This pattern clearly indicates a synergistic effect of the two agents. A further finding was that the characteristic deficit in verbal memory and symbolic processing (especially spelling) emerged for all children treated on this protocol, regardless of whether they had received CRT. This finding reinforces our previous speculation that some agent other than CRT, possibly corticosteroid, is responsible for the observed deficits in rote memory and symbolic processing. One caveat, however, is the underrepresentation of children treated at young ages, who may be especially sensitive to toxicity associated with CRT. As these children become available for evaluation, we will be able to construct a more complete picture of the potential for late effects related to CRT.

The current version of the model (see Table 13.4), which continues to conceptualize the sequelae of ALL treatment in terms of two distinct cognitive processes, can be summarized as follows: First, the Global process, which is presumed to represent toxicity to white matter and affects females disproportionately, results from a synergistic interaction of MTX and CRT. To account for the considerable cognitive toxicity seen on the earlier protocols, which included 2,400 cGy of CRT but only the CD of systemic MTX, we hypothesize that

TABLE 13.4. Findings from Study III

Cognitive function	Finding	Sex affected	Agent
Global: IQ	Females who received HD-MTX *with* CRT scored lower than other females and all males	Females	HD MTX + CRT
Specific: Verbal memory/ coding	Males and females scored below expectations whether or not they received CRT	Both	Steroid

an increase in the intensity of either agent will potentiate the toxicity of the combination. In the earlier protocols, the CRT dose was substantially higher, and in the later ones, toxicity was evident only in those girls who received a very high MTX dose prior to the lower CRT dose (1,800 cGy).

Second, there is a persistent pattern of deficits in the Specific process, as manifested on tests of both rote verbal memory (as measured by the Digit Span) and symbolic, possibly phonological, processing (manifested most prominently in spelling). This pattern is seen in both sexes, and, as our most recent study indicates, occurs even when CRT is not included in the protocol. Since the results of the latter study (Waber et al., 1995) have excluded CRT as the effective agent, the most likely candidate is steroid. Reports of adverse effects of dexamethasone on declarative memory in adult volunteers (Newcomer, Craft, Hershey, Askins, & Bardgett, 1994) support the plausibility of this hypothesis. Examining potential dose and intensity effects of corticosteroids on cognitive outcomes in pediatric ALL patients will be a central focus of future studies.

Generational Changes: Decrease in Severity of Outcomes across Protocols

As indicated earlier, the trend in leukemia treatment has been to decrease the intensity of treatment where feasible. In the case of CRT, for example, the standard dose for even the highest-risk patients has been reduced to 1,800 cGy. CRT has also been eliminated for patients whose risk for relapse is thought to be low. For example, SR females on DF/CH protocols are now treated without CRT.

A descriptive comparison of the neuropsychological findings for patients in the three studies (Waber, Urion, et al., 1990; Waber et al., 1992, 1995) indicates a corresponding trend for less severe treatment effects over time. The children in all three studies had been in continuous complete remission since diagnosis, and all were between 7 and 16 years of age. Median elapsed times from diagnosis for the three studies were 7, 7, and 4 years for Studies I, II, and III, respectively. A severity rating based on IQ and achievement scores, which was used in the initial study (Waber, Urion, et al., 1990), was applied to children from all three cohorts.

Figure 13.1 shows frequencies of individuals in each severity category for males and females separately for each of the three studies described above, demonstrating a general decrease in the severity of adverse outcomes across the three cohorts. Of interest, males showed relatively low levels of significant impairment in all three studies. By contrast, the rate of significant impairment was highest among females in the earliest cohort and declined across successive cohorts. Males and females had comparable outcomes in the most recent study (Protocol 87–01).

Thus, although neuropsychological late effects continue to be an important consideration in ALL treatment, the severity of these outcomes has diminished as treatment protocols have evolved, particularly for female patients. Reduced intensity of treatment has been associated with improved neurobehavioral outcomes. At the same time that rates of neurotoxicity have declined over time on the DF/CH protocols, overall survival rates have improved. The 5-year event-free survival rates of the three cohorts, considered chronologically, were 53%, 74%, and 76% (see Figure 13.2). Thus mitigation of late effects has been achieved without compromising efficacy.

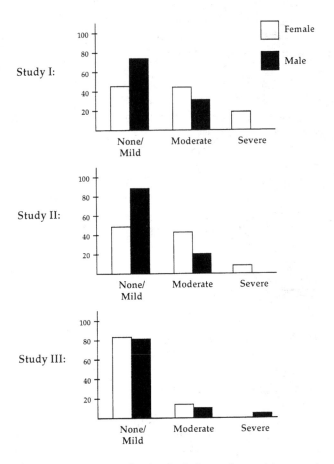

FIGURE 13.1. Distribution (percentage) of individuals for each cognitive severity rating by sex for Studies I, II, and III. None/Mild, estimated IQ greater than or equal to 90, and within 1 *SD* of mean on at least two of the four academic tests (single-word reading, reading comprehension, spelling, calculation); Moderate, either (a) IQ greater than or equal to 90, and 1 *SD* below mean on at least three academic measures, or (b) IQ less than 90, and 1 *SD* below mean on three or fewer academic tests; Severe, IQ less than 90, and 1 *SD* below mean on all four academic tests.

ANIMAL STUDIES

As previously indicated, our program has had the benefit of companion experimental animal studies. These have allowed us to test hypotheses that could not be examined in the clinical context. Moreover, the animal model allows us to detect late effects of treatment in a relatively brief time frame.

The behavioral measure used in our animal model is based on spontaneous activity—specifically, naturally occurring sequences of motor acts. Although rat behaviors per se do not have human equivalents, temporal organization of rat behaviors directed by the CNS is generic. Behavioral analysis of rat behavior thus consists of the time structure of single acts and sequences of acts (a K-function calculation for 2-, 5-, 10-, 20-, 30-, 45-, 100-, and 200-second time bins), in addition to measures of motor act initiation (total number of initiations of an act) and total times (total number of seconds for which a behavioral act

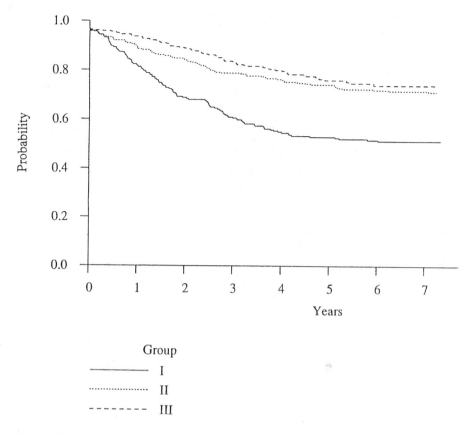

FIGURE 13.2. Event-free survival curves for treatment groups represented by Study I (Protocols 73-01, 77-01, and 80-01), Study II (Protocol 81-01), and Study III (Protocol 87-01). The data are from Clavell et al. (1986) and Tarbell et al. (1991), as updated by Richard Gelber, PhD.

continues, including the seconds of initiation). To conduct behavioral testing, one experimental and one sham-treated animal matched for sex, age, and experience in the test environment are placed simultaneously on opposite sides of a partition dividing a Plexiglas box. The animals explore the environment for 15 minutes while video cameras record behavior in 1-second time frames. The cameras are linked to computers located outside the observation room, and the computers, not humans, identify the motor acts of each rat and analyze these data (Kernan, Mullenix, & Hopper, 1987). Thus neurotoxicity is measured quantitatively in terms of deviation of behavioral time structure in exposed versus control animals (Kernan, Mullenix, Kent, Hopper, & Cressie, 1988; Mullenix & Kernan, 1989).

In the series of studies undertaken to date to examine treatment toxicity, immature rats were exposed to agents commonly used in CNS therapy, and their growth and behavioral outcomes were evaluated. The agents examined included MTX, steroids, and CRT in various doses, combinations, and sequences. Exposures were calculated to mimic clinical doses, without being lethal or inducing gross neurotoxicity in immature rats. CRT was given as a single whole-brain dose of 1,000 cGy (the approximate biological equivalent of a clinical dose of 2,400 cGy given to children in 12 to 14 fractions). One or two intraperitoneal injections of <4 mg/kg MTX and/or <36 mg/kg steroid (prednisolone) were given

1 to 3 hours prior to or after CRT. Growth and behavior were then monitored as the animals matured, to examine effects similar to those observed in children given CNS therapy. Assessments of growth included measures of body weight and length, and body and craniofacial proportions. Behavioral assessments included measures of spontaneous act initiations, total times, and time structure, determined via the computer pattern recognition system.

The initial studies confirmed that agents used in CNS therapy were associated with neurotoxicity; they thus established the feasibility of the animal model (Mullenix et al., 1990; Schunior et al., 1990). Growth failure and craniofacial abnormalities, which can be seen in children treated for ALL, were directly linked to a single agent, CRT (Schunior et al., 1990). Permanent behavioral changes induced by a combination of MTX, prednisolone, and CRT and were far more dramatic than those induced by CRT alone (Mullenix et al., 1990). The overall pattern of changes observed with the combined agents was the same as that seen with CRT alone, the difference being one of magnitude only (Mullenix, 1995). Qualitative changes in behavioral patterns, however, emerged when the model was expanded to include other single-agent exposures and agent combinations (Mullenix et al., 1994; Mullenix, 1997; Schunior et al., 1994).

The collective findings of these studies have direct applicability to clinical treatment of children with ALL. First, behavior was more likely to be affected by agent combinations than by single-agent therapies. Behavioral time structure was at greater risk when CRT was a component of the combination than when combinations did not include CRT. The only single agent that resulted in a statistically significant alteration of overall behavior was steroid. CRT given as a single 1,000-cGy dose did not result in such changes.

Second, behavioral change was sensitive to variation in MTX and prednisolone doses within combinations. As the MTX dose (in combination with constant 1,000-cGy CRT) increased, behavioral and growth deficits became more apparent. There was an optimal MTX dose level, however, where the two agents apparently interacted antagonistically and where behavioral and growth deficits were less apparent. Mitigation of such deficits was not observed when MTX doses were lower or higher than this optimal dose range, indicating that the neurotoxicity was not linearly related to drug dose; rather, the relationship was U-shaped.

Third, outcome depended on the sex of the animals. Females were more susceptible to combined MTX and CRT, and the optimal drug dose was lower for females than for males. In contrast, however, males exhibited greater sensitivity to steroids.

Finally, the sequence by which agents are administered in combination therapy affected outcome (Mullenix et al., 1999). For example, in order to achieve the optimal MTX-CRT combination to minimize behavioral and growth deficits, it was necessary that the MTX be given prior to CRT. The same MTX dose administered after CRT was likely to result in severe behavioral disruption, and it consistently produced growth deficits. This result is consistent with the clinical findings of Balsam et al. (1991), who reported that MTX given before CRT mitigated late cognitive effects, most prominently among girls who were less than 5 years of age when irradiated.

The finding of greater sensitivity of females to the MTX-CRT combination is also consistent with the clinical findings. Although the mechanism underlying this phenomenon (which is probably endocrine-related) is not understood, sex differences in toxicity have also been observed in other organ systems. Female patients, for example, are more likely to suffer anthracycline-induced cardiac toxicity (Lipshultz et al., 1995). Antileukemic treatment efficacy is likewise sex-dependent. In our Protocol 87-01, in which SR patients were treated without CRT, the rate of CNS relapse was considerably higher for male than for female patients (Billett et al., 1993). This sex effect may well occur at the cellular level, since it does not appear to be CNS-specific.

In sum, the animal model has revealed important parallels to the findings of systematic clinical observations and has provided clearer delineation of variables important to the cause and prevention of neurotoxicity associated with agents used in CNS therapy in children. The striking parallels include (1) relatively mild behavioral effects of CRT given at therapeutic doses as a single agent; (2) synergistic interaction of MTX and CRT in inducing behavioral changes; (3) a potentially protective effect of MTX given at an optimal dose prior to irradiation (Balsam et al., 1991); and (4) a striking sex specificity of outcomes, particularly the vulnerability of females to the MTX-CRT combination. It also raises some concerns in areas where clinical investigation has not yet taken place, most prominently with respect to potential neurotoxicity of steroids for male patients.

Although the mechanisms of action for these various treatment effects have not been proved, Mullenix (1997) has proposed possibilities that are worthy of further exploration. Whatever the reasons for treatment effects, a major implication of the animal findings is that simply deleting CRT from CNS therapy, which for some patients may jeopardize efficacy of treatment (Nachman et al., 1994), will not necessarily preclude treatment toxicity. Safe treatment of the developing CNS will entail a tailored approach, including considerations of factors such as agent combinations, their doses and sequences of administration, and especially the sex of the patient—all of which must be balanced against any potential compromise of treatment efficacy.

CONCLUSION

We have summarized a research program for investigating late neurobehavioral effects of ALL treatment and have presented a neuropsychological model that has proven highly consistent in predicting treatment effects across independent cohorts. This model has considerable specificity and is supported by findings from experimental laboratory studies. The model not only accounts for existing findings, but can also serve as a basis for predicting outcomes of proposed treatment protocols.

Predictions made by the model include the following:

1. Females are highly vulnerable to MTX-CRT combinations. In particular, when CRT is used, MTX dose should be monitored carefully. (At the lower doses, however, the adverse effects of the MTX-CRT combination can be mitigated when MTX is given prior to CRT rather than concurrently; Balsam et al., 1991.)

2. By the same token, males tolerate more intensive doses of MTX-CRT better than females. Since males have a somewhat greater mortality from ALL than females, this finding suggests that males may be treated more intensively without concern about significant added neurotoxicity (with a caveat about steroids, as indicated below).

3. Corticosteroids should be employed with care in the treatment of ALL (and indeed in all pediatric settings). Although there is not yet direct evidence for a link between steroids and learning difficulties, the use of higher doses or more potent forms of these drugs should be carefully monitored. The animal data suggest that for these agents, males may be the more vulnerable sex.

Reference to the model can also be useful in resolving apparent contradictions in the research literature. For example, we (Waber et al., 1995) reported that for most ALL patients, CRT does not increase the neurocognitive burden beyond that observed with drug therapy alone. This finding is consistent with reports of some groups (Halberg et al., 1991; Mulhern et al., 1991), but at variance with those of others (Anderson, Smibert, Ekert, & Godber, 1994; Jankovic et al., 1994), who conclude that CRT is associated with increased neurotoxicity.

In the Jankovic et al. (1994) study, the reported adverse effect of CRT on IQ was apparently accounted for by the youngest group of patients (under 3 years of age at diagnosis). Underrepresentation of children diagnosed at very young ages in our study (due to inapplicability of test procedures) could partially account for the divergent findings. Moreover, the group that received CRT in the Jankovic et al. study was disproportionately female (55% CRT vs. 38% in the no-CRT group). The model would predict that such a distribution would increase vulnerability to CRT. Since the investigators did not include sex as a factor in their analyses, it is not possible to evaluate the extent to which the preponderance of females contributed to the overall outcome.

Although the Anderson et al. (1994) study compared children treated with and without CRT, the CRT group was made up of children who had received either 1,800 cGy or 2,400 cGy. The model would predict that only females treated with 2,400 cGy would show adverse outcomes, and this subgroup may in fact have accounted for the CRT effect reported by the authors. Radiation dose was not included in the analysis, however, nor were crucial variables such as sex and age at diagnosis. As a consequence, the impact of these factors is difficult to evaluate.

Given the considerable specificity of treatment toxicity, researchers should acknowledge contributing factors (e.g., patient characteristics, components of therapy) in study design and statistical analysis. The completeness of the analytic model is important, because the specificity can have direct implications for clinical care. On the one hand, beneficial treatment should not be withheld from one subgroup of patients (e.g., children older than 3 years at diagnosis, males) because of the special sensitivity of other subgroups (e.g., younger children, females). Nor would it be appropriate to withhold the 1,800-cGy dose of CRT because of adverse outcomes associated with the 2,400-cGy dose.

A further consideration, highlighted by the animal studies, is the relevance of agent combinations in predicting treatment toxicity. Our clinical data indicate quite clearly that for female patients, the combined impact of MTX and CRT eventuates in the poorest neurobehavioral outcomes. Apparently a high dose of either agent, in combination with the other, can lead to this type of synergy. Data from the animal studies parallel these findings. Although treatment combinations are sometimes methodologically difficult to accommodate, it is necessary to evaluate the effects of such combinations rather than to focus on a single agent (e.g., CRT) or even a restricted component of treatment (e.g., CNS therapy), in order to obtain an accurate appreciation of the impact of these agents on children's development.

A final issue is that nearly all the studies of late effects have focused on CRT as the primary toxic agent, with secondary consideration given to the possible role of MTX. Our data, which are consistent with those of Mulhern, Wasserman, Fairclough, and Ochs (1988), indicate that deficits in verbal memory and symbolic processing are prevalent even among children treated for ALL without CRT. Our animal studies have motivated us to consider the role of a third agent, corticosteroids, as a source of toxicity. Although we do not yet have probative evidence that steroids cause late cognitive effects, the existing laboratory and clinical data are highly suggestive. Here again, without critical examination of the effects of this treatment agent, one runs the risk of excluding one potentially beneficial agent (e.g.,

CRT) from treatment protocols due to an adverse outcome actually stemming from another (steroids).

Future studies in our program will evaluate the potential for mitigating late effects while preserving efficacy by using a hyperfractionation strategy to deliver the CRT (smaller radiation fractions twice a day) (Tarbell et al., 1991). We will also evaluate potential late toxicity associated with the introduction of dexamethasone, a more potent steroid than prednisone, as the glucocorticoid component of therapy.

Progress in this research area is necessarily slow. Many years are often required to evaluate a protocol adequately, and hypotheses regarding treatment effects continue to be more speculative than many would like to admit. Still, as treatment protocols have evolved and become less intensive, late neurocognitive effects have tended to become less severe. Emphasis on the consequences of specific treatment agents will allow us to tailor treatment protocols more precisely. In this way, children at greatest risk for late cognitive sequelae can be treated more cautiously, while those children at lower risk are not unnecessarily denied effective treatment. The overriding goal of neuropsychological research is not to determine whether a particular agent is toxic, but to clarify the factors to be considered in specifying the costs and benefits of treatment. Decisions regarding treatment should be based on a set of complex considerations having to do with the age and sex of the child, as well as the effects of particular combinations (and even timing of combinations) of treatment agents.

ACKNOWLEDGMENTS

We gratefully acknowledge the guidance and collaboration of Stephen E. Sallan, MD, who directs the Dana–Farber/Children's Hospital Consortium ALL Program, and Nancy J. Tarbell, MD, of the Department of Radiation Oncology, Children's Hospital, in the studies described in this chapter. We are also grateful to Richard Gelber, PhD, for providing Figure 13.2.

REFERENCES

Altman, J., Anderson, W. J., & Wright, K. A. (1968). Gross morphological consequences of irradiation of the cerebellum in infant rats with repeated doses of low-level X-ray. *Experimental Neurology, 21,* 69–91.

Anderson, V., Smibert, E., Ekert, H., & Godber, T. (1994). Intellectual, educational, and behavioural sequelae after cranial irradiation and chemotherapy. *Archives of Disease in Childhood, 70,* 476–483.

Balsam, W. R., Bleyer, W. A., Robison, L. L., Heyn, R. M., Mendros, A. T., Sitarz, A., Blatt, J., Sather, H. N., & Hammond, G. D. (1991). Intellectual function in long-term survivors of childhood leukemia: Protective effect of pre-irradiation methotrexate? A Children's Cancer Study Group study. *Medical and Pediatric Oncology, 19,* 486–492.

Billett, A. L., Gelber, R. D., Tarbell, N. J., Barr, R., Blattner, S., Clavell, L., LeClerc, J. M., Lipton, J., Schwenn, M., Schorin, M., Cohen, H. J., & Sallan, S. E. (1993). Sex differences in the risk of central nervous system (CNS) relapse in childhood acute lymphoblastic leukemia (ALL) [Abstract]. *Proceedings of the American Society of Clinical Oncology, 12,* 317.

Bleyer, W. A. (1988). Central nervous system leukemia. *Pediatric Clinics of North America, 35,* 789–814.

Brown, R. T., Madan-Swain, A., Pais, R., Lambert, R. G., Sexson, S., & Ragab, A. (1992). Chemotherapy for acute lymphocytic leukemia: Cognitive and academic sequelae. *Journal of Pediatrics, 121,* 885–890.

Butler, R. W., & Copeland, D. R. (1993). Neuropsychological effects of central nervous system prophylactic treatment in childhood leukemia: Methodological considerations. *Journal of Pediatric Psychology, 18,* 319–338.

Clavell, L. A., Gelber, R. D., Cohen, H. J., Hitchcock-Bryan, S., Cassady, R., Tarbell, N. J., Blattner, S. R., Tantravahi, R., Leavitt, P., & Sallan, S. E. (1986). Four-agent induction and intensive asparaginase therapy for treatment of childhood acute lymphoblastic leukemia. *New England Journal of Medicine, 315,* 657–663.

Cousens, P., Waters, B., Said, J., & Stevens, M. (1988). Cognitive effects of cranial irradiation in leukaemia: A survey and meta-analysis. *Journal of Child Psychology and Psychiatry, 29,* 839–852.

Drigan, R., Spirito, A., & Gelber, R. D. (1992). Behavioral effects of corticosteroids in children with acute lymphoblastic leukemia. *Medical and Pediatric Oncology, 20,* 13–21.

Eiser, C. (1978). Intellectual abilities among survivors of childhood leukaemia as a function of CNS irradiation. *Archives of Disease in Childhood, 53,* 391–395.

Fletcher, J. M., & Copeland, D. R. (1988). Neurobehavioral effects of central nervous system prophylactic treatment of cancer in children. *Journal of Clinical and Experimental Neuropsychology, 10,* 495–538.

Gamis, A. S., & Nesbit, M. E. (1991). Neuropsychologic (cognitive) disabilities in long-term survivors of childhood cancer. *Pediatrician, 18,* 11–19.

Gurney, J. G., Severson, R. K., Davis, S., & Robison, L. L. (1995). Incidence of cancer in children in the United States: Sex-, race-, and 1 year age-specific rates by histologic type. *Cancer, 75,* 2186–2198.

Halberg, F. E., Kramer, J. H., Moore, I. M., Wara, W. M., Matthay, K. K., & Ablin, A. R. (1991). Prophylactic cranial irradiation dose effects on late cognitive function in children treated for acute lymphoblastic leukemia. *International Journal of Radiation Oncology, Biology, Physics, 22,* 13–16.

Hicks, S. P., & D'Amato, C. J. (1966). Effects of ionizing radiations on mammalian development. In D. H. M. Woollan (Ed.), *Advances in teratology* (pp. 195–250). London: Logos Press.

Jankovic, M., Browers, P. Valsecchi, M. G., Van Veldhuizen, A., Huisman, J., Kamphuis, R., Kingma, A., Mor, W., Van Dongen-Milman, J., Ferronato, L., Mancini, M., Spinetta, J. J., & Masera, G. (1994). Association of 1800 cGy cranial irradiation with intellectual function in children with acute lymphoblastic leukemia. *Lancet, 344,* 224–227.

Katz, J. A., Pollock, R. H., Jacaruso, D., & Morad, A. (1993). Final attained height in patient successfully treated for childhood acute lymphoblastic leukemia. *Journal of Pediatrics, 123,* 546–552.

Kaufmann, P. M., Moore, I. M., Espy, K. A., & Hutter, J. J. (1994). Attention and learning strategies following triple intrathecal chemotherapy for childhood leukemia. *Journal of the International Neuropsychology Society, 1,* 324.

Kernan, W. J., Mullenix, P. J., & Hopper, D. L. (1987). Pattern recognition of rat behavior. *Pharmacology, Biochemistry and Behavior, 27,* 559–564.

Kernan, W. J., Mullenix, P. J., Kent, R., Hopper, D. L., & Cressie, N.A.C. (1988). Analysis of the time distribution and time sequence of behavioral acts. *International Journal of Neuroscience, 43,* 35–51.

Kleinman, S. N., & Waber, D. P. (1994). Prose memory strategies of children treated for leukemia: A story grammar analysis of the Anna Thompson passage. *Neuropsychology, 8,* 464–470.

Lipshultz, S. E., Lipsitz, S. R., Mone, S. M., Goorin, A. M., Sallan, S. E., Sanders, S. P., Orav, E. J., Gelber, R. D., & Colan, S. D. (1995). Female sex and drug dose as risk factors for late cardiotoxic effects of doxorubicin therapy for childhood cancer. *New England Journal of Medicine, 332,* 1738–1743.

Madan-Swain, A., & Brown, R. T. (1991). Cognitive and psychosocial sequelae for children with acute lymphocytic leukemia and their families. *Clinical Psychology Review, 11,* 267–294.

Mildenberger, M., Beach, T. G., McGeer, E. G., & Ludgate, C. M. (1990). An animal model of prophylactic cranial irradiation: histologic effects at acute, early and delayed stages. *International Journal of Radiation Oncology, Biology, Physics, 18,* 1051–1060.

Mulhern, R. K., Fairclough, D., & Ochs, J. (1991). A prospective comparison of neuropsychologic performance of children surviving leukemia who received 18-Gy, 24-Gy, or no cranial irradiation. *Journal of Clinical Oncology, 9,* 1348–1356.

Mulhern, R. K., Wasserman, A. L., Fairclough, D., & Ochs, J. (1988). Memory function in disease-free survivors of childhood acute lymphocytic leukemia given CNS prophylaxis with or without 1,800 cGy cranial irradiation. *Journal of Clinical Oncology, 6,* 315–320.

Mullenix, P. J. (1996). The computer pattern recognition system for study of spontaneous behavior of rats: A diagnostic tool for damage in the central nervous system? In P. R. Sanberg, K.-P. Ossenkopp, & M. Kavaliers (Eds.), *Motor activity and movement disorders: Research issues and applications* (pp. 243–268). Clifton, NJ: Humana Press.

Mullenix, P. J. (1997). Radiation protection in the developing central nervous system: Investigation of a biological approach. In E. A. Bump & K. Malaker (Eds.), *Radioprotectors: Chemical, biological and clinical perspectives* (pp. 349–371). Boca Raton, FL: CRC Press.

Mullenix, P. J., & Kernan, W. J. (1989). Extension of the analysis of the time structure of behavioral acts. *International Journal of Neuroscience, 44,* 251–262.

Mullenix, P. J., Kernan, W. J., Schunior, A., Howes, A., Waber, D. P., Sallan, S. E., & Tarbell, N. J. (1994).

Interactions of steroid, methotrexate, and radiation determine neurotoxicity in an animal model to study therapy for childhood leukemia. *Pediatric Research*, 35, 171–178.

Mullenix, P. J., Kernan, W., Tassinari, M., Schunior, A., Waber, D. P., Howes, A., & Tarbell, N. J. (1990). An animal model to study toxicity of CNS therapy for childhood acute lymphoblastic leukemia: Effects on behavior. *Cancer Research*, 50, 6461–6465.

Mullenix, P. J., Mulkern, R., Schunior, A., Kernan, W. J., Howes, A., Waber, D. P., Sallan, S. E., & Tarbell, N. J. (1999). *Protection by pre-irradiation methotrexate in rats*. Unpublished data.

Nachman, J., Sather, H., Lukens, J., Gaynon, P., Wolff, L., Arthur, D., Cherlow, J., & Trigg, M. (1994). Cranial radiation improves event free survival for high risk patients with acute lymphoblastic leukemia showing a rapid response to BFM induction chemotherapy [Abstract]. *Proceedings of the American Society of Clinical Oncology*, 13, 317.

Neglia, J. P., Meadows, A. T., Robison, L. L., Kim, T. H., Newton, W. A., Ruymann, F. B., Sather, H. N., & Hammond, G. D. (1991). Second neoplasms after acute lymphoblastic leukemia in childhood. *New England Journal of Medicine*, 325, 1330–1336.

Newcomer, J. W., Craft, S., Hershey, T., Askins, K., & Bardgett, M. E. (1994). Glucocorticoid-induced impairment in declarative memory performance in adult humans. *Journal of Neuroscience*, 14, 2047–2053.

Peckham, V. C., Meadows, A. T., Bartel, N., & Marrero, O. (1988). Educational late effects in long-term survivors of childhood acute lymphocytic leukemia. *Pediatrics*, 81, 127–133.

Pui, C.-H. (1997). Acute lymphoblastic leukemia. *Pediatric Clinics of North America*, 44, 831–846.

Ries, L. A. G., Miller, B. A., & Hankey, B. F. (Eds.). (1994). *SEER cancer statistic review 1973–1991: Tables and graphs* (DHHS Publication No. NIH-2789). Bethesda, MD : National Cancer Institute.

Roman, D. D., & Sperduto, P. W. (1995). Neuropsychological effects of cranial radiation: Current knowledge and future directions. *International Journal of Radiation Oncology, Biology, Physics*, 31, 983–998.

Rourke, B. P. (1987). Syndrome of non-verbal learning disabilities: The final common pathway of white matter disease/dysfunction? *Clinical Neuropsychologist*, 1, 209–234.

Schunior, A., Mullenix, P. J., Zengel, A. E., Landy, H., Howes, A., & Tarbell, N. J. (1994). Radiation effects on growth are altered in rats by prednisolone and methotrexate. *Pediatric Research*, 35, 416–423.

Schunior, A., Zengel, A. E., Mullenix, P. J., Tarbell, N. J., Howes, A., & Tassinari, M. W. (1990). An animal model to study toxicity of central nervous system therapy for childhood acute lymphoblastic leukemia: Effects on growth and craniofacial proportion. *Cancer Research*, 50, 6461–6465.

Smith, M., Arthur, D., & Camitta, B. (1996). Uniform approach to risk-classification and treatment assignment for children with acute lymphoblastic leukemia. *Journal of Clinical Oncology*, 14, 18–24.

Tarbell, N. J., Waber, D. P., Cohen, H., Gelber, R., & Sallan, S. E. (1991). Hyperfractionated cranial irradiation (HCI) in childhod acute lymphoblastic leukemia (ALL): Rationale and preliminary results [Abstract]. *Proceedings of the American Society of Clinical Oncology*, 10, 239.

Waber, D. P., Gioia, G., Paccia, J., Sherman, B., Dinklage, D., Sollee, N., Urion, D. K., & Sallan, S. E. (1990). Sex differences in cognitive processing in children treated with CNS prophylaxis for acute lymphoblastic leukemia. *Journal of Pediatric Psychology*, 15, 105–122.

Waber, D. P., Isquith, P. K., Kahn, C. M., Romero, I., Sallan, S. E., & Tarbell, N. J. (1994). Metacognitive factor si the visuospatial skills of long-term survivors of acute lymphoblastic leukemia (ALL): An experimental approach to the Rey–Osterrieth Complex Figure Test (ROCF). *Developmental Neuropsychology*, 10, 349–367.

Waber, D. P., Tarbell, N. J., Kahn, C. J., Gelber, R. D., & Sallan, S. E. (1992). The relationship of sex and treatment modality to neuropsychologic outcome in childhood acute lymphoblastic leukemia. *Journal of Clinical Oncology*, 10, 810– 817.

Waber, D. P., Tarbell, N. J., Fairclough, D., Atmore, K., Castro, R., Isquith, P., Lussier, F., Romero, I., Carpenter, P. J., Schiller, M., & Sallan, S. E. (1995). Cognitive sequelae of treatment in childhood acute lymphoblastic leukemia: Cranial radiation requires an accomplice. *Journal of Clinical Oncology*, 13, 2490–2496.

Waber, D. P., Urion, D. K., Tarbell, N. H., Niemeyer, C., Gelber, R. N., & Sallan, S. E. (1990). Late effects of central nervous system treatment of acute lymphoblastic leukemia in childhood are sex-dependent. *Developmental Medicine and Child Neurology*, 32, 238–248.

14

SICKLE CELL DISEASE

M. DOUGLAS RIS
ROYAL GRUENEICH

BACKGROUND

About 2,000 years ago, a technological development was introduced that eventuated in the disease we now refer to as sickle cell anemia (SCA): Metal tools made possible the clearing of large tracts of land in the tropical rain forests of West Africa. Removal of the natural drainage system provided by the trees, and irrigation of root crops such as yams, produced areas of standing water exposed to sunlight—an optimal breeding ground for the malaria-bearing *Anopheles* mosquito. With an estimated mortality rate as high as 20% in some areas of Africa (Livingston, 1971), malaria may be responsible for more human deaths than any other disease. Thus there emerged a potent selection force in regional human evolution (Eaton, 1994). A biological threat of this magnitude would call for an extreme genetic remedy. Such is the reasoning behind the putative "balanced polymorphism" of SCA, in which the lethality of the homozygous state is balanced by the survival advantage of the heterozygous state (by selective sickling and removal from the bloodstream of parasitized red blood cells). The responsible gene therefore persists in great numbers, with a carrier rate in parts of West Africa as high as 20–30%.

Research into the West African origins of SCA suggests that many aspects of the affliction were recognized and "codified" in the mythology and customs of several ethnic groups. Edelstein (1986) provides an insightful account of what are referred to in traditional African medicine as *ogbanje*, or "repeater children." This notion may have originated from the common experience that several children in the same families would die soon after birth. It was believed that such children were inhabited by a spirit taking on the likeness of a beautiful child, only to die in infancy and be reborn in subsequent children. Achebe (1969) gives a touching account of this in *Things Fall Apart*:

> As she buried one child after another her sorrow gave way to despair and then to grim resignation. The birth of her children, which should be a woman's crowning glory, became for Ekwefi mere physical agony devoid of promise. The naming ceremony after seven market weeks

320

became an empty ritual. Her deepening despair found expression in the names she gave her children. One of them was a pathetic cry, Onwumbiko—"Death, I implore you." But death took no notice: Onwumbiko died in his fifteenth month. The next child was a girl Ozoemena— "May it not happen again." She died in her eleventh month.

Such traditional beliefs are common in those parts of Africa where there is a known concentration of the sickle cell gene. The death of many infants in the same families may have been the result of infections to which children with SCA are highly susceptible.

Early case reports of probable SCA appeared in the North American medical literature in the mid-19th century. Lebby (1846) described the postmortem of a runaway slave executed for murder who had a full chest, narrow hips, spare build, no spleen, and remittent fevers during life. The first description of the hematological features of the disease was provided by an eminent Chicago cardiologist, James Herrick. Herrick (1910) related the case of a dental student from Grenada who was found to have oddly sickle-shaped red blood cells. Additional cases appeared in the medical literature in the ensuing years, including a case by Mason (1922) of Johns Hopkins, who coined the term *sickle cell anemia.*

Following the discovery by Herrick of the red blood cell basis of SCA, the next major landmark discovery was that of Linus Pauling (Pauling, Itano, Singer, & Wells, 1949), who described the abnormal hemoglobin molecule (HbS) in the disease. Pauling and colleagues went on to demonstrate that carriers had both normal and abnormal hemoglobin (Hb), although they bore no clinical manifestations of the disease. By the mid-1950s, the scientific investigation of the genetic basis of SCA had advanced to the point that Ingram (1956) could identify the specific amino acid substitution (valine for glutamic acid) at position 6 of the β-globulin chain in the HbS molecule. Research and clinical management of SCA were given further impetus by President Nixon's pronouncement in his 1971 address to Congress that SCA was a neglected health condition. This was followed by the National Sickle Cell Anemia Control Act passed by Congress in 1972, and by the establishment of comprehensive sickle cell centers throughout the country.

EPIDEMIOLOGY AND GENETICS

Screening of newborns for hemoglobinopathies began in the United States in the early 1970s. Through such efforts, it has been estimated that SCA occurs in 1 in 600 African American newborns, with 8 in 100 being carriers (sickle cell trait) of the disease. The abnormal sickle cell gene conforms to a Mendelian recessive pattern of inheritance and seems to have originated at least four times in Africa, crossing into many ethnic groups through population expansion (Nagel, 1994). The presence of the gene in African Americans is a result of 400 years of slave trade involving various points in West Africa.

Despite the high frequency of the disease in parts of Africa, SCA is not recognized as a major public health problem and is not listed as one of the major killers in Africa. Most children inheriting the disease live in remote rural areas, are undiagnosed, and die at an early age, often as a result of infection. Thus the natural history of SCA in Africa is not well documented (Ohene-Frempong, 1991).

Inconsistent terminology has complicated epidemiological investigations of the disease. SCA refers to the homozygous (HbSS) state that results from inheritance of the HbS gene from both parents. Sickle cell disease (SCD) refers to a range of conditions, including SCA as well as less common compound heterozygous states. The latter conditions typically have less severe clinical courses and involve pairing of HbS with another abnormal Hb: sickle cell–HbC disease (HbSC disease), sickle cell–β^0 thalassemia (HbSβ^0 thalassemia), sickle cell–$\beta^\pm$ thalassemia (HbS$\beta^\pm$ thalassemia), and sickle cell–β^+ thalassemia (HbSβ^+ thalassemia). Because the mechanism of inheritance is autosomal recessive, in a family with two carrier parents there will be a 25% risk of SCD in offspring, with 50% of the offspring being clinically asymptomatic carriers. Characterization of both patients with SCD and individuals with sickle cell trait as "sicklers" has added further confusion, as persons with the trait are asymptomatic and do not have a disease per se.

NATURAL HISTORY

A high proportion of fetal Hb in newborns acts to protect infants with SCD from early manifestations of the disease. By about the second month of life, anemia, colic-like symptoms, and feeding problems become evident. In the first decade of life, periods of well-being are punctuated by acute illness and pain episodes precipitated by infectious febrile illnesses. These pain episodes increase in length and frequency with age (Powars, 1994). *Streptococcus pneumoniae*, causing septicemia and meningitis, constitutes the major risk in infancy; in the past, it accounted for most infant deaths. Prophylactic treatment with penicillin has successfully prevented most pneumococcal infections in infants and young children.

Cerebral vasculopathy and infarction, the major concerns of early and middle childhood, are given more extensive treatment in a subsequent section of this chapter. Splenic sequestration syndrome, in which the spleen becomes massively enlarged with the entrapment of blood, is a life-threatening complication that often follows an infectious illness. By age 6 years, 90% of children with SCA have splenic hypofunction, eventuating in a mere fibrous remnant of the spleen in 85–90% of African American adults with SCA (Yam & Li, 1994).

Problems associated with infection and cerebral infarction give way in late adolescence and adulthood to chronic organ damage as the principal challenge in managing the disease. The effects of SCA are ubiquitous and involve most systems of the body. There may be progressive loss of bony tissue and joint destruction; kidney, liver, and cardiac disease; retinal lesions; ankle ulcers; gout; and acute chest syndrome (due to infarction or infection) leading to adult respiratory distress syndrome (Charache, 1994).

Owing to improved methods of detection, prevention, and treatment, 90% of children with SCA born after 1980 in developed countries will reach the third decade of life. Eighty-two percent of deaths in adults with SCA are related to complications, with renal failure, acute cardiovascular event, and congestive heart failure being the most common causes. Males have a somewhat shorter life expectancy than females (42 years and 48 years, respectively) (Charache, 1994).

PATHOPHYSIOLOGY

The central mechanism in the pathophysiology of SCD is the sickling of red blood cells, which involves a change from the normal biconcave disc to the sickle form (Scott-Conner & Brunson, 1994; Platt, 1994). When HbS is deoxygenated, it becomes polymerized as long, thin, parallel bundles of HbS fibers. These long strands of polymerized Hb cause sickling, or deformation in shape, of the red blood cells. Sickling increases the viscosity of blood and may result in the formation of masses of red blood cells that occlude small vessels. Polymerization is a complex process that depends on such factors as changes in oxygen level, temperature, and pH. Polymerization is also critically affected by HbF (i.e., fetal Hb) and HbA (i.e., normal child and adult Hb), both of which significantly reduce HbS polymer content in cells, with HbF having a substantially greater effect than HbA. Because of the protective effect of HbF, newborn infants with SCD are generally asymptomatic. However, as HbS production increases and HbF levels decrease, clinical symptoms may begin to emerge.

Initially, the sickling process is reversible when the red blood cells are reoxygenated (Platt, 1994). These "reversibly sickled cells" have the normal biconcave shape and also have normal viscosity. The process that underlies the vaso-occlusive episodes in SCD may be one in which reversibly sickled cells enter into the small blood vessels in the oxygenated state because of their normal rheological properties and then occlude the vessels as they become distorted in shape after deoxygenation. After repeated episodes of sickling and reversal to the normal shape, the membrane of the red cell is damaged, and the cell becomes irreversibly sickled. These effects on the membrane properties of red blood cells appear to play an integral role in the disease process; in particular, it has been found that HbS red blood cells adhere more readily to endothelial surfaces than do normal cells, with the degree of adherence being closely related to severity of clinical symptoms (Platt, 1994).

Vaso-occlusive episodes are common in SCD and can affect all major organs, including the central nervous system. Although the reported risk of stroke in children with SCD is variable, in most studies it falls in the range of 5–10% in children with HbSS disease (i.e., SCA), which is 225 to 400 times the risk in the general population (Ohene-Frempong, 1991; Balkaran et al., 1992; Powars, Wilson, Imbus, Pegelow, & Allen, 1978). It has been estimated that approximately a third of patients with HbSS disease will be affected by a cerebrovascular accident (CVA) by their 30th birthday. Although the risk for stroke is highest for patients with HbSS disease, strokes have been reported in patients with HbSC disease and the various types of HbSβ thalassemia as well (Ohene-Frempong, 1991; Powars et al., 1978). Ischemic stroke is most common in children, whereas hemorrhagic stroke is most common in adults—a reversal of the usual age pattern for CVAs (Powars et al., 1978). The most common symptoms are hemiplegia, language disturbances, seizures, coma, and visual disturbances. In untreated patients, recurrent strokes are common, one estimate being that 70% of such patients will suffer a second stroke within 3 years (Platt, 1994).

It was initially thought that the strokes in SCD were related to occlusion of small blood vessels. However, since the work of Stockman, Nigro, Mishkin, and Oski (1972), evidence from (1) postmortem exams, (2) angiographic studies, and (3) computed tomography (CT), magnetic resonance imaging (MRI), and transcranial Doppler ultrasound studies has consistently shown that the majority of cases involve multiple stenoses of the distal internal carotid and proximal anterior and middle cerebral arteries (Adams et al., 1992; Adams, Nichols, McKie, Milner, & Gammal, 1988; Kugler et al., 1993; Rothman, Fulling, & Nelson, 1986). The blood vessels usually show evidence of intimal proliferation, fibrosis, and fragmentation, and in some cases there is formation of thrombi. The study by Adams et al. (1988) is particularly illustrative of the neuropathological findings regarding stroke in SCD. These investigators classified a total of 34 strokes in 25 patients with SCD, of whom 22 had a prior history of ischemic stroke. Eighty percent of the strokes were classified as being most consistent with large-vessel disease; the other 20% were consistent with other mechanisms of infarction, such as small-vessel disease or embolism. Border zone or watershed infarctions were common in cases where large-vessel disease was implicated. The results demonstrated that although large-vessel disease appears to account for the majority of stroke episodes in SCD, small-vessel disease may account for a significant percentage of incidents.

Transfusion therapy appears to reduce the rate of stroke recurrence substantially, as indexed by a markedly lower rate of recurrence compared to that for untransfused stroke patients (Ohene-Frempong, 1991). One regimen for transfusion therapy is to make two to four exchange transfusions in the acute phase, then to lower the HbS levels to below 30% of the total Hb with partial exchanges or simple transfusions every 3–5 weeks. Unfortunately, transfusion therapy is not effective for all patients; it is uncertain how long the therapy needs to be continued; and long-term transfusion therapy carries risks such as iron overload and, at least in the past, compromise of the immune system from contaminated blood (Platt, 1994).

Further elucidation of the pathophysiology of SCD is provided by research regarding cerebral blood flow (CBF) dynamics. This research has consistently documented an increased rate of CBF in patients with SCD, both children and adults. A strong inverse relation between cerebral perfusion and hematocrit values has also been shown (Prohovnik et al., 1989; Herold et al., 1986; Brass et al., 1991; Adams et al., 1992). In addition, patients who have suffered a stroke have *lower* CBF rates than patients who have no history of stroke, and the perfusion rate is lower in stroke patients who have been transfused than in those who have not been transfused (Prohovnik et al., 1989; Venketasubramanian, Prohovnik, Hurlet, Mohr, & Piomelli, 1994). The effect of transfusion on CBF is immediate, and Venketasubramanian et al. (1994) found that reductions in flow resulting from transfusion were comparable in infarcted and noninfarcted areas of the brain. Prohovnik et al. (1989) suggest that the most likely mechanism for the relationship of hematocrit value to CBF rate is that low hematocrit increases perfusion because of limited oxygen delivery, thus requiring dilatation of the blood vessels. According to this model, the reduction of flow observed with transfusion is probably a function of improved oxygenation of tissue, both through an increase in hematocrit and replacement of HbS cells with HbA cells. In the case of stroke, it may be that cerebral tissue initially reacts to reduced perfusion pressure with dilatation of blood vessels, but that this adaptation fails, resulting in reduced CBF. Prohovnik et al. (1989) speculate that the chronic state of dilatation of cerebral blood vessels may involve lowered cerebrovascular reserve capacity. With a significant drop in perfusion pressure or increase in metabolic demand, the system fails because it has exceeded its reserve capacity.

NEUROPSYCHOLOGICAL DEVELOPMENT

Patients with Strokes

Several studies have documented severe neuropsychological deficits following stroke (defined clinically, not radiographically) in children with SCD. Powers et al. (1978) performed psychometric testing on 10 of 15 long-term survivors of stroke. Four of the remaining 5 patients were so neurologically handicapped that testing could not be carried out, and 7 of the 10 who were tested had IQs less than 70 on the Wechsler scales. Wilimas, Goff, Anderson, Lengston, and Thompson (1980) evaluated the cognitive functioning of 10 children with SCD (9 with HbSS disease and 1 with HbSC disease) who experienced strokes and were subsequently placed on a transfusion protocol. Testing was conducted following an initial stroke and was repeated up to three times at 6-month intervals. On the Wechsler scales, the children's Full Scale IQ (FSIQ) scores at initial evaluation ranged from 45 to 79, with a median value of 67. There was usually some improvement in children's scores on evaluation 6 months later, but five of six patients who experienced a second stroke showed a decrease in their scores over follow-up.

Hariman, Griffith, Hurtig, and Keehn (1991) evaluated the functional and psychometric status of 14 children with SCD who had suffered strokes. These children were compared to age- and gender-matched children with SCD who had not suffered strokes. Children in the stroke group exhibited only mild or minimal functional motoric deficits, except that fine motor hand functions were moderately impaired on the hemiparetic side. Only a few children in this group demonstrated mild difficulties in performance of activities of daily living. Eleven of the 14 children with strokes, however, had estimated IQ scores below 80 on an abbreviated Wechsler Intelligence Scale for Children—Revised (WISC-R), and the mean estimated IQ score for the children with stroke was 68, compared to 91 for the control group.

Cohen, Branch, McKie, and Adams (1994) investigated neuropsychological functioning in children with HbSS disease who were undergoing chronic transfusion therapy after having a single stroke. Their sample was divided into a group of four children who had experienced a single left-hemisphere stroke and six children who had sustained a single right-hemisphere stroke. The left-hemisphere group tended to have global impairments of verbal and nonverbal abilities, including deficits in general intellectual skills (mean WISC-R FSIQ = 62, Verbal IQ [VIQ] = 62, Performance IQ [PIQ] = 67), auditory/verbal memory abilities, visual–spatial skills, and academic achievement. Visual-perceptual abilities, as measured by the Kaufman Assessment Battery for Children (K-ABC) Gestalt Closure subtest and the Test of Visual Perceptual Skills, were spared. In contrast, the right-hemisphere group tended to demonstrate more selective deficits, primarily in the areas of visual–spatial abilities (e.g., WISC-R FSIQ = 73, VIQ = 82, and PIQ = 69) and arithmetic achievement.

A recent article from the Cooperative Study of Sickle Cell Disease (Armstrong et al., 1996) reported an incidence of 6.6% for strokes in 105 subjects with the HbSS genotype. None of the 56 subjects with the HbSC genotype suffered clinical strokes. Children with strokes had a mean WISC-R FSIQ of 70.8 (VIQ = 72.1, PIQ = 74.1) and exhibited comparable academic deficiencies.

Taken together, studies on children with strokes related to SCD consistently document low borderline to mildly (and in some cases, moderately) retarded levels of functioning. Neurocognitive deficits are often broad-ranging, although some lateralizing patterns corresponding to the affected hemisphere have been reported.

Patients without Strokes

Several other studies have examined children without histories of clinical neurological events, although these samples probably included patients with subclinical strokes. Indeed, it is only recently that investigators have further divided their samples on the basis of the presence or absence of imaging abnormalities (see "Neuroimaging Correlates," below). Early studies of patients without strokes failed to detect significant developmental effects of SCD on IQ. For example, Chodorkoff and Whitten (1963) found no differences in IQ between 19 children with SCD and their unaffected siblings. In subsequent studies, Kosacoff, Seligman, and Dosik (1974) and Allen (1983) arrived at the same conclusion. The results of these studies were limited by their small sample sizes, broad age ranges, failure to report genotype, restricted battery of cognitive measures, and (in two cases) the use of test norms rather than comparison to a matched control group.

Four later, better-controlled studies have reported neuropsychological dysfunction in patients with SCD and no history of CVAs (Wasserman, Wilimas, Fairclough, Mulhern, & Wang, 1991; Swift et al., 1989; Fowler et al., 1988; Brown et al., 1993). Some of these studies found lower overall IQs in patients with SCD. Swift et al. (1989) reported a mean WISC-R FSIQ of 77.7 in patients with SCD, compared to 94.3 in healthy sibling controls. Wasserman et al. (1991) found a smaller but statistically significant difference between patients with SCD (FSIQ = 82.7) and sibling controls (FSIQ = 88). Other researchers have found evidence of more specific deficits in academic skills. Brown et al. (1993) found group differences in reading decoding, but not math, while Fowler et al. (1988) reported significant differences in both reading and spelling. Deficits in attention (Fowler et al., 1988; Brown et al., 1993) and visual–motor coordination (Fowler et al., 1988) have also been described. The studies by Swift et al. (1989) and Fowler et al. (1988) included only patients with the HbSS genotype. Wasserman et al. (1991) studied a more genotypically heterogeneous sample, but did not report the results by genotype. Brown et al. (1993) did not find a difference in intellectual performance between children with the HbSS genotype and other genotypes.

Neuroimaging Correlates

Research on the correlation between neuroimaging and neuropsychological studies in children with SCD has focused on the phenomenon of *silent strokes*, defined in terms of abnormalities on neuroimaging studies without overt clinical symptoms (Craft, Schatz, Glauser, Lee, & DeBaun, 1993). There appears to be a high rate of silent strokes in children with SCD; they occurred in 14% of one sample (Pavlakis et al., 1988) and in 35% of another sample (Craft et al., 1993). Studies of the relationship between silent strokes and neuropsychological deficits in children with SCD have yielded inconsistent findings. Kugler et al. (1993) did not find significant differences on a variety of neuropsychological measures between a group of eight patients with abnormal MRI scans and a matched control group of eight patients with normal MRI scans. In contrast, Craft et al. (1993) found that three patients with silent strokes involving anterior lesions made significantly more intrusion errors on the Children's Auditory Verbal Learning Test than did a sibling control group. Three children with silent strokes involving diffuse lesions scored significantly lower than the sibling controls on WISC-R Block Design and Object Assembly.

In the only study with *concurrent* imaging findings, Armstrong et al. (1996) were able to show that patients with silent strokes (12.4% of the total sample) had lower IQs than those with normal MRIs (WISC-R FSIQ = 82.8 vs. 90). Since normal controls were not included in this study, it is unclear whether the intellectual development of patients with normal scans was adversely affected by their disease. However, these findings argue that the intellectual deficits in children with SCD can be accounted for largely or exclusively by these subclinical CVAs. A similar conclusion was reached by Craft et al. (1993), who found that in the absence of clinical or subclinical strokes, children with SCD did not differ on a battery of neuropsychological tests from sibling controls. More recently, Watkins et al. (1998) also found no difference between sibling controls and patients with SCD who had not suffered either clinical or subclinical strokes.

Although these recent investigations are consistent in finding increased neuropsychological risk in children with SCD (at least those with clinical or radiographic neurological abnormalities), it remains unclear whether these deficits represent diffuse impairment or a more localized/lateralized pattern of neuropsychological dysfunction. Swift et al. (1989)

interpreted their results as reflecting generalized impairment, while Brown et al. (1993) suggested that the weaknesses they discovered on measures of attention indicated more specific involvement of the frontal lobes. However, a subsequent study by Goonan, Goonan, Brown, Buchanan, and Eckman (1994) failed to reveal differences between patients with SCD and sibling controls on laboratory and behavioral measures of attention and impulse control.

Differential impairment across age groups has been examined in these cross-sectional studies, with mixed results. This issue may be important, as it has implications for the underlying pathophysiological mechanism(s) responsible for these deficits. Some studies report that older children are at greater risk than younger children (Brown et al., 1993; Fowler et al., 1988), consistent with the hypothesis of progressive cerebrovascular disease (e.g., distal insufficiency or accrual of microinfarcts). Other investigators, however, have failed to find age differences in outcomes (Swift et al., 1989), or have found that older patients function at *higher* levels than younger patients (Wasserman et al., 1991). Studies of the early development of children with SCD are generally lacking, but a report from the Cooperative Study of Sickle Cell Disease (Wang, Grover, Gallagher, Espeland, & Fandal, 1993) indicates progressive impairment with age. For children under 3 years of age, questionable or abnormal outcomes on the Denver Developmental Screening Test were rare (3.6%); in children in the 3- to 5-year-old range, these outcomes were significantly more common (12%).

One shortcoming of many of these studies has been an overreliance on "level-of-performance" analytic strategies. In a disease characterized by heterogeneity of lesion size, location, and chronicity, differences between SCD and control groups may be obscured, particularly when omnibus IQ indices are used. Investigations of the effects of localized lesions on specific neuropsychological dimensions identified *a priori* would appear to be a more promising research strategy (Craft et al., 1993). Furthermore, as will be argued later, other indices, such as greater intraindividual variability across neuropsychological domains, may prove to be more sensitive than level-of-performance measures to the developmental aberrations found in children with SCD.

In sum, children with SCD who have not suffered overt clinical strokes may nevertheless exhibit compromised neurocognitive development. Our understanding of the underlying pathophysiology of such impairment is incomplete. It may be that such developmental deviations and clinical strokes have a common basis in large-vessel disease. It is also possible that alternate mechanisms, such as chronic anemia (Brown et al., 1993) and small-vessel disease/occlusion (operating independently, additively, or interactively), are important in understanding neuropsychological risk in these patients.

School Performance, Absenteeism, and Achievement Test Performance

Some reports indicate greater academic difficulties in children with SCD, as measured by rates of grade repetitions and special services received (Fowler et al., 1988). This has not been a consistent finding, however, as Brown et al. (1993) found no significant differences in rates of special education placement between children with SCD and unaffected siblings. Wasserman et al. (1991) found no differences between children with SCD and controls in grade placement, grade point average, and frequency of special education placement. Although it is tempting to link the school problems of children with SCD to frequent absences caused by their illness, there appears to be no relationship between number of days absent and academic achievement scores (Brown et al., 1993).

Scores on standardized achievement tests do not always correspond to classroom performance, and so both indices must be considered when one is examining academic performance in children with SCD. Fowler et al. (1988) reported poorer performance on school-administered achievement tests in children with SCD than in controls. The group with SCD also obtained lower Wide Range Achievement Test scores on Reading and Spelling, but not on Arithmetic. Similarly, Brown et al. (1993) found that children with SCD scored lower than controls on K-ABC Reading Decoding but not on K-ABC Math. Swift et al. (1989) found deficits in both reading and math. The limited evidence available thus far therefore suggests that reading ability is more affected in these children. The reason for this is unclear, but it may provide a clue as to the timing of neuropathological changes in children with SCD.

Behavioral/Psychosocial Morbidity

Studies using parent and teacher reports of psychological maladjustment have also yielded somewhat inconsistent results. Swift et al. (1989) found no more difficulties in patients than controls on the Social Competence scale of the Child Behavior Checklist, whereas in an uncontrolled study of children with SCD, Iloeje (1991) reported significant psychiatric morbidity on the Rutter Scales. Neurotic symptoms were more prevalent than antisocial behaviors. However, Iloeje did not exclude patients with a positive neurological history; hence this sample may have been more neurologically compromised than the samples of patients without histories of discrete neurological events. Hurtig and White (1986) reported increased internalizing symptoms in male adolescents with SCD relative to test norms, although patients who had suffered strokes were not excluded. A subsequent study by this group (Hurtig, Koepke, & Park, 1989) reported no relationship between psychosocial adjustment and various measures of disease severity.

THE CINCINNATI SICKLE CELL DISEASE STUDY

A cohort of 32 children with SCD has been followed at Children's Hospital Medical Center in Cincinnati since 1993. These children, who were 8 to 14 years of age and had no known cerebrovascular events at the time of enrollment in the study, have been compared to 32 matched normal classroom controls in regard to their neuropsychological and socio-emotional development. In addition, the relationship of disease factors (genotype, severity of illness) and neuroimaging studies (conventional MRI, MRI perfusion) to neuropsychological functioning in the children with SCD has been examined. This is an ongoing study, though to date only data from the initial assessment have been analyzed.

Neuropsychological Development

The children with SCD performed moderately lower than the control children on several neuropsychological measures, including overall IQ (WISC-R FSIQ = 86 for the SCD group compared to FSIQ = 92 for controls), composite measures of verbal skills and attention and memory skills, and a measure of impulsivity that controlled for IQ. However, there were no significant differences between the groups on composite measures of academic achievement, visual–spatial skills, and fine motor skills. Children with SCD and controls did not differ, either, in terms of composite score discrepancies (e.g., verbal minus visual–spatial composites) or on indices of scatter across tests. No consistent relationship was found between neuropsychological performance and genotype (18 children had HbSS disease or HbSβ^0 thalassemia [the most severe forms of SCD], 10 had HbSC disease, and 6 had Hbβ$^+$ thalassemia). Furthermore, measures of disease severity (Hb levels, composite disease severity ratings) were unrelated to neuropsychological status (Ris, Grueneich, & Kalinyak, 1995).

Neuroimaging Correlates

Conventional MRI and MRI perfusion studies were obtained for 22 of the children with SCD. Perfusion-weighted MRI is a relatively new procedure that involves administration of a rapid and compact intravenous bolus of MRI contrast agent. Analysis of the diffusion of the contrast provides relevant information about blood perfusion in the brain (Tzika et al., 1993). The imaging data were scored by a pediatric neuroradiologist and a neuroradiology fellow, using a quantitative system that evaluated the degree of structural and functional cortical and white matter abnormalities (Grueneich, Ball, Ris, & Kalinyak, 1998). Ten children (45% of the sample) exhibited abnormalities on the neuroimaging studies; two had structural abnormalities only, five had perfusion abnormalities only, and three had both structural and perfusion abnormalities. The structural abnormalities consisted primarily of small but numerous and diffuse punctate lesions in the white matter, and the perfusion abnormalities consisted primarily of areas of hypoperfusion, especially in the frontal lobes.

The presence of neuroimaging abnormalities was strongly correlated with greater clinical disease severity. In addition, patients who exhibited neuroimaging abnormalities were at increased risk for clinical stroke, with all three patients who demonstrated both structural and perfusion abnormalities subsequently developing overt symptoms of stroke. However, neuroimaging abnormalities were not significantly correlated with *level* of neuropsychological performance (e.g., IQ, test composites), but were associated with greater *variability or unevenness* in performance across different neuropsychological domains (as measured by discrepancies in scores and indices of test scatter). Thus there was a high rate of imaging abnormalities and neuropsychological dysfunction in our sample of children with SCD, despite their having been selected on the basis of an absence of clinical neurological events. Moreover, MRI abnormalities were associated with *irregularities* in neuropsychological development, rather than with a distinct profile or a deficit in overall level of performance

The complexities of relating imaging data to neuropsychological variables are further illustrated in a case report we published of a child with SCD who had suffered a stroke (Ris et al., 1996). Since this patient was part of the Cincinnati cohort, we had completed neuropsychological and MRI studies shortly before the stroke, and these procedures were repeated after the stroke. There were no obvious neuropsychological manifestations of the numerous prestroke imaging abnormalities (widening of the extra-axial fluid spaces frontally, areas of increased signal within the white matter, decreased perfusion in both frontal lobes). Furthermore, whereas neurological deficits (including left hemiparesis and left visual neglect) were evident after the stroke, neurocognitive impairment was most apparent in *discrepancies* between different types of ability (e.g., verbal vs. nonverbal memory), although even these symptoms were quite subtle. The child's poststroke WISC-R FSIQ of 103 was not significantly different from her prestroke FSIQ of 99—a pattern that contrasts with the typical borderline to mildly mentally retarded level of functioning in SCD patients who have suffered strokes. One possibility is that this patient's stroke altered her developmental trajectory, such that longer-term follow-up would have demonstrated more divergence from normality. However, increased functional morbidity over time may also be related to neurological progression.

Behavioral/Psychosocial Morbidity

The Cincinnati SCD Study employed sociometric ("best friend" and "like" ratings), peer nomination (Revised Class Play [RCP]), projective, and self-report measures. The only difference between children with SCD and matched classroom controls was in regard to their social relationships (Noll, Vannatta, Koontz, & Kalinyak, 1996). Males with SCD were perceived as less aggressive on the RCP than controls, and females with SCD were seen as less sociable and less well accepted. Therefore, like Hurtig and White (1986), we found an interaction involving gender. It was proposed that symptoms, such as chronic fatigue, may divert males away from externalizing and toward internalizing adjustment patterns. Girls, on the other hand, may be more affected by disease-related curtailment of social opportunities and/or physical changes associated with SCD (e.g., late maturation, small stature) that may decrease their social appeal. Consistent with the neuropsychological findings, there was also no relationship between peer adjustment and disease severity, nor did we find increased emotional problems in the SCD group. The absence of group differences in emotional functioning is contrary to the findings of Hurtig and White (1986), but may be related to the fact that we studied an older cohort of children. We also failed to find a significant relationship between measures of peer adjustment and neuropsychological variables.

The common finding of white matter lesions on MRI in patients with SCD prompted us to look for evidence of nonverbal learning disabilities (NLDs; Rourke, 1987) in our cohort (Stith et al., in press). More specifically, we examined whether children with SCD presented with the triad of cognitive, academic, and socioemotional deficits described by Rourke. The cognitive and academic manifestations of NLDs were assessed in two ways. First we calculated a composite defined in terms of verbal domain scores minus spatial/constructional domain scores plus the average of reading and spelling minus arithmetic ([V – S/C] + [(R + S)/2 – A]). This composite produced a continuous variable with values ranging from most NLD-like to least NLD-like. A second, more straightforward method that did not take into account academic performance was simply to subtract PIQ from VIQ. The two NLD variables correlated highly, and yielded similar results in the subsequent data analyses.

On the basis of these continuous scores, three subgroups of children with SCD were formed. An NLD group (n = 14) consisted of those subjects who scored more than a standard deviation above the mean and whose performance therefore most resembled the NLD pattern. A non-NLD group (n = 39) consisted of those subjects who fell within one standard deviation above or below the mean. Finally, a verbal disability group (n = 11) consisted of those patients who scored greater than one standard deviation below the mean (and whose performance was therefore least NLD-like). Our hypothesis was not fully supported, in that we found no significant correlation between NLD scores and social isolation on the RCP. However, the means of the three groups were in the expected direction, with the NLD group showing the most (z = .38) and the verbal disability group showing the least (z = –.29) social isolation. It is possible that with a larger sample and more purely defined groups, the model would have been supported. This finding is noteworthy—not only because SCD is a disease in which the NLD pattern has not been examined, but also because, to our knowledge, peer nomination methods have not been used to measure the psychosocial deficits in children with NLDs.

CONCLUSIONS

SCD is a genetic disorder with potentially devastating neuropsychological consequences. Children with the most common genotype, HbSS, are at greatest risk for sequelae. Clinical strokes, which occur in approximately 10% of children with SCD, are associated with marked declines in intellectual/neuropsychological functioning. Evidence of subclinical ischemic changes is found in from 12% to 44% of children with SCD, depending upon sampling methods (e.g., age, genotype) and measurement/technical methods (e.g., conventional MRI vs. MRI perfusion). As we refine our ability to characterize both imaging abnormalities and neuropsychological functioning, more reliable behavior–imaging relationships are likely to emerge. Inconsistent findings in this regard can be attributed to ignorance about the underlying pathophysiology and its developmental time course. MRI abnormalities often precede the clinical strokes, which occur at a mean age of 7.7 years. Indeed, one can postulate that ischemic changes in the brain may be evident much earlier than this, on the basis of evidence suggesting deviations from the normal developmental trajectory as early as 3–5 years of age. If so, then it may be that the intellectual deficits documented in children with SCD who have not had clinical strokes originate early in life. One implication of this would be that research, like the Cincinnati SCD Study, sampling an older cohort will not find robust age effects (i.e., greater impairment with increased age), except perhaps for a specific class of later-maturing neuropsychological functions (e.g., executive functions). Using cross-sectional methodology to study older children with SCD may be easier, but it may be too far downstream from the critical neuropathological processes to yield clear-cut findings.

As a group, children with SCD may be at higher risk for academic problems, depending upon how this is measured. Achievement test performance may offer the most consistent evidence of this, with reading appearing to be most at risk. Research on the socioemotional adjustment of children with SCD indicates that they are at risk for such problems, although it appears unlikely that outcomes can be satisfactorily modeled without taking into account both environmental/psychological *and* neuropathological/neuropsychological risk factors. Too often, investigators have focused on one set of variables to the exclusion of the other.

CRITIQUE OF EXISTING RESEARCH ON SEQUELAE

Clarification of the neurodevelopmental effects of SCD has proved to be a challenging enterprise. As is often the case, existing research provides more questions than answers. Inconsistencies across studies are common, whether the focus is on neuropsychological development, academic performance, socioemotional adjustment, or relationships among these domains. These inconsistencies can probably be attributed in part to the methodological shortcomings of this literature, which include (1) overreliance on cross-sectional rather than prospective, longitudinal designs; (2) failure to differentiate between patients who have and have not suffered overt or radiographic strokes; (3) inclusion of patients with different genotypes, or failure to specify genotypes; (4) use of global measures, such as IQ and behavior checklists; and (5) lack of control groups. The age range of children studied is often large, with some samples including children ranging from preschoolers to older adolescents. Research findings on the developmental course of children with SCD are potentially affected by sample rates of clinical or subclinical CVAs, the ages at which developmental evaluations are conducted, and the types of outcomes measured. Depending on these factors, results may alternately depict stable development, progressive decline, or accelerated development.

Variations in sampling methods may also contribute to contradictory results. Whereas larger studies can claim greater power, these investigations have also been plagued by attrition and ascertainment bias. Neuropsychological investigations have been thwarted by overreliance on analyses of level of performance. Irregularities in children's performances across domains may be signs of adverse developmental impact, but are often overlooked. Studies investigating behavior–imaging correlations have generally failed to use sophisticated clinical coding or quantitative methodologies (e.g., volumetrics), thereby potentially limiting analysis of relationships between these variables.

In addition, neurodevelopmental difficulties in children with SCD occur in the context of family environment and sociodemographic influences. Families of children with SCD are often socioeconomically disadvantaged, yet environmental factors receive surprisingly little attention in the SCD literature. Three of the four studies to date that have examined both socioeconomic/family variables and neuropsychological functioning have found significant correlations between these variables (Swift et al., 1989; Fowler et al., 1988; Brown et al., 1993; Armstrong et al., 1996). In one case (Brown et al., 1993), socioeconomic status was a better predictor of intellectual functioning than the best medical/biological variable (Hb level). Ultimately, the lion's share of variance in developmental outcome may be claimed by such contextual factors. Minimally, they limit us to "see through a glass, darkly," making it difficult to discern relationships of interest. We have clearly arrived at a point in the evolution of this literature where we can begin to test more elaborate models of outcome that consider a fuller range of both risk and protective factors in the development of these children (Masten et al., 1995).

FUTURE DIRECTIONS

Multi-institutional collaborative studies, such as the Cooperative Study of Sickle Cell Disease, promise to remedy some of the deficiencies of research on SCD. Through collaborative efforts, large enough samples can be recruited to investigate the complex matrix of biological and nonbiological factors influencing the neurodevelopmental course of children with SCD. Advances in MRI technology and systems for quantification of imaging parameters hold promise in furthering our understanding of the neuropathology of this disease. Building on the less focused studies of the past, further refinement of neurobehavioral measurement is also possible. For example, it is becoming increasingly apparent from functional imaging and blood flow studies that frontal areas of the brain are at risk; this provides guidance in the selection of measures used in the search for behavioral correlates of neuropathological changes.

Future research may have direct implications for treatment of this disease. For example, at least for certain subgroups of patients, the risk for neurodevelopmental problems may more than offset the risks associated with chronic transfusions and thus may justify this approach as a prophylaxis. Similarly, recent studies showing the promising effects of hydroxyurea therapy in increasing fetal hemoglobin and decreasing vaso-occlusive events may lead to treatments that decrease neurodevelopmental morbidity (Jayabose et al., 1996). Finally, as we try to specify the degree and nature of the sequelae of SCD, we have yet to determine the efficacy of nonmedical interventions in promoting improved neuro-developmental outcomes.

Research into SCD is challenging in multiple respects (biological, psychosocial, and methodological). It serves as an exemplar of how medical and behavioral research must proceed hand in hand—each informing the other—in order to capture the full range of morbidity and its complex interactions, and to gauge treatment effects. There are few genetic diseases producing such devastating effects with such a high incidence, and therefore with such a high payoff for significant advances in treatment.

REFERENCES

Achebe, C. (1969). *Things fall apart.* New York: Fawcett Crest.

Adams, R. J., McKie, V., Nichols, F., Carl, E., Zhang, D. L., McKie, K., Figueroa, R., Litaker, M., Thompson, W., & Hess, D. (1992). The use of transcranial ultrasonography to predict stroke in sickle cell disease. *New England Journal of Medicine, 326*(9), 605–610.

Adams, R. J., Nichols, F., McKie, V., Milner, P., & Gammal, T. E. (1988). Cerebral infarction in sickle cell anemia: Mechanism based on CT and MRI. *Neurology, 38,* 1012–1017.

Allen, P. (1983). The psychoeducational effects of sickle cell anemia: An analysis of school success, nonsuccess in a group of children with sickle cell anemia. *Dissertation Abstracts International, 44,* 1727A. (University Microfilms No. 83-24872)

Armstrong, F. D., Thompson, R. J. J., Wang, W., Zimmerman, R., Pegelow, C. H., Miller, S., Moser, F., Bello, J., Hurtig, A., & Vass, K. (1996). Cognitive functioning and brain magnetic resonance imaging in children with sickle cell disease: Report of the Neuropsychology Committee of the Cooperative Study of Sickle Cell Disease. *Pediatrics, 97*(6, Pt. 1), 864–870.

Balkaran, B., Char, G., Morris, J. S., Thomas, P. W., Serjeant, B. E., & Serjeant, G. R. (1992). Stroke in a cohort of patients with homozygous sickle cell disease. *Journal of Pediatrics, 120*(3), 360–366.

Brass, L. M., Prohovnik, I., Pavlakis, S. G., DeVivo, D. C., Piomelli, S., & Mohr, J. P. (1991). Middle cerebral artery blood velocity and cerebral blood flow in sickle cell disease. *Stroke, 22,* 27–30.

Brown, R. T., Buchanan, I., Doepke, K., Eckman, J. R., Baldwin, K., Goonan, B., & Schoenherr, S. (1993). Cognitive and academic functioning in children with sickle-cell disease. *Journal of Clinical Child Psychology, 22*(2), 207–218.

Charache, S. (1994). Natural history of disease: Adults. In S. H. Embury, R. P. Hebbel, N. Mohandas, & M. H. Steinberg (Eds.), *Sickle cell disease: Basic principles and clinical practice.* New York: Raven Press.

Chodorkoff, J., & Whitten, C. F. (1963). Intellectual status of children with sickle cell anemia. *Journal of Pediatrics, 63,* 29–35.

Cohen, M. J., Branch, W. B., McKie, V. C., & Adams, R. J. (1994). Neuropsychological impairment in children with sickle cell anemia and cerebrovascular accidents. *Clinical Pediatrics, 33*(9), 517–524.

Craft, S., Schatz, J., Glauser, T. A., Lee, B., & DeBaun, M. R. (1993). Neuropsychologic effects of stroke in children with sickle cell anemia. *Journal of Pediatrics, 123*(5), 712–717.

Eaton, J. W. (1994). Malaria and selection of the sickle gene. In S. H. Embury, R. P. Hebbel, N. Mohandas, & M. H. Steinberg (Eds.), *Sickle cell disease: Basic principles and clinical practice.* New York: Raven Press.

Edelstein, S. J. (1986). *The sickled cell: From myths to molecules.* Cambridge, MA: Harvard University Press.

Fowler, M. G., Whitt, J. K., Lallinger, R. R., Nash, K. B., Atkinson, S. S., Wells, R. J., & McMillan, C. (1988). Neuropsychological and academic functioning of children with sickle cell anemia. *Journal of Developmental and Behavioral Pediatrics, 9,* 213–220.

Goonan, B. T., Goonan, L. J., Brown, R. T., Buchanan, I., & Eckman, J. R. (1994). Sustained attention and inhibitory control in children with sickle cell syndrome. *Archives of Clinical Neuropsychology, 9*(1), 89–104.

Grueneich, R., Ball, W. S., Ris, M. D., & Kalinyak, K. (1998). *MRI clinical coding system for sickle cell disease.* Manuscript submitted for publication.

Hariman, L. M. F., Griffith, E. R., Hurtig, A. L., & Keehn, M. T. (1991). Functional outcomes of children with sickle-cell disease affected by stroke. *Archives of Physical Medicine and Rehabilitation, 72,* 498–502.

Herold, S., Brozovic, M., Gibbs, J., Lammertsma, A. A., Leenders, K. L., Carr, D., Fleming, J. S., & Jones, T. (1986). Measurement of regional cerebral blood flow, blood volume and oxygen metabolism in patients with sickle cell disease using positron emission tomography. *Stroke, 17,* 692–698.

Herrick, J. B. (1910). Peculiar elongated and sickle-shaped red blood corpuscles in a case of severe anemia. *Archives of Internal Medicine, 6,* 517–521.

Hurtig, A. L., Koepke, D., & Park, K. B. (1989). Relation between severity of chronic illness and adjustment in children and adolescents with sickle cell disease. *Journal of Pediatric Psychology, 14,* 117–132.

Hurtig, A. L., & White, L. S. (1986). Psychosocial adjustment in children and adolescents with sickle cell disease. *Journal of Pediatric Psychology, 11,* 411–427.

Iloeje, S. O. (1991). Psychiatric morbidity among children with sickle-cell disease. *Developmental Medicine and Child Neurology, 33,* 1987–1994.

Ingram, V. M. (1956). A specific chemical difference between the globins of normal human and sickle-cell anemia hemoglobin. *Nature, 178,* 792–794.

Jayabose, S., Tugal, O., Sandoval, C., Patel, P., Puder, D., Lin, T., & Visintainer, P. (1996). Clinical and hematologic effects of hydroxyurea in children with sickle cell anemia. *Journal of Pediatrics, 129,* 559–565.

Kosacoff, M. I., Seligman, B. R., & Dosik, H. (1974). Psychological aspects of sickle cell anemia and its variants. In J. I. Hercules, A. N. Schechter, W. A. Eaton, & R. E. Jackson (Eds.), *Proceedings of the First National Symposium on Sickle Cell Disease.* Washington, DC: Department of Health, Education and Welfare.

Kugler, S., Anderson, B., Cross, D., Sharif, Z., Sano, M., Haggerty, R., Prohovnik, I., Hurlet-Jensen, A., Hilal, S., Mohr, J. P., & DeVivo, D. C. (1993). Abnormal cranial magnetic resonance imaging scans in sickle-cell disease: Neurological correlates and clinical implications. *Archives of Neurology, 50*(6), 629–635.

Lebby, R. (1846). Case of absence of the spleen. *Southern Journal of Medical Pharmacology, 1,* 481–483.

Livingston, F. B. (1971). Malaria and human polymorphisms. *Annual Review of Genetics, 5,* 33–64.

Mason, V. R. (1922). Sickle cell anemia. *Journal of the American Medical Association, 79,* 1318–1320.

Masten, A. S., Coatsworth, J. D., Neeman, J., Gest, S. D., Tellegen, A., & Garmezy, N. (1995). The structure and coherence of competence from childhood through adolescence. *Child Development, 66,* 1635–1659.

Nagel, R. L. (1994). Origins and dispersion of the sickle gene. In S. H. Embury, R. P. Hebbel, N. Mohandas, & M. H. Steinberg (Eds.), *Sickle cell disease: Basic principles and clinical practice.* New York: Raven Press.

Noll, R. B., Vannatta, K., Koontz, K., & Kalinyak, K. (1996). Peer relationships and emotional well-being of youngsters with sickle cell disease. *Child Development, 67,* 423–436.

Ohene-Frempong, K. (1991). Stroke in sickle cell disease: Demographic, clinical, and therapeutic considerations. *Seminars in Hematology, 28*(3), 213–219.

Pauling, L., Itano, H., Singer, S. J., & Wells, I. C. (1949). Sickle cell anemia: A molecular disease. *Science, 110,* 543–548.

Pavlakis, S. G., Bello, J., Prohovnik, I., Sutton, M., Ince, C., Mohr, J. P., Piomelli, S., Hilal, S., & DeVivo, D. C. (1988). Brain infarction in sickle cell anemia: Magnetic resonance imaging correlates. *Annals of Neurology, 23,* 125–130.

Platt, O. (1994). Membrane proteins. In S. H. Embury, R. P. Hebbel, N. Mohandas, & M. H. Steinberg (Eds.), *Sickle cell disease: Basic principles and clinical practice.* New York: Raven Press.

Powars, D. (1994). Natural history of the disease: The first two decades. In S. H. Embury, R. P. Hebbel, N. Mohandas, & M. H. Steinberg (Eds.), *Sickle cell disease: Basic principles and clinical practice.* New York: Raven Press.

Powars, D., Wilson, B., Imbus, C., Pegelow, C. H., & Allen, J. L. (1978). The natural history of stroke in sickle cell disease. *American Journal of Medicine, 65,* 461–470.

Prohovnik, I., Pavlakis, S. G., Piomelli, S., Bello, J., Mohr, J. P., Hilal, S., & DeVivo, D. C. (1989). Cerebral hyperemia, stroke, and transfusion in sickle cell disease. *Neurology, 39,* 344–348.

Ris, M. D., Grueneich, R., & Kalinyak, K. (1995). Neuropsychological risk in children with sickle cell disease [Abstract]. *Journal of the International Neuropsychological Society, 1,* 360.

Ris, M. D., Kalinyak, K. A., Ball, W. S., Noll, R. B., Wells, R. J., & Rucknagel, D. (1996). Pre- and poststroke MRI and neuropsychological studies in sickle cell disease: A case study. *Archives of Clinical Neuropsychology, 11*(6), 481–490.

Rothman, S. M., Fulling, K. H., & Nelson, J. S. (1986). Sickle cell anemia and central nervous system infarction: A neuropathological study. *Annals of Neurology, 20,* 684–690.

Rourke, B. P. (1987). Syndrome of nonverbal learning disabilities: The final common pathway of white-matter disease/dysfunction? *The Clinical Neuropsychologist, 1*, 209–234.

Scott-Conner, C. E., & Brunson, C. D. (1994). The pathophysiology of the sickle hemoglobinopathies and implications for perioperative management [Review]. *American Journal of Surgery, 168*(3), 268–274.

Stith, L. E., Garstein, M. A., Ris, M. D., Grueneich, R., Vannatta, K., Kalinyak, K., & Noll, R. B (in press). Neuropsychological functioning of youth with sickle cell disease. *Journal of Pediatric Psychology.*

Stockman, J. A., Nigro, M. A., Mishkin, M. M., & Oski, F. A. (1972). Occlusion of large cerebral vessels in sickle-cell anemia. *New England Journal of Medicine, 287*, 846–850.

Swift, A. V., Cohen, M. J., Hynd, G. W., Wisenbaker, J. M., McKie, K. M., Makari, G., & McKie, V. C. (1989). Neuropsychological impairment in children with sickle cell anemia. *Pediatrics, 84*, 1077–1085.

Tzika, A. A., Massoth, R. J., Ball, W. S., Majumdar, S., Dunn, R. S., & Kirks, D. R. (1993). Cerebral perfusion in children: Detection with dynamic contrast-enhanced T2*-weighted MR images. *Radiology, 187*, 449–458.

Venketasubramanian, N., Prohovnik, I., Hurlet, A., Mohr, J. P., & Piomelli, S. (1994). Middle cerebral artery velocity changes during transfusion in sickle cell anemia. *Stroke, 25*, 2153–2158.

Wang, W., Grover, R., Gallagher, D., Espeland, M., & Fandal, A. (1993). Developmental screening in young children with sickle cell disease: Results of a cooperative study. *American Journal of Pediatric Hematology/Oncology, 15*, 87–91.

Wasserman, A. L., Wilimas, J. A., Fairclough, D. L., Mulhern, R. K., & Wang, W. (1991). Subtle neuropsychological deficits in children with sickle cell disease. *American Journal of Pediatric Hematology/Oncology, 13*(1), 14–20.

Watkins, K. E., Hewes, D. K. M., Connelly, A., Kendall, B. E., Kingsley, D. P. E., Evans, J. E. P., Gadian, D. G., Vatzgha-Khadem, F., & Kirkham, F. J. (1998). Cognitive deficits associated with frontal-lobe infarction in children with sickle cell disease. *Developmental Medicine and Child Neurology, 40*, 536–543.

Wilimas, J. A., Goff, J. R, Anderson, H. R., Lengston, J. W., & Thompson, E. (1980). Efficacy of transfusion therapy for one to two years in patients with sickle cell disease and cerebrovascular accidents. *Journal of Pediatrics, 96*, 205–208.

Yam, L. T., & Li, C. Y. (1994). The spleen. In S. H. Embury, R. P. Hebbel, N. Mohandas, & M. H. Steinberg (Eds.), *Sickle cell disease: Basic principles and clinical practice.* New York: Raven Press.

15

DIABETES

JOANNE F. ROVET

Insulin-dependent diabetes mellitus (IDDM) is an autoimmune disease with serious and lifelong implications, including effects on brain and behavior. IDDM follows destruction of pancreatic beta cells, where insulin, an essential hormone for glucose metabolism, is produced. Because IDDM has a slow and insidious course, it is typically not recognized and diagnosed until beta cell function has been nearly totally destroyed and levels of endogenous insulin completely depleted. The diagnosis is usually based on symptoms of polydypsia (thirst), polyuria (frequent urination), and fatigue, although some children may be much sicker when they are diagnosed. Treatment requires daily injections of insulin, which are adjusted according to food intake and level of activity. With the exception of needing to follow a tedious and relentless treatment regimen for life, affected children are generally healthy and develop normally once their diabetes is stabilized. However, because their levels of exogenous insulin do not perfectly mimic normal physiological production, children with diabetes are continuously exposed to blood glucose perturbations outside the normal range.

Because glucose is an essential fuel for brain metabolism, any excursions in blood glucose concentrations can disrupt central nervous system (CNS) function transiently (Hume, McGeechan, & Burchell, 1999) and permanently (Amiel, 1996; Lucas, Morley, & Cole, 1988). Recent studies show that in diabetes, brain dysfunction arises from abnormal levels of either glucose or insulin, both of which vary considerably in pediatric patients. Extremely high or extremely low glucose levels can lead to convulsions or ischemia. Frequent hyperglycemia may be associated with delayed myelination, while frequent hypoglycemia affects cerebral blood flow and neurotransmission.

In diabetes, not only are children exposed to a number of adverse events associated with this disease, some events, such as convulsions from severe hypoglycemia, may be more prevalent in children (particularly very young children) than in adults. In addition, because children are still undergoing major brain development at the time of diagnosis and over the course of childhood, they may be more vulnerable than adults to diabetes-associated brain damage. The type of damage will depend on the nature of the event and its timing.

For the past 15 years, my research program has focused on identifying critical disease factors in pediatric diabetes and their specific neurobehavioral manifestations. Our goal has been to plot the trajectory of diabetes-related events on the developing CNS. In this chapter, I describe some of this work. I begin with an overview of the disease, its treatment, and complications; a description of associated psychosocial issues; and a review of some of the major diabetes-related effects on the brain. This is followed by a description of the neurological and neurobehavioral aspects of diabetes from a lifespan perspective (including pregnancy) and the findings from five studies conducted in my lab on children and adolescents with diabetes. These studies concern (1) the role of age of onset of diabetes on specific cognitive dysfunctions; (2) changes in cognitive abilities from diagnosis of diabetes through the first 3 years; (3) puberty as a potential trigger for selective neuropsychological complications; (4) long-term effects of diabetes on cognitive functions; and (5) effects of diabetes on attentional processing. I conclude by integrating these findings in light of what is known about diabetes and insulin on the brain, and by pointing to avenues for future research. Throughout the chapter, a major theme is the unique effects of different diabetes-related events and their timing on specific brain–behavior relations.

INSULIN-DEPENDENT DIABETES MELLITUS: AN OVERVIEW

IDDM is one of the most common chronic diseases of childhood. In North America, IDDM affects about 1 in every 600 children under the age of 12. The incidence, which varies considerably by geographic region, is much higher in countries in northern Europe—especially Finland, where as many as 1 in 250 children may have diabetes (Reunanen, Äkerblom, & Käär, 1982). There is the added concern that the incidence of IDDM may be increasing world-wide, (especially in children under the age of 5 years) (Gardner, Bingley, Sawtell, Weeks, & Gale, 1997).

Diabetes occurs when the body lacks insulin, which is a hormone needed to metabolize glucose. Without insulin, glucose accumulates in the urine and bloodstream (hyperglycemia), while the body draws on other energy sources until it literally starves. Exceedingly high levels of blood sugar lead to unconsciousness, coma, and ultimately death. However, prompt and continuous treatment with insulin allows affected children to lead long and productive lives.

Insulin therapy involves two or three daily injections of exogenous insulin and a strict diet to control for insulin needs. The dosage of insulin is monitored according to concurrent levels of blood glucose (assessed with a glucose meter several or more times daily) and is regulated in accordance with daily food intake, activity, and factors such as stress or illness. However, in spite of this close control, this regimen poorly mimics normal physiology; an affected child often experiences episodes when blood sugars are mild to moderately elevated (hyperglycemia) or reduced (hypoglycemia). Severe hyperglycemia can lead to diabetic ketoacidosis, a condition that contributes to permanent neurological dysfunction (Tsalikian, Daneman, Becker, Crumrine, & Drash, 1980) and can be fatal. Severe hypoglycemia, which leads to unconsciousness and seizures, can also be associated with permanent brain damage.

Because the effects of blood glucose elevations are cumulative, chronic hyperglycemia is associated with a variety of physical complications (e.g., nephropathy, retinopathy, neuropathy, and vascular disease). Although these complications are rarely seen in children, they appear to have their beginnings during puberty, which is thought to serve as a trigger (Kostraba et al., 1989). In order to prevent these complications, it is of paramount importance for patients with diabetes to maintain their blood glucose levels constantly in the normal range; this assumes continuous, tight glycemic control. However, the cost associated with tight control is an increased risk of hypoglycemia. In addition, because very small children are less able to communicate sensations of physiological change in blood glucose levels and it is more difficult to make dosage adjustments for them, children below the age of 5 are at very high risk of hypoglycemia and associated seizures.

PSYCHOSOCIAL MANIFESTATIONS OF DIABETES

Diabetes places a tremendous burden on the child and the family because of the daily insulin injections and blood glucose monitoring, and because of the need to adhere continuously to a restricted diet and to adjust insulin levels to activity, food, stress, and so forth. Behavioral and psychosocial problems are thus very common in children with IDDM and their families, and these have been attributed to the difficulties in living with this disease (Johnson, 1980). Among children with diabetes, there are both age- and gender-specific problems, and some groups appear to be more susceptible than others at certain ages. For example, in one of our earliest studies (Rovet, Ehrlich, & Hoppe, 1988a), boys who acquired their diabetes during middle childhood (i.e., past age 5) were observed to be at increased risk of behavior problems, whereas boys who developed diabetes prior to age 5 were relatively unaffected. This reflected the elevated anxiety levels and body image distortions of the boys with later-developing diabetes, and was attributed to an incompatibility between their diabetes (which fostered dependent behavior for effective metabolic control) and normal male psychological development during latency (which assumes increasing independence and a strong physical sense of self). Presumably, the boys who developed diabetes earlier had come to see diabetes as a normal part of life, with no imminent threat to their growing independence during latency. Although our study did not show an increased incidence of behavior problems in girls who developed diabetes before or after age 5, studies of female adolescents have revealed that they are quite vulnerable (Anderson, Miller, Auslander, & Santiago, 1981; Johnson, 1980; La Greca, Swales, Klemp, Madigan, & Skyler, 1995), including being at greater risk of anorexia nervosa (Rydall, Rodin, Olmsted, Devenyit, & Daneman, 1997).

There is considerable individual variation in adaptation to diabetes, adherence to dietary and exercise requirements, and psychosocial adjustment (Rovet & Fernandes, 1999). Indeed, a child's temperament (as measured by temperament questionnaires) may play a critical role in the levels of blood glucose that are achieved. We previously reported that children who achieved better glycemic control were those with a constellation of temperament characteristics reflecting high activity levels, regularity in daily routines, mild reactivity to external stimulation, increased distractibility, and a negative disposition (Rovet & Ehrlich, 1988). Consequently, we proposed that individual differences in behavioral organization, energy consumption, and stress modulation affected normal levels of blood glucose levels and interacted with treatment requirements.

DIABETES AND THE BRAIN

In the last 20 years, several studies have served to demonstrate both transient and permanent effects of diabetes on the brain. This research has indicated adverse sequelae associated with either an excess or a lack of glucose. Structural damage of neurons has been attributed to glucose toxicity, whereas functional changes have been related to altered vascularity and neurotransmission.

There are also adverse sequelae associated with too little or too much insulin. Studies identifying insulin receptors in brain regions critical for cognitive functioning, such as the cortex, hippocampus, and cerebellum (Baskin, Figlewicz, Woods, Porte, & Dorsa, 1987; Havrankova, Roth, & Brownstone, 1983; Kappy, Sellinger, & Raizada, 1984), suggest a mode for insulin involvement in both brain and cognitive functions. However, although considerable attention has been directed to the role of insulin receptors in the hypothalamus and their relationship to eating (Schwartz, Figlewicz, Woods, Porte, & Baskin, 1993), very little is known about their role in the other structures that mediate cognitive function.

In addition, there appear to be different consequences of diabetes if abnormal glucose levels are acute and severe as opposed to chronic and mild (Holmes, 1990), and different mechanisms are proposed for these different clinical circumstances (McCall & Figlewicz, 1997). This section reviews the findings based on both animal- and patient-based studies on the effects of hyperglycemia and hypoglycemia on brain and behavior.

Effects of Hyperglycemia

Hyperglycemia can cause brain dysfunction via multiple routes. These include (1) abnormalities in fuel metabolism, (2) changes in cerebral blood flow, (3) abnormal vascularity, and (4) altered nutrient transport. Glucose toxicity associated with severe hyperglycemia can damage neurons and vasculature directly (McCall & Figlewicz, 1997), but there are also indirect effects of hyperglycemia associated with altered cell signaling and neurotransmission. In addition, permanent brain damage can arise from diabetes ketoacidosis, a severe and debilitating condition associated with prolonged and excessively high blood glucose levels (Tsalikian et al., 1980). Finally, because the effects of frequent mild hyperglycemia episodes are cumulative, brain functioning is also impaired if glucose levels are frequently elevated to a moderate degree.

Excess levels of blood glucose can also affect the developing brain by altering the synthesis of structural compounds (including myelin), as well as affecting fuel production. Although some have argued that a young child's brain is protected to a greater degree than an adult's because of its greater flexibility in using nonglucose fuels (such as lactate) for energy production (Amiel, 1996; McCall & Figlewicz, 1997), adverse effects of hyperglycemia on developing structures are known to occur.

Electrophysiological Studies

Electroencephalographic (EEG) alterations have long been observed in children and adults with diabetes (Eeg-Olofsson & Petersen, 1966), suggestive of diabetic encephalopathy in brain stem and midbrain regions (Donald et al., 1981). A recent study using event-related potentials in adolescents showed that despite the lack of difference between diabetic subjects and controls on psychometric tasks, adolescents with diabetes characteristically had significantly longer P300 latencies (Uberall, Renner, Edl, Parzinger, & Wenzel, 1996), which suggested diabetes-related changes in brain functioning.

Neuropathological Studies

Structural changes have been observed in the CNS of diabetic patients (Mooradian, 1988). Although various pathologies have been described, these are usually subtle unless a vascular accident or an acute alteration in plasma glucose has occurred. The primary manifestations include cerebral infarction, hemorrhage, degeneration of ganglion cells, demyelination, and loss of axons (DeJong, 1977).

In animals with induced diabetes, cerebral cortex weight is reduced; there is a significant loss of neocortical neurons; and the density of cortical capillaries is diminished (Jakobsen, Sidenius, Gundersen, & Osterby, 1987). These changes are associated with poorer performance on memory tasks (Flood, Mooradian, & Morley, 1990). Diabetes also produces biochemical changes in the CNS, including altered serotonin levels and decreased norepinephrine and dopamine content, particularly in the hippocampus (Merali & Ahmad, 1986).

Effects of Hypoglycemia

Hypoglycemia is an iatrogenic consequence of insulin therapy and is more common in patients with better-controlled than poorly controlled diabetes. Hypoglycemia is associated with biochemical changes in brain function, including altered neurotransmission, energy failure, and membrane depolarization (McCall, 1992). Hypoglycemic episodes can cause seizures and lead to permanent brain damage resulting from neuronal shrinkage and swelling (Auer & Siesjo, 1990; Brierley, Brown, & Meldrum, 1971) and from necrosis (Mooradian, 1988). The cortex, caudate, and hippocampus are especially vulnerable to the effects of hypoglycemia (McCall, 1992), whereas the cerebellum is relatively spared. Chronic hypoglycemia also alters the blood–brain barrier transport of glucose and microvascular metabolism (McCall, 1992). Like glucose, insulin alters CNS signaling through its direct action on brain neurotransmitters, and mild hypoglycemia has been associated with the altered synthesis, release, and synapse reuptake of norepinephrine, dopamine, and serotonin.

One of the major complications of hypoglycemia is a condition known as *hypoglycemia unawareness*, which is a type of brain-signaling dysfunction. As a result of frequent hypoglycemia, some patients experience a complete absence of the physiological warning symptoms of a forthcoming hypoglycemic episode; consequently, they do not take corrective measures to counteract its effects. These individuals are therefore at even greater risk of developing very severe hypoglycemia and associated brain damage.

Electrophysiological and neuroimaging studies using event-related potentials have shown that in normal individuals without diabetes, altered P300 latencies were associated with insulin-induced hypoglycemia (Blackman, Towle, Lewis, Spire, & Polonsky, 1989; Pozzessere, et al., 1991) and altered cerebral blood flow (Tallroth, Ryding, & Agardh, 1992). In children with diabetes, EEG abnormalities have been observed in as many as 25% of cases between 1 and 21 years of age (Haumont, Dorch, & Pelc, 1979). Of these, 60% had poor metabolic control, and 80% had a history of more than five episodes of severe hypoglycemia. Similar rates were reported by Soltéz and Acsadi (1989), who observed EEG abnormalities in 26% of their diabetic sample (most of whom were diagnosed prior to age 5) versus 7% of controls.

In adult patients, a history of prior hypoglycemia has its most pronounced effects on brain function during a hypoglycemic episode. In a study by Amiel (1996), the EEGs of diabetic patients with and without previous hypoglycemia were compared during the use of a glucose clamp technique. Although the groups did not differ in the euglycemic state, individuals with a prior history of hypoglycemia showed more atypical EEG parameters and a greater degree of cortical slowing when their blood glucose levels first entered the hypoglycemic range. Similar findings have been reported by Tribl et al. (1996), who found a stronger effect during slight hypoglycemia in patients with hypoglycemia unawareness.

In patients with diabetes subjected to studies of regional cerebral blood flow via single-photon emission computed tomography, repeated episodes of severe hypoglycemia were associated with greater tracer uptake in the prefrontal cortex and reduced uptake in the calcarine cortex (Macleod et al., 1994; Tallroth et al., 1992). MRI findings showed a patient who developed severe amnesia after hypoglycemic coma had a marked lesion in the left temporal lobe (Chalmers, Risk, Kean, Grant, Ashworth, & Campbell, 1991).

Effects of Altered Insulin Levels

Insulin has been implicated as a crucial regulator in neurotransmitter pathways. Several different insulin receptors have been identified (Sesti et al., 1991), and these have been localized in the synapses of such brain regions as the cortex, the hippocampus, the cerebellum, and the arcuate nucleus of the hypothalamus (Baskin et al., 1987; Havrankova et al., 1983; Kappy et al., 1984). Although the implications of these findings for insulin-regulated hypothalamic control of feeding are well studied (Schwartz et al., 1993), little if anything is known about the role of insulin in mediating cognitive functioning.

Amine reuptake transporters may be specific targets for insulin action in the CNS (Figlewicz, Szot, Chavez, Woods, & Veith, 1994). Studies using rats showed that when insulin was directly infused into the brain, norepinephrine content was decreased and dopamine increased, whereas experimentally induced hypoinsulinism was associated with increased norepinephrine and decreased dopamine (McCall & Figlewicz, 1997). Using the hypoglycemic clamp technique, which involves experimentally manipulating blood glucose levels via intravenous catheterization, several studies of humans have also shown that insulin directly influences catecholamine levels (Amiel, Simonson, Sherwin, Lauritano, & Tamborlane, 1987; Borg, Borg, & Tamborlane, 1997) and regulates tyrosine hydroxylase activity (Kono & Takada, 1994).

Recent advances in insulin therapy allow for a closer approximation to the normal state and may lead to fewer neuropsychological sequelae (Sesti et al., 1992). These advances include pumps that continuously infuse insulin into the bloodstream, intensive management involving multiple daily injections, and newly manufactured insulins that allow a slower rate of release and action.

NEUROPSYCHOLOGICAL SEQUELAE OF DIABETES

Child Studies

Previous Studies

The earliest studies of children with diabetes demonstrated few associated neuropsychological impairments. In fact, some of the first investigations reported above-average intelligence levels in pediatric patients (Brown & Thompson, 1940; Kubany, Danowski, & Moses, 1956). However, more recent research has indicated cognitive and psychoeducational disabilities in selective subgroups of pediatric diabetes patients (Northam, 1996; Rovet, Ehrlich, Czuchta, & Akler, 1993; Sansbury, Brown, & Meacham, 1997). Particularly affected are children who developed their diabetes prior to age 5 (Ack, Miller, & Weil, 1961; Bjorgaas, Gimse, Vik, & Sand, 1997; Hagen et al., 1990; Holmes & Richman, 1985;

Rovet, Ehrlich, & Hoppe, 1988b), who have experienced frequent or severe hypoglyce-mia (Golden et al., 1989; Rovet, Ehrlich, & Hoppe, 1987), or who have diabetes of long-standing duration (Holmes & Richman, 1985; see also Puczynski, 1997, for a review).

In children, diabetes has selective versus global effects on neurocognitive abilities, with visual–motor, memory, and attentional skills being especially vulnerable (Hagen et al., 1990; Wolters, Yu, Hagen, & Kail, 1996; Northam, 1996; Rovet et al., 1988b; Ryan & Wil-liams, 1993). The specfic types of deficits also reflect the nature of the associated diabetes-related events. For example, poorer visual abstract reasoning abilities have been associated with more frequent episodes of mild hypoglycemia (Golden et al., 1989), whereas poorer attention shifting has been associated with chronic hyperglycemia (Ryan, Longstreet, & Morrow, 1985).

Holmes, Cornwell, Dunlap, Chen, and Lee (1992) reported an anomalous Wechsler Intelligence Scale for Children—Revised (WISC-R) factor structure for children with IDDM. Whereas a three-factor solution typically characterizes children's WISC-R per-formance (i.e., Verbal Comprehension, Perceptual Organization, and Freedom from Distractibility), children with diabetes demonstrated two visual-perceptual ability fac-tors (i.e., four factors in all). In these children, visual discrimination abilities were dis-tinct from spatial/conceptual abilities, whereas they were combined in children without diabetes. This dichotomization of visual-perceptual abilities in the diabetes group was attributed to their reduced visual discrimination abilities as a result of retinal nerve damage or retinopathy, and was assumed to have a greater impact on tasks with high visual dis-crimination and minimal motor demands than on those with greater motor and minimal scanning and discrimination demands.

With regard to school performance, poorer reading and arithmetic achievement were observed in children with early-onset diabetes (Rovet et al., 1988b; Ryan, Vega, & Drash, 1985), who were also more likely to have learning disabilities (Gath, Smith, & Baum, 1980; Rovet et al., 1993) and a greater need for remedial services (Anderson et al., 1984; Rovet et al., 1988b). School learning problems were associated with a history of hypoglycemic convulsions, at least 5 years' duration of illness, and frequent school absenteeism stem-ming from clinic appointments and hospitalizations (Rovet et al., 1993; Ryan, Longstreet, & Morrow, 1985).

The effects of hypoglycemia on cognitive functioning have been directly studied by several groups. To evaluate hypoglycemia in a controlled naturalistic environment, Reich et al. (1990) studied children who reported to the diabetes camp infirmary whenever they experienced a mild or a more severe hypoglycemic episode. Each child, on each occasion, was assessed at the time of the episode as well as several hours later and was given a vari-ety of neuropsychological tasks. During hypoglycemia, transient changes were observed in motor performance, attention, and memory, and these decrements did not resolve once blood glucose levels had returned to normal.

In a more controlled study, Ryan, Atchison, et al. (1990) examined children's neuro-cognitive abilities following induction of a hypoglycemic episode via the insulin glucose clamp technique. When blood glucose levels were in the mildly hypoglycemic range, men-tal efficiency was significantly lower on tests of flexibility, planning, decision making, at-tention to detail, and rapid responding. Complete recovery of cognitive functioning was not contemporaneous with restoration of euglycemia, particularly for tests of rapid respond-ing and attention.

Hershey, Craft, Bhargava, and White (1997) directly compared children with IDDM who had or did not have severe hypoglycemic episodes. The results showed that the pa-tients who had had severe hypoglycemia had selective verbal memory deficits.

Age-at-Onset Study

Our first study of children with diabetes examined whether early age at diabetes onset was associated with specific neurocognitive impairment. This study followed directly from the observations of Ryan, Vega, and Drash (1985) that adolescents with diabetes had poorer outcomes only if they developed their disease prior to age 5. As their study was correlational and investigated subjects long after they developed their disease, we proposed directly comparing early- and late-onset child groups.

The design of our study entailed a direct comparison of 6- to 13-year-old children, of whom 27 had developed diabetes prior to age 4, 24 had developed diabetes past age 5, and 30 were sibling controls. The age range was 6.1 to 13.9 years, and subjects received a comprehensive battery of psychometric tests that included multiple WISC-R subtests, two Science Research Associates Primary Mental Abilities Test subtests (Verbal Meaning and Spatial Relations), the Beery Developmental Test of Visual–motor Integration, and the Wide Range Achievement Test. Parents were additionally assessed for intelligence and socioeconomic status (SES), and they received a detailed semistructured interview on their child's diabetic history. The children's medical charts were also reviewed for hemoglobin A_1 levels and further medical data.

Following factor analysis, test results were summarized in terms of spatial and verbal composite scores. Only children with early-onset diabetes had poorer scores than siblings, performing worse on the spatial but not on the verbal, composite (Figure 15.1). This was observed mainly for girls with early diabetes onset, whereas boys with early diabetes onset performed poorly only if they had had a hypoglycemic convulsion at a young age (data not shown, Rovet et al., 1987). There were no adverse effects of ketoacidosis or duration of illness on any performance indices of neurocognitive abilities, and, unexpectedly, better current glycemic control was associated with lower Performance IQ levels. The latter was attributed to an increased risk of hypoglycemia, as a consequence of overall better control.

The findings from this study suggested that among children with diabetes, those who developed diabetes at an early age were at increased risk of subsequent neurocognitive impairment. The results also indicated that there were independent effects of age of onset and hypoglycemic convulsions, which affected males and females differently.

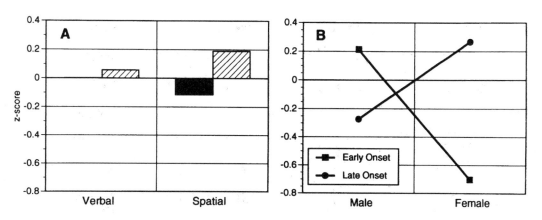

FIGURE 15.1. Verbal and spatial composite scores for diabetes versus control subjects (panel A), and spatial composite scores for male and female subjects with early- and late-onset diabetes (panel B). The data are from Rovet, Ehrlich, and Hoppe (1987).

Prospective Study of Newly Diagnosed Diabetes

Because the study described above was cross-sectional and retrospective in design, we did not know whether the deficits in children with early-onset diabetes preceded their disease or were acquired as a result of it. Also, since information on diabetic control was collected retrospectively and depended on parent recall, it was not possible to evaluate precisely the exact contributions of the different diabetes-related factors.

We next conducted a prospective study of 63 consecutive newly diagnosed pediatric patients with diabetes, who were followed through the first 3 years of illness. Children were initially assessed within 3 months of diagnosis (most within the first month) and subsequently at 1 and 3 years. Controls consisted of 40 nondiabetic siblings under the age of 12 years, and each control was seen twice only (at the initial visit of the diabetic sibling and 3 years later). All subjects received a comprehensive battery of age-appropriate psychometric tasks, which included a test of intelligence and achievement (when appropriate) and multiple tests of language, spatial ability, and memory. For children with diabetes, information was regularly collected from their diabetes diaries at each trimonthly clinic visit. These diaries contained daily information on blood glucose levels and on specific diabetes-related events. The diary data were subsequently transcribed and recoded to provide indices of (1) monthly asymptomatic low blood sugar episodes; (2) monthly low blood sugar episodes with symptoms of dizziness, sweating, or shaking; (3) episodes of severe hypoglycemia (convulsions, fainting, coma) and ketoacidosis; and (4) monthly episodes of high blood sugars with ketones in urine (ketonuria). Trimonthly glycosylated hemoglobin levels, and information on hospitalizations and diabetes-specific adverse events, were also obtained from the medical record.

For the data analyses, composite scores were determined for each major ability area, which served as the primary dependent variables. Table 15.1 shows that the diabetes group did not differ from controls at diagnosis and that there were no specific impairments pre-

TABLE 15.1. Mean Scores for Groups in the Prospective Study

	Diagnosis		1 year	3 years	
	Diabetes	Control	Diabetes[a]	Diabetes	Control
Full Scale IQ	115.6	111.4	115.7	113.8	106.5***
Verbal IQ	113.2	109.1	113.1	108.0	101.1***
Performance IQ	115.1	109.1	116.2	118.2	111.3*
Beery VMI (%ile)	64.1	63.3	61.0	57.5	69.3†
WRAT					
Reading	48.8	39.7	53.3	57.4	48.5
Arithmetic	36.6	40.7	43.0	44.9	38.8
Composite scores					
Verbal	−.020	−.075	—	.174	−.253**
Spatial	.061	−.120	—	.080	−.187
Memory	−.148	.138	—	.090	−.159
Attention	.057	.006	—	.182	−.209**

Note. The diagnosis and 1-year data are from Rovet, Ehrlich, and Czuchta (1990); the 3-year data are from Rovet, Ehrlich, Czuchta, and Akler (1993). VMI, Beery Developmental Test of Visual–Motor Integration; WRAT, Wide Range Achievement Test.

[a]Only diabetes subjects were tested at this session.

†$p = .07$. *$p < .05$. **$p = .01$. ***$p < .001$.

dating diagnosis. After 1 year of illness, there was no evidence of any acquired impairments in the group of children with diabetes as a whole (Rovet, Ehrlich, & Czuchta, 1990). However, children with onset before 5 years of age scored below those with later-onset diabetes in spatial ability, whereas children with later-onset diabetes scored lower in verbal ability (data not shown, Rovet et al., 1990). After 3 years of illness, the diabetes group scored *higher* than sibling controls in IQ measures and in the verbal and attention domains; however, they did show a trend toward poorer visual–motor abilities than controls. As the groups did not differ in their school achievement, the first 3 years of diabetes did not appear to be associated with any increased risk of learning disabilities (Rovet et al., 1993).

Within the diabetes group, children with early-onset diabetes scored significantly higher than those with later-onset illness in the verbal domain, and to a lesser degree in the memory and attention domains. In contrast, children with later-onset diabetes scored higher than those with early-onset illness in the spatial domain. These findings suggest specific effects depending on age at onset, with the development of visual–spatial abilities being more sensitive to diabetes beginning in the very early years, and the development of language, memory, and attention to diabetes beginning later in childhood.

The results of this study were also examined in terms of change over time. Change scores were defined in terms of residualized change from baseline to 3-year performance. Overall, relatively little change was observed for either the diabetes group or the control group. In the verbal area, the diabetes group demonstrated more change than controls, which reflected improved performance (Figure 15.2). Of the children with diabetes, 5% declined significantly, 20% displayed mild declines, and 25% improved. However, rather than attributing the improved performance of these children to real improvements due to diabetes, we attributed it to their suboptimal performance at diagnosis because the children were ill and were adjusting emotionally to the disease and its demands. Premorbid values were obviously not available.

Correlations were computed between major biomedical variables and primary factor scores. The results revealed a positive association between verbal ability and better glycemic control. Also, better verbal ability, and to a lesser degree better memory and attention

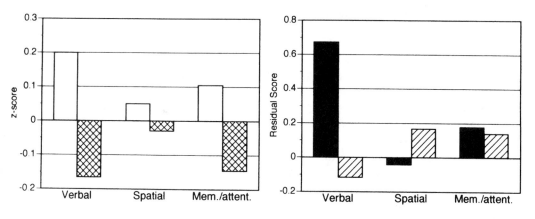

FIGURE 15.2. Composite scores after 3 years of diabetes in children with early (white bars) and late (hatched bars) disease onset (left panel); 3-year change scores in children with diabetes from time of disease onset (black bars) and sibling controls (striped bars) (right panel). The data are from Rovet, Ehrlich, Czuchta, and Akler (1993).

skills, were associated with a greater (not lower) incidence of asymptomatic low blood sugar levels. This anomalous finding was interpreted as a by-product of better diabetic control contributing to more low readings, rather than as a positive effect of below-normal blood sugars. In the spatial domain, poorer performance was not associated with any diabetes-related parameters. With respect to school achievement, poorer arithmetic and (to a lesser degree) poorer reading were associated with a greater number of mild hypoglycemic episodes that needed intervention, such as juice.

Among the participants with diabetes, only 3 of 63 experienced one or more hypoglycemic convulsions during the first 3 years of illness, and only 1 child experienced ketoacidosis. However, these 4 children did not show any declines in ability over the first 3 years that could be attributed to these adverse events.

The results of this prospective study therefore suggest that children with diabetes neither had deficits predating their illness nor developed neurocognitive impairment within the first 3 years of illness. In some children, poorer performance was associated with certain diabetes-related factors, with poorer verbal, attention, memory, and arithmetic abilities being associated with less adequate glycemic control and more frequent hyperglycemia. Asymptomatic low blood sugars and mild to moderate hypoglycemia reactions did not adversely affect neurocognitive abilities, whereas poorer arithmetic was associated with frequent episodes of mild to moderate hypoglycemia. The improved performance in certain domains associated with frequent episodes of hypoglycemia has been replicated by Northam, Anderson, Werther, Adler, and Andrewes (1995), and is considered to be a marker of more assiduous metabolic control rather than a benefit of having hypoglycemia. There were too few children in our study who had convulsions or ketoacidosis over the first 3 years of illness to study their effects properly.

Adolescent Studies

Previous Studies

Ryan, Vega, Longstreet, and Drash (1984) conducted the first comprehensive investigation of the neuropsychological characteristics of adolescents with diabetes. Compared to their siblings who served as controls, subjects with diabetes as a group indicated problems on tests of visual–motor coordination and short-term memory. Poorer verbal and conceptual abilities were also seen in older teenagers with diabetes, whereas younger patients were unaffected.

Subsequently, Ryan, Vega, and Drash (1985) reported that adolescents who developed diabetes prior to age 5 did more poorly than those who developed diabetes later on tests of executive functioning, fine motor skills, visual–spatial abilities, memory, and motor speed, with 24% of the early-onset group meeting criteria for neurological impairment (compared with 6% for the later-onset group and for controls). The deficits of the early-onset group were attributed to organic disturbance from multiple episodes of hypoglycemia (Ryan, Vega, & Drash, 1985), which were known to be more frequent and difficult to control in very small children (Eeg-Olofsson & Petersen, 1966; Ternand, Go, Gerich, & Haymond, 1982). However, as Ryan and colleagues did not obtain information on hypoglycemia directly, they were not able to test this hypothesis.

More recently, Northam, Bowden, Anderson, and Court (1992) studied the relationship between neuropsychological performance and retrospectively collected disease-related information in a group of 85 young adolescents (14 to 16.5 years of age). Unfortunately, as there were no control subjects in this study, it was not possible to identify areas of specific impairment. Nevertheless, female subjects performed below age expectations on tests of verbal ability, whereas their performance on tests of nonverbal ability was at or above age standards. There were no significant relationships between neuropsychological functioning and disease-related factors such as age at onset, chronic poor control, or major metabolic crises.

One explanation for the different findings reported by these two research groups is that Ryan and colleagues studied both younger and older adolescents, whereas Northam and colleagues studied only younger ones. If neuropsychological sequelae of diabetes become manifest *during* adolescence, these sequelae may be more pronounced in the older age group only, as observed by Ryan et al. (1984). Another explanation concerns secular improvements in diabetes management that transpired in the decade between the two studies; these include blood glucose self-monitoring with glucometers (Skyler, 1989), improved insulins, and overall better management practices. Thus the better performance of subjects in more recent studies may reflect fewer adverse events and hence fewer neuropsychological sequelae as a result of better diabetes control.

The Diabetes and Puberty Study

In an effort to reconcile the different findings of the studies described above, we sought to examine whether something unique happens during puberty that contributes to the increased number of neurocognitive deficits in late adolescence and in adulthood (see below). Several studies have demonstrated that puberty is an independent risk factor for the physical complications of diabetes (Lingren, Dahlquist, Efendic, Persson, & Skottner, 1990; Rogers et al., 1986), due to the increased insulin resistance that is normally associated with the gonadal and adrenal hormone changes of puberty (Caprio et al., 1989; Bloch, Clemons, & Sperling, 1987). Consistent with this possibility was the finding that complication severity was correlated only with duration of diabetes from onset of puberty and not overall diabetes duration, which included the prepubertal duration (Kostraba et al., 1989; Krolewski, Laffel, Krolewski, Quinn, & Warram, 1995). Because puberty was thought to trigger the physical complications, including peripheral nervous system complications (Donaghue et al., 1993), we asked whether the CNS could be similarly affected.

We knew from studies on autopsy material (Yakovlev & Lecours, 1975) and magnetic resonance imaging (Jernigan et al., 1991; Pfefferbaum et al., 1994) that the timing of myelination varies across different brain regions. The frontal lobes and reticular formation, for example, have protracted periods of myelination, which extend into the second and third decades of life (Yakovlev & Lecours, 1975), whereas the parietal lobes and cerebellum are fully myelinated by age 5. Also, it was known that the pattern of development advances within regions from central to peripheral areas (Grodd, 1993). Given *in vitro* evidence showing that myelin production is impeded in the presence of excess glucose (Vlassara, Brownlee, & Cerami, 1983), we questioned whether the cerebral structures myelinating later would be more vulnerable to diabetes in adolescence than those myelinating earlier.

Our primary hypothesis was that the cognitive functions subserved by later-myelinating neural substrates (viz., attention, executive processing) would be compromised by diabetes in puberty, whereas the cognitive functions subserved by earlier-myelinating structures (viz., spatial and motor abilities), would be affected by earlier-occurring disease-related events, particularly hypoglycemic convulsions. We proposed that with advancing pubertal stage, the difference between diabetic and control subjects would increase, but only for executive processing and attention tasks. Visual–spatial deficits would continue to be associated with early disease onset and/or a history of hypoglycemic convulsions.

The study design involved a cross-sectional comparison of preadolescent and adolescent subjects, who were equally stratified by pubertal stage and sex. There were 103 preadolescent and adolescent subjects with diabetes, and 100 controls matched for age (± 3 months) and sex. Subjects with diabetes had had their disease for at least 3 years and were ascertained through the Diabetes Clinic at the Hospital for Sick Children. They ranged in age from 9.3 to 18.3 years and had had their diabetes for an average of 6.8 years, developing it at an average age of 6.4 years. Controls were recruited from children and friends of hospital employees ($n = 53$), friends of probands ($n = 34$), and siblings and cousins of probands ($n = 13$). For both the diabetes and control groups, there were a minimum of 20 subjects at each of the five Tanner pubertal stages, as determined by self-report in both groups and also validated against the medical records in the diabetes group. There were no differences between groups as to SES.

Subjects were assessed with a comprehensive day-long battery of neuropsychological tests, consisting of multiple measures of language, visual–spatial processing, motor skills, memory and learning, attention, and executive processing (see Table 15.2). For subjects with diabetes, blood glucose measurements were also obtained at five regular intervals during the course of the assessment, and the children and/or their parents were subsequently interviewed about diabetes history and metabolic control. Medical charts were also reviewed for information on current and long-term glycemic control, complications, and hospitalizations.

To reduce the number of variables, correlations and factor analyses were conducted. Within the verbal, spatial, and perceptual domains, all tasks within each domain were highly correlated with each other. For these tasks, composite scores were derived as domain scores. For the memory and motor domains, several clusters of correlations were observed (e.g., visual–motor, fine motor, and graphomotor skills; rote memory, working memory, and visual memory), necessitating computation of subdomain composite scores. As none of the tasks assessing attention and executive functions were correlated with each other, the results from these tasks were examined individually. Pubertal status effects were determined via significant interactions between pubertal stage and group or between pubertal stage, sex, and group.

The results are presented in Table 15.3. As a group, subjects with diabetes did more poorly than controls only on indices of spatial and graphomotor abilities and on selective aspects of attention and executive processing. Significant pubertal status effects were observed for measures of attention (Matching Familiar Figures Test [MFFT] errors), spatial processing (mental rotation task), executive processing (Stroop interference, males only), and visual memory (Rey–Osterreith Complex Figure Recall, females only). Figure 15.3 shows that for the MFFT (panel A) but not the Wisconsin Card Sorting Test (WCST, panel B), the number of errors between diabetes and control groups increased with advancing pubertal stage.

When subgroups of diabetes subjects were compared, those developing diabetes prior to age 5 performed more poorly than either those developing it later or controls in the following aspects: verbal, perceptual, and fine motor domains; visual memory and working memory subdomains; and verbal fluency. Similarly, subgrouping subjects by seizure history revealed that diabetes subjects with a positive history had poorer spatial, working memory, and attention abilities.

Blood glucose levels obtained at time of testing were shown to be correlated with levels of ability in the following domains: language comprehension and visual–motor skills,

TABLE 15.2. Tests Used in the Puberty Study

Domain	Subdomain	Test(s)
Intelligence		WISC-R/WAIS-R
Language		TOAL Listening Vocabulary
		TOAL Speaking Grammar
		Token Test
		Verbal Fluency ("F"-"A"-"S")
		WISC-R/WAIS-R Vocabulary
		WISC-R/WAIS-R Similarities
Visual–spatial		Judgment of Line Orientation Test
		Mental rotations
		Visual search task
		WISC-R/WAIS-R Block Design
Motor	Perceptual–motor	Tactile Performance Test
		Trail Making Test A
		WISC-R/WAIS-R Coding
	Motor coordination and strength	Finger Tapping Test
		Grip Strength Test
		Grooved Pegboard Test
	Graphomotor	Beery Developmental Test of Visual–Motor Integration
		Rey–Osterrieth Complex Figure Copy
Memory and learning	Rote memory	Denman Immediate Story Recall
	Working memory	WISC-R Digit Span (backward)
	Visual memory	Memory for Human Faces
		Rey–Osterrieth Complex Figure Recall
	Learning	Paired-associates learning
		Digit–Symbol Paired Associates Test
		Tactile Performance Test Memory
Attention	Attention I	Modified Matching Familiar Figures Test
	Attention II	Continuous-performance test
Executive processing	Exec. pro. I	Stroop Color–Word Test
	Exec. pro. II	Wisconsin Card Sorting Test
	Exec. pro. III	Trail Making Test B
Achievement		Wide Range Achievement Test—Revised

Note. WISC-R, Wechsler Intelligence Scale for Children—Revised; WAIS-R, Wechsler Adult Intelligence Scale—Revised; TOAL, Test of Adolescent Language.

visual search speed, and executive processing (based on WCST performance only). As a rule, performance was better when blood glucose levels were higher, although the subjects with blood glucose levels in the hypoglycemic range did not perform atypically. As can be seen in Figure 15.4, subjects with higher blood glucose levels at time of testing made fewer perseverative errors on the WCST. They also had shorter visual search reaction times (data not shown).

These results therefore indicate there are both structural and functional effects of diabetes on the developing brain in childhood and adolescence. The observations of pubertal status effects for some (but not all) indices of executive processing and attention, and of

TABLE 15.3. Mean z Scores from the Puberty Study

	Effect of diabetes			Effect of age at onset			Effect of seizures		
	Diabetes (D)	Control (C)	Signif. gp. diff.	Early (E)	Late (L)	Signif. gp. diff.	Seizures (S)	No seizures (NS)	Signif. gp. diff.
Verbal	-.04	.07		-.10	.00		-.27	.04	S < C*
Perceptual	-.06	.07	D < C†	-.19	.03	E < C*	-.35	-.02	S < NS, S < C**
Spatial	-.06	.09	D < C†	-.24	.04	E < C*	-.36	-.03	S < C*
Motor									
Visual–motor	.01	-.01		-.05	.05	E < L*	-.07	-.00	S < NS*, S < C*
Fine motor	-.04	.04		-.17	.05	E < C**	-.22	-.03	
Graphomotor	-.12	.09	D < C*	-.04	-.17	L < C*	-.03	-.19	NS < C*
Memory									
Rote	.05	-.05		.10	.02		-.10	.03	S < NS*
Working	.04	-.04		-.17	.17	E < L*	-.39	.14	S < NS*, S < C*
Recognition	-.02	.02		-.31	.15	E < L,C*	-.47	.04	S < NS*, S < C*
Attention									
MFFT (mean errors)[a]	.10	-.11	D > C†	.18	.03	E > C*	.46	.10	S > NS*, S > C**
CPT (commission errors)[a]	.16	-.10	D > C*	.32	.01	E > C	.74	.03	S > NS*, S > C**
Executive processing									
WCST (perseverative errors)[a]	.02	-.02		.06	-.10		.13	-.00	
Stroop interference	-.11	.11		-.13	.09		.12	-.20	
Trail Making Test B	-.04	.04							

Note. MFFT, Matching Familiar Figures Test; CPT, continuous-performance test; WCST, Wisconsin Card Sorting Test. (These apply to subsequent tables as well.)

[a]Positive score signifies more errors.

†p < .10. *p < .05, **p < .01, based on analysis of variance (one-tailed test).

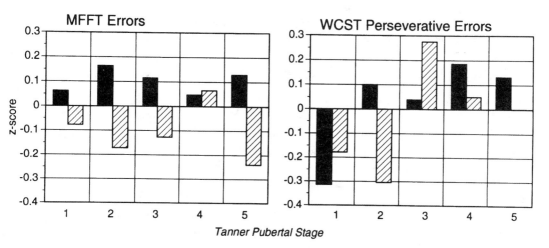

FIGURE 15.3. Error rates as a function of pubertal stage on the modified Matching Familiar Figures Test (left panel) and Wisconsin Card Sorting Test (right panel). Subjects with diabetes are represented by the black bars, and controls by the striped bars.

the influence of early age at onset or hypoglycemic convulsions on other abilities, suggest that different brain systems may be influenced by different diabetes-related events and their timing. Abilities subserved by posterior brain regions (e.g., spatial and perceptual abilities) were found to be more sensitive to earlier diabetes events, whereas abilities subserved by anterior brain regions (executive processing and attention) were found to be sensitive to later-occurring, pubertal-stage events. The finding that certain aspects of attentional and spatial processing were poorer in the presence of lower blood glucose concentrations

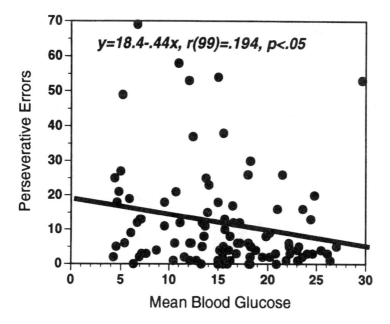

FIGURE 15.4. Relationship between diabetes subjects' mean blood glucose concentrations at time of testing and Wisconsin Card Sorting Test perseverative errors.

at time of testing also suggests that the frontal lobes may be particularly sensitive to ambient hypoglycemia, even when the set point is in the normal range.

Long-Term Follow-Up Study

A major limitation of most prospective studies on diabetes is the relatively short period of time during which subjects have actually been followed. In the diabetes and puberty study described just above, we had the unique opportunity to evaluate 16 subjects who had also participated much earlier in the prospective study, the majority of whom acquired diabetes at an early age. Because of the detailed evaluations that were provided to these subjects in the puberty study, we were in an ideal position to examine the long-term course of diabetes on *specific* neuropsychological functions (Rovet & Ehrlich, 1999).

These 16 children were studied at four time intervals: diagnosis, 1 and 3 years after diagnosis (prospective study), and 7 years after diagnosis (puberty study). As shown in Figure 15.5, they demonstrated significant declines in Verbal but not Performance IQ (panel A) and on tests of vocabulary knowledge and rote memory (panel B), as well as on tests of visual–motor integration and academic achievement (not shown).

Subjects' individual Verbal IQ scores are plotted in Figure 15.6 as a function of age at diabetes onset and seizure history. It can be seen that the subjects with the largest declines were those who either developed diabetes early or had one or more seizures (or both), whereas those with later-onset diabetes and no seizures showed minimal change.

For the 7-year postdiagnosis neuropsychological assessment, pair matches were formed according to sex, age (± 3 months), and SES (same level) with subjects from the control pool of the diabetes and puberty study. Comparisons between diabetes and control groups overall revealed few significant differences and only a difference in fine motor skills for children with early-onset diabetes (Table 15.4). However, diabetes children with a positive seizure history had significantly poorer scores in the language, perceptual, fine motor, visual–motor, memory, and attention areas than the other groups. For memory, the results revealed a larger effect for visual ($p < .05$) than for verbal ($p < .10$) working memory, and no effect for immediate or delayed recall.

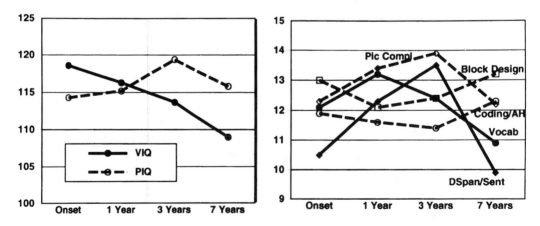

FIGURE 15.5. Changes in ability over first 7 years of diabetes. Left panel presents results by IQ scale, and right panel presents results by individual subtests. Data from Rovet and Ehrlich (1999).

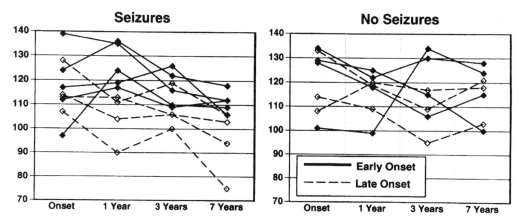

FIGURE 15.6. Changes in Verbal IQ for individual subjects according to age at onset of diabetes and whether or not they had had hypoglycemic seizures. Data from Rovet and Ehrlich (1999).

These findings therefore indicate few long-term effects of diabetes on children's neuro-cognitive abilities *unless* they experienced hypoglycemic seizures. Over the 7-year interval spanned by the two studies, the diabetic subjects' verbal abilities declined steadily, whereas their nonverbal abilities remained relatively stable. This decline was associated with both early age at onset and/or a history of seizures from hypoglycemia. Comparisons of these subjects with closely matched controls revealed no major group differences except for children with a history of hypoglycemic seizures, who did more poorly in a number of domains. This signifies that having hypoglycemic seizures during childhood is a major risk factor for cognitive impairment. As their pattern of deficit is consistent with children with memory problems associated with documented hippocampal damage (Vargah-Khadem, Gadian, Watkins, Connelly, Paesschen, & Mishkin, 1997), this suggests hypoglycemic insufficiency may target the hippocampus, which is known to have an abundance of insulin receptors (Schwartz, Figlewicz, Woods, Porte, & Baskin, 1993) and be damaged by insulin excess (Auer, 1986).

Diabetes and Attention Study

Problems in attention have long been recognized in patients with diabetes. Among adults, attention problems have been related to chronic hyperglycemia, long disease duration (Ryan, Williams, Finegold, & Orchard, 1993), and recurrent severe hypoglycemia (Langan, Deary, Hepburn, & Frier, 1991; Wredling, Levander, Adamson, & Lins, 1990). In children and adolescents, poorer attention has been observed using clinical instruments (Rovet et al., 1987), experimental paradigms (Hagen et al., 1990), and questionnaires given to teachers (Northam et al., 1992) and parents (Ryan, 1990). Children's attention problems have been associated with early age at onset and hypoglycemia (Holmes & Richman, 1985).

Using glucose–insulin infusion techniques, several investigators have also reported that attention is especially sensitive to low blood glucose concentrations (Holmes, Hayford, Gonzalez, & Weydert, 1983; Widom & Simonson, 1990). This has been observed in children (Ryan, Adams, & Heaton, 1990) and adults with diabetes (Gonder-Frederick, Cox, Driesen, Ryan, & Clarke, 1994; Mitrakou et al., 1991) and in individuals without

TABLE 15.4. Mean z Scores from the Long-Term Follow-Up Study

	Effect of diabetes		Effect of age at onset		Effect of seizures	
						No
	Diabetes (n = 16)	Control (n = 16)	Early (n = 10)	Late (n = 6)	Seizures (n = 9)	seizures (n = 7)
Verbal	.09	.18	.18	−.07	−.15	.39†
Perceptual	−.21	−.24	−.22	−.20	−.57	.24*
Spatial	.08	−.14	−.11	.33	−.16	.32
Motor						
Visual–motor	−.09	−.36	−.19	.06	−.52	.45*
Fine motor	−.01	−.18	−.19	.28*	−.24	.29**
Graphomotor	−.02	.06	.00	−.05	−.17	.20
Memory						
Rote	−.07	.01	.08	−.33	−.22	.13
Working	.25	−.16	.12	.48	−.39	.29†
Recognition	−.09	−.27	−.15	.01	−.03	.62†
Attention						
MFFT (Mean errors)[a]	.45	.13	.29	.71	.89	−.11**
CPT (commission errors)[a]	.68	.08	1.13	−.05	1.44	−.43**
Executive processing						
WCST (perseverative errors)[a]	.39	.24	−.32	−.52	−.60	.13**
Stroop interference	−.06	.30	−.03	−.10	.10	−.25
Trail Making Test B[b]	−.24	.19	−.21	−.29	−.36	−.15

[a]Positive score signifies more errors.

[b]Positive score signifies faster performance.

†p < .10. *p < .05. **p < .01.

diabetes as well (Ipp & Forster, 1987; Stevens et al., 1989). Vigilance and the ability to sustain attention are two aspects of attention most sensitive to low blood sugars (Holmes, Koepke, Thompson, Gyves, & Weydert, 1984; Pramming, Thorsteinsson, Stigsby, & Binder, 1988), and there is an inverse relationship between attention task demands and degree of blood glucose lowering needed to produce dysfunction (Holmes, Koepke, & Thompson, 1986). Several studies have shown a lag in recovery of attention following return to euglycemia (Gschwend, Ryan, Atchison, Arslanian, & Becker, 1995; Reich et al., 1990).

There is growing evidence in the neuropsychological literature showing that attention is not a unitary process, but is instead a multicomponential set of abilities (Cooley & Morris, 1990), which appear to be localized in different neuroanatomical regions (Mirsky, 1995; Stuss, Shallice, Alexander, & Picton, 1995) or to involve different brain systems (Posner & Petersen, 1990). Commonly studied attention subcomponents are the abilities to focus, select, share, shift, inhibit, suppress, and switch attention. Although several different tasks have been used to investigate attention in individuals with diabetes, few studies have involved administering more than one attention task to the same group (Gschwend et al., 1995; Holmes et al., 1984), and none have examined multiple facets of attention in children. To determine how diabetes affects attentional processing in children and adolescents, Miguel Alvarez and I reexamined the attention test findings from the diabetes and puberty study. Our goal was to identify the components most affected by diabetes in the pediatric population and the contributing factors (Rovet & Alvarez, 1997).

Subjects for this study were the same groups of 103 preadolescent and adolescent children with diabetes and 100 controls described earlier. The tasks and processes are listed in Table 15.5. Composite scores for each attention process were defined by averaging z scores for the various test parameters. Although variable combinations were determined on an *a priori* basis, support for combining variables in this fashion was later provided by correlations and factor analyses.

The results revealed that the diabetes group overall performed more poorly than controls only on the select component of attention (Table 15.6). When subjects were subgrouped by age at diabetes onset, the early-onset group had poorer select and focus abilities than the late-onset group or controls. Subgrouping subjects by history of hypoglycemic seizures revealed that children with a positive seizure history performed more poorly on the select, focus, and inhibit attentional processes than did those who had never experienced seizures from hypoglycemia (see Table 15.6).

These results therefore suggest selective effects of diabetes on attention. Diabetes per se was associated with poorer performance on only the select component; early-onset diabetes was linked with poorer performance on two components (focus and select); and hypoglycemic convulsions were associated with poorer performance on three (focus, select, and inhibit). The sustain, suppress, shift, and switch processes were unaffected in our sample. According to recent theories of attention (e.g., Stuss et al., 1995), those processes that are subserved by the cingulate (focus) and left dorsolateral prefrontal cortex (select, inhibit) appear to be most affected by diabetes, especially when hypoglycemic seizures occur. In contrast, the processes mediated by the right dorsolateral, medial, and orbital frontal cortices (e.g., switch, shift, suppress) appear to be less affected. Because seizures occurred in our sample mostly between 7 and 10 years of age, this suggests that the compromised neural substrates (particularly those subserving inhibitory skills) may

TABLE 15.5. Attention Processes Assessed and Proposed Associated Neural Substrates

Process	Task(s)	Measure[a]	Proposed substrate(s)
Sustain	CPT	Change in errors over blocks	Right dorsolateral frontal cortex[b]; thalamus and reticular formation[c]
Focus/set	MFFT Visual search task CPT Trail Making Test A	Errors Mean reaction time Omission errors Reaction time	Inferior parietal, superior temporal[c]
Concentrate/select	MFFT	Error slope	Anterior cingulate[c]
Inhibit	CPT	Commission errors	Medial and dorsolateral frontal cortex[b]
Suppress	Stroop	Interference score	Dorsolateral frontal cortex[b]
Shift/alternate	Trail Making Tests A and B	Reaction times	Prefrontal cortex, anterior cingulate[c]
Switch/disengage	WCST	Perseverative errors	Medial and dorsolateral frontal cortex[b]

[a]Operational definitions for all of the measures are given in Rovet and Alvarez (1997).
[b]Based on Stuss et al. (1995).
[c]Based on Mirsky (1995).

TABLE 15.6. Mean *z* Scores from the Attention Study

Process	Effect of diabetes		Effect of age at onset		Effect of seizures	
	Diabetes	Control	Early	Late	Seizures	No seizures
Sustain	.070	−.025	−.054	.085	−.017	.127
Focus	−.063	.011	−.120	.000	−.300	−.041*
Select	−.119	.123*	−.226	.164***	−.369	−.119*
Inhibit	−.137	.015	−.304	.046	−.662	−.018**
Suppress	−.108	.112	−.131	−.086	.120	−.202
Switch	−.021	.022	.058	−.098	.05	.10
Shift	−.020	.031	−.003	−.042	−.141	.001

Note. The data are from Rovet and Alvarez (1997).
*$p < .05$. **$p < .01$. ***$p < .001$.

have been undergoing active development at this time, thereby placing the children at additional risk for attentional and other neuropsychological impairment. Further research may address whether selective attentional processes are differentially sensitive to the timing of seizure episode and whether seizures at an older age disrupt the processes that were not affected in our sample, which are subserved by more medial and orbitofrontal sites.

Adult Studies

Studies of adults with diabetes include not only patients with IDDM or type I diabetes, but patients with type II diabetes or non-insulin-dependent diabetes mellitus (NIDDM). Patients with NIDDM secrete insulin (i.e., their pancreatic function is intact), but because they have insulin resistance, the amount produced is insufficient for their bodily needs. In many individuals, insulin insufficiency is associated with obesity and old age. Although NIDDM is uncommon in children, the number of adolescents with this type of diabetes appears to be increasing (Pinhas-Hamiel et al., 1996).

Neuropsychological studies on mature patients (with both kinds of diabetes) have identified a number of associated impairments. These have include moderate to severe difficulties in learning and memory among individuals with IDDM (Franceschi et al., 1984; Skenazy & Bigler, 1984) and NIDDM (Dey, Misra, Desai, Mahapatra, & Padma, 1995; Lichty & Connell, 1988; Mooradian, Perryman, Fitten, Kavonian, & Morley, 1988; Perlmuter, Anderson, Fan, & Tabanico, 1997; Perlmuter et al., 1984). Psychomotor skills have also been shown to be affected (Meuter, Thomas, Gurneklee, Gries, & Lohmann, 1980; Skenazy & Bigler, 1984; Ryan & Williams, 1993). Ryan and Williams (1993) have suggested that these deficits may reflect the differential sensitivities of specific neural systems (in the aging brain) to the "toxic" effects of chronic hyperglycemia. Further, elderly patients may also be especially susceptible to hypoglycemia, due to progressive lack of symptom awareness and slowed self-remediation (Meneilly, Cheung, Tessier, Yakura, & Tuokko, 1994).

Adults with IDDM, who have a history of recurrent and severe hypoglycemia perform more poorly than controls on tests of motor ability, short-term and associated memory, visual–spatial ability, problem solving, and reaction time (Langan et al., 1991; Sachon et al., 1992; Wredling et al., 1990; Wirsen, Tallroth, Lindren, & Agardh, 1991). Because the

Langan et al. (1991) study controlled for the effects of premorbid IQ, age, and duration of diabetes, their findings signify that recurrent severe hypoglycemia is indeed a risk factor for cumulative cognitive impairment in adult diabetic patients treated with insulin.

In the study by Ryan et al. (1993), diabetes subjects with a long duration of illness and one or more complications (suggestive of frequent hyperglycemia) performed more poorly on tests of sustained attention, rapid analysis of visual–spatial detail, and eye–hand coordination than did patients without complications. In this study, attention and executive function skills were more sensitive to chronic hyperglycemia, and motor and memory skills were more sensitive to hypoglycemia. These findings therefore indicate a variety of subtle cognitive abnormalities in adults with diabetes, reflecting either chronic and long-term elevations in blood glucose or frequent episodes of severe hypoglycemia.

One of the largest controlled treatment trials ever conducted, known as the Diabetes Control and Complications Trial (DCCT; see DCCT Research Group, 1993), involved 1,422 patients ranging in age from 13 to 39 years who were ascertained through multiple centers throughout the United States and Canada. The purpose of the DCCT was to determine whether intensive diabetes management (more than three injections and more than four blood glucose measurements daily) could reduce the complications of diabetes relative to conventional therapy (one or two injections daily). As part of this study, the effects of different management approaches on neuropsychological functioning were evaluated at baseline and repeatedly throughout the trial.

In a report on the preliminary baseline findings, Ryan, Adams, and Heaton (1990) found that the diabetes group generally showed normal neurobehavioral scores and only performed below average on tests requiring rapid motor or mental responses. Poorer performance on motor tasks was associated with less adequate glycemic control (suggesting hyperglycemia), whereas poorer performance on tests of rapid mental processing was associated with a history of severe hypoglycemia. After 5 years of either intensive or conventional therapy, relatively few new neuropsychological sequelae were observed among either group; the two no-treatment groups differed only on a test of rapid motor responding (finger tapping), which was associated with poorer glycemic control. Although hypoglycemia was significantly increased in the group receiving intensive therapy, it was not associated with poorer ability on any task (DCCT Research Group, 1996). These results are similar to the findings of a comparable study in Stockholm (Reichard, Berglund, Britz, Levander, & Rosenqvist, 1991), which showed no effects of intensive therapy and no relationship between number of episodes and outcome or change in performance over a 3-year interval, despite increased hypoglycemia. Overall, both of these large-scale studies indicated little direct effect of hypoglycemia on the adult brain, although the interpretation has been challenged because of serious methodological shortcomings (Deary, 1997). The baseline findings from these studies suggest that the adverse effects of hypoglycemia occur much earlier in development (Langan et al., 1991).

Diabetes in Pregnancy

Because glucose is critically necessary for early brain development, it is not surprising that maternal diabetes may have untoward effects on fetal brain development and subsequent neurocognitive functioning. Both maternal diabetes predating pregnancy and diabetes that develops during pregnancy (gestational diabetes) can adversely affect the fetus. Gestational diabetes is usually of the NIDDM variety as a result of the increased metabolic demands on insulin production, which disappears following pregnancy in most (but not all) women.

Maternal diabetes is associated with higher rates of fetal loss, neonatal death, and congenital malformations (Coustan, Berkowitz, & Hobbins, 1980), particularly if the blood glucose levels were elevated during pregnancy and ketoacids (which are toxic for the fetal brain) were present (Churchill, Berendes, & Nemores, 1969; Stehbens, Baker, & Mitchell, 1977). Altered maternal metabolism during pregnancy and the associated by-products are thought to be teratogenic, especially early in pregnancy (Rizzo, Metzler, Burns, & Burns, 1991).

Several studies have been conducted on the offspring of mothers with both IDDM and gestational diabetes, to establish when and to what degree fetuses are affected. Several studies are based on large perinatal collaborative projects of pregnancy outcome. As a rule, offspring IQs were in the normal range, but significantly lower than average (Churchill et al., 1969; Haworth, McRae, & Dilling, 1976; Stehbens et al., 1977), while language and psychomotor skills were poorer (Churchill et al., 1969; Petersen, Pedersen, Greisen, Pedersen, & Mølsted-Pedersen, 1988). Associations between severity and duration of diabetes and neuropsychological outcome of offspring were also observed (Churchill et al., 1969; Stehbens et al., 1977).

Unfortunately, most of the research on diabetes and pregnancy to date has been methodologically flawed because of small samples or samples that included children with both types of diabetes, as well as a lack of appropriate controls, inadequate metabolic information, and the absence of longitudinal follow-up. One exception is a study by Sells, Robinson, Brown, and Knopp (1994), who evaluated 109 offspring of IDDM mothers on multiple occasions in infancy and early childhood. These children demonstrated no decrements in intelligence or motor or language deficits, if their mothers' diabetes was well controlled during pregnancy. By contrast, the offspring of mothers whose diabetes was poorly controlled during pregnancy displayed less than optimal cognitive and language skills, suggesting that inadequate glycemia and ketoacids can affect the fetal brain. More research is clearly needed to determine how disease timing and severity affect clinical outcome, and to compare the developmental consequences of pregestational versus gestational diabetes. Blood glucose levels that are critical for normal brain development should also be identified.

CONCLUSIONS AND FUTURE DIRECTIONS

Diabetes has a number of neurocognitive manifestations in both pediatric and adult populations. Since diabetes is lifelong, some of the disease sequelae are cumulative and can arise from multiple episodes of hyperglycemia; this is illustrated by diabetes-related insults to non-CNS systems, such as the heart and kidneys. This means that children will be affected to a lesser degree than adults, but that the effects will be progressive, as we have observed in our extended prospective study. Although the specific effects of chronic hyperglycemia are not yet clear, attention, visual–spatial processing, eye–hand coordination, and verbal skills appear to be particularly vulnerable in diabetic children.

There are also adverse effects of insulin therapy and, in particular, exposure to hypoglycemia, especially hypoglycemic convulsions. However, very little information exists as to the nature and character of the seizure activity itself in this population (Foster & Hart, 1987; Wayne, Dean, Booth, & Tenenbein, 1990), which may have specific implications for outcome. Very young children are especially susceptible to permanent damage from severe hypoglycemia, and possibly from chronic mild episodes as well (e.g., Golden et al., 1989), whereas older children and adults are generally less severely affected. Although the earlier studies showed that seizures were more common in children below age 5 and affected visual–spatial abilities, our more recent findings suggest that seizures may now be occurring at a later age and are manifested in poorer verbal and working memory abilities (Rovet & Ehrlich, 1999). In addition, certain functional abilities appear to be transiently vulnerable to declines in blood glucose, as has been demonstrated in the experimental glucose clamp studies and more naturalistic paradigms, as well as in our puberty study.

Much of the evidence with regard to the neuropsychological consequences of diabetes is based on adults with long-standing disease and relatively complete brain development. Children, who are especially vulnerable to hypoglycemia, have been studied by only a few research teams, primarily in North America and Australia. Research on the childhood sequelae of diabetes, moreover, has been often hampered by methodological weaknesses, including samples of children ranging widely in age (necessitating different test measures for different groups), improper or no controls, small sample sizes, and single measurements. This research has typically been descriptive, with few attempts to link the full panoply of diabetes-related events to specific outcomes. In order to specify more exactly how the developing brain may be affected from a neuropsychological point of view, there is a pressing need for more detailed studies of the pediatric population. Even though diabetes is a relatively prevalent disease, a multicenter collaborative study may be required to control for the many relevant disease-related factors that can affect the developing brain. Efforts should be made to utilize a common set of measures appropriate across age groups and settings, and these should include both procedures with demonstrated clinical value and laboratory-based methods. It is also important that neurocognitive skills be examined componentially and systematically via process-based approaches. Finally, because of potential associations between insulin therapy and performance, controlled studies employing repeated measures and balanced crossover designs should be considered for children with diabetes.

In conclusion, diabetes provides a theoretically interesting and promising model for the study of neurocognitive processing in children. Because the timing of specific diabetes-specific events can be recorded with relative precision, future studies of pediatric diabetes patients will not only clarify more about the disease and its impact on the brain; they may also increase our understanding of the developing brain itself.

ACKNOWLEDGMENTS

The work described in this chapter has been generously supported since its inception by several operating grants from the Canadian Diabetes Association and supplementary funds from the Banting and Best Diabetes Foundation. I am especially grateful to Robert Ehrlich for introducing me to diabetes and for his long-standing collaborative support and interest in the psychological aspects of diabetes. I also appreciate the assistance of the diabetes team at The Hospital for Sick Children (HSC), who so willingly assisted us at every stage possible. Marla Hoppe, Deborah Altman, and Min-Na Hockenberry were integral to this research in recruiting, testing, and coordinating the various studies. Without them, the work would not have been possible. Miguel Alvarez is a dedicated scientist who, during his two visits from Cuba, helped to unravel some of the mysteries of endocrinopathies and attention. His stay in Toronto was generously supported by the HSC Foundation and a RESTRACOM Visiting Scientistship. Jennifer Rovet assisted with the bibliography and final editing. Finally, I want to thank all of the participants (with and without diabetes), who helped so generously to advance our understanding of this disease.

REFERENCES

Ack, M., Miller, I., & Weil, W. (1961). Intelligence of children with diabetes mellitus. *Pediatrics, 28,* 764–770.

Amiel, S. A. (1996). Studies in hypoglycaemia in children with insulin-dependent diabetes mellitus. *Hormone Research, 45,* 285–290.

Amiel, S. A., Simonson, D. C., Sherwin, R. S., Lauritano, A. A., & Tamborlane, W. V. (1987). Exaggerated epinephrine responses to hypoglycemia in normal and insulin-dependent diabetic children. *Journal of Pediatrics, 110,* 832–837.

Anderson, B. J., Hagen, J., Barclay, C., Goldstein, G., Kandt, R., & Bacon, G. (1984). Cognitive and school performance in diabetic children. *Diabetes, 33*(Suppl. 1), 8.

Anderson, B. J., Miller, J. P., Auslander, W. F., & Santiago, J. (1981). Family characteristics of diabetic adolescents: Relations to metabolic control. *Diabetes Care, 4,* 586–594.

Auer, R. N. (1986). Hypoglycemic brain damage. *Stroke, 17,* 488–496.

Auer, R. N., & Siesjo, B. K. (1988). Biological differences between ischemia, hypoglycemia, and epilepsy. *Annals of Neurology, 24,* 699–707.

Baskin, D. G., Figlewicz, D. P., Woods, S. C., Porte, D., & Dorsa, D. M. (1987). Insulin in the brain. *Annual Review of Physiology, 49,* 335–347.

Bjorgaas, M., Gimse, R., Vik, T., & Sand, T. (1997). Cognitive function in type 1 diabetic children with and without episodes of severe hypoglycaemia. *Acta Paediatrica, 86,* 148–153.

Blackman, J. D., Towle, V. L., Lewis, G. F., Spire, J. P., & Polonsky, K. S. (1989). Hypoglycemic thresholds for cognitive dysfunction in humans. *Diabetes, 39,* 828–835.

Bloch, C. A., Clemons, P., & Sperling, M. A. (1987). Puberty decreases insulin sensitivity. *Journal of Pediatrics, 110,* 481–487.

Borg, W. P., Borg, M. A., & Tamborlane, W. V. (1997). The brain and hypoglycemic counterregulation: Insights from hypoglycemic clamp studies. *Diabetes Spectrum, 10,* 33–38.

Brierley, J. B., Brown, A. W., & Meldrum, B. S. (1971). The nature and time course of the neuronal alterations resulting from oligaemia and hypoglycaemia in the brain of *Macacamulatta. Brain Research, 25,* 483–499.

Brown, G. D., & Thompson, W. H. (1940). The diabetic child: An analytic study of his development. *American Journal of Diseases of Children, 59,* 238–254.

Caprio, S., Plewe, G., Diamond, M. P., Simonson, D. C., Boulwar, S. D., Sherwin, R. S., & Tamborlane, W. V. (1989). Increased insulin secretion in puberty: A compensatory response to reductions in insulin sensitivity. *Journal of Pediatrics, 114,* 963–967.

Chalmers, J., Risk, M. T., Kean, D. M., Grant, R., Ashworth, B., & Campbell, I. W. (1991). Severe amnesia after hypoglycemia. *Diabetes Care, 14,* 922–925.

Churchill, J. A., Berendes, H. W., & Nemores, J. (1969). Neuropsychological deficits in children of diabetic mothers. *American Journal of Obstetrics and Gynecology, 105,* 257–268.

Cooley, E., & Morris, R. (1990). Attention in children: A neuropsychologically based model for assessment. *Developmental Neuropsychology, 6,* 239–274.

Coustan, D. R., Berkowitz, R. L., & Hobbins, J. C. (1980). Tight metabolic control of overt diabetes in pregnancy. *American Journal of Medicine, 68,* 845–852.

Deary, I. J. (1997). Hypoglycemia-induced cognitive decrements in adults with type I: A case to answer? *Diabetes Spectrum, 10,* 42–47.

DeJong, R. N. (1977). CNS manifestation of diabetes mellitus. *Postgraduate Medical Journal, 61,* 101–107.

Dey, J., Misra, A., Desai, N. G., Mahapatra, A. K., & Padma, M. V. (1997). Cognitive function in younger type II diabetics. *Diabetes Care, 20,* 32–35.

Diabetes Control and Complications Trial (DCCT) Research Group. (1993). The effect of intensive treatment of diabetes on the development and progression of long-term complications in insulin-dependent diabetes mellitus. *New England Journal of Medicine, 329,* 977–986.

Diabetes Control and Complications Trial (DCCT) Research Group. (1996). Effects of intensive diabetes therapy on neuropsychological function in adults in the diabetes control and complications trial. *Annals of Internal Medicine, 124,* 379–388.

Donaghue, K. C., Bonney, M., Simpson, J., Schingshadl, J., Fung, A. T. W., Howard, N. J., & Silink, M. (1993). Autonomic and peripheral nerve function in adolescents with and without diabetes. *Diabetes Medicine, 10,* 664–671.

Donald, M. W., Bird, C. E., Lawson, J. S., Letemendia, F. J. J., Monga, T. N., Surridge, D. H. C., Varette-Cerre, P., Williams, D. L., Williams, D. M. L., & Wilson, D. L. (1981). Delayed auditory brainstem responses in diabetes mellitus. *Journal of Neurology, Neurosurgery and Psychiatry, 44,* 641–644.

Eeg-Olofsson, O., & Petersen, I. (1966). Childhood diabetic neuropathy: A clinical and neuropsychological study. *Acta Pediatrica Scandinavica, 55,* 163–176.

Figlewicz, D. P., Szot, P., Chavez, M., Woods, S. C., & Veith, R. C. (1994). Intraventricular insulin increases dopamine transporter mRNA in rate VTA/substantia nigra. *Brain Research, 644,* 331–334.

Flood, J. F., Mooradian, A. D., & Morley, J. E. (1990). Characteristics of learning and memory in streptozocin-induced diabetic mice. *Diabetes, 39,* 1391–1398.

Foster, J., & Hart, R. (1987). Hypoglycemic hemiplegia: Two cases and a clinical review. *Stroke, 18,* 944–946.

Franceschi, M., Cecchetto, R., Minicucci, F., Smizne, S., Baio, G., & Canal, N. (1984). Cognitive processes in insulin-dependent diabetes. *Diabetes Care, 7,* 228–231.

Gardner, S. G., Bingley, P. J., Sawtell, P. A., Weeks, S., & Oak, C. A. (1997). Rising incidence of insulin dependent diabetes in children aged 5 years in the Oxford region: Time analysis trend. The Bart's-Oxford Study Group. *British Medical Journal, 315,* 713–717.

Gath, A., Smith, M. A., & Baum, J. D. (1980). Emotional behavioral and educational disorders in diabetic children. *Archives of Disease in Childhood, 55,* 371–375.

Golden, M. P., Ingersoll, G. M., Brack, C. J., Russell, B. A., Wright, J. C., & Huberty, T. J. (1989). Longitudinal relationship of asymptomatic hypoglycemia to cognitive function in IDDM. *Diabetes Care, 12,* 89–93.

Gonder-Frederick, L. A., Cox, D. J., Driesen, N. R., Ryan, C. M., & Clarke, W. L. (1994). Individual differences in neurobehavioral disruption during mild and moderate hypoglycemia in adults with IDDM. *Diabetes, 43,* 1407–1412.

Grodd, W. (1993). Normal and abnormal patterns of myelin development of the fetal and infantile human brain using magnetic resonance imaging. *Current Opinion in Neurology and Neurosurgery, 6,* 393–397.

Gschwend, S., Ryan, C., Atchison, J., Arslanian, S., & Becker, D. (1995). Effects of acute hyperglycemia on mental efficiency and counterregulatory hormones in adolescents with insulin-dependent diabetes mellitus. *Journal of Pediatrics, 126,* 178–184.

Hagen, J. W., Barclay, C. R., Anderson, B. J., Freeman, D. J., Segal, S. S., Bacon, G., & Goldstein, G. W. (1990). Intellectual functioning and strategy use in children with insulin-dependent diabetes mellitus. *Child Development, 61,* 1714–1727.

Haumont, D., Dorch, H., & Pelc, S. (1979). EEG abnormalities in diabetic children. *Clinical Pediatrics, 18,* 750–752.

Havrankova, J., Roth, K., & Brownstone, M. J. (1983). Insulin receptors in brain. *Advances in Metabolic Disorders, 10,* 259–268.

Haworth, J. C., McRae, K. N., & Dilling, L. A. (1976). Prognosis of infants of diabetic mothers in relation to neonatal hypoglycemia. *Developmental Medicine and Child Neurology, 18,* 471–479.

Hershey, T., Craft, S., Bhargava, N., & White, N. H. (1997). Memory and insulin dependent diabetes mellitus (IDDM): Effects of childhood onset and severe hypoglycemia. *Journal of the International Neuropsychological Society, 3,* 509–520.

Holmes, C. S. (1990). Neuropsychological sequelae of acute and chronic blood glucose disruption in adults with insulin-dependent diabetes. In C. Holmes (Ed.), *Neuropsychological and behavioral aspects of diabetes* (pp. 122–154). New York: Springer-Verlag.

Holmes, C. S., Cornwell, J., Dunlap, W., Chen, R., & Lee, C. (1992). Anomalous factor structure of the WISC-R for diabetic children. *Neuropsychology, 6,* 341–350.

Holmes, C. S., Hayford, J. T., Gonzalez, J. L., & Weydert, J. A. (1983). A survey of cognitive functioning at different glucose levels in diabetic persons. *Diabetes Care, 6,* 180–185.

Holmes, C. S., Koepke, K. M., & Thompson, R. G. (1986). Simple versus complex performance impairments at three blood glucose levels. *Psychoneuroendocrinology, 11,* 353–357.

Holmes, C. S., Koepke, K. M., Thompson, R. G., Gyves, P. W., & Weydert, J. A. (1984). Verbal fluency and naming performance in type 1 diabetes at different blood glucose concentrations. *Diabetes Care, 7,* 454–459.

Holmes, C. S., & Richman, L. C. (1985). Cognitive profiles of children with insulin-dependent diabetes. *Journal of Developmental and Behavioral Pediatrics, 6,* 323–326.

Hume, R., McGeechan, A., & Burcheil, A. (1999). Failure to detect preterm infants at risk of hypoglycemia before discharge. *Journal of Pediatrics, 134,* 499–502.

Ipp, E., & Forster, B. (1987). Sparing of cognitive function in mild hypoglycemia: Dissociation from the neuroendocrine response. *Journal of Clinical Endocrinology and Metabolism, 65,* 806–810.

Jakobsen, J., Sidenius, P., Gundersen, H. J. G., & Osterby, R. (1987). Quantitative changes of cerebral neocortical structure in insulin-treated long-term streptozocin-diabetic rates. *Diabetes, 36,* 597–601.

Jernigan, T. L., Archibald, S. L., Berhow, M. T., Sowell, E. R., Foster, D. S., & Hesselink, J. R. (1991). Cerebral structure on MRI: Part I. Localization of age-related changes. *Biological Psychiatry, 29,* 55–67.

Johnson, S. B. (1980). Psychosocial factors in juvenile diabetes: A review. *Journal of Behavioral Medicine*, *3*, 95–116.

Kappy, M., Sellinger, S., & Raizada, S. (1984). Insulin binding in four regions of the developing rat brain. *Journal of Neurochemistry*, *42*, 198–203.

Kono, T., & Takada, M. (1994). Dopamine depletion in nigrostriatal neurons in the genetically diabetic rat. *Brain Research*, *634*, 155–158.

Kostraba, J. N., Dorman, J. S., Orchard, T. J., Becker, D. J., Ohki, Y., Ellis, D., Doft, B. H., Lobes, L. A., Laporte, R. E., & Drash, A. L. (1989). Contribution of diabetes duration before puberty to development of microvascular complications in IDDM subjects. *Diabetes Care*, *12*, 686–693.

Krolewski, A. S., Laffel, L. M. B., Krolewski, M., Quinn, M., & Warram, J. H. (1995). Glycosylated hemoglobin and the risk of microalbuminuria in patients with insulin-dependent diabetes mellitus. *New England Journal of Medicine*, *332*, 1251–1255.

Kubany, A. J., Danowski, T. S., & Moses, C. (1956). The personality and intelligence of diabetes. *Diabetes*, *5*, 462–467.

La Greca, A. M., Swales, T., Klemp, S., Madigan, S., & Skyler, J. (1995). Adolescents with diabetes: Gender differences in psychosocial functioning and glycemic control. *Children's Health Care*, *24*, 61–78.

Langan, S. J., Deary, I. J., Hepburn, D. A., & Frier, B. M. (1991). Cumulative cognitive impairment following recurrent severe hypoglycemia in adult patients with insulin-treated diabetes mellitus. *Diabetologia*, *34*, 337–344.

Lichty, W., & Connell, C. (1988, August). *Cognitive functioning of diabetics versus nondiabetics.* Paper presented at the 96th Annual Meeting of the American Psychological Association, Atlanta, GA.

Lingren, F., Dahlquist, G., Efendic, S., Persson, B., & Skottner, A. (1990). Insulin sensitivity and glucose-induced insulin response changes during adolescence. *Acta Pediatrica Scandinavica*, *79*, 431–436.

Lucas, A., Morley, R., & Cole, T. J. (1988). Adverse neurodevelopmental outcome of moderate neonatal hypoglycaemia. *British Medical Journal*, *297*, 1304–1308.

Macleod, K. M., Hepburn, D. A., Deary, I. J., Goodwin, G. M., Dougall, N., Ebmeier, K. P., & Frier, B. M. (1994). Regional cerebral blood flow in IDDM patients: Effects of diabetes and recurrent severe hypoglycaemia. *Diabetologia*, *37*, 257–263.

McCall, A. L. (1992). The impact of diabetes on the CNS. *Diabetes*, *31*, 557–570.

McCall, A. L., & Figlewicz, D. P. (1997). How does diabetes mellitus produce brain dysfunction? *Diabetes Spectrum*, *10*, 25–32.

Meneilly, G. S., Cheung, E., Tessier, D., Yakura, C., & Tuokko, H. (1994). The effect of improved glycemic control on cognitive functions in the elderly patient with diabetes. *Journal of Gerontology*, *48*, M117–M121.

Merali, Z., & Ahmad, Q. (1986). Diabetes-induced alterations in brain monoamine and metabolite levels: Effects of insulin replacement. *Society for Neuroscience Abstracts*, *12*, 125.

Meuter, F., Thomas, W., Gurneklee, D., Gires, F., & Lohmann, R. (1980). Psychometric evaluation of performance in diabetes mellitus. *Hormone and Metabolic Research Supplement*, *9*, 9–17.

Mirsky, A. (1995). Perils and pitfalls on the path to normal potential: The role of impaired attention. *Journal of Clinical and Experimental Neuropsychology*, *17*, 481–498.

Mitrakou, A., Ryan, C., Veneman, T., Mokan, M., Jenssen, T., Kiss, I., Durrant, J., Cryer, P., & Gerich, J. (1991). Hierarchy of glycemic thresholds for counterregulatory hormone secretion, symptoms, and cerebral dysfunction. *American Journal of Physiology*, *260*, E67–E74.

Mooradian, A. D. (1988). Diabetic complications of the central nervous system. *Endocrine Reviews*, *9*, 346–356.

Mooradian, A., Perryman, K., Fitten, J., Kavonian, G., & Morley, J. (1988). Cortical function in elderly non-insulin dependent diabetic patients. *Annals of Internal Medicine*, *110*, 2369–2372.

Northam, E. (1996). *Neuropsychological changes in children with insulin dependent diabetes mellitus.* Unpublished doctoral dissertation, University of Melbourne, Parkville, Victoria, Australia.

Northam, E., Anderson, P., Werther, G., Adler, R., & Andrewes, D. (1995). Neuropsychological complications of insulin dependent diabetes in children. *Child Neuropsychology*, *1*, 74–87.

Northam, E., Bowden, S., Anderson, V., & Court, J. (1992). Neuropsychological functioning in adolescents with diabetes. *Journal of Clinical and Experimental Neuropsychology*, *14*, 884–900.

Perlmuter, L. C., Anderson, K. S., Fan, X., & Tabanico, F. (1997). Does cognitive function decline in type II diabetes? *Diabetes Spectrum*, *10*, 57–62.

Perlmuter, L. C., Hakami, M., Hodgson-Harrington, C., Ginsberg, J., Katz, J., Singer, D. E., & Nathan, D. M. (1984). Decreased cognitive function in aging non-insulin-dependent diabetic patients. *American Journal of Medicine*, *77*, 1043–1048.

Petersen, M. B., Pedersen, S. A., Greisen, G., Pedersen, J. F., & Mølsted-Pedersen, L. (1988). Early growth delay in diabetic pregnancy: Relation to psychomotor development at age 4. *British Medical Journal, 296*, 598–600.

Pfefferbaum, A., Mathalon, D. H., Sullivan, E. V., Rawles, J. M., Zipursky, R. B., & Lim, K. O. (1994). A quantitative magnetic resonance image study of changes in brain morphology from infancy to late adulthood. *Archives of Neurology, 51*, 874–887.

Pinhas-Hamiel, O., Dolan, L. M., Daniels, S. R., Standiford, D., Khoury, P. R., & Zietler, P. (1996). Increased incidence of non-insulin-dependent diabetes mellitus among adolescents. *Journal of Pediatrics, 128*, 608–615.

Posner, M. I., & Petersen, S. E. (1990). The attentional system of the human brain. *Annual Review of Neuroscience, 13*, 25–42.

Pozzessere, G., Valle, E., Crignis, S. D., Cordischi, V. M., Fattapposta, F., Rizzo, P. A., Pietravalle, P., Cristina, G., Morano, S., & Di Mario, U. (1991). Abnormalities of cognitive functions in IDDM revealed by P300 event-related potential analysis. *Diabetes, 40*, 952–958.

Pramming, S., Thorsteinsson, B., Stigsby, B., & Binder, C. (1988). Glycaemic threshold for changes in electroencephalograms during hypoglycaemia in patients with insulin dependent diabetes. *British Medical Journal, 292*, 665–667.

Puczynski, S. (1997). Neurocognitive effects of diabetes in children and adolescents: Disease-related and psychosocial effects on cognitive function and class room performance. *Diabetes Spectrum, 10*, 51–57.

Reich, J. N., Kaspar, J. C., Puczynski, M. S., Puczynski, S., Cleland, J. W., Dell'Angela, K., & Emanuele, M. A. (1990). Effect of a hypoglycemic episode on neuropsychological functioning in diabetic children. *Journal of Clinical and Experimental Neuropsychology, 12*, 613–626.

Reichard, P., Berglund, A., Britz, A., Levander, S., & Rosenqvist, U. (1991). Hypoglycaemic episodes during intensified insulin treatment: Increased frequency but no effect on cognitive function. *Journal of Internal Medicine, 229*, 9–16.

Reunanen, A., Åkerblom, H. K., & Käär, M. L. (1982). Prevalence and ten year (1970–1979) incidence of insulin-dependent diabetes mellitus in children and adolescents in Finland. *Acta Pediatrica Scandinavica, 71*, 893–899.

Rizzo, T., Metzger, B. E., Burns, W. J., & Burns, K. (1991). Correlations between antepartum maternal metabolism and intelligence of offspring. *New England Journal of Medicine, 325*, 911–916.

Rogers, D. G., White, N. H., Santiago, J. V., Miller, J. P., Weldon, V. V., Kilo, C., & Williamson, J. R. (1986). Glycemic control and bone age are independently associated with muscle capillary basement membrane width in diabetic children after puberty. *Diabetes Care, 9*, 453–459.

Rovet, J. F., & Alvarez, M. (1997). Attentional functioning in children and adolescents with IDDM. *Diabetes Care, 11*, 77–82.

Rovet, J. F., & Ehrlich, R. M. (1988). Effect of temperament on metabolic control in children with diabetes mellitus. *Diabetes Care, 11*, 77–82.

Rovet, J. F., & Ehrlich, R. M. (1999). The effect of hypoglycemic seizures on cognitive function in children with diabetes: A 7-year prospective study. *Journal of Pediatrics, 34*, 503–506.

Rovet, J. F., Ehrlich, R. M., & Czuchta, D. (1990). Intellectual characteristics of diabetic children at diagnosis and one year later. *Journal of Pediatric Psychology, 15*, 775–788.

Rovet, J. F., Ehrlich, R. M., Czuchta, D., & Akler, M. (1993). Psychoeducational characteristics of children and adolescents with insulin-dependent diabetes mellitus. *Journal of Learning Disabilities, 26*, 7–22.

Rovet, J. F., Ehrlich, R. M., & Hoppe, M. (1987). Intellectual deficits associated with early onset of insulin-dependent diabetes mellitus in children. *Diabetes Care, 10*, 510–515.

Rovet, J. F., Ehrlich, R., & Hoppe, M. (1988a). Behaviour problems in children with diabetes as a function of sex and age of onset of disease. *Journal of Child Psychology and Psychiatry, 28*, 477–491.

Rovet, J. F., Ehrlich, R. M., & Hoppe, M. (1988b). Specific intellectual deficits in children with early onset diabetes mellitus. *Child Development, 59*, 226–234.

Rovet, J., & Fernandes, C. (1999). Insulin-Dependent Diabetes Mellitus. In R. T. Brown (Ed.), *Cognitive aspects of chronic illness* (pp. 142–171). New York: Guilford Press.

Ryan, C. M. (1990). Neuropsychological consequences and correlates of diabetes in childhood. In C. S. Holmes (Ed.), *Neuropsychological and behavioral aspects of diabetes* (pp. 58–84). New York: Springer-Verlag.

Ryan, C. M., Adams, K., & Heaton, R. (1990). Baseline neurobehavioral evaluation of adults in the Diabetes Control and Complications Trial (DCCT). *Diabetes, 39*(Suppl.), 7A.

Ryan, C. M., Atchison, J., Puczynski, S., Puczynski, M., Arslanian, S., & Becker, D. (1990). Mild hypoglycemia associated with deterioration of mental efficiency in children with insulin-dependent diabetes mellitus. *Journal of Pediatrics, 117*, 32–38.

Ryan, C. M., Longstreet, C., & Morrow, L. (1985). The effects of diabetes mellitus on the school attendance and school achievement of adolescents. *Child: Care, Health and Development, 11,* 229–240.

Ryan, C. M., Vega, A., & Drash, A. (1985). Cognitive defects in adolescents who developed diabetes early in life. *Pediatrics, 75,* 921–927.

Ryan, C. M., Vega, A., Longstreet, C., & Drash, A. (1984). Neuropsychological changes in adolescents with insulin dependent diabetes. *Journal of Consulting and Clinical Psychology, 52,* 335–342.

Ryan, C. M., & Williams, T. M. (1993). Effects of insulin-dependent diabetes on learning and memory efficiency in adults. *Journal of Clinical and Experimental Neuropsychology, 15,* 685–700.

Ryan, C. M., Williams, T. M., Finegold, D. N., & Orchard, T. J. (1993). Cognitive dysfunction in adults with type 1 (insulin-dependent) diabetes mellitus of long duration: Effects of recurrent hypoglycaemia and other chronic complications. *Diabetologia, 36,* 329–334.

Rydall, A. C., Rodin, G. M., Olmsted, M. P., Devenyl, R. G., & Daneman, D. (1997). Disordered eating behavior and microvascular complications in young women with insulin-dependent diabetes mellitus. *New England Journal of Medicine, 336,* 1849–1854.

Sansbury, L., Brown, R. T., & Meacham, L. (1997). Predictors of cognitive functioning in children and adolescents with insulin-dependent diabetes mellitus: A preliminary investigation. *Children's Health Care, 26*(3), 197–210.

Sachon, C., Grimaldi, A., Digy, J., Pillon, B., Dubois, B., & Thervet, P. (1992). Cognitive function, insulin-dependent diabetes and hypoglycaemia. *Journal of Internal Medicine, 231,* 471–475.

Schwartz, M. W., Figlewicz, D. P., Woods, S. C., Porte, D., & Baskin, D. G. (1993). Insulin, neuropeptide Y, and food intake. *Annals of the New York Academy of Sciences, 692,* 60–71.

Sells, C. J., Robinson, N. R., Brown, Z., & Knopp, R. H. (1994). Long-term developmental follow-up of infants of diabetic mothers. *Journal of Pediatrics, 125,* S9–S17.

Sesti, G., Marini, M. A., Montemurro, A., Borboni, P., Di Cola, G., Bertoli, A., De Pirro, R., & Lauro, R. (1991). Evidence that human and porcine insulin differently affect the human insulin receptor: Studies with monoclonal anti-insulin receptor antibodies. *Journal of Endocrinological Investigation, 14,* 913–918.

Sesti, G., Marini, M. A., Montemurro, A., Condorelli, L., Borboni, P., Haring, H., Ullrich, A., Goldfine, I. D., de Pirro, R., & Lauro, R. (1992). Evidence that two naturally occurring human insulin receptor α-subunit variants are immunologically distinct. *Diabetes, 41,* 6–10.

Skenazy, J., & Bigler, E. (1984). Neuropsychological findings in diabetes mellitus. *Journal of Clinical Psychology, 40,* 246–258.

Skyler, J. S. (1989). Intensive insulin therapy: A personal and historical perspective. *Diabetes Educator, 15,* 33–39.

Soltéz, G., & Acsadi, G. (1989). Association between diabetes, severe hypoglycaemia and electroencephalographic abnormalities. *Archives of Disease in Childhood, 64,* 992–996.

Stehbens, J. A., Baker, G. L., & Mitchell, M. (1977). Outcome of ages 1, 3, and 5 years of children born to diabetic women. *American Journal of Obstetrics and Gynecology, 127,* 408–413.

Stevens, A. V., McKane, W. R., Bell, P. M., Bell, P., King, D. J., & Hayes, J. R. (1989). Psychomotor performance and counterregulatory responses during mild hypoglycemia in healthy volunteers. *Diabetes Care, 12,* 12–17.

Stuss, D. T., Shallice, T., Alexander, M. P., & Picton, T. W. (1995). A multidisciplinary approach to anterior attentional functions. *Annals of the New York Academy of Sciences, 769,* 191–211.

Tallroth, G., Ryding, E., & Agardh, C. D. (1992). Regional cerebral blood flow in normal man during insulin-induced hypoglycemia and in the recovery period following glucose infusion, *Metabolism, 41,* 717–721.

Ternand, C., Go, V. L. W., Gerich, J. E., & Haymond, M. W. (1982). Endocrine pancreatic response of children with onset of insulin-requiring diabetes before age 3 and after age 5. *Pediatrics, 101,* 36–39.

Tribl, G., Howorka, K., Heger, G., Anderer, P., Thomas, H., & Zeitlhofer, J. (1996). EEG topography during insulin-induced hypoglycemia in patients with insulin-dependent diabetes mellitus. *European Neurology, 36,* 303–309.

Tsalikian, E., Daneman, D., Becker, D. J., Crumrine, P. K., & Drash, A. L. (1980). EEG changes during therapy of diabetic ketoacidosis in children. *Journal of Pediatrics, 96,* 1115–1116.

Uberall, M. A., Renner, C., Edl, S., Parzinger, E., & Wenzel, D. (1996). VEP and ERP abnormalities in children and adolescents with prepubertal onset of insulin-dependent diabetes mellitus. *Neuropediatrics, 27,* 88–93.

Vargah-Khadem, F., Gadian, D. G., Watkins, K. E., Connelly, A., Van Paesschen, W., & Mishkin, M. (1997). Differential effects of early hippocampal pathology on episodic and semantic memory. *Science, 277,* 376–380.

Vlassara, H., Brownlee, M., & Cerami, A. (1983). Excessive nonenzymatic glycoslyation of peripheral and central nervous system myelin components in diabetic rats. *Diabetes, 32,* 670–674.

Wayne, E., Dean, H., Booth, F., & Tenenbein, M. (1990). Focal neurologic deficits associated with hypoglycemia in children with diabetes. *Journal of Pediatrics, 117,* 575–577.

Widom, B., & Simonson, D. C. (1990). Glycemic control and neuropsychologic function during hypoglycemia in patients with insulin-dependent diabetes mellitus. *Annals of Internal Medicine, 112,* 904–912.

Wirsen, A., Tallroth, G., Lingren, M., & Agardh, C. (1991). Neuropsychological performance differences between type 1 diabetic and normal men during insulin-induced hypoglycaemia. *Diabetic Medicine, 9,* 156–165.

Wolters, C. A., Yu, S. L., Hagen, J. W., & Kail, R. (1996). Short term memory and strategy use in children with insulin-dependent diabetes mellitus. *Journal of Consulting and Clinical Psychology, 64,* 1397–1405.

Wredling, R., Levander, S., Adamson, U., & Lins, P. E. (1990). Permanent neuropsychological impairment after recurrent episode of severe hypoglycaemia in man. *Diabetologia, 33,* 152–157.

Yakovlev, P. I., & Lecours, A. (1975). The myelogenetic cycles of regional maturation of the brain. In A. Minkowski (Ed.), *Regional development of the brain in early life* (pp. 3–64). Oxford: Blackwell.

16

END-STAGE RENAL DISEASE

EILEEN B. FENNELL

Chronic renal failure and end-stage renal disease affect about 3–4 children per 1,000,000 per year in the United States. The causes of renal failure are varied, but the progression to renal failure results in an increasingly debilitating illness. Renal failure affects a child's growth and development, often produces neurobehavioral and neurological complications, can result in psychological and psychiatric disorders in the affected child and his or her family, and eventually may require complex medical treatments. Treatments such as dialysis or kidney transplantation are instituted in order for the child to survive the disorder and obtain a reasonable quality of life. With advances in the management of renal diseases, as well as the availability of treatment options such as dialysis or kidney transplantation, the pediatric neuropsychologist is likely to be confronted with questions regarding the effects of renal disease and its treatment on the developing brain.

In this chapter, relevant issues in the neuropsychological and psychological/psychiatric assessment of children are discussed. The chapter includes three sections. The first of these is an overview of kidney anatomy and function, causes of kidney disease, systemic effects of chronic renal failure and end-stage renal disease, and issues in dialysis and renal transplantation. In the second section, neuropsychological research on the cognitive effects of chronic renal failure, dialysis, and renal transplantation is reviewed; psychological problems encountered in this patient group are also discussed. The final section summarizes the relevant findings of this literature review and addresses future directions in research.

RENAL FUNCTION, RENAL DISEASES, AND TREATMENT CONSIDERATIONS

Anatomy and Physiology of the Kidneys

The kidneys are a pair of organs that lie in the retroperitoneal space above the level of the umbilicus. Each kidney consists of an outer layer (cortex) and an inner layer (medulla). Each kidney contains millions of nephrons, the basic processing unit of the kidney. Each nephron consists of (1) a glomerulus for initial filtration of the blood; (2) the proximal tubule, through which the filtered blood and filtrate pass and where the blood is partially resorbed; (3) the loop of Henle, where sodium and chloride are preferentially resorbed; (4) the distal tubule, through which the ultrafiltrate passes and where acid (H ion) and potassium are secreted and sodium is resorbed; and (5) the collecting ducts, where water is resorbed.

The kidneys' major function is to provide a filtering mechanism for the by-products of protein metabolism that collect in the blood. Electrolyte balance, water conservation and excretion, and buffering of the acid–base (pH) balance of blood serum by sodium bicarbonate all take place in the kidneys (Baron, Fennell, & Voeller, 1995). In addition to this filtering and secretory function of the kidneys, they also produce hormones and thus have an endocrine function as well. The hormones erythropoietin and Vitamin D_3 are both secreted by the kidneys. Erythropoietin stimulates the bone marrow to produce red blood cells. Vitamin D_3 is necessary for adequate intestinal absorption of minerals (calcium, magnesium, and phosphorus). Inadequate production of Vitamin D_3 can cause the kidneys to take up necessary calcium from resorption of bone and thus to reduce bone densities, in order to maintain adequate serum levels of calcium and phosphorus (Baron et al., 1995; Lum, 1995).

The physiological mechanisms that underlie normal kidney function are quite complex. These mechanisms can be altered by numerous congenital and acquired disorders. Table 16.1 lists possible adverse events that can result in loss of normal kidney function. As this table suggests, many different conditions can affect kidney functioning, including disorders related to the structure of the kidneys and urinary system, the adverse effects of infections or autoimmune processes, blunt trauma to the kidneys, renal disease resulting from toxins or chemotherapeutic agents, and kidney dysfunction arising as a secondary effect of a different primary disease (e.g., diabetes) or other condition (e.g., hypoxia) (Bergstein, 1996; Lum, 1995). Regardless of the etiology of renal failure, many typical medical problems emerge as kidney function decreases (Holliday, Bryant, & Avner, 1994).

Renal Failure and End-Stage Renal Disease

Renal failure is defined as a loss of normal kidney function, as measured by the rate of creatinine clearance. *Moderate renal failure* is present when a child has less than 35% of normal creatinine clearance—an index of the rate of plasma clearance of creatinine by the glomeruli of the kidneys, referred to as the *glomerular filtration rate* (GFR). The label of *end-stage renal disease* is applied to a child (or adult) whose GFR is 10% or less of the normal rate. At this point, dialysis may be instituted to assist the failing kidneys, and the

TABLE 16.1. Types of Disorders that Adversely Affect Kidney Function

Congenital disorders/anomalies	Acquired disorders
Renal agenesis	Trauma
Malformations of the kidney	Hypoxia
Polycystic kidney disease	Infection
Urethral malformations	Acute nephritis
Vascular malformations	Glomerulonephritis
	Drug toxicity
	Immunological disorders (e.g., systemic lupus erythematosus)
	Diabetes

child may be placed on a waiting list for renal transplantation. Table 16.2 lists some of the potential causes of renal failure.

As the kidneys' ability to filter the protein metabolism waste products effectively from the blood or to secrete erythropoietin and/or vitamin D_3 is reduced, the patient develops chronic renal disease. Problems associated with chronic renal failure include hypertension, growth retardation or failure, anemia, chronic edema, congestive heart failure, metabolic/electrolyte imbalances, hyperparathyroidism, bleeding tendencies, chronic infections and slow healing of lacerations, neurological disorders, elevated serum triglycerides, cardiac myopathies, and glucose intolerance (Bergstein, 1996; Frauman & Myers, 1994; Geary & Haka-Ikse, 1989; Lum, 1995). The neurological complications may involve changes in mental alertness and concentration, headaches, muscle weakness, peripheral neuropathies, amnesias, seizures, and encephalopathies (Baron et al., 1995; Bergstein, 1996; Trompeter, Polinsky, Andreoli, & Fennell, 1986; Geary et al., 1980; Uysal, Renda, Saatci, & Yaiaz, 1990).

Neuroimaging studies of patients with chronic renal failure and end-stage renal disease report generalized changes; however, the possibility that these studies were prompted by symptoms of brain pathology raises questions with regard to the representativeness of the findings (Menkes, 1995; Steinberg, Efrat, Pomeranz, & Drukker, 1985). Reductions in head circumference, an index of brain development, have been reported in children with chronic renal failure since infancy (McGraw & Haka-Ikse, 1985). Changes in electroencephalograms, electromyograms, and evoked potentials have also been reported in children with chronic renal failure (Berretta, Holbrook, & Haller, 1986; Menkes, 1995).

A rare complication referred to as *dialysis dementia* has been reported in both children and adults who undergo hemodialysis. This condition includes progressive loss of speech and other cognitive functions, myoclonus, seizures and personality changes. It is often progressive and can be fatal. Although the precise cause of this syndrome is unknown, aluminum toxicity from the dialysate may be a contributing factor (Andreoli, Bergstein, & Sherrard, 1984).

Treatment

Medical Management of Renal Failure

Before a patient reaches end-stage renal disease, medical management is instituted to treat the side effects of decreasing renal function. Medical management includes pharmacological interventions to reduce hypertension (antihypertensive medications); dietary restrictions to reduce intake of sodium, potassium, or phosphate; use of dietary phosphate binders to re-

TABLE 16.2. Potential Causes of Renal Failure

Primary renal disease	Nonrenal disorders
Anomalous kidney structures or vessels	Obstructive uropathies
Cortex	Burns
Medulla	Blood loss due to hemorrhage
Acute/chronic infections	Hypotensive crises
Renal tumors	Cardiac failure
Acute tubular necrosis	Hypoxic events
Hemorrhagic ischemia	
Vascular coagulation of cortex or venous supply	

Note. Data from Lum (1995).

duce elevated serum phosphate levels; dietary restriction of protein intake when blood uria nitrogen levels are elevated; restrictions in fluid intake; treatment of anemias with recombinant human erythropoietin; and management of urinary tract infections (Baron et al., 1995; Lum, 1995; Sinaiko, 1994). A particular difficulty in treating children is to ensure that dietary restrictions and other management procedures do not compromise growth (Kohaut, 1995). This task is somewhat easier with infants and young children, whose food intake is more easily provided by the family; dietary compliance often becomes problematic in school-age children and adolescents. Parent education regarding compliance with both medications and dietary restrictions is an essential part of treatment (Johnson, 1991; Beck et al., 1980).

Dialysis

When renal failure progresses to the point at which child has less than 10% of normal GFR, the typical treatment involves institution of one of several types of dialysis. Dialysis essentially provides an alternate means of kidney function. Two types of dialysis procedures are currently available for infants, children, and adolescents in end-stage renal disease: *hemodialysis* and *peritoneal dialysis*. Therapies instituted recently for children and adults on dialysis include erythropoietin therapy to treat associated anemias (Nissenson, 1994), as well as low doses of growth hormone therapy to improve the velocity of height growth (Fine, 1997; Schwartz et al., 1995).

Hemodialysis is a procedure involving circulation of the child's blood through an artificial kidney. The artificial kidney filters excess water and waste products across a semipermeable membrane into a solution called the *dialysate*, which is designed to match the electrolyte balance of the patient's blood. In this procedure, a surgical fistula is created to provide access to an artery and a vein via a cannula. An alternate method is to insert a semipermanent catheter into a large vein, typically the subclavian. The typical hemodialysis session lasts between 3 and 4 hours. During this time, the child may eat food that is prohibited in his or her routine diet (e.g., potato chips). The child may also sleep, visit with other patients, or play quietly. Despite these opportunities, the child may be tired following completion of a dialysis session. Medical complications of hemodialysis include pain at the site of cannulation of the fistula, infections or clotting of the fistula or semipermanent catheter, and a metabolic dialysis disequilibrium (which on rare occasions can precipitate seizures). Other medical treatments are designed to promote growth in height, to manage chronic fatigue related to anemia, and to maintain the child's health while he or she awaits an organ transplant (Kaiser, Polinsky, Stover, Morgenstern, & Baluarte, 1994). Family stress can result from the need to travel to a dialysis center three or four times per week. Because one parent often takes on this role, economic consequences may result from the loss of this parent's income. Siblings may also be stressed by frequent travel or role changes (Foulkes, Boggs, Fennell, & Skibinski, 1993).

Peritoneal dialysis involves the use of the peritoneal cavity as the filter. Typically, a catheter is surgically placed through the abdominal wall into the peritoneum. Dialysate is then infused into the peritoneal cavity via this catheter. When the dialysate is removed, excess water and waste products (which have diffused across the peritoneal membrane) are removed. A machine is often used to flush the dialysate into the peritoneum across the peritoneal membrane and to extract the filtered dialysate. The latter procedure, referred to as *continuous cycling peritoneal dialysis* (CCPD), is frequently carried out at night while the patient is asleep. If the procedure is performed manually, it is referred to as *continuous ambulatory peritoneal dialysis* (CAPD). The major advantages of these continuous methods of dialysis are that the vascular complications of hemodialysis are avoided, infections are less frequent, the need for medications to slow blood clotting (e.g., heparin) is avoided, and the method can be adapted to younger children and infants. Typically, peritoneal dialysis is performed at home and requires parent training both in the dialysis procedures and in infection control. Parental difficulties with these aspects of treatment preclude some children from receiving CCPD or CAPD.

Transplantation

Whereas the goal of dialysis is to provide a substitute for failing kidneys, the goal of renal transplantation is to replace the failed kidneys with a new kidney in order to promote cognitive and physical development (Davis, Chang, & Nevins, 1990). A suitable replacement kidney is obtained from one of two sources: a living related donor (typically a member of the immediate family) or a cadaver donor. Kidney transplantation is most likely to be successfully when the donated kidney is immunologically compatible with the recipient, and compatibility is typically highest with living related donors. The donated kidney is surgically removed, leaving the donor with one functioning kidney. After immunological assays are completed, the donor is carefully screened for any medical conditions that might compromise life with one kidney.

The donated kidney, which is typically placed into the abdominal cavity of the recipient, will change in size to accommodate the body mass of the recipient (Urizar, 1996). Prior to receipt of the donor organ, the failed kidneys are removed, and the patient is fully dependent on dialysis. Once transplantation occurs, the recipient is placed on immunosuppressant medication to prevent organ rejection and is closely monitored for signs of rejection of the donated kidney. Immunosuppressant medications typically utilized to prevent rejection are prednisone, cyclosporine, and azathioprine. These medications are delivered systemically and can often have troublesome side effects, such as those listed in Table 16.3 (see also Grimm & Ettenger, 1992).

TABLE 16.3. Common Side Effects of Immunosuppressant Medications

Medication	Side effects
Steroids	Truncal obesity
	Hypertension
	Hirsutism
	Osteopenia
	Osteonecrosis
	Growth failure
	Cataracts
Azathioprine	Decreased white blood cell production
	Anemia
	Alopecia
	Liver dysfunction
Cyclosporine	Hypertension
	Gastroenteritis
	Hirsutism
	Renal dysfunction
	Headaches
	Seizures (rarely)

Note. Data from Baron, Fennell, and Voeller (1995).

The donated kidney may be rejected despite immunosuppressant treatment. Rejection either can occur acutely, or can take a chronic course involving gradual reduction in renal function, hypertension, and increased spilling of protein into the urine. Most rejections appear to be consequences of immunological factors. Occasionally, however, the vascular supply to the donated kidney is the primary site of rejection. When rejection occurs, dialysis will need to be resumed, the rejected organ must be surgically removed, and the child must again be placed on a waiting list to receive a second donor organ. When rejection is taking place (whether on an acute or a chronic basis), both the patient and family are under a great deal of stress, and supportive family or individual therapy may be necessary. Anxiety and depression following renal rejection are commonly encountered by the attending physician and other medical or transplant team members. For this reason, many dialysis centers and kidney transplant teams routinely include social workers, psychiatrists, and psychologists to provide the needed interventions prior to, during, and following organ transplantation (Berger, 1978; Paluszny, DeBeukelaer, & Rowane, 1991; Rodrigue et al., 1997).

NEUROPSYCHOLOGICAL AND PSYCHOLOGICAL STUDIES OF CHRONIC RENAL FAILURE, DIALYSIS, AND TRANSPLANTATION

Overview

Although renal dialysis and kidney transplantation have been available to the pediatric age group since the 1960s, few studies have examined the neuropsychological effects of chronic renal failure and its treatment. The lack of research in this area is unfortunate, especially given clear indications that renal disease can exert direct negative effects on brain functioning, can induce a variety of neurological complications, and can indirectly alter brain functioning as a secondary consequence of systemic disease (Baron et al., 1995; Berg & Linton, 1989; Frauman & Myers, 1994; Lawry, Brouhard, & Cunningham, 1994). Initial studies of children undergoing dialysis focused primarily on psychological adjustment to the rigors of treatment. By the mid-1970s, however, researchers also began to examine intellectual functioning in this patient group. Some of the first neuropsychological studies of more specific areas of cognitive functioning, such as attention, memory, visual–spatial skills, and speed of responding, were undertaken in the mid-1980s and early 1990s. A summary of the neuropsychological deficits documented in these and more recent studies is given in Table 16.4. Research that has examined the neuropsychological effects of chronic renal failure, dialysis treatment, and transplantation is reviewed in greater detail below. The section ends with a consideration of psychosocial effects.

Cognitive Effects of Chronic Renal Failure

Chronic renal failure has a variety of adverse consequences for the developing brain (Bergstein, 1996). In one study of developmental outcomes, Geary and Hoka-Ikse (1989) followed the development of very young children (mean age 1 year, 11 months) over the course of about 1½ years. They found that 10 of the 33 children studied were developmentally delayed (8 mildly and 2 moderately). Growth and development in these children were correlated with their degree of renal dysfunction.

In a more recent study of school-age children, Lawry et al. (1994) compared the IQ scores of children and adolescents ($n = 11$) undergoing dialysis to those of children who had received renal transplantation. Although these researchers failed to detect group dif-

TABLE 16.4. Common Neuropsychological Problems Reported in Children with End-Stage Renal Disease

Intellectual impairments
   Lower performance IQ
   Lower Full Scale IQ

Developmental delays in infants
   Mental
   Motor

Memory disorders
   Impaired short-term memory
   Verbal learning problems

Attentional dysfunction
   Impaired immediate span
   Slowed reaction times
   Errors of impulsivity on vigilance tests
   Errors of inattention on vigilance tests

Visuospatial and Visuoconstructional disorders
   Impaired two-dimensional construction
   Impaired two-dimensional copying

ferences in IQ, they found that the dialysis patients performed more poorly than the transplant group on standardized achievement tests of written language. Other investigators have reported mean IQ scores in the low-average range for groups of children with end-stage renal disease (Bock et al., 1989; Crittenden, Holliday, Potter, Piel, & Salvatierra, 1980; Crittenden, Holliday, Piel, & Potter, 1985; Fennell, Rasbury, Fennell, & Morris, 1984).

The members of an identical twin pair discordant for renal disease ("prune belly syndrome") also differed on standardized intellectual testing, with the sick twin scoring significantly below the healthy twin (Fennell & Rasbury, 1980). Later follow-up of the twin pair revealed that the affected twin had continuing problems in intellectual functioning, attention, memory, visuospatial, and visuomotor skills. The latter impairments were evident even after the affected twin received a successful transplant (Morris, Fennell, Fennell, & Rasbury, 1985).

Cognitive deficits have also been reported in studies comparing children with chronic renal failure to normal children matched on age, sex, and socioeconomic status. These deficits include delayed visuomotor copying skills and visuospatial constructional skills, impaired verbal learning, and problems in short-term memory (Fennell, Fennell, Mings, & Morris, 1986; Fennell et al., 1989, 1990a, 1990b, 1990c).

Cognitive Effects of Dialysis

Although studies of the effects of dialysis on intellectual and other neuropsychological functions have been conducted since the 1970s, most research in this area has focused on adult patients. In general, studies of pediatric patients have not included children whose renal disease involved significant neurological complications, such as cerebral hemorrhage, embolic infarcts, dialysis encephalopathy, or dialysis disequilibrium (Baron et al., 1995). In one such study, Bird and Semmler (1986) examined 10 infants who were placed on CAPD/CCPD for congenital renal disease and found that all 10 patients had significant developmental delays (Bayley Scales of Infant Development indices below 60).

Children who do not have significant complications and who are treated with hemodialysis may have more positive outcomes. We (Rasbury, Fennell, Fennell, & Morris, 1986) compared 18 children undergoing hemodialysis to 18 age- and IQ-matched normal controls. The children on hemodialysis were tested after dialysis. The investigation failed to find group differences either on measures of verbal learning and immediate memory for a 10-item word list, or on two subtests of the Cattell Culture Fair Test of intelligence (Lezak, 1995). These results are contrary to reports of improved memory and attention in adult patients following hemodialysis (Heilman, Moyer, Melendez, Schwartz, & Miller, 1975). The Rasbury et al. (1986) findings, however, are similar to those of an earlier study by our group (Rasbury, Fennell, Eastman, Gavin, & Richards, 1979). In this study, the same group of 14 children undergoing hemodialysis were compared to 14 sex- and race-matched normal controls. The groups were not equated on IQ, and measures included the Culture Fair Test, a verbal learning measure similar to the one used in the Rasbury et al. (1986) study, and an auditory continuous-performance test (CPT) to assess vigilance. As in the Rasbury et al. (1986) study, the results failed to reveal any group differences on pre- and posttesting of the dialysis patients and the normal control group.

Studies comparing children treated with CAPD to children treated with hemodialysis have suggested that CAPD patients perform better on selected neuropsychological measures (Baum et al., 1982). In a series of studies of different treatments for end-stage renal disease by our own research group at the University of Florida (Fennell et al., 1986, 1989, 1990a, 1990b, 1990c), children on CAPD performed better than children on hemodialysis on tests of immediate memory for digits and word lists. Children on CAPD also showed higher levels of verbal learning on a verbal selective reminding task and made fewer errors of omission and commission on a visual CPT. The two treatment groups did not differ in visuospatial skills, although both groups were impaired on these measures. The difference between the findings of this series of studies and the earlier results of Baum et al. (1982) may lie in the different and more comprehensive neuropsychological battery employed by our University of Florida group.

In addition to possible cognitive benefits obtained with CAPD as compared to intermittent hemodialysis, CAPD may have physical benefits for the child. Several recent studies suggest that children on CAPD maintain a better growth rate than children on hemodialysis, have lower blood urea nitrogen levels, and show improved metabolic acidosis (Kaiser et al., 1994; Warady, Kriley, Lovell, Farrell, & Hellerstein, 1988).

Cognitive Effects of Renal Transplantation

Kidney transplantation has been available to infants, children, and adolescents since the mid-1960s. It is one of the most frequently employed types of organ transplant procedures, and lessons learned in managing allograft rejection following kidney transplantation were subsequently applied to children undergoing heart, lung, and liver transplants. The effects of kidney transplantation on cognition, growth, and development of motor skills, academic achievement, and social functioning have been summarized in several previous reviews (Bock et al., 1989; Frauman & Myers, 1994; Hobbs & Sexson, 1993; So et al., 1987; Stewart, Kennard, Waller, & Fixler, 1994). According to these reviews, successful renal transplant improves growth; maintains normal mental and motor development; and improves performance on neuropsychological measures of memory and learning, attention, simple and choice reaction time, and visual vigilance (Davis et al., 1990; Najarian et al., 1990; Fennell et al., 1990a, 1990b, 1990c).

The findings of our own research group at the University of Florida have been more mixed. In one study (Fennell et al., 1990a), for example, we found persistent problems in visuospatial constructional skills (as assessed by the Object Assembly subtest of the Wechsler scales and a visuomotor task) following successful renal transplantation in a cohort of pediatric patients. Potential participants in the Florida series were excluded if any known neurological events had occurred in the course of illness or treatment. Since many of the children in this series of studies had been suffering from kidney failure since early childhood, a two-stage model was proposed to account for the effect of successful renal transplantation on neuropsychological functioning. In this model, effective dialysis or restoration of near-normal renal functioning via CAPD or renal transplantation was most likely to restore functions that were relatively state-dependent (e.g., attention, memory, reaction time, and vigilance). In contrast, early-onset renal disease was hypothesized to have permanently altered the course of normal development of some brain functions, resulting in more stable developmental delays that would not be as readily altered by the improved physiological functioning provided by CAPD or renal transplantation (Fennell et al., 1990a). The persistent deficits in visuospatial and visuomotor functioning observed in the Fennell et al. (1990a) study were interpreted as providing support for this model.

Correlations between neuropsychological performance and medical variables were also examined in the Florida series (Fennell et al., 1990b). Performance on tests of verbal memory and learning was significantly correlated with measures of blood urea nitrogen, creatinine clearance, and systolic blood pressure. Age at onset of renal failure was not related to any of the neuropsychological measures.

Patterns of neuropsychological performance were examined as well (Fennell et al., 1990c). In this study, treatment groups (hemodialysis, CAPD, renal transplant) were followed every 6 months for 24 months. Each patient was matched to a normal control on the basis of age, sex, IQ, and socioeconomic status, and the control subject was tested over the same intervals as the patient. According to correlational analyses, patterns of associations among test scores were different in some of the treatment groups compared to their controls. For example, errors of omission on the visual CPT and speed of choice reaction time were significantly related to immediate and short-term memory scores for the renal patients, but not for the normal controls. We suggested that several domains of neuropsychological functioning in children with renal disease were more interdependent than in normal children and more affected by level of arousal. Thus even successful renal transplantation may have subtle effects on neuropsychological performance.

The recent findings that neither hemodialysis or CAPD can fully prevent cognitive or other developmental delays (e.g., growth, sexual maturation) has led to the suggestion that children in chronic renal failure or end-stage renal disease might fare better if they received transplants sooner. As yet, however, there are no published studies comparing the efficacy of early versus late renal transplantation on later neuropsychological functioning. The feasibility of undertaking longitudinal studies of this nature in the future will depend in part on the availability of suitable donor kidneys.

Psychosocial Functioning in Chronic Renal Failure and Its Treatment

Despite the frequency of dialysis treatments and renal transplantation in the pediatric age group, relatively few recent studies have focused on the psychosocial functioning of these children (Baron et al., 1995). As noted earlier, medical management of chronic renal failure, dialysis treatments, and renal transplantation are all complex processes that can place a burden on the patient's and family's coping resources. Psychological responses to renal failure and to its therapy may result in the development of behavioral disorders such as noncompliance (Johnson, 1991; La Greca, 1988; Beck et al., 1980), or even in frank psychiatric symptomatology (Breslau, 1985; Marshall, 1979).

A child who suffers from chronic renal failure or who undergoes renal transplantation is required to adhere to a difficult medical regimen; this often leads to periodic or chronic problems in compliance (Varni & Babani, 1986). Noncompliance in turn may adversely affect the child's health and precipitate increased stress among family members, including parents and siblings (Foulkes et al., 1993; Shulman, 1983). In a recent review of studies of compliance within the pediatric age group, Bearison (1994) noted that noncompliance with medical treatments, even in cases of serious chronic illnesses in children (e.g., cancer, renal disease, asthma), occurs in about 50% of individuals participating in published studies. This high rate of noncompliance is observed whether medications are self-administered or are given by parents to younger children. Bearison argues that there is no compelling evidence for a relationship between the degree of medical noncompliance and such factors as illness severity, lack of education about the need for medical treatment, the scheduling of doctors' visits, the need for medication administration, adverse side effects of therapy, or even demographics. His conclusions are consistent with findings from studies of compliance among pediatric renal patients, as well as with the relatively small effects of parent education programs, age, sex, and social supports on compliance with medical care (Beck et al., 1980; Kaplan & DeNour, 1979; Korsch, Fine, & Francis-Negrete, 1978; Foulkes et al., 1993).

Families of children with chronic medical conditions such as renal disease are confronted with numerous stressors. Medical crises, medical compliance, financial and role strains, educational needs, and changes in social support can all lead to disruptions in family life (Cole, 1991; Drotar, 1981; La Greca, 1990; Paluszny et al., 1991; Siegal & Hudson, 1992). Studies of the psychosocial consequences of illness for the child and family thus require consideration of multiple and potentially interactive influences on outcome. Although several multidimensional models have been proposed (Daniels, Moos, Billings, & Miller, 1987; Foulkes et al., 1993), various methodological problems continue to impede research in this area (Stewart et al., 1994). Harper (1991) notes that most studies of childhood chronic illness focus only on psychopathological responses to illness and tend to overlook responses that fail to meet predetermined classification schemes. The effects of a child's age at the time of illness onset or subsequent psychosocial development is also rarely studied. Harper argues for more studies of adaptation to the chronic illness, as well as for a greater focus on social interactions with peers as determinants of a child's coping skills.

In parallel with studies of psychological or psychiatric disorders in adults with chronic renal failure (Marshall, 1979; Sampson, 1975), children with this condition have higher than normal rates of depression and anxiety disorders. In one exemplary investigation, Van der vlist, Woeff, Nanta, and Van de Ven (1989) utilized drawings to solicit responses from children undergoing treatment with hemodialysis. Children's responses included feelings of being physically different from other children and of lowered self-esteem, anxiety, and sad mood. These findings are similar to those of earlier studies of psychological disorders among pediatric hemodialysis patients (Korsch, Fine, Grushkin, & Negrete, 1971; Korsch et al., 1978).

More recently, Fukunishi, Honda, Kamiyama, and Ito (1993) compared a group of 23 pediatric patients on CAPD to a matched sample of 23 healthy controls. Using a structured diagnostic psychiatric interview for the children and a family environment self-report measure completed by the mothers, they found that the CAPD group showed a significantly higher rate of separation anxiety disorder. Mothers of CAPD patients reported lower rates of independence and achievement for their children than did mothers of the healthy controls.

In a follow-up study, Fukunishi and Kudo (1995) compared these same 23 CAPD patients and 27 pediatric renal transplant patients to 27 age-matched healthy controls. Separation anxiety disorder was diagnosed in 17 of the CAPD patients and in 5 of the transplant patients. School maladjustment problems were also more common among the CAPD patients. Again, families of the renal patients had lower scores on tests assessing orientation to independence and achievement, compared to the healthy control families. In contrast to the latter results, the sample of 17 CAPD patients examined retrospectively by Hulstijn-Dirkmaat (1989) adapted well to their treatment. The families studied by Hulstijn-Dirkmaat did, however, report increased levels of stress related to the patients' eating problems and difficulties adhering to medication regimens.

Although depressive symptoms have been reported among pediatric patients who are undergoing treatment for end-stage renal disease (Shulman, 1983), a potential confound in these clinical reports is the effect of chronic illness per se on many of the neurovegetative symptoms of depression. For example, fatigue, appetite, and sleep disturbances; cognitive slowing; and attentional problems are common side effects of diminished renal functioning and the uremic state (Bergstein, 1996; Menkes, 1995). To date, however, no published studies of children with end-stage renal disease have attempted to disentangle these potential confounds. Management of the anemia associated with dialysis therapy, and the attendant improvement in energy levels and in growth and development, may well diminish the frequency of perceived depressive disorders in these patients (Nissenson, 1994). Similarly, depressive or anxiety disorders related to *specific* aspects of treatment, such as allograft rejection, hospitalization for transplantation, and initiation of dialysis therapy, have not been well studied in children (Baron et al., 1995). Studies to date have also failed to examine interactions of neuropsychological deficits with the development of behavioral or psychological disorders in either pediatric or adult renal patients (Hart & Kreutzer, 1988). Finally, there have been no longitudinal studies of psychosocial adjustment in children who undergo dialysis and successful renal transplantation. The relationship of age-related factors to psychosocial outcomes in these patients is largely unknown.

SUMMARY OF RESEARCH FINDINGS AND FUTURE DIRECTIONS

The preceding review reveals a relatively small literature on the neuropsychological and psychological functioning of children and adolescents with chronic renal failure who undergo dialysis treatments or receive renal transplants. Although this research permits few firm conclusions, several findings are worthy of special emphasis:

1. Chronic renal failure can lead to a number of serious systemic medical problems, placing the brain and central nervous system at risk for metabolic toxicities, vascular disease, retarded growth, and development of premature encephalopathy with atrophic changes.

2. Congenital renal disease seems to be especially disadvantageous to neuropsychological development.

3. The cognitive problems found in infants and young children with chronic renal failure, including delays in mental and motor development, coincide with problems in general physical growth.

4. School-age children and adolescents with chronic renal failure also experience a higher rate of intellectual impairment compared to siblings and to normal controls. Specific neuropsychological sequelae of chronic renal failure in older school-age samples include weaknesses in verbal memory and learning, slowed reaction times, attentional disorders, and visuospatial constructional difficulties. Whether nonverbal memory and learning are affected has yet to be determined in this patient group.

5. Children and adolescents treated with chronic hemodialysis generally perform less well on neuropsychological tests than do children receiving other forms of dialysis (CAPD, CCPD).

6. Successful transplantation appears to provide the best outcome for children of all ages. Fewer cognitive and neuropsychological problems are noted in these patients than in either children who receive conventional medical management of chronic renal failure or children who enter some type of dialysis treatment.

7. Although psychological adjustment problems have been reported for children undergoing hemodialysis, CAPD, and renal tranplantation, the prevalence of specific psychiatric diagnoses (e.g., depressive or anxiety disorders) is in large part unknown.

8. Noncompliance with the medical regimens associated with the various modes of therapy for end-stage renal disease is a common problem for both the patient and family. It has proved difficult, moreover, to improve compliance rates in this and other types of chronic childhood illness.

9. Finally, there have been no studies of the long-term psychosocial impact of chronic renal failure in the pediatric age group. Information about age-related changes in coping and adaptation is sparse, and any conclusions in this regard would have to be based upon cross-sectional studies of collections of renal patients with varying degrees of neurological and neuropsychological dysfunction.

More research is needed to replicate and clarify many of the findings reported to date on the development of children with chronic renal failure. Studies examining the relationship of neuropsychological outcomes to age at onset of illness and to duration and severity of illness would be especially helpful. The influence of transient versus more permanent neuropsychological dysfunction on coping and adaptation in these children would be another direction for future research. Longitudinal studies of brain structure via nuclear magnetic imaging or functional nuclear magnetic imaging are also needed, to give us a better understanding of the long-term outcome in early-onset chronic renal failure. Models of adaptation and coping developed for other pediatric medical conditions should be systematically tested in studies of renal patients. Lastly, future studies need to examine the quality of life in long-term survivors of childhood renal transplantation. As the age of organ transplant recipients is lowered and the time period between dialysis and transplantation is shortened, longitudinal follow-up of pediatric patients through adolescence and into adulthood becomes even more critical. To date, knowledge of longer-term outcomes of transplantation has been based primarily on retrospective case studies. Larger and more systematic investigations are required to determine how children with transplants progress through these later developmental stages.

REFERENCES

Andreoli, S. P., Bergstein, J. M., & Sherrard, D. J. (1984). Aluminum intoxication from aluminum-containing phosphate binders in children with azotemia not undergoing dialysis. *New England Journal of Medicine, 310,* 1079–1084.

Baron, I. S., Fennell, E. B., & Voeller, K. K. S. (1995). *Pediatric neuropsychology in the medical setting*. New York: Oxford University Press.

Baum, M., Powell, D., Calvin, S., McDaid, T., McHenry, K., Mar, H., & Potter, D. (1982). Continuous ambulatory peritoneal dialysis in children: Comparisons with hemodialysis. *New England Journal of Medicine, 307*, 1537–1542.

Bearison, D. J. (1994). Medical compliance in pediatric oncology. In D. J. Bearison & R. K. Mulhern (Eds.), *Pediatric psychooncology* (pp. 84–98). New York: Oxford University.

Beck, D. D., Fennell, R. S., Yost, R. L., Robinson, J. D., Geary, M. B., & Richard, G. A. (1980). Evaluation of an educational program on compliance with medication regimens in pediatric patients with renal transplants. *Journal of Pediatrics, 96*, 1094–1097.

Berg, R. A., & Linton, J. C. (1989). Neuropsychological sequelae of chronic medical disorders. In C. R. Reynolds & E. Fletcher-Janzen (Eds.), *Handbook of clinical child neuropsychology* (pp. 107–128). New York: Plenum Press.

Berger, M. (1978). The role of the clinical child psychologist in an endstage renal disease program. *Journal of Clinical Child Psychology, 7*, 17–18.

Bergstein, J. M. (1996). Nephrology (sections 1–5). In R. E. Behrman, R. M. Kleigman, & A. M. Arvin (Eds.), *Nelson textbook of pediatrics* (15th ed., pp. 1480–1521). Philadelphia: W. B. Saunders.

Berretta, J. S., Holbrook, C. T., & Haller, J. S. (1986). Chronic renal failure presenting as proximal muscle weakness in a child. *Journal of Child Neurology, 1*, 50–52.

Bird, A. K., & Semmler, C. J. (1986). The early developmental and neurologic sequelae of children with renal failure treated with CAPD/CCPD [Abstract]. *Pediatric Research, 20*, 446.

Bock, G. H., Conners, K., Ruley, J., Samango-Sprouse, C. A., Conry, J. A., Weiss, I., Eng, G., Johnson, E. L., & David, C. T. (1989). Disturbances of brain maturation and neurodevelopment during chronic renal failure in infancy. *Journal of Pediatrics, 114*, 231–238.

Breslau, N. (1985). Psychiatric disorders in children with physical disabilities. *Journal of the American Academy of Child Psychiatry, 24*, 87–94.

Cole, B. R. (1991). The psychosocial implications of pre-emptive transplantation. *Pediatric Nephrology, 5*, 158–161.

Crittenden, M. R., Holliday, M. A., Piel, C. F., & Potter, D. E. (1985). Intellectual development of children with renal insufficiency and end stage renal disease. *International Journal of Pediatric Nephrology, 6*, 275–280.

Crittenden, M. R., Holliday, M. A., Potter, D. E., Piel, C. F., & Salvatierra, O. (1980). IQ in children with renal failure [Abstract]. *Pediatric Research, 14*, 617.

Daniels, D., Moos, R. H., Billings, R. H., & Miller, J. J. (1987). Psychosocial risk and resistance factors among children with chronic illness, healthy siblings and healthy controls. *Journal of Abnormal Child Psychology, 15*, 295–308.

Davis, I. D., Chang, P., & Nevins, T. E. (1990). Successful renal transplantation accelerates development in young uremic children. *Pediatrics, 86*, 594–600.

Drotar, D. (1981). Psychological perspectives in chronic illnesses. *Journal of Pediatric Psychology, 6*, 211–228.

Fennell, E. B., Fennell, R. S., Mings, E., & Morris, M. K. (1986). The effect of various modes of therapy on cognitive performance in a pediatric population: Preliminary data. *International Journal of Pediatric Nephrology, 7*, 107–112.

Fennell, R. S., Fennell, E. B., Carter, R. L., Mings, E., Klausner, A. B., & Hurst, J. R. (1989). Effects of changing therapy on cognition of children in renal failure. *Child Nephrology and Urology, 9*, 211–219.

Fennell, R. S., Fennell, E. B., Carter, R. L., Mings, E., Klausner, A. B., & Hurst, J. R. (1990a). A longitudinal study of the cognitive function of children with renal failure. *Pediatric Nephrology, 4*, 11–15.

Fennell, R. S., Fennell, E. B., Carter, R. L., Mings, E., Klausner, A. B., & Hurst, J. R. (1990b). Association between renal function and cognition in childhood chronic renal failure. *Pediatric Nephrology, 4*, 16–20.

Fennell, R. S., Fennell, E. B., Carter, R. L., Mings, E., Klausner, A. B., & Hurst, J. R. (1990c). Correlations between performance on neuropsychological tests in children with chronic renal failure. *Child Nephrology and Urology, 10*, 199–204.

Fennell, R. S., & Rasbury, W. C. (1980). Cognitive functioning of identical twins discordant for prune belly syndrome and end stage renal failure. *Journal of Pediatrics, 90*, 41–44.

Fennell, R. S., Rasbury, W. C., Fennell, E. B., & Morris, M. K. (1984). The effects of kidney transplantation on cognitive performance in a pediatric population. *Pediatrics, 74*, 273–278.

Fine, R. N. (1997). Growth hormone treatment of children with chronic renal insufficiency, end-stage renal disease and following renal transplantation: Update 1997. *Journal of Pediatric Endocrinology and Metabolism, 10*(4), 361–370.

Foulkes, L. M., Boggs, S. R., Fennell, R. S., & Skibinski, R. (1993). Social support, family variables, and compliance in renal transplant children. *Pediatric Nephrology, 7*, 185–188.

Frauman, A. C., & Myers, J. T. (1994). Cognitive, psychosocial and physical development in infants and children with end stage renal disease. *Advances in Renal Replacement Therapy, 1*, 49–54.

Fukunishi, I., Honda, M., Kamiyama, Y., & Ito, A. (1993). Anxiety disorders and pediatric continuous ambulatory peritoneal dialysis. *Child Psychiatry and Human Development, 24*, 59–64.

Fukunishi, I., & Kudo, H. (1995). Psychiatric problems of pediatric end-stage renal failure. *General Hospital Psychiatry, 17*, 32–36.

Geary, D. F., Fennell, R. S., III, Andriola, M., Gudat, J., Rodgers, B. M., & Richard, G. A. (1980). Encephalopathy in children with chronic renal failure. *Journal of Pediatrics, 90*, 41–44.

Geary, D. F., & Halka-Ikse, K. (1989). Neurodevelopmental progress of young children with chronic renal disease. *Pediatrics, 84*(1), 68–72.

Grimm, P. C., & Ettenger, R. (1992). Pediatric renal transplantation. *Advances in Pediatrics, 39*, 441–493.

Harper, D. (1991). Paradigms for investigating rehabilitation and adaptation to childhood disability and chronic illness. *Journal of Pediatric Psychology, 16*, 533–542.

Hart, R. P., & Kreutzer, J. S. (1988). Renal system. In R. E. Tarter, D. H. Van Thiel, & K. L. Edwards (Eds.), *Medical neuropsychology* (pp. 99–120). New York: Plenum Press.

Heilman, K. M., Moyer, R. S., Melendez, F., Schwartz, H. D., & Miller, B. D. (1975). A memory defect in uremic encephalopathy. *Journal of Neurological Science, 26*, 245–249.

Hobbs, S. A., & Sexson, S. B. (1993). Cognitive development and learning in the pediatric organ transplant recipient. *Journal of Learning Disabilities, 26*, 104–113.

Holliday, M. A., Bryant, T. M., & Avner, E. D. (1994). *Pediatric nephrology* (4th ed.). Baltimore: Williams & Wilkins.

Hulstijn-Dirkmaat, I. (1989). Continuous ambulatory peritoneal dialysis in children and family stress. *International Journal of Adolescent Medicine and Health, 4*, 19–25.

Johnson, S. B. (1991). Compliance in pediatric psychology. In J. H. Johnson & S. B. Johnson (Eds.), *Advances in child health psychology* (pp. 249–264). Gainesville: University of Florida Press.

Kaiser, B. A., Polinsky, M. S., Stover, J., Morgenstern, B. Z., & Baluarte, H. J. (1994). Growth of children following the initiation of dialysis: A comparison of three dialysis modalities. *Pediatric Nephrology, 8*, 733–738.

Kaplan De-Nour, A. (1979). Adolescents' adjustments to chronic hemodialysis. *American Journal of Psychiatry, 136*, 430–433.

Kohaut, E. C. (1995). Chronic renal disease and growth in childhood. *Current Opinion in Pediatrics, 7*, 171–175.

Korsch, B. M., Fine, R. N., & Francis-Negrete, V. (1978). Noncompliance in children with renal transplants. *Pediatrics, 61*, 872–876.

Korsch, B., Fine, R. N., Grushkin, C. M., & Negrete, V. F. (1971). Experiences with children and their families during extended hemodialysis and kidney transplantation. *Pediatric Clinics of North America, 18*, 625–636.

La Greca, A. M. (1988). Adherence to prescribed medical regimens. In D. K. Routh (Ed.), *Handbook of pediatric psychology* (pp. 299–320). New York: Guilford Press.

La Greca, A. M. (1990). Social consequences of pediatric conditions: Fertile soil for future investigations and interventions. *Journal of Pediatric Psychology, 15*, 185–307.

Lawry, K. W., Brouhard, B. H., & Cunningham, R. J. (1994). Cognitive functioning and school performance in children with renal failure. *Pediatric Nephrology, 8*, 326–329.

Lezak, M. (1995). *Neuropsychological assessment* (3rd ed.). New York: Oxford University Press.

Lum, G. M. (1995). Kidney and urinary tract. In W. W. Hay, J. R. Groothuis, A. R. Hayward, & M. J. Levin (Eds.), *Current pediatric diagnosis and treatment* (12th ed., pp. 683–709). Norwalk, CT: Appleton & Lange.

Marshall, J. (1979). Neuropsychiatric aspects of renal failure. *Journal of Clinical Psychiatry, 40*, 81–85.

McGraw, M. S., & Haka-Ikse, K. (1985). Neurologic–developmental sequelae of chronic renal failure in infancy. *Journal of Pediatrics, 106*, 579–583.

Menkes, J. H. (1995). *Textbook of child neurology* (5th ed.). Baltimore: Williams & Wilkins.

Morris, M. K., Fennell, E. B., Fennell, R. S., & Rasbury, W. C. (1985). A case study of identical twins discordant for renal failure: Longterm neuropsychological deficits. *Developmental Neuropsychology, 1*, 81–92.

Najarian, J. S., Frey, D. J., Matas, A. J., Gillingham, K. J., So, S. S. K., Cook, M., Chavers, B., Mauer, S. M., & Nevins, T. E. (1990). Renal transplantation in infants. *Annals of Surgery, 212*, 353–365.

Nissenson, A. R. (1994). Erythropoietin treatment in peritoneal dialysis patients. *Peritoneal Dialysis International*, *14*(Suppl. 3), 563–569.

Paluszny, M. J., DeBeukelaer, M. M., & Rowane, W. A. (1991). Families coping with the multiple crises of chronic illness. *Loss, Grief and Care*, *5*, 15–26.

Rasbury, W. C., Fennell, R. S., Eastman, B. G., Garin, E. H., & Richards, G. (1979). Cognitive performance of children with renal disease. *Psychological Reports*, *45*, 231–239.

Rasbury, W. C., Fennell, R. S., III, Fennell, E. B., & Morris, M. K. (1986). Cognitive functioning in children with end stage renal disease, pre- and post-dialysis sessions. *International Journal of Pediatric Nephrology*, *7*, 45–50.

Rodrigue, J. R., MacNaughton, K., Hoffman, R., Graham-Pole, J., Andres, J. M., Novak, D. A., & Fennell, R. S. (1997). Transplantation in children: A longitudinal assessment of mothers' stress, coping and perceptions of family functioning. *Psychosomatics*, *38*(5), 478–486.

Sampson, T. F. (1975). The child in renal failure: Emotional impact of treatment on the child and his family. *Journal of the American Academy of Child Psychiatry*, *14*, 462–476.

Schwartz, I. D., Warady, B. A., Buchanan, C. L., Reed, L., Hussey, L. M., Howard, C. P., Hellerstein, S., & Grunt, J. A. (1995). "Low-dose" growth hormone therapy during peritoneal dialysis or following renal transplantation. *Pediatric Nephrology*, *9*, 320–324.

Shulman, J. L. (1983). Coping with major disease—child, family and pediatrician. *Pediatrics*, *102*, 988–991.

Siegel, L. J., & Hudson, B. O. (1992). Hospitalization and medical care of children. In C. E. Walker & M. C. Roberts (Eds.), *Handbook of clinical child psychology* (2nd ed., pp. 845–858). New York: Wiley.

Sinaiko, A. (1994). Treatment of hypertension in children. *Pediatric Nephrology*, *8*, 603–609.

So, S. K., Chang, P. N., Najarian, J. S., Mauer, S. M., Simmons, R. L., & Nevins, T. E. (1987). Growth and development in infants after renal transplantation. *Journal of Pediatrics*, *110*, 343–350.

Steinberg, A., Efrat, R., Pomeranz, A., & Drukker, A. (1985). Computerized tomography of the brain in children with chronic renal failure. *International Journal of Pediatric Nephrology*, *6*, 121–126.

Stewart, S. M., Kennard, B. D., Waller, D. A., & Fixler, D. (1994). Cognitive function in children who receive organ transplantation. *Health Psychology*, *13*, 3–13.

Trompeter, R. S., Polinsky, M. S., Andreoli, M., & Fennell, R. S. (1986). Neurological complications of renal failure. *American Journal of Kidney Disease*, *7*, 318–328.

Urizar, R. E. (1996). Renal transplantation. In R. E. Behrman, R. M. Kliegman, & A. M. Arvin (Eds.), *Nelson textbook of pediatrics* (15th ed., pp. 1522–1526). Philadelphia: W. B. Saunders.

Uysal, S., Renda, Y., Saatci, U., & Yaaz, K. (1990). Neurological complications in chronic renal failure: A retrospective study. *Clinical Pediatrics*, *29*(9), 510–514.

Van der vlist, E., Wolff, E. D., Nanta, J., & Van de Ven, A. P. (1989). Psychosocial experiences of children on dialysis and other renal transplantation illustrated by picture drawing. *International Journal of Adolescent Medicine and Health*, *4*, 45–50.

Varni, J. W., & Babani, L. (1986). Long-term adherence to health care regimens in pediatric chronic disorders. In N. A. Krasnegor, J. D. Arasteh, & M. F. Cataldo (Eds.), *Child health behavior: A behavioral pediatrics perspective* (pp. 502–520). New York: Wiley.

Warady, B. A., Kriley, M., Lovell, H., Farrell, S. E., & Hellerstein, S. (1988). Growth and development of infants with end-stage renal disease receiving long-term peritoneal dialysis. *Journal of Pediatrics*, *112*, 714–719.

17

HUMAN IMMUNODEFICIENCY VIRUS

MARGARET B. PULSIFER
ELIZABETH H. AYLWARD

The first pediatric case of human immunodeficiency virus (HIV) infection was reported to the Centers for Disease Control (CDC) in 1982, about 18 months after the first case report in adults (Rogers et al., 1987). Thus, in comparison with many other pediatric diseases and developmental disorders, HIV is relatively new, and research regarding its effects on development is still evolving. Over the course of the epidemic, the impact of HIV and acquired immune deficiency syndrome (AIDS) on development has been changing—both as the nature of the epidemic has changed (e.g., an increased proportion of infants infected perinatally vs. the proportion of children infected via transfusion), and as treatment has been introduced to postpone the appearance of symptoms in some children and to alleviate or even reverse symptoms in others. As a result, findings from the earliest studies regarding the prevalence and severity of neurodevelopmental impairment in HIV-infected infants and children may not be applicable to the current population of HIV-infected children. In addition to the changing face of the epidemic, changes in diagnostic criteria and terminology (e.g., use of such terms as *AIDS*-related complex) make it difficult to apply findings from earlier studies to our current situation. Despite these and many other obstacles to research in this population, our understanding of neurodevelopment in HIV-infected infants and children is becoming increasingly clear, as are the implications of this devastating epidemic for the children, their families, and society as a whole.

CHARACTERISTICS OF PEDIATRIC HIV INFECTION

Incidence/Prevalence

As of December 1998, 8,461 children under the age of 13 years had been diagnosed with AIDS, accounting for approximately 1% of the total number of reported AIDS cases in the United States (CDC, 1998). Most of these children were African American (58%) or Hispanic (23%). The majority (85%) resided in large metropolitan areas (≥500,000 population), and 57% of cases were reported from New York, Florida, New Jersey, and California (CDC, 1998). As of December 1998, 91% of children with AIDS had been infected through mother-to-infant (vertical) transmission, 7% through contaminated blood or blood products (horizontal transmission), and 2% with no specific risk factor (CDC, 1998). When present, maternal HIV infection was associated most often with injection drug use (36%) or sexual contact with an at-risk partner (33%) (CDC, 1998).

During 1998, the rates of reported pediatric AIDS cases from all causes were 3.2 for African Americans, 0.9 for Hispanics, and 0.3 for other racial/ethnic groups per 100,000 children (CDC, 1998). This represents a dramatic reduction in incidence from 1996 and previous years. Prior to 1985, a major source of HIV infection for both children and adults was through blood transfusion or replacement coagulation factor, which resulted in 12,000 cases of HIV infection. After 1985, implementation of HIV-1 antibody testing of the blood supply caused a steep decline in such horizontal HIV transmission. At present, the majority of all new pediatric cases of HIV infection have involved mother-to-infant transmission either *in utero*, intrapartum, or through breast feeding. There is some evidence that most perinatal transmission occurs around the intrapartum or very late prenatal period, and 12–14% may be related to breastfeeding (Fowler, 1997). Perinatal transmission of HIV infection was substantially reduced subsequent to 1994–1995, with the publication in 1994 by the Public Health Service of guidelines for treatment with zidovudine (an antiretroviral drug formerly called azidothymidine or AZT), and of recommendations in 1995 for HIV counseling and voluntary testing of pregnant women. Partially as a result of these measures, the incidence of perinatally acquired AIDS in the United States declined 43% between 1992 and 1996, from 8.4 to 4.8 per 100,000 births (CDC, 1997). The 1992 rate represents the peak rate of perinatal transmission to date. Incidence figures for cases of pediatric AIDS undoubtedly under represent overall HIV infection rates, as many HIV-infected infants and children may not show symptoms severe enough to warrant a diagnosis of AIDS.

In the absence of zidovudine treatment (prior to 1994), data have suggested vertical transmission rates of about 15–30% (CDC, 1995). If the prevalence of HIV infection among childbearing women is relatively stable at 1.6–1.7 per 1,000 (CDC, 1995), and approximately 7,000 infants are born each year to HIV-infected mothers, then it can be estimated that approximately 1,000–2,000 infected infants would be born to untreated mothers each year. Multi-center treatment studies by the Pediatric AIDS Clinical Trials Group have found that administration of zidovudine during pregnancy can reduce the mother-to-infant transmission rate of HIV infection from 25.5% to 8.3% (Connor et al., 1994). Under ideal conditions, universal zidovudine treatment could eliminate as many as two-thirds (1,200) of vertically acquired HIV infections annually in the United States (Davis et al., 1995).

Several risk factors have been found to increase the likelihood of perinatal transmission of HIV. Such factors include decreased gestational age (Goedert et al., 1989), low infant birth weight <2,500 g (Landesman et al., 1996), increased maternal viral load (Fowler, 1997; Pitt et al., 1997), and obstetrical risk factors such as illicit drug use during pregnancy, fetal membrane rupture of more than four hours (Landesman et al., 1996; Fowler, 1997), and mode of delivery. Recent studies have found that elective cesarean section is associated with lower perinatal HIV transmission rate than emergency cesarean or vaginal delivery (Mandelbrot et al., 1998).

While there have been significant reductions in both vertical and horizontal transmission of HIV in the United States in recent years, the problem is still a major pediatric health care issue both here and in other countries. As of December 1998, 12.1 million women and 1.2 million children worldwide were living with HIV infection; of these, approximately 95% live in developing countries (UNAIDS, 1998). In 1998, 2.5 million people worldwide died from HIV infection, including 2 million adults and 510,000 children younger than 15 years of age (UNAIDS, 1998).

Diagnosis

It is important to note that all infants born to HIV-infected women carry passively acquired maternal HIV antibodies; as a result, they almost always present with a positive test for antibodies during the neonatal period (Mellins et al., 1994). Thus a positive test for antibodies is not necessarily indicative of infection in infants younger than 15 months. Infants who initially test seropositive and then revert to seronegative status are termed seroreverters. Several studies have demonstrated no developmental abnormalities in seroreverters when these are compared to seronegative controls who are appropriately matched on socioeconomic variables (Aylward, Butz, Hutton, Joyner, & Vogelhut, 1992; Nozyce et al., 1994; Msellati et al., 1993; Wachtel et al., 1993). As will be discussed later, infants who are seroreverters often serve as control subjects in studies of development in HIV-infected children. Until recently, it was difficult to ascertain an infant's infection status before 15 months of age. It is now possible to measure HIV directly by culture for the virus or by polymerase chain reaction (PCR) for HIV-1 DNA sequences, in order to diagnose infants younger than 15 months of age. HIV infection is classified as transfusion-associated if there is a history of having received a transfusion of blood, blood components, or tissue between 1977 and 1985 without other reported risk factors.

Natural History

When socioeconomic variables are controlled for, HIV-infected infants do not differ at birth from seronegative infants on clinical measures such as gestational age, birthweight, and head circumference (European Collaborative Study, 1991; Johnson et al., 1989; Pollack et al., 1996), and most infants have no disease manifestations at birth (Falloon, Eddy, Wiener, & Pizzo, 1989). Both growth and neurodevelopment have been found to be correlated with HIV viral load; infants with high plasma HIV RNA copies at 6 months of age were more likely to exhibit severe growth and developmental delay than infants with lower viral burden (Pollack et al., 1996). Furthermore, plasma RNA and CD4+ lymphocyte count have been found to be good predictors of clinical course among HIV-infected children (Palumbo et al., 1998).

The progression of AIDS, and in particular the time between infection and diagnosis, varies depending on the mode of transmission. In general, the interval between infection with HIV and development of AIDS is longer in children infected through transfusion (median = 3.5 years) than in those infected via perinatal viral exposure (median = 1.75 years), but shorter than for adults infected through transfusion (median = 4.5 years) (Jones, Byers, Bush, Oxtoby, & Rogers, 1992). The interval between infection and diagnosis of AIDS does not differ between children transfused before 1 month of age and those transfused after that age. After onset of symptoms, survival time does not differ between cases who were neonatally transfused and those who were vertically infected (Frederick, Mascola, Eller, O'Neil, & Byers, 1994).

Age of onset at first symptoms appears to be related to progression of the illness in infants infected through vertical transmission: Those with onset of symptoms before 1 year of age often demonstrate rapid progression and death, whereas those with symptom onset after 1 year of age usually show slower disease progression. Blanche et al. (1990) found that one-third of vertically infected infants had an early onset and severe disease progression, exhibiting opportunistic infections and encephalopathy before 12 months, and death by age 5. The remaining two-thirds had a later onset of symptoms, without either opportunistic infections or encephalopathy in the first year, and were still alive at age 5.

It has been suggested that the two patterns of disease progression (early symptom onset and rapid progression vs. later symptom onset and slower progression) may be related to different viral strains or host-related factors (Dickson et al., 1989). Route of transmission may also result in differences in disease progression, with infants who are infected through neonatal blood transfusion demonstrating the pattern of later onset and slower progression, in comparison with those infected perinatally (Frederick et al., 1994). Frederick et al. (1994) and others have suggested that the infants infected perinatally who develop symptoms at a later age, and have less rapid deterioration, may represent those with intrapartum HIV transmission as opposed to interuterine transmission. Because disease progression appears to be different for children infected *in utero* versus those infected at the time of birth, there have been recent attempts to distinguish between these two groups. Bryson, Luzuriaga, and Wara (1992) proposed that exposure should be considered *in utero* if the HIV genome is detected by PCR or if HIV-1 is isolated from blood within 48 hours of birth. Among non-breastfed infants, intrapartum infection should be assumed if blood samples obtained during the first week are negative for the virus, but those obtained from 7 to 90 days following birth are positive.

According to the American Academy of Pediatrics (1999), many children with perinatally acquired HIV infection and AIDS are now surviving to middle childhood and some to adolescence. The median lifespan for children with perinatal HIV infection has been reported to be between 8.6 to 13 years, and between 36% to 61% of infants with perinatally acquired HIV are expected to survive to age 13 years (American Academy of Pediatrics, 1999).

NEUROPATHOLOGY/PATHOPHYSIOLOGY OF NEURODEVELOPMENTAL ABNORMALITIES

Gross postmortem examination of brains of children with HIV infection and progressive encephalopathy reveals diminished brain weight for age (Epstein, Sharer, & Goudsmit, 1988). Epstein and Gelbard (1999) described several characteristic features of HIV infection in infants, including impaired brain growth leading to microcephaly with onset between 2 and 4 months of age, and chronic inflammation of the brain. Microscopic inspection reveals inflammatory cell infiltrates with macrophages and multinucleated giant cells, white matter changes including pallor and astrocytosis, and calcification and inflammation of blood vessels in the basal ganglia and deep cerebral white matter (Dickson et al., 1989; Epstein et al., 1988). On electron microscopy, characteristic lentivirus particles typical of HIV are found within macrophages and multinucleated cells (Epstein et al., 1988).

As with adults, cortical atrophy and ventricular enlargement are the most common neuroradiological findings in children with HIV infection (Belman et al., 1985, 1986; Epstein et al., 1986; DeCarli, Civitello, Brouwers, & Pizzo, 1993). White matter hyperintensities and basal ganglia calcification are also often observed (Bradford, Abdenour, Frank, Scott, & Beerman, 1988; Roy, Geoffroy, Lapointe, & Michaud, 1992; DeCarli et al., 1993; Wiley,

Belman, Dickson, Rubinstein, & Nelson, 1990; Epstein et al., 1987; Price et al., 1988; Belman et al., 1986). DeCarli et al. (1993) found one or more of these abnormalities in 86% of the pediatric HIV cases studied. They reported that all patients with cerebral calcification were encephalopathic and had acquired HIV through vertical transmission. In general, abnormalities are noted on computed tomography (CT) in symptomatic children, particularly those with neurological and/or neuropsychological impairment (Roy et al., 1992; DeCarli et al., 1993; Epstein et al., 1986), although CT changes can be evident before the loss of developmental milestones (Epstein et al., 1986).

Brouwers, DeCarli, et al. (1995) found significant associations between ratings of CT abnormalities (ventricular size, cerebral atrophy, white matter attenuation, intracerebral calcifications and other lesions) and measures of cognitive and behavioral functioning in a sample of 92 children with symptomatic HIV disease. Significant correlations were also demonstrated between ratings of CT abnormalities and measures of disease severity (cluster designation 4 [CD4] leukocyte measures, elevations of p24 antigen) (Brouwers, Tudor-Williams, et al., 1995). Studies involving serial CT scans have found more marked and progressive neuroradiological changes in children with cognitive decline (Belman et al., 1986; Wiley et al., 1990). Furthermore, reduction in brain atrophy has been observed in children treated with zidovudine (Pizzo et al., 1988; DeCarli et al., 1991).

The pathophysiology of neurodevelopmental deterioration in children with AIDS (or of HIV dementia in adults) is not well understood. However, because central nervous system (CNS) opportunistic infections are rare in children, it is assumed that infection of the brain by the virus itself must be responsible for many of the neurodevelopmental abnormalities. There is considerable interest in whether either host- or virus-mediated neurotoxins are involved in producing neuronal dysfunction and nerve cell death (Brouwers et al., 1993; Epstein & Gelbard, 1999). Brouwers et al. (1993) reported significantly higher age-adjusted cerebrospinal fluid (CSF) concentrations of quinolinic acid in HIV-infected encephalopathic children than in those without encephalopathy. They also found significant correlations between these concentrations and measures of general intelligence in 40 symptomatic HIV-infected children. Furthermore, treatment with zidovudine lowered CSF quinolinic acid concentrations and simultaneously improved cognitive functioning. Mintz et al. (1989) found elevated serum levels of tumor necrosis factor, a macrophage/monoctye-derived immunomediator, in 79% of pediatric patients with progressive encephalopathy, compared with 8% of children without neurological involvement. The latter finding suggests that circulating tumor necrosis factor may be responsible for the myelin damage that occurs in HIV-associated encephalopathy.

NEUROLOGICAL EFFECTS: OVERVIEW

From very early in the epidemic, it has been recognized that neurological symptoms are common and are often early signs of HIV infection in children. For example, Belman et al. (1988) found evidence of CNS dysfunction in 90% of infants and children with symptomatic HIV infection. More recently, Englund et al. (1996) identified CNS abnormality in 65.9% of infants and children (N=839) with HIV infection. The most frequent neurological abnormality found was motor dysfunction; nearly half of children less than 12 months of age had motor abnormalities, most commonly increased muscle tone, and 20% had cerebral atrophy on CT or MRI. Motor abnormalities were found to decrease with age.

The most common neurological symptoms in pediatric HIV infection include progressive encephalopathy, developmental delay and even loss of developmental milestones, and signs of pyramidal dysfunction (Belman et al., 1988; Fowler, 1994). Although the term *encephalopathy* is often used in describing CNS manifestations of HIV in children, there are as yet no generally accepted criteria for this diagnosis (Brouwers et al., 1993). The term is used loosely to refer to a decline in motor or mental status, but is often applied as well to describe cases in which there is additional direct evidence of CNS involvement, such as neuroradiological abnormalities; electroencephalographic abnormalities; CSF abnormalities; cerebral atrophy; and/or the pathological features of severe white matter degeneration, inflammatory cell infiltrates with macrophages, and multinucleated giant cells (Brouwers et al., 1990; Mintz et al., 1989). The manifestations of severe HIV encephalopathy in children are quite pervasive and chronic, often involving deficits in the cognitive, motor, and behavioral domains. It is assumed that encephalopathy in most pediatric cases is the result of direct infection of the CNS, as it is unusual for children to develop CNS opportunistic infections, malignancies, or other viral CNS infections of the sort frequently observed in adults with HIV-related cognitive declines (Brouwers, Belman, & Epstein, 1990; DeCarli et al., 1993). It is also generally agreed that the incidence and magnitude of HIV-related behavioral and neurological deficits are greater in the pediatric population than in adults (Belman et al., 1985, 1988) and that the most severe and pervasive neurological problems occur in those children who have serious HIV disease in the first 2 years of life (Belman et al., 1996).

Unlike adults, children with HIV infection often demonstrate neurological deficits early in the course of the disease. The degree of neurological deficit generally parallels the degree of immunodeficiency (Epstein et al., 1988), and severe encephalopathy is highly correlated with the occurrence of opportunistic infections (Blanche et al., 1990). It is not uncommon, however, to observe progressive encephalopathy in children with minimal immunological abnormalities (Epstein et al., 1986, 1988). Scott et al. (1989) reported that 12% of their pediatric cases with HIV presented with encephalopathy as the first symptom. Even in children without obvious encephalopathy, cognitive decline may be one of the earliest manifestations of infection (Pizzo et al., 1988). Because of the high prevalence of neurodevelopmental impairments in infants and children, neurocognitive status is often considered an important indication of therapeutic efficacy (Wachtel, McGrath, Houck, Chmielewski, & Tepper, 1994).

Prevalence rates for neurological involvement in HIV-infected infants and children vary considerably, depending on the stage of illness of the samples being studied, on the definition of *neurological involvement*, and (in more recent studies) on utilization of antiretroviral treatment. The European Collaborative Study (1991), for example, reported encephalopathy or other neurological abnormality in only 3 of 64 (5%) HIV-infected infants who were "pre-AIDS," whereas Epstein et al. (1988) reported some form of neurological involvement in 57 of 79 (72%) HIV-infected children.

When present, the progression of encephalopathy can take one of several courses in HIV-infected infants and children. Figure 17.1 shows several possible courses of encephalopathic development (Brouwers, Belman, & Epstein, 1990). Belman et al. (1988) described the longitudinal course of encephalopathy in 61 infants and children. In 11 of these, the encephalopathy was categorized as "subacute, progressive," with relentless deterioration of play, loss of previously acquired developmental milestones, progressive apathy, and progressive bilateral pyramidal tract signs. Another 31 cases, whose encephalopathy was categorized as at a "plateau," demonstrated variable periods of time in which there was little or no cognitive development, a failure to attain new milestones, and/or a rate of development that was slowed in comparison to previous developmental progress. Thirteen of these 31 children demonstrated further neurological deterioration with loss of

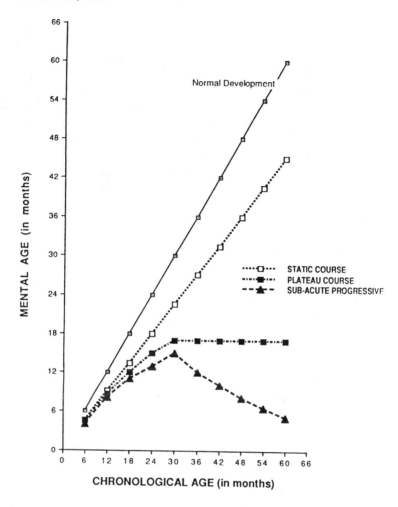

FIGURE 17.1. Different encephalopathic courses in HIV-infected infants and children. From "Central Nervous System Involvement: Manifestations, Evaluation, and Pathogenesis" by P. Brouwers, A. L. Belman, and L. G. Epstein, 1990, in P. A. Pizzo and C. M. Wilfert (Eds.), *Pediatric AIDS: The Challenge of HIV Infection in Infants, Children, and Adolescents* (pp. 433–454). Baltimore: Williams & Wilkins. Copyright 1990 by Williams & Wilkins. Reprinted by permission.

cognitive skills and were classified as at a "plateau, subacute," while the other 18 children retained skills. Finally, 17 cases showed a "static" course, with steady acquisition of cognitive and motor skills, although not necessarily at a normal rate. Other investigators have used modifications of this classification system (e.g., Epstein et al., 1988), with most studies at least making the distinction between a static and a progressive course of neurodevelopmental impairment. In the earliest studies, a prevalence rate of 50–62% was reported for progressive encephalopathy in patients with advanced symptomatic HIV-1 disease. A 30–40% rate was estimated in a later study (Roy et al., 1992). In a series that included children whose disease ranged from asymptomatic[1] to advanced, a 19.6% prevalence rate was reported (Brouwers, Belman, & Epstein, 1990). Tardieu et al. (1995) reported that most cases of progressive encephalopathy were observed before the age of 3 years, with most of these children dying before the age of 6. Patients alive at 6 years of age, however, were usually neurologically normal and able to attend elementary school.

COGNITIVE DEVELOPMENT

The earliest studies that alerted investigators to the neurodevelopmental effects of HIV were descriptive case studies (Belman et al., 1985) and descriptions of small samples of patients at various stages of disease progression (e.g., Epstein et al., 1986; Ultmann et al., 1985, 1987; Diamond, 1989). In general, these studies indicated that symptomatic HIV-infected children often had significant cognitive impairment; that children with AIDS had more severe neuropsychological impairments than did children who were HIV-infected but without AIDS; and that the greatest impairments were in psychomotor skills, perceptual and visual integration, and perceptual–motor skills, as opposed to language or verbally mediated skills (Belman et al., 1988; Ultmann et al., 1985, 1987; Diamond et al., 1987; Diamond, 1989; Epstein et al., 1986).

Many recent investigations have now greatly increased our understanding of the cognitive, the motor, and (more recently) the social and emotional consequences of HIV infection in children through the use of appropriate control groups, administration of standardized instruments, and careful descriptions of samples. In studying the neuropsychological effects of HIV infection in children, there are many confounding variables that must be considered. HIV-infected children are often born to mothers with low levels of education and socioeconomic status. In many instances, the children's mothers received poor prenatal care, sometimes abused alcohol or drugs during pregnancy, and may be unable to provide a stimulating environment. In addition, it is assumed that children who are HIV-infected are exposed to more environmental stress, sometimes including parental death, foster care placement, frequent hospitalizations, and the stigma associated with HIV status. For these reasons, it is essential to use appropriate control groups rather than to make reference to published developmental norms, in an attempt to isolate the effect of the disease from the effects of other factors that may have contributed to neuropsychological impairment. One of the most common research designs used with this population involves comparison of the development of HIV-infected children to that of children who were born to HIV-seropositive mothers, but who did not become infected. This type of design generally allows for control of such variables as prenatal care, maternal drug and alcohol abuse, low socioeconomic status, and factors associated with having an ill parent. Other designs involving comparison of HIV-infected children to children who have other chronic diseases allow for control of such variables as frequent hospitalization, school absence, and stress of treatment. No design, however, can control for all of the variables that distinguish HIV-infected infants and children from their seronegative counterparts. Consequently, confounding factors must be kept in mind when one is interpreting results from studies of the neuropsychological effects of HIV infection. Other factors to consider in interpreting research findings include the severity of non-neurological symptoms (e.g., lymphoid interstitial pneumonitis, hepatomegaly, candidiasis), the children's age at evaluation, age at infection, sample selection (random vs. clinic referral), route of infection, and treatment with antiretroviral or other medications.

Infant Cognitive Development

Most studies of HIV-infected children, especially those under 3 years of age, have assessed overall cognitive ability rather than discrete areas of neuropsychological functioning. In studies comparing infants (2 to 24 months) who were infected through vertical transmission with well-matched groups of HIV-seronegative and/or seroreverter infants, significant group differences have been found on the Mental Development Index (MDI) of the Bayley Scales of Infant Development (Nozyce et al., 1994; Wachtel et al., 1993; Aylward et al., 1992). Mellins et al. (1994) found that infected infants scored approximately 10 points below seroreverter and seronegative infants on the Bayley MDI, although this difference also failed to reach significance. It is possible that the lack of significant group differences in this study was due to the fact that the seroreverter group and seronegative groups had higher incidence of prenatal drug exposure than did the seropositive group (62% exposure for the seropositive children vs. 70% for the seroreverter children and 100% for the seronegative children). Mellins et al. (1994) concluded that HIV-infected children with prenatal drug exposure demonstrated significantly poorer cognitive performance than infants who had only one of these risk factors.

A large (N=839) multi-site study found that 33.7% of HIV infected infants (3-12 months of age) showed cognitive delay (Bayley MDI<70) compared to 21.3% of older children (1 to 18 years of age) (McCarthy General Cognitive Index/WISC-R IQ<70); the odds of having a low cognitive score was significantly higher in children with low CD4 lymphocyte percentages of <15 (Englund et al., 1996). A study conducted in Uganda (Drotar et al., 1997) found that by 12 months of age, 26% of HIV infected infants had cognitive abnormalities, compared to 6% abnormalities among seroreverters and seronegative infants. A later follow-up (Drotar et al., 1999) found similar results at ages birth to 24 months of age.

Whereas Wachtel et al. (1993) did not describe the level of symptom severity in their HIV-infected sample, the Aylward et al. (1992) and Mellins et al. (1994) studies included no infants with AIDS. Similarly, Nocyze et al. (1994) examined infants with a serious AIDS-defining illness separately from those without AIDS or those with a less severe AIDS-defining illness (i.e., lymphoid interstitial pneumonitis[2]). Aylward et al. (1992) noted that many of the HIV-infected infants, even those who were symptomatic, performed well within the normal range. In addition, the HIV-infected infants with the lowest scores on developmental assessment were not necessarily those with the most severe and/or greatest number of non-neurological symptoms. Nocyze et al. (1994) reported that the cognitive impairments observed in their sample appeared to be present predominantly, although not exclusively, in those HIV-infected children who developed a serious AIDS-defining condition in the first 2 years of life.

It can be concluded, then, that HIV-infected infants as a group generally demonstrate delayed cognitive development compared to seronegative infants of the same sociodemographic cohort, and that the children with the most severe delays show higher viral loads and are generally, but not always, those with the most severe non-neurological symptoms.

Cognitive Development in School Age Children

Studies with school-age children have been less well controlled than investigations of sequelae in infants. Levenson, Mellins, Zawadzki, Kairam, and Stein (1992) reported that 44% of a sample of HIV-infected children (aged 2.5 to 8.5 years) referred for neuropsychological evaluation performed in the mentally retarded range on the McCarthy Scales' General Cognitive Index. However, neither symptomatic nor asymptomatic HIV-infected children scored at significantly lower levels than a small group of seroreverter children. Tardieu et al. (1995) found more positive outcomes in a non-referred sample of school-age children (mean age of 6.8 (±1.0) years) infected through vertical transmission. The mean IQ of this sample on the French version of the Stanford–Binet was 95. Only one child scored below 75, and about two-thirds of the patients had normal school achievement. Whereas performance on most tests was within normal limits, about half of the subjects had scores indicating impairment on visual–spatial and time orientation tests, and 44% had speech and/or language difficulties. In this study, 58% of the children were asymptomatic or had only mild HIV-related symptoms, and all were ambulatory. In a study of children aged 5 to 12 years, Havens, Whitaker, Feldman, Alvarado, and Ehrhardt (1993) found that HIV-infected children scored significantly lower than HIV seronegative children on the Stanford–Binet (Fourth Edition) Short Term Memory, Quantitative Reasoning, and Total Composite scales. However, the two groups did not differ on the Expressive One-Word Picture Vocabulary Test or the Receptive One-Word Picture Vocabulary Test. It is not clear whether all of the children were infected through vertical transmission. The infected children were at different stages of the illness, but all were relatively healthy. Thus, although studies of HIV-infected school-age children have yielded less conclusive findings than studies of infants, it appears that there is at least a subset of HIV-infected children who perform within normal limits even into the school-age years. There is no consensus with regard to which areas of cognitive ability are most impaired in HIV-infected children within this age group.

Cognitive Development in Children Infected through Transfusion of Blood or Blood Products

Several studies of cognitive development in HIV-infected children have specifically addressed the issue in hemophiliac children or children infected through transfusion of blood. These children are less often affected by many of the factors that confound studies of cognitive development in children who acquire the disease through vertical transmission (e.g., prenatal drug exposure, poor prenatal care, poor socioeconomic environment, stress from parental illness or death). In addition, the prenatal effects of HIV infection on the developing CNS can be eliminated from consideration. Investigations involving these populations are often strengthened by the availability of good control groups (i.e., children who received transfusions but did not become affected).

Cohen et al. (1991) compared a group of children who became infected through neonatal blood transfusion with a group of seronegative children who had also received transfusions as neonates. The children were 3.2 to 9.2 years of age at testing, and none of the HIV-infected children had AIDS (67% asymptomatic). Using an extensive neuropsychological battery, the investigators found few significant group differences. The groups did not differ on overall IQ or measures of auditory memory, visual–motor integration, or attention. Seronegative children did perform better than HIV-infected children on tests of visual–sequential memory, reading, and arithmetic. Cohen et al. noted that other significant group differences were observed on tasks that require motor speed, visual scanning, and cognitive flexibility—the very tasks that are most consistently depressed in symptomatic HIV-infected adults males. Within the infected group, symptomatic children performed consistently less competently than non-symptomatic children on all measures, but these differences were statistically significant for only a few specific tests.

In a well-controlled study of hemophiliac children (aged 4 to 19 years), Whitt et al. (1993) found no significant differences between those children who had become infected through HIV-contaminated blood/blood products and those who were seronegative, on six domains of neuropsychological functioning: motor, language, memory, attention, visual processing, and problem solving. However, a high incidence of subtle neuropsychological deficits relative to age norms and individual cognitive potential was found on measures of motor performance, attention, and speeded visual processing within both infected and uninfected groups. HIV-infected children were generally asymptomatic. The authors concluded that subtle neuropsychological deficits in relatively healthy HIV-infected children with hemophilia cannot be attributed to CNS effects of HIV infection.

Comparing cognitive development in perinatal and nonperinatal transmission in children ages >6 to 18 years, Englund et al. (1996) found that those with nonperinatal acquired HIV had lower incidence of cognitive impairment (IQ<70) than children with perinatally acquired HIV (3.7% vs. 8.8%), but generally the same amount of CNS abnormality (33.3% vs. 29.8%).

Results of studies from children infected through transfusion of HIV-contaminated blood or blood products reveal that neuropsychological effects are less severe than in the children infected through vertical transmission and may in fact show a pattern of onset and progression of neuropsychological symptoms that is more similar to that observed in HIV-infected adults.

Language Development

Several studies have specifically assessed language development in HIV-infected infants. Using standardized administration of a set of language items, Wachtel et al. (1994) found significantly poorer performance by HIV-infected infants at ages 12 and 18 months, but not 6 months, in comparison with seronegative and seroreverter infants. In a similar study with children in Rwanda, Msellati et al. (1993) found that infected children performed more poorly than controls at all ages (6, 12, 18, and 24 months), but that scores were significantly different only at 24 months. Johnson et al. (1989) found no language differences between HIV-infected and uninfected infants on the Denver Developmental Screening Test. Condini et al. (1991), working with infants who were 18 to 30 months of age, found that HIV-infected infants had significantly shorter mean length of utterance. The infected children also performed at lower levels on production and comprehension tasks at 2 years of age, but seemed to catch up with uninfected peers by age 3. More recently, Coplan et al. (1998) found that HIV infected children (N = 9), ages 6 weeks to 45 months, performed significantly lower on the Early Language Milestone Scale-2nd Edition compared with infected children (N = 69) (Global Language score 89.3 vs. 96.2). Seven of the 9 HIV infected children demonstrated language delays, although MRI or CT of the brain were normal in 6 of the 7 children. Thus it appears that language delays can be observed in HIV-infected infants but may be most pronounced between 12 and 24 months of age.

In older children, both expressive and receptive language appear to be negatively affected by HIV infection, with expressive language being most impacted. Wolters et al. (1995) assessed receptive and expressive language functioning in 36 children with symptomatic HIV infection (58% classified as encephalopathic; mean age = 5.5 years) and 20 uninfected siblings (mean age = 7.8 years). The infected children scored significantly lower than the unaffected siblings on both receptive and expressive language measures, and expressive language functioning was significantly lower than receptive language functioning in the infected children, but not in the siblings. The encephalopathic group scored significantly lower than the non-encephalopathic group on both receptive and expressive measures, but did not differ in degree or direction of discrepancy between the receptive and expressive language scores, and greater severity of CT scan abnormalities was significantly correlated with poorer receptive and expressive language functioning in the HIV-infected children. A follow-up study of these subjects (Wolters et al., 1997) 24 months later confirmed these results and, in addition, found a decline in both receptive and expressive language (despite antiretroviral therapy), although overall cognitive functioning remained stable. Thus HIV infection, at least in children who are symptomatic, is associated with language deficits, particularly in expressive language. While some expressive language problems may be attributable to oral-motor difficulties related to basal ganglia insult, the presence of both expressive and receptive language dysfunction suggests a more fundamental impairment.

MOTOR DEVELOPMENT

Given the widespread presence of basal ganglia abnormalities in children with HIV infection, it is not surprising to find motor dysfunction in many of these children. In the earliest group of descriptive studies, psychomotor delays were portrayed as being more severe than cognitive delays in young children, and deterioration of motor skills was often observed with disease progression (Ultmann et al., 1987; Epstein et al., 1986; Belman et al., 1988). Belman et al. (1988) noted a high incidence of bilateral pyramidal tract signs, mild to moderate spastic paresis, and generalized muscle weakness in symptomatic HIV-infected children. Both motor delays and cognitive deficits were observed more often in children with progressive encephalopathy than in children with less severe symptoms.

In studies comparing HIV-infected infants (aged 2 to 36 months) to well-matched seronegative or seroreverter controls, investigators have found significantly lower scores for the infected group on the Psychomotor Development Index of the Bayley Scales of Infant Development (Aylward et al., 1992; Wachtel et al., 1993; Mellins et al., 1994; Nozyce et al., 1994), the Fine Motor Developmental Quotient of the Peabody Developmental Motor Scales (Wachtel et al., 1994), and other standardized assessments of gross and fine motor development (Msellati et al., 1993; Johnson et al., 1989). Wachtel et al. (1994) found that HIV-infected children, ranging in age from 6 to 36 months, had poorer fine motor skills than controls when tested at baseline, but that this difference was no longer present at follow-up testing 12 months later. They concluded that the improvement observed in the infected children's scores might be the result of medical and developmental intervention. A cross-sectional comparison by Msellati et al. (1993) failed to yield differences between HIV-infected and uninfected children in fine motor skills at either 18 or 24 months of age. Many of the HIV-infected infants in these studies still functioned well within the normal range on psychomotor tasks. Aylward et al. (1992) noted that the poorest Psychomotor Development Index scores were not always attained by the children with the greatest number or severity of symptoms. Nozyce et al. (1994), however, observed motor impairments predominantly, although not exclusively, in those HIV-infected children who developed a serious AIDS-defining condition (i.e., a condition other than lymphoid interstitial pneumonitis) in the first 2 years of life. In a study conducted in Zaire, Boivin et al. (1995) identified motor deficits in asymptomatic HIV-infected children under two years of age on the Denver Developmental Screening Test, compared to HIV-negative children born to HIV-infected mothers. Drotar et al. (1997) found that HIV-infected infants (6 to 24 months of age) in Uganda had greater deficits in motor development than seroreverters and uninfected infants. By 12 months, 30% of HIV-infected infants demonstrated motor abnormalities compared to 11% of seroreverters and 5% among seronegative infants. A later study with this sample (Drotar et al. 1999) confirmed these results, particularly among those HIV-infected infants with abnormal neurological exams.

In older children, Levenson et al. (1992) found HIV-infected children aged 2.5 to 8.5 years to score in the low average range on the Motor scale of the McCarthy Scales of

Children's Abilities. Boivin et al. (1995), in a study of vertically infected children (>2 years of age) in Zaire, found sequential motor deficits on the Kaufman Assessment Battery for Children and motor deficits on the Childhood Screening Profiles. Cohen et al. (1991) found that children who were infected through neonatal blood transfusion (aged 3.2 to 9.2 years) performed more poorly on fine motor tasks than a group of seronegative children who had also received transfusions as neonates. Tardieu et al. (1995), however, found no delays on tests of fine motor abilities in a group of vertically infected children (mean age = 6.8 years).

Thus it can be concluded that HIV-infected infants as a group have significant delays in gross motor development compared to their uninfected peers. Early delays in fine motor development may or may not be sustained. Like delays in cognitive development, motor delays are more common in children with more severe symptoms, and many infected children continue to develop normally. Motor delays are more consistently observed in infants than in older children.

SOCIAL AND EMOTIONAL DEVELOPMENT

It is easy to understand that children with HIV infection are at high risk for social, emotional, and behavioral problems. For many who contracted the disease vertically, the effects of illness may be compounded by the effects of prenatal drug exposure, poor prenatal care, impoverished environment, death or chronic illness of a parent, and instability of living arrangements. For children who acquired the disease through transfusion of contaminated blood or blood products, behavioral adjustment and cognitive and academic functioning may be affected by the concomitant disorders or illnesses that led to the transfusion. For all HIV-infected children, there are the stresses of stigma (and sometimes secrecy), frequent medical contacts and possible hospitalizations, and school absence. Parents' response to the disease state (e.g., overprotection or leniency in discipline) can also contribute to behavior problems. In addition to these "by-products" of HIV infection, the disease can affect behavior through its direct effect on the brain, as well as through other physical symptoms (e.g., fatigue, weakness, sensory impairment). Because of the complexity of the relationship between the disease and environmental stresses, it is very difficult to determine which social and emotional problems are the direct effects of infection and which problems result from secondary disease consequences or comorbid conditions.

A large multi-site study ($N = 839$) found that 13.3% of HIV infected children, ages 3 months to 18 years, exhibited abnormalities in behavior or affect, a percentage that was independent of the child's age. The most common behavioral abnormalities were difficulty with social interaction such as apathy and withdrawal, and emotional lability (Englund et al., 1996).

Severely encephalopathic children have been described as unable to engage in purposeful, "expressive" social, emotional, and motivational behavior (Moss et al., 1994). Other abnormal behaviors observed in HIV-infected children include vacant staring, flattened affect, lethargy, lack of social interest, agitation, poor attention and concentration, diminished purposeful goal-directed behavior, decreased motor activity, or increased impulsivity (Moss et al., 1989). Few studies have examined the effects of HIV infection on social and emotional development in infants. Msellati et al. (1993) rated infants on items related to "social contacts," and found that HIV-infected infants performed significantly more poorly than uninfected infants at 6 and 24 months. These differences were not significant, however, at 12 and 18 months of age. Moss et al. (1994) used a Q-sort procedure to assess social, emotional, and motivational behavior in encephalopathic and nonencephalopathic infants. In children under 2 years of age, patients with HIV-associated encephalopathy were rated as more apathetic and nonsocial in their behavior than nonencephalopathic patients. In a later study, Moss et al. (1996) compared behaviors between encephalopathic and nonencephalopathic HIV-infected children in two age groups, infants (mean = 1.8 years) and older children (mean = 5.15 years). In both groups, encephalopathic children showed lower activity levels and less social and emotional responsiveness than the nonencephalopathic groups.

In older children, Moss et al. (1994) found that encephalopathic children (mean age = 7.8 years) had significantly higher scores than nonencephalopathic patients on scales measuring depression, autism, and irritability. Other studies with school-age children have found high rates of emotional and behavioral problems in HIV-infected children, but little convincing evidence that these problems are direct results of the infection. Papola, Alvarez, and Cohen (1994) found that 42% of HIV-infected children assessed in their clinic had formal psychiatric diagnoses, including attention-deficit/hyperactivity disorder, depression, anxiety disorders, and adjustment disorder, while many others had symptoms insufficient to warrant formal diagnoses. Tardieu et al. (1995) found that none of the HIV-infected children in their sample had severe psychoaffective symptoms, but about 30% had moderate symptoms, including anxiety, depression, behavioral problems, or pervasive developmental disorders. Havens et al. (1993), in examining a group of 5- to 12-year-old HIV-infected children, found high rates of psychiatric disorders, including attention-deficit/hyperactivity disorder (58%) and oppositional defiant disorder (25%); however, they did not find significantly higher rates of these disorders in the HIV-infected children than in seronegative and seroreverter children. In India, Khan (1992) also found high rates of behavior problems (rocking, head banging, temper tantrums, teeth grinding, anger, nail biting, and thumb sucking) among both HIV-infected and noninfected multiple-transfused thalassemic children. In another study of children infected through blood transfusion, Cohen et al. (1991) failed to find differences between HIV-infected and uninfected groups on teacher and parent ratings of attention/hyperactivity, problem behavior, and social competence.

It is not surprising that high rates of social and emotional dysfunction and behavior problems have been observed in children with HIV infection, given the environmental stresses encountered by these children and their families. There is some evidence, however, that at least some of the behavior problems may be directly associated with the infection of the CNS and not simply the results of secondary factors. Moss et al. (1994) found that a score reflecting overall severity of behavioral problems was significantly correlated with a global measure of CNS disease based on CT scan ratings (e.g., measures of ventricular enlargement, white matter abnormalities, calcifications). On the other hand, studies demonstrating a lack of group differences between HIV-infected children and appropriate controls suggest that some of the emotional and behavioral problems may be due to the secondary effects of HIV (e.g., stigma, frequent medical contacts, hospitalizations, school absence, parents' response to the disease), and that these problems may therefore be lessened if efforts are made to reduce the presence and/or impact of these conditions. For example, a 2-year longitudinal study by Moss et al. (1998) found that overall psychological adjustment was stable in HIV infected school-age children, although negative life events were associated with greater psychological and behavioral problems.

MEDICATION EFFECTS ON NEURODEVELOPMENT

Pizzo et al. (1988) published one of the first reports regarding the effectiveness of zidovudine (by continuous intravenous infusion) for treatment of HIV infection in infants and children. Subjects were 21 symptomatic HIV-infected children, ranging in age from 14 months to 12 years. Sixty-two percent had neurological symptoms or evidence of HIV-associated encephalopathy at the initiation of treatment. In addition to improvements in clinical measures (e.g., weight, immunoglobulin levels, CD4 cell count), all 13 children who had presented with encephalopathy before treatment showed neurodevelopmental improvements. Serial IQ testing conducted before therapy and after 3 and 6 months of continuous therapy with zidovudine revealed improved follow-up scores on both verbal and nonverbal tasks for the 13 encephalopathic children, as well as for 5 other children who had no evidence of encephalopathy before treatment (Pizzo et al., 1988; Brouwers, Moss, et al., 1990). The Adaptive Behavior Composite score from the Vineland scales also showed significant increments from baseline to follow-up, as did the Communication, Daily Living, and Socialization subscales (Brouwers, Moss, et al., 1990). Similar improvement was noted in gait and coordination (Pizzo et al., 1988). Neuropsychological improvement appeared to be independent of other clinical changes, but was mirrored by reductions over time in brain atrophy on CT scans (DeCarli et al., 1991). The effectiveness of zidovudine treatment for HIV-infected children was confirmed by a larger study (McKinney et al., 1991), using oral administration (180 mg/m^2) in a group of children with advanced HIV disease or AIDS. Cognitive improvements were especially marked for children less than 3 years of age. More recently, investigators in a large multicenter trial demonstrated that oral administration of a low dose of zidovudine (90 mg/m^2) was as effective as the higher dose in children with mild to moderate disease (Brady et al., 1996).

Moss et al. (1994) demonstrated a significant decrease in behavior problems for HIV-infected children after a 6-month course of treatment with zidovudine, especially on scales assessing depression and autism. Behavioral improvements were primarily observed in children with encephalopathy. Over the follow-up period, the scores of these children became very similar to those obtained by the nonencephalopathic children. In the same sample, Wolters, Brouwers, Moss, and Pizzo (1994) demonstrated improvements on the Communication, Daily Living, and Socialization domains of the Vineland Adaptive Behavior scales, as well as on the overall Adaptive Behavior Composite, for both encephalopathic and nonencephalopathic children. No improvement was observed, however, for the Motor domain score. Some success in improving motor function in HIV-infected children has been found with Levodopa therapy, where children, ages 4 to 13 years old, with extrapyramidal dysfunction, showed promise (Mintz et al., 1996).

Less evidence for improvement in neuropsychological function was found in a trial of dideoxycytidine alone and in an alternating schedule with zidovudine in symptomatic HIV-infected children (Pizzo et al., 1990). However, the authors of this study noted that lack of deterioration in neurocognitive performance might be viewed as a positive treatment outcome, given the natural history of cognitive decline in these cases. Dideoxycytidine had antiretroviral activity in some children, and it was concluded that the alternating regimen of dideoxycytidine and zidovudine might be beneficial for patients who have hematological intolerance to zidovudine alone.

CONCLUSIONS

Children with HIV infection are at risk for neuropsychological and neurological abnormalities. Specifically, difficulties in cognitive functioning, language development, motor skills, and emotional and behavioral functioning are often observed in children with HIV infection, particularly those with symptomatic HIV infection. Infants with vertically transmitted HIV are particularly vulnerable to delays in mental and motor development and to

CNS abnormalities because it appears that their perinatal exposure to the virus can have dramatic effects on the developing brain. In older HIV infected children and adolescents, neuropsychological effects appear to be more subtle and often do not appear until the later stages of the disease process. Neuroimaging and neuropathology studies have shown that cortical atrophy, white matter hyperintensities, and basal ganglia calcifications are commonly found in children with HIV infection. These brain abnormalities are consistent with the neuropsychological deficits seen in HIV-infected children, including delayed cognitive development and motor dysfunction. Although recent advances in antiretroviral therapy and treatment of opportunistic infections have lengthened the life span of HIV-infected children, HIV infection remains a significant public health issue in the United States and the incidence of HIV infection among children in developing countries is increasing. A longer life span for children with HIV infection is likely to make neuropsychological and neurological problems more apparent and increase the importance of quality of life issues. As suggested by the preceding review of studies, there are many methodological obstacles in conducting research on the neuropsychological effects of pediatric HIV infection. In addition to the difficulty encountered in attempting to control for the great number of confounding factors, research in this area is plagued with various other problems, some of which are unique to this disease.

Patients with pediatric HIV/AIDS are a difficult population to follow. Those who acquired the infection through vertical transmission often reside in unstable, transient home situations. Caregivers (often not parents) may not consistently bring the children in for appointments, especially if the visits only involve collection of data for research. When children move from one home environment to another, it is often difficult to track them for longitudinal follow-up. It is also difficult to follow children when they are hospitalized or are too sick to be tested. Even when they can be tested, results may not be valid if the children are not feeling well.

Many children with HIV infection are from backgrounds in which English is not the predominant language. Even if translators can be found to assist in test administration, many of the instruments have not been validated for non-English administration. Even for cases in which English is the first language, the children's sociocultural background may prevent valid use of available norms. For this reason, it is generally necessary for investigators studying the neuropsychological effects of pediatric HIV to employ appropriate control groups, rather than relying on a published norming sample as a comparison group.

In longitudinal studies of pediatric HIV, a problem that is frequently encountered involves the lack of single test procedures for following children over a wide age span. For example, since many investigators are interested in following children from birth, it is often necessary to begin assessment with a test of infant development (e.g., the Bayley Scales) and then to switch to a different test (e.g., the Stanford–Binet, the Wechsler Scales of Preschool and Primary Intelligence) when children reach preschool age. Because it is not known how scores from one test correspond to scores on other tests, especially for this population, it is difficult to determine whether a child's rate of development has changed over time. Longitudinal studies can also be confounded by practice effects. Fletcher et al. (1991) describe the use of individual change models to overcome some of the difficulties in analyzing and interpreting longitudinal data, especially in studies of the effectiveness of treatments for HIV-infected children.

Changes in treatment can also make the results of longitudinal studies difficult to interpret. Even in well-designed drug trials, there are always some children who cannot tolerate the medication and must be switched to other forms of treatment. In addition, it is often difficult to determine how well families have complied with the drug regimen. Assessing the effectiveness of a treatment becomes highly problematic when children who are not doing well are taken off treatment or when it is unclear whether all children are following the protocol. Inevitable problems are also encountered in data analysis due to attrition resulting from either death or loss to follow-up.

Interpretation of published studies is sometimes difficult because of the authors' failure to specify the nature of the sample. For example, studies involving the neuropsychological effects of HIV infection sometimes fail to describe the severity of symptoms in the group being studied. As noted earlier, the extent of neuropsychological impairment appears to be closely related to symptom severity in many cases. Route of infection, age at infection, and types of treatment (dosage and length) to which the subjects have been exposed need to be clarified. Failure to describe these factors makes it difficult to interpret and apply research findings. Investigators also need to specify confounding factors that are known to affect neurodevelopment (e.g., prenatal drug exposure, prematurity, instability of living situation), and must describe the procedures used to take these factors into account. To reiterate, many of the negative outcomes associated with pediatric HIV infection may be due to factors associated with the disease rather than to the disease itself.

Investigators must also carefully describe the diagnostic procedures and criteria used to classify children (e.g., they must operationally define such terms as *encephalopathic* and *symptomatic*). Evidence must be presented regarding the validity of neuropsychological tests for the population being studied. Finally, investigators must discuss the extent to which results may be generalized to other populations; they must especially consider the need for data that can be applied to patients in developing countries, as well as in the United States.

FUTURE RESEARCH

Although the pediatric HIV epidemic is relatively new, we have made good progress in understanding the neuropsychological effects of this devastating disease. Several areas of research still need further exploration. First, we now know that there is a sizable subset of HIV-infected children who develop relatively well and who for many years do not experience the cognitive and motor delays that were originally believed to be an integral part of the disease process. Further study of this group of children may lead to insights regarding the genetic and environmental factors that mediate the effects of the infection. Second, because many HIV-infected children are living longer and developing more normally than investigators originally believed possible, it will be important to determine how HIV infection affects school performance and what types of interventions will assist infected children in having successful academic careers. Third, more research is needed to distinguish between the direct and indirect effects of HIV infection on neuropsychological development. If we can determine which impairments are primarily the result of secondary effects (e.g., stress, instability of home situation), we may be able to determine strategies for eliminating or alleviating some of the negative impact of the disease. Fourth, neuropsychologists can assist in the assessment of treatment efficacy by determining which neurodevelopmental outcomes are most affected by the infection at different ages and stages of illness. Children in treatment trials are now exposed to many hours of neuropsychological testing over the course of the trials. By pinpointing more precisely which cognitive and motor skills are most closely associated with disease progression, we may be able to make more efficient use of time and resources. Finally, neuropsychologists, in conjunction with health psychologists and educators, can play an important role in determining what strategies may be most effective in preventing the spread of HIV infection. By developing appropriate educational programs for children and adolescents, we may be able to have a most important impact on the prevention of future transmission of this devastating illness.

NOTES

1. The term *asymptomatic* is not used consistently across studies of children with HIV infection. In general, however, studies done between 1987 and 1994 used a classification system devised by the CDC (1987), whereby children could be classified as having "asymptomatic infection" if their immune function was normal or abnormal (i.e., hypergammaglobulinemia, T-helper lymphopenia, decreased T-helper-to-T-suppressor ratio, absolute lymphopenia), but they did not have other HIV-associated symptomatic infections or conditions (e.g., progressive neurological disease, lymphoid interstitial pneumonitis, secondary infectious diseases, secondary cancers, hepatitis, cardiopathy, nephropathy, hematological disorder, dermatological disease). These guidelines remained in place until 1994, when a revised system for classifying severity of HIV infection in children was published (CDC, 1994). According to these guidelines, children can be considered "nonsymptomatic" if they have no signs or symptoms considered to be the result of HIV infection or who have only one of the following conditions: lymphadenopathy, hepatomegaly, splenomegaly, dermatitis, parotitis, recurrent or persistent upper respiratory infection, sinusitis, or otitis media. Not all studies, however, have used CDC guidelines in defining the symptom severity of their subjects.

2. Several reports indicate that the prognosis for children with lymphoid interstitial pneumonitis is substantially better than that for children who have other AIDS-defining conditions (CDC, 1994).

REFERENCES

American Academy of Pediatrics (1999). Disclosure of illness status to children and adolescents with HIV infection. *Pediatrics, 103*(1), 164–166.

Aylward, E. H., Butz, A. M., Hutton, N., Joyner, M. L., & Vogelhut, J. W. (1992). Cognitive and motor development in infants at risk for human immunodeficiency virus. *American Journal of Diseases of Children, 146,* 218–222.

Belman, A. L., Diamond, G., Dickson, D., Horoupian, D., Llena, J., Lantos, G., & Rubinstein, A. (1988). Pediatric acquired immunodeficiency syndrome: Neurologic syndromes. *American Journal of Diseases of Children, 142,* 29–35.

Belman, A. L., Lantos, G., Horoupian, D., Novick, B. E., Ultmann, M. H., Dickson, D. W., & Rubinstein, A. (1986). AIDS: Calcification of the basal ganglia in infants and children. *Neurology, 36,* 1192–1199.

Belman, A. L., Muenz, L. R., Marcus, J. C., Goedert, J. J., Landesman, S., Rubenstein, A., Goodwin, S., Durako, S., & Willoughby, A. (1996). Neurologic status of human immunodeficiency virus 1-infected infants and their controls: A prospective study from birth to 2 years. Mother and Infants Cohort Study. *Pediatrics, 98,* 1109–1118.

Belman, A. L., Ultmann, M. H., Horoupian, D., Novick, B., Spiro, A. J., Rubinstein, A., Kurtzberg, D., & Cone-Wesson, B. (1985). Neurological complications in infants and children with acquired immune deficiency syndrome. *Annals of Neurology, 18,* 560–566.

Blanche, S., Tardieu, M., Duliege, A., Rouzioux, C., Le Deist, F., Fukunaga, K., Caniglia, M., Jacomet, C., Messiah, A., & Griscelli, C. (1990). Longitudinal study of 94 symptomatic infants with perinatally acquired human immunodeficiency virus infection. *American Journal of Diseases of Children, 144,* 1210–1215.

Boivin, M. J., Green, S. D., Davies, A. G., Giordani, B., Mokili, J. K., & Cutting, W. A. (1995). A preliminary evaluation of the cognitive and motor effects of pediatric HIV infection in Zairian children. *Health Psychology, 14*(1), 13–21.

Bradford, B. F., Abdenour, G. E., Frank, J. L., Scott, G. B., & Beerman, R. (1988). Usual and unusual radiologic manifestations of acquired immunodeficiency syndrome (AIDS) and human immunodeficiency virus (HIV) infection in children. *Radiologic Clinics of North America, 26,* 341–353.

Brady, M. T., McGrath, N., Brouwers, P., Gelber, R., Fowler, M. G., Yogev, R., Hutton, N., Bryson, Y. J., Mitchell, C. D., Fikrig, S., Borkowsky, W., Jimenez, E., McSherry, G., Rubinstein, A., Wilfert, C. M., McIntosh, K., Elkins, M. M., Weintrub, P. S., & the Pediatric AIDS Clinical Trials Group. (1996). Randomized study of the tolerance and efficacy of high- versus low-dose zidovudine in human immunodeficiency virus-infected children with mild to moderate symptoms (AIDS Clinical Trials Group 128). *Journal of Infectious Diseases, 173,* 1097–1106.

Brouwers, P., Belman, A. L., & Epstein, L. G. (1990). Central nervous system involvement: Manifestations, evaluation, and pathogenesis. In P. A. Pizzo & C. M. Wilfert (Eds.), *Pediatric AIDS: The challenge of HIV infection in infants, children, and adolescents* (pp. 433–454). Baltimore: Williams & Wilkins.

Brouwers, P., DeCarli, C., Civitello, L., Moss, H., Wolters, P., & Pizzo, P. (1995). Correlation between computed tomographic brain scan abnormalities and neuropsychological function in children with symptomatic human immunodeficiency virus disease. *Archives of Neurology, 52,* 39–44.

Brouwers, P., Heyes, M., Moss, H., Wolters, P., Poplack, D., Markey, S., & Pizzo, P. (1993). Quinolinic acid in the cerebrospinal fluid of children with symptomatic human immunodeficiency virus type 1 disease: Relationships to clinical status and therapeutic response. *Journal of Infectious Diseases, 168,* 1380–1386.

Brouwers, P., Moss, H., Wolters, P., Eddy, J., Balis, F., Poplack, D., & Pizzo, P. (1990). Effect of continuous-infusion zidovudine therapy on neuropsychologic functioning in children with symptomatic human immunodeficiency virus infection. *Journal of Pediatrics, 117,* 980–985.

Brouwers, P., Tudor-Williams, G., DeCarli, C., Moss, H., Wolters, P., Civitello, L., & Pizzo, P. (1995). Relation between stage of disease and neurobehavioral measures in children with symptomatic HIV disease. *AIDS, 9,* 713–720.

Bryson, Y. J., Luzuriaga, K., & Wara, D. (1992). Proposed definitions for in utero versus intrapartum transmission of HIV-1. *New England Journal of Medicine, 327,* 1246–1247.

Bryson, Y. J., Pang S., Wei, L. S., Dickover, R., Diagne, A., & Chen, I. S. Y. (1995). Clearance of HIV infection in a perinatally infected infant. *New England Journal of Medicine, 332,* 833–838.

Centers for Disease Control (CDC). (1987). Classification system for human immunodeficiency virus (HIV) infection in children under 13 years of age. *Morbidity and Mortality Weekly Report, 36,* 225–230, 235.

Centers for Disease Control (CDC). (1994). 1994 revised classification system for human immunodeficiency virus infection in children less than 13 years of age. *Morbidity and Mortality Weekly Report, 43,* 1–10.

Centers for Disease Control (CDC). (1995). Update: AIDS among women—United States, 1994. *Morbidity and Mortality Weekly Report, 44,* 81–84.

Centers for Disease Control and Prevention (CDC) (1997). Update: Perinatally acquired HIV/AIDS-United States, 1997. *Morbidity and Mortality Weekly Report, 46,* 1086–1092.

Centers for Disease Control and Prevention (CDC) (1998). *HIV/AIDS Surveillance Report, 10(2),* 1–43.

Cohen, S., Mundy, T., Karrasik, B., Lieb, L., Ludwig, D., & Ward, J. (1991). Neuropsychological functioning in human immunodeficiency virus type 1 seropositive children infected through neonatal blood transfusion. *Pediatrics, 88,* 58–68.

Condini, A., Axia, G., Cattelan, C., D'Urso, M. R., Laverda, A. M., Viero, F., & Zacchello, F. (1991). Development of language in 18–30-month-old HIV-1-infected but not ill children. *AIDS, 5,* 735–739.

Connor, E. M., Sperling, R. S., Gelber, R., Kiselev, P., Scott, G., O'Sullivan, M. J., VanDyke, R., Bey, M., Shearer, W., Jacobson, R. L., Jimenez, E., O'Neill, E., Bazin, B., Delfraissy, J. F., Culnane, M., Coombs, R., Elkins, M., Moye, J., Stratton, P., & Balsley, J. (1994). Reduction of maternal–infant transmission of human immunodeficiency virus type 1 with zidovudine treatment. *New England Journal of Medicine, 331,* 1173–1180.

Coplan, J., Contello, K. A., Cunningham, C. K., Weiner, L. B., Dye, T. D., Roberge, L., Wojtowycz, M. A., & Kirkwood, K. (1998). Early language development in children exposed to or infected with human immunodeficiency virus. *Pediatrics, 102(1),* E8.

Davis, S. F., Byers, R. H., Lindegren, M. L., Caldwell, B., Karon, J. M., & Gwinn, M. (1995). Prevalence and incidence of vertically acquired HIV infection in the United States. *Journal of the American Medical Association, 247,* 952–955.

DeCarli, C., Civitello, L. A., Brouwers, P., & Pizzo, P. A. (1993). The prevalence of computed axial tomographic abnormalities of the cerebrum in 100 consecutive children symptomatic with the human immunodeficiency virus. *Annals of Neurology, 34,* 198–205.

DeCarli, C., Fugate, L., Falloon, J., Eddy, J., Katz, D. A., Friedland, R. P., Rapoport, S. I., Brouwers, P., & Pizzo, P. A. (1991). Brain growth and cognitive improvement in children with human immunodeficiency virus-induced encephalopathy after 6 months of continuous infusion zidovudine therapy. *Journal of Acquired Immune Deficiency Syndromes, 4,* 585–592

Diamond, G. W. (1989). Developmental problems in children with HIV infection. *Mental Retardation, 27,* 213–217.

Diamond, G. W., Kaufman, J., Belman, A. L., Cohen, L., Cohen, H. J., & Rubinstein, A. (1987). Characterization of cognitive functioning in a subgroup of children with congenital HIV infection. *Archives of Clinical Neuropsychology, 2,* 245–256.

Dickson, D. W., Belman, A. L., Park, Y. D., Wiley, C., Horoupian, D. S., Llena, J., Kure, K., Lyman, W. D., Morecki, R., Mitsudo, S., & Cho, S. (1989). Central nervous system pathology in pediatric AIDS: An autopsy study. *Acta Pathologica, Microbiologica, et Immunologica Scandinavica, 8*(Suppl.) 40–57.

Drotar, D., Olness, K., Wiznitzer, M., Guay, L., Marum, L., Svilar, G., Hom, D., Fagan, J. F., Ndugwa, C., & Kiziri-Mayengo, R. (1997). Neurodevelopmental outcomes of Ugandan infants with human immuno-deficiency virus type 1. *Pediatrics, 100*(1), E5.

Drotar, D., Olness, K., Wiznitzer, M., Schatschneider, C., Marum, L., Guay, L., Fagan, J., Hom, D., Svilar, G., Ndugwa, C., & Mayengo, R. K. (1999). Neurodevelopmental outcomes of Ugandan infants with HIV infection: An application of growth curve analysis. *Health Psychology, 18*(2), 114–121.

Englund, J. A., Baker, C. J., Raskino, C., McKinney, R. E., Lifschitz, M. H., Petrie, B., Fowler, M. G., Connor, J. D., Mendez, H., O'Donnell, K., Wara, D. W., & the AIDS Clinical Trail Group Protocol 152 Study Team. (1996). Clinical and laboratory characteristics of a large cohort of symptomatic, human immunodeficiency virus-infected infants and children. *Pediatric Infectious Disease Journal, 15*(11), 1025–1036.

Epstein, L. G., & Gelbard, H. A. (1999). HIV-1 induced neuronal injury in the developing brain. *Journal of Leukocyte Biology 65*(4), 453–457.

Epstein, L. G., Sharer, L. R., & Goudsmit, J. (1988). Neurological and neuropathological features of human immunodeficiency virus infection in children. *Annals of Neurology, 23*(Suppl.), S19–S23.

Epstein, L. G., Goudsmit, J., Paul, D. S., Morrison, S. H., Connor, E. M., Oleske, J. M., & Holland, B. (1987). Expression of human immunodeficiency virus in cerebrospinal fluid of children with progressive encepha-lopathy. *Annals of Neurology, 21,* 397–401.

Epstein, L. G., Sharer, L. R., Oleske, J. M., Connor, E. M., Goudsmit, J., Bagdon, L., Robert-Guroff, M., & Koenigsberger, M. R. (1986). Neurologic manifestations of human immunodeficiency virus infection in children. *Pediatrics, 78,* 678–687.

European Collaborative Study. (1991). Children born to women with HIV-1 infection: Natural history and risk of transmission. *Lancet, 337,* 253–260.

Falloon, J., Eddy, J., Wiener, L., & Pizzo, P. A. (1989). Human immunodeficiency virus infection in children. *Journal of Pediatrics, 114,* 1–30.

Fletcher, J. M., Francis, D. J., Pequegnat, W., Raudenbush, S. W., Bornstein, M. H., Schmitt, F., Brouwers, P., & Stover, E. (1991). Neurobehavioral outcomes in diseases of childhood. *American Psychologist, 46,* 1267–1277.

Fowler, M. G. (1994). Pediatric HIV infection: Neurologic and neuropsychologic findings. *Acta Paediatr Supplement, 400,* 59–62.

Fowler, M. G. (1997). Update: Transmission of HIV-1 from mother to child. *Current Opinion in Obstetrics and Gynecology, 9*(6), 343–348.

Frederick, T., Mascola, L., Eller, A., O'Neil, L., & Byers, B. (1994). Progression of human immunodeficiency virus disease among infants and children infected perinatally with human immunodeficiency virus or through neonatal blood transfusion. *Pediatric Infectious Disease Journal, 13,* 1091–1097.

Goedert, J., Mendez, H., Drummond, J., Robert-Guroff, M., Minkoff, H., Holman, S., Stevens, R., Rubinstein, A., Blattner, W., Willoughby, A., & Landesman, S. (1989). Mother-to-infant transmission of human immu-nodeficiency virus type 1: Association with prematurity or low anti-gp 120. *Lancet, ii,* 1351–1354.

Havens, J., Whitaker, A., Feldman, J., Alvarado, L., & Ehrhardt, A. (1993). A controlled study of cognitive and language function in school-aged HIV-infected children. *Annals of the New York Academy of Sciences, 693,* 249–251.

Johnson, J. P., Nair, P., Hines, S. E., Seiden, S. W., Alger, L., Revie, D. R., O'Neil, K. M., & Hebel, R. (1989). Natural history and serologic diagnosis of infants born to human immunodeficiency virus-infected women. *American Journal of Diseases of Children, 143,* 1147–1153.

Jones, D. S., Byers, R. H., Bush, T. J., Oxtoby, M. J., & Rogers, M. F. (1992). Epidemiology of transfusion-associated acquired immunodeficiency syndrome in children in the United States, 1981 through 1989. *Pediatrics, 89,* 123–127.

Khan, M. A. (1992). Psycho-social aspects of HIV infection and AIDS in multiple transfused thalassemic children. *Indian Journal of Pediatrics, 59,* 429–434.

Landesman, S. H., Kalish, L. A., Burns, D. N., Minkoff, H., Fox, H. E., Zorrilla, C., Garcia, P., Fowler, M. G., Mofenson, L., & Tuomala, R. (1996). Obstetrical factors and the transmission of human immunode-ficiency virus type 1 from mother to child. *New England Journal of Medicine, 334*(25), 1617–1623.

Levenson, R. L., Mellins, C. A., Zawadzki, R., Kairam, R., & Stein, Z. (1992). Cognitive assessment of human immunodeficiency virus-exposed children. *American Journal of Diseases of Children, 146,* 1479–1483.

Mandelbrot, L., LeChenadec, J., Berrebi, A., Bongain, A., Benifla, J. L., Delfraissy, J. F., Blanche, S., & Mayaux, M. J. (1998). Perinatal HIV-1 transmission: Interaction between zidovudine prophylaxis and mode of delivery in the French Perinatal Cohort. *Journal of the American Medical Association 280*, 55–60.

Marion, R. W., Wiznia, A. A., Hutcheon, R. G., & Rubinstein, A. (1986). Human T-cell lymphotropic virus type III (HTLV-III) embryopathy. *American Journal of Diseases of Children, 140*, 638–640.

McKinney, R. E., Maha, M. A., Connor, E. M., Feinberg, J., Scott, G. B., Wulfsohn, M., McIntosh, K., Borkowsky, W., Modlin, J. F., Weintrub, P., O'Donnell, K., Gelber, R. D., Rogers, G. K., Lehrman, S. N., & Wilfert, C. M. (1991). A multicenter trial of oral zidovudine in children with advanced human immunodeficiency virus disease. *New England Journal of Medicine, 324*, 1018–1025.

Mellins, C. A., Levenson, R. L., Zawadzki, R., Kairam, R., & Weston, M. (1994). Effects of pediatric HIV infection and prenatal drug exposure on mental and psychomotor development. *Journal of Pediatric Psychology, 19*, 617–628.

Mintz, M., Rapaport, R., Oleske, J. M., Connor, E. M., Koenigsberger, M. R., Denny, T., & Epstein, L. G. (1989). Elevated serum levels of tumor necrosis factor are associated with progressive encephalopathy in children with acquired immunodeficiency syndrome. *American Journal of Diseases of Children, 143*, 771–774.

Mintz, M., Tardieu, M., Hoyt, L., McSherry, G., Mendelson, J., & Oleske, J. (1996). Levodopa therapy improves motor function in HIV-infected children with extrapyramidal syndromes. *Neurology, 47*(6), 1583–1585.

Mok, J., DeRossi, A., Ades, A., Giaquinto, C., Grosch-Worner, L., & Peckham, C. (1987). Infants born to mothers seropositive for human immunodeficiency virus. *Lancet, i*, 1164–1168.

Moss, H. A., Bose, S., Wolters, P., & Brouwers, P. (1998). A preliminary study of factors associated with psychological adjustment and disease course in school-age children infected with the human immunodeficiency virus. *Journal of Developmental and Behavioral Pediatrics, 19*(1), 18–25.

Moss, H. A., Brouwers, P., Wolters, P. L., Wiener, L., Hersh, S., & Pizzo, P. A. (1994). The development of a Q-sort behavioral rating procedure for pediatric HIV patients. *Journal of Pediatric Psychology, 19*, 27–46.

Moss, H. A., Wolters, P. L., Brouwers, P., Hendricks, M. L., & Pizzo, P. A. (1996). Impairment of expressive behavior in pediatric HIV-infected patients with evidence of CNS disease. *Journal of Pediatric Psychology, 21*(3), 379–400.

Moss, H., Wolters, P., Eddy, J., Weiner, L., Pizzo, P., & Brouwers, P. (1989). The effects of encephalopathy on the social and emotional behavior of pediatric AIDS patients [Abstract]. *Proceedings of the Fifth International Conference on AIDS, 328.*

Msellati, P., Lepage, P., Hitimana, D. G., Van Goethem, C., Van de Perre, P., & Dabis, F. (1993). Neurodevelopmental testing of children born to human immunodeficiency virus type 1 seropositive and seronegative mothers: A prospective cohort study in Kigali, Rwanda. *Pediatrics, 92*, 843–848.

Nozyce, M., Hittelman, J., Muenz, L., Durako, S. J., Fischer, M. L., & Willoughby, A. (1994). Effect of perinatally acquired human immunodeficiency virus infection on neurodevelopment in children during the first two years of life. *Pediatrics, 94*, 883–891.

Palumbo, P. E., Raskino, C., Fiscus, S., Pawha, S., Fowler, M. G., Spector, S. A., Englund, J. A., & Baker, C. J. (1998). Predictive value of quantitative plasma HIV RNA and CD4+ lymphocyte count in HIV-infected infants and children. *Journal of the American Medical Association, 279*(10), 756–761.

Papola, P., Alvarez, M., & Cohen, H. J. (1994). Developmental and service needs of school-age children with human immunodeficiency virus infection: A descriptive study. *Pediatrics, 94*, 914–918.

Pitt, J., Brambilla, D., Reichelderfer, P., Landay, A., McIntosh, K., Burns, D., Hillyer, G. V., Mendez, H., & Fowler, M. G. (1997). Maternal immunologic and virologic risk factors for infant human immunodeficiency virus type 1 infection: Findings from the Women and Infants Transmission Study. *Journal of Infectious Diseases, 175*(3), 567–575.

Pizzo, P., Butler, K., Balis, F., Brouwers, P., Hawkins, M., Eddy, J., Einloth, M., Falloon, J., Husson, R., Jarosinski, P., Meer, J., Moss, H., Poplack, D., Santacroce. S., Wiener, L., & Wolters, P. (1990). Dideoxycytidine alone and in an alternating schedule with zidovudine in children with symptomatic human immunodeficiency virus infection. *Journal of Pediatrics, 117*, 799–808.

Pizzo, P., Eddy, J., Falloon, J., Balis, F., Murphy, R., Moss, H., Wolters, P., Brouwers, P., Jarosinski, P., Rubin, M., Broder, S., Yarchoan, R., Brunetti, A., Maha, M., Nusinoff-Lehrman, S., & Poplack, D. (1988). Effect of continuous intravenous infusion of zidovudine (AZT) in children with symptomatic HIV infection. *New England Journal of Medicine, 319*, 889–896.

Pollack, H., Kuchuk, A., Cowan, L., Hacimamutoglu, S., Glasberg, H., David, R., Krasinski, K., Borkowsky, W., & Oberfield, S. (1996). Neurodevelopment, growth, and viral load in HIV-infected infants. *Brain, Behavior, & Immunology, 10*(3), 298–312.

Price, D. B., Inglese, C. M., Jacobs, J., Haller, J. O., Kramer, J., Hotson, G. C., Loh, J. P., Schlusselberg, D., Menez-Bautista, R., Rose, A. L., & Fikrig, S. (1988). Pediatric AIDS: Neuroradiological and neuro-developmental findings. *Pediatric Radiology, 18*, 445–448.

Rogers, M. F., Thomas, P. A., Starcher, E. T., Noa, M. C., Bush, T. J., & Jaffe, H. W. (1987). Acquired immunodeficiency syndrome in children: Report of the Centers for Disease Control National Surveillance, 1982 to 1985. *Pediatrics, 79*, 1008–1014.

Roy, S., Geoffroy, G., Lapointe, N., & Michaud, J. (1992). Neurological findings in HIV-infected children: A review of 49 cases. *Canadian Journal of Neurological Sciences, 19*, 453–457.

Rubinstein, A., & Bernstein, L. (1986). The epidemiology of pediatric acquired immunodeficiency syndrome. *Clinical Immunology and Immunopathology, 40*, 115–121.

Scott, G. B., Hutto, C., Makuch, R. W., Mastrucci, M. T., O'Connor, T., Mitchell, C. D., Trapido, E. J., & Parks, W. P. (1989). Survival in children with perinatally acquired human immuno-deficiency virus type 1 infection. *New England Journal of Medicine, 321*, 1791–1796.

Tardieu, M., Mayaux, M. J., Seibel, N., Funck-Brentano, I., Straub, E., Teglas, J. P., & Blanche, S. (1995). Cognitive assessment of school-age children infected with maternally transmitted human immunodeficiency virus type 1. *Journal of Pediatrics, 126*, 375–379.

Ultmann, M. H., Belman, A. L., Ruff, H. A., Novick, B. E., Cone-Wesson, B., Cohen, H. J., & Rubinstein, A. (1985). Developmental abnormalities in infants and children with acquired immune deficiency syndrome (AIDS) and AIDS-related complex. *Developmental Medicine and Child Neurology, 27*, 563–571.

Ultmann, M. H., Diamond, G. W., Ruff, H. A., Belman, A. L., Novick, B. E., Rubinstein, A., & Cohen, H. J. (1987). Developmental abnormalities in children with acquired immunodeficiency syndrome (AIDS): A follow up study. *International Journal of Neuroscience, 32*, 661–667.

UNAIDS. (1998). *AIDS epidemic update: December 1998.*

Wachtel, R. C., McGrath, C., Houck, D., Chmielewski, D., & Tepper, V. J. (1994). Fine motor testing in children: Not fine. *Pediatric AIDS and HIV Infection: Fetus to Adolescent, 5*, 86–88.

Wachtel, R. C., Tepper, V. J., Houck, D. L., Nair, P., Thompson, C., & Johnson, J. P. (1993). Neurodevelopment in pediatric HIV-1 infection: A prospective study. *Pediatric AIDS and HIV Infection: Fetus to Adolescent, 4*, 198–203.

Whitt, J. K., Hooper, S. R., Tennison, M. B., Robertson, W. T., Gold, S. H., Burchinal, M., Wells, R., McMillan, C., Whaley, R. A., Combest, J., & Hall, C. D. (1993). Neuropsychologic functioning of human immunodeficiency virus-infected children with hemophilia. *Journal of Pediatrics, 122*, 52–59.

Wiley, C. A., Belman, A. L., Dickson, D. W., Rubinstein, A., & Nelson, J. A. (1990). Human immunodeficiency virus within the brains of children with AIDS. *Clinical Neuropathology, 9*, 1–6.

Wolters, P. L., Brouwers, P., Civitello, L., & Moss, H. A. (1997). Receptive and expressive language function of children with symptomatic HIV infection and relationship with disease parameters: A longitudinal 24-month follow-up study. *AIDS, 11*(9), 1135–1144.

Wolters, P. L., Brouwers, P., Moss, H. A., & Pizzo, P. A. (1994). Adaptive behavior of children with symptomatic HIV infection before and after zidovudine therapy. *Journal of Pediatric Psychology, 19*, 47–61.

Wolters, P. L., Brouwers, P., Moss, H. A., & Pizzo, P. A. (1995). Differential receptive and expressive language functioning of children with symptomatic HIV disease and relation to CT scan brain abnormalities. *Pediatrics, 95*, 112–119.

PART IV

Clinical Implications and Applications

18

DEVELOPMENTAL NEUROPSYCHOLOGICAL ASSESSMENT

JANE HOLMES BERNSTEIN

Ideas are the glue that holds facts together in comprehensible structures. (Rapp, 1997, p. xi)

This book contributes to the rapidly expanding base of knowledge about children's neuropsychological functioning. The development of such a knowledge base is of intrinsic scientific value, inasmuch as it increases our understanding of neurobehavioral development. It is also fundamental to the effective evaluation and management of the child with a neurobehavioral problem. However, although neuropsychological functioning in children has been studied intensively in recent years, as reflected in the establishment of journals focused on pediatric neuropsychology (and the increased number of child-based studies in previously adult-focused general neuropsychology publications), the implications of this increased knowledge for clinical practice have received far less scrutiny. But ethical practice in clinical work requires that the clinical analysis of a child's behavior be informed by, and incorporate, relevant new knowledge that contributes to the improved well-being of the child. In addition, clinicians rigorously applying new techniques and principles make a unique contribution to the science of pediatric neuropsychology in their analysis of the manner in which the individual child actually functions in the natural environment. Such detailed clinical observations prompt new questions and lead to the generation of hypotheses that can be systematically tested in the research setting (McKenna & Warrington, 1986), further increasing and enriching the knowledge base.

The premise underlying the present discussion is that advances in our understanding of the relationship between brain and behavior in the child oblige clinicians to scrutinize their diagnostic and prescriptive thinking and mandate a complementary update in clinical methods. Currently, the most salient "missing element" in the practice of assessment in pediatric neuropsychology remains that of the integration of *development*, in spite of Tramontana and Hooper's (1988) clear identification of the lack. The most dramatic new knowledge with specific relevance to pediatric practice in neuropsychology comes from the neurosciences and throws light specifically on biological variables in the context of

development (Deacon, 1997; Edelman, 1987; Elman et al., 1996; Greenough, Black, &
Wallace, 1987; Segalowitz & Hiscock, 1992; Thatcher, 1992). Armed with principles derived from these new analyses, neuropsychologists are now increasingly able to apply their
expertise to, and learn from, populations of patients with neurological or systemic disorders that influence biological variables and have an impact on brain function (Taylor &
Fletcher, 1995). To take advantage of new knowledge and apply it to patients' benefit
requires that neuropsychological practitioners integrate both biology and development in
their models of assessment.

Unfortunately, development cannot simply be sprinkled, like a seasoning, into the gently
simmering stew of the traditional test-based assessment of the child. Nor is it appropriately viewed as a backdrop (albeit a crucial one) against which the child's cognitive skills,
separately measured, are viewed. Development is not a backdrop to the organism; it defines the organism in its current state. Nor, as highlighted by Tramontana and Hooper
(1988, p. 30), does applying a developmental perspective mean "simply assuring that the
tests and measures are appropriate for the age range of children being assessed" or only
"utilizing measures that are sensitive to the child's increasing competence over time." They
argue that its core requirement is an "understanding [of] how brain functions develop
normally as well as under various pathological conditions." Providing a comprehensive,
biologically referenced description of neurobehavioral functioning in the individual child
will thus necessitate a reconceptualization of the assessment process—one that has development at its core.

Such a reconceptualization is not a trivial undertaking. I believe that it is, importantly,
an issue of investigative design (research or clinical) and cannot be addressed by constructing
more refined tests or even collecting normative data. It requires a "top-down" analysis of
the whole assessment process in pediatric neuropsychology—from the theoretical foundations of neurobehavioral development and assessment practice itself, to the implications
for data collection and management, to the impact on diagnostic formulations and management strategies. The goal of this chapter is to highlight some of the issues that I believe
will need to be taken into consideration in this endeavor.

BASIC ASSUMPTIONS OF DEVELOPMENTAL
NEUROPSYCHOLOGICAL ASSESSMENT

The basic assumptions that frame the discussion of developmental neuropsychological
assessment to be outlined here (see also Bernstein, Kammerer, Prather, & Rey-Casserly,
1998) have important implications for theory, for method, and for the definition of what
precisely constitutes the nature of a neurobehavioral "problem" and therefore what the
goal of assessment is taken to be. They are as follows:

1. The primary goal of the clinical assessment is to promote the development of independence, competence, and well-being at the maximum level for the child being assessed,
now and in the future. The clinical assessment cannot be restricted to, or unduly focused
upon, academic skills or school performance. School is a critical part of a child's life, but
the skills needed for adult adjustment are not all developed or practiced there. Comprehensive clinical assessment must promote optimal functioning in all adaptive domains.

2. The criterial feature of the child is that he or she develops; the child's behavioral
repertoire changes over time. To do justice to the child's experience, assessment methodology must be *developmentally* referenced.

3. The necessary substrate for behavioral function of all types is *brain*. This is as true for social, emotional, and/or regulatory behaviors as it is for cognitive skills. Developmental outcome is a "neuropsychological/psychological layercake" (M. B. Denckla, personal communication, 1981). Invoking brain variables is not, however, sufficient to explain a given observed behavior.

4. The brain does not operate in isolation. Both the structure of the brain and its development depend on the context in which it operates. How brain function is manifested in behavior at any given moment is determined as much by contextual variables as by brain structures. Observed behavior is the product of transactions between the organism and its environment. Assessment of behavior must therefore be based on close scrutiny of the *context* in which the brain operates and behavior is observed.

5. The theoretical matrix within which developmental neuropsychological assessment takes place is therefore conceptualized as one whose interacting variables are BRAIN, CONTEXT, and DEVELOPMENT. All behaviors are scrutinized within this matrix. No behavioral outcome can be understood in terms of only one of the variables in the matrix.

Given the fifth point, incorporating DEVELOPMENT into clinical assessment models within this overall framework requires the scrutiny of both BRAIN and CONTEXT as well. (Throughout the chapter, I maintain the use of capital letters for the three components of the theoretical matrix; I employ this form of representation as a shorthand to refer to the range of concepts cued by these constructs.)

This chapter is not intended to be exhaustive, but to highlight a variety of issues pertinent to the construction of models of neuropsychological assessment that incorporate development. I first examine different ideas about the nature of the clinical assessment process itself (including, importantly, the overall stance of the clinician toward the assessment activity). I then review each of the components of the theoretical matrix, delineating some of their implications. Although, given the assumptions stated above, it is not possible to separate BRAIN, CONTEXT, and DEVELOPMENT from one another, each section is focused to the extent possible on one of the matrix components. These sections highlight aspects of the approach with regard to theoretical, methodological, and management implications. They are followed by a discussion of the link between the evaluative and management components of assessment.

THE NATURE OF CLINICAL ASSESSMENT

To incorporate the developmental perspective into clinical assessment requires, first, scrutiny of the nature of clinical assessment itself. What does a clinical assessment entail? What are the formal theoretical assumptions that govern this type of endeavor? What are its methods—its modes of practice and of interpretation? What is special about the assessment of children? How these questions are answered by individual clinicians determines to a great extent how they practice.

Goals and Purposes of Clinical Assessment

It may be helpful to start by reviewing some assumptions about the goals and purposes of clinical assessment. The clinical assessment is the primary means by which the products of research are utilized in the service of the individual. It is the primary professional activity of the clinician, the overriding goal of which is to promote the optimal adaptation and well-being of the person being assessed. *Assessment* is not coterminous with *evaluation* or *testing*, although these terms are frequently used as though they were synonymous. Assessment is a "complex clinical activity" (Vanderploeg, 1994, p. 38) that cannot simply be equated with testing (Matarazzo, 1990). Nor is it finished once a child has been assigned to a diagnostic category; it also requires the formulation of a coherent management strategy. Thus, assessment subsumes evaluation and management as two sides of the same coin and, importantly, entails that the same theoretical principles that govern the evaluative process (the child in the clinician's office) also direct the management plan (the child's adaptation, now and in the future, in his or her own world).

Assessment as Investigation

The clinical assessment is approached as an experiment with an n of 1. This means that the clinical investigation must fulfill the same formal requirements as the research investigation (Bernstein & Weiler, in press). Reexamining the nature of assessment thus does not mean bemoaning the lack of specific tests or of normative data (although improved tests and wider-ranging norms would certainly be desirable). It means starting "at the top": identifying what questions should be asked, determining whether the investigative design can respond to the questions being posed, querying the methodology, analyzing the potential biases that may influence data collection and interpretation, and exploring the implications of different strategies for diagnostic decision making.

Clinical versus Standardized Assessment

As suggested above, the primary goal of a comprehensive clinical assessment is, in an important sense, to produce a comfortable, competent 25-year-old—that is, an adult who can take his or her place in society. Comprehensive clinical assessment must promote optimal functioning in all adaptive domains. This entails, of necessity, a longitudinal and developmental perspective. This goal is entirely congruent with the view of parents, who are necessarily in for the long haul; it need not, however, be the goal of educators, whose mandate (somewhat facetiously stated) is "to produce the world's best third—or sixth—grader" (Bernstein, 1998, p. 3).

From the longitudinal viewpoint, an important part of the clinician's role is to foster, to the extent possible, maximum independence and maximum social acceptance over time in the youngster who presents for evaluation. To promote this larger goal, the evaluative or diagnostic component of the assessment requires the clinician not to "paint by numbers" (K. O. Yeates, personal communication, 1996), but rather to paint "the psychological portrait" (Matarazzo, 1990, p. 1016) of the child. This entails both an intraindividual and a broad-based analysis, encompassing in one integrated assessment emotional, regulatory, motor, and sensory capacities, as well as cognitive abilities and social, societal, and academic achievement (Bornstein, 1990). These requirements dovetail perfectly with the neuropsychological perspective on behavior. Not only does clinical neuropsychology by its very nature as a clinical discipline focus on the individual; it is also inherently integrative in its fundamental reliance on knowledge of brain as the necessary, albeit not sufficient, substrate for *all* behavior. Thus the challenge is to describe this child's unique neurobehavioral repertoire—a description that entails scrutiny and understanding of all categories of behavior in light of all the others.

The premises of longitudinal perspective and broad-based description are not fundamental to the conduct of more traditional analyses of children's abilities based on standardized assessment models. The assumptions underlying the use of standardized tests, even in the neuropsychological context, are not the assumptions of assessment in the clinical setting. Clinical assessment is a wider-ranging endeavor than that provided by psychological testing alone (Matarazzo, 1990). Traditional assessment relies heavily, and in some settings exclusively, on standardized tests. Such tests were developed with the primary goal of *interindividual ranking*, in order to assign children to appropriate educational settings and services. They were not designed primarily for *intraindividual analysis*, which requires that the clinician respond to the child individually. Thus the clinician is obligated to contravene a basic premise of the standardized assessment (i.e., that all children be responded to equally; see Ginsburg, 1997, for an elegant analysis of the challenge to be faced here). Of note in this regard is the concept of *rapport*, as discussed in the manuals for even our most prestigious psychological tests and test batteries. Rapport is typically presented as if it is some sort of static entity that is established once and for all before testing proceeds. But rapport, by its very nature, depends on the individualized and ongoing response of the clinician to the child, and vice versa. There is thus an inherent contradiction in the juxtaposition of the requirement for rapport and the requirements for standardization!

An additional limitation of psychological tests is their inability to "model adequately the underlying neural substrate . . . [or to] . . . situate the behavior in the context of the specific characteristics of childhood neural pathology" (Holmes-Bernstein & Waber, 1990, p. 317). Although specific patterns of psychological test performance may have neurological validity, in that they suffice to predict group membership in neurologically involved versus noninvolved youngsters (Fletcher, Taylor, Levin, & Satz, 1995), no pattern of psychological test performance can "diagnose" a brain system in a single individual without the intermediation of the trained clinician, who has the skills and expertise needed to make a judgment linking the behavioral profile to a specified neural substrate. It is the inference drawing that is neuropsychological, not the test performance (Taylor, 1988). This is as true of actuarially based assessment strategies as of "clinically framed" approaches (Willis, 1986).

This is not to say, of course, that the tools and techniques of standardized assessment methodologies cannot be employed for the individualized clinical assessment. They are and should be. What it does entail, however, is an examination of the goals and purposes of the clinical assessment, of the theoretical framework governing the assessment activity, of the methodology to be employed, and (only then) of the role of the tests and techniques in the overall assessment strategy.

The Theoretical Framework for Assessment

Assessment of a child's repertoire of behavioral capacities does not take place in a theoretical vacuum, but is undertaken in the context of the clinician's particular set of beliefs (theory) as to how this particular organism behaves—its capabilities and limitations. The theory of neurobehavioral functioning held by the clinician determines (1) what the clinician chooses to assess and how he or she goes about doing it (the evaluative component), and (2) how the resulting data are interpreted and used as the basis for intervention (the management component). The clinical assessment process can be understood as the method by which the clinician attempts to map a theory of a specific child (derived from the individual assessment procedure) onto a more general theory of the developing child derived from the neurobehavioral knowledge base (taken to include, for the well-trained neuro-psychological clinician, knowledge of psychology and education as well as neuropsychology and neurology). The theoretical framework for assessment must thus include this more general *theory of the organism*.

A theory of the organism, however, is not enough in and of itself. Clinicians do their work in the context of perceived dysfunction or disability. For pediatric neuropsychologists, the continuum of dysfunction/disability ranges from behavioral and learning disorders (which may not involve documentable brain lesions but are nonetheless presumed to be dependent on brain functioning) to specific examples of biological breakdown (whose impact on brain function and/or development can be clearly demonstrated). Clinical analysis of a child's behavioral function must be undertaken in the context of the *theory or theories of the potential disorders* that affect children at different ages.

In addition, the means whereby the clinical analysis is undertaken requires a *theory of the assessment process* itself. This is not a fixed entity. Both new knowledge of the organism to be measured and the availability of new methodologies—new models of test construction (Lowman, 1996), as well as new tests (Das, Naglieri, & Kirby, 1994; Korkman, Kemp & Kirk, 1998; Kaplan, Fein, Delis, & Morris, 1999)—can lead to changes in what and how we measure. They therefore require diagnostic thinking, and the assumptions and methodology of the assessment process, to be continually reviewed and updated.

The theoretical framework for assessment is thus, at a minimum, tripartite: It includes (1) a theory of the organism, (2) a theory or theories of potential disorders, and (3) a theory of the assessment process. In some views (including my own), it includes a further component: (4) a theory of pedagogy.[1]

Current Models of Neuropsychological Assessment

The models addressed here are deliberately characterized as models of assessment, in line with my earlier definition of the two necessary components of the assessment process. The discussion does not address different approaches to measurement of neuropsychological functions as exemplified in fixed versus flexible batteries (see, e.g., Bornstein, 1990, for a review). The discussion focuses on different approaches to the integrated process of diagnosis, evaluation, and management that constitutes assessment in its full (and proper) sense.

The approach to the clinical assessment of the child advocated here is characterized as the *systemic developmental approach* or the *neurodevelopmental systems approach*. This should be differentiated from two other approaches to the clinical assessment of children that have been informed by neuropsychology—namely, *normative developmental approaches* and the *process approach*.

Normative Developmental Approaches

First, although the neurodevelopmental systems approach (Bernstein et al., 1998; Bernstein, Prather, & Rey-Casserly, 1995; Bernstein & Waber, 1997; Bernstein & Weiler, in press; Holmes-Bernstein & Waber, 1990) recognizes the importance of biology, behavior, and context, the approach is not the type of "biobehavioral–contextual" model formulated by Fletcher and Taylor (Taylor & Fletcher, 1990; Fletcher et al., 1995) or, in broadly similar terms, by Rourke and his colleagues (Rourke, Bakker, Fisk, & Strang,

1983; Rourke, Fisk, & Strang, 1986). The assessment approaches of Fletcher and Taylor and their colleagues, and of Rourke and his colleagues, are similar in their organization in terms of the child's cognitive ability structure and the context in which this is analyzed. They differ markedly, however, in how they integrate the BRAIN variable. Based on their elegant review of the "fallacies" that result from an unconsidered application of adult neuropsychological principles to the evaluation of children's behavior, Fletcher and Taylor (1984) explicitly eschewed BRAIN as a core premise of the assessment strategy and argued for a function–function approach. In contrast, Rourke (1975, 1982) equally explicitly chose in favor of BRAIN, and has continued to make application to brain-referenced constructs to explain clinical profiles (Rourke, 1989; Rourke et al., 1983, 1986). Most of Rourke and colleagues' research investigations have nonetheless been driven by group selection on the basis of contrasting patterns of academic or cognitive performance profiles.

A colleague and I (Bernstein and Weiler, in press) have characterized the core assessment strategy of the Fletcher/Taylor and Rourke approaches as representative of "normative developmental" models. These are distinguished from the neurodevelopmental systems/systemic developmental model by the fact that in the former, the unit of analysis at the core of the clinical strategy is the child's *cognitive ability structure*. The clinical meaning of the cognitive ability structure is subsequently interpreted in relation to the biobehavioral context appropriate to the child in question. The normative developmental models clearly incorporate developmental principles; the clinician has a sophisticated understanding of the developmental differences in the biobehavioral contexts of children of different ages. Nonetheless, the core unit of analysis is the child's *current presentation*. That is, it is a "horizontal" analysis, with the biobehavioral and developmental factors being incorporated in the role of moderator variables that weigh the observations in the interpretive process.

The Systemic Developmental/Neurodevelopmental Systems Approach

In contrast, the systemic developmental/neurodevelopmental systems approach takes *the child himself or herself* as the core unit of analysis. To many readers, this may appear to be a distinction that is not immediately meaningful. Doesn't everyone work with the child? Don't we all have the child's welfare at heart? The distinction is, however, not initially one that applies to the actual interaction with the child in the office (although it has specific implications even for this). Instead, it is one of method—a critical building block in the investigative design.

In developing one's clinical strategy, what one chooses to put first—that is, the core unit of analysis—reflects the theoretical framework within which the data will be collected and interpreted; it thus both frames the overall investigative design and shapes the subsequent collection of data. Putting the child first situates our approach squarely in the developmental psychology tradition, highlighting the child as a constructor of knowledge (Piaget, 1936/1952) and a "behaver" in the environment (Vygotsky, 1978, 1986). In contrast, starting with the cognitive ability structure as the core unit of analysis sends a different message—one that focuses on cognition and academic skills/adjustment. The difference in fundamental approach will have different implications. Methodologically, the clinical strategies will be subject to different biases and will require different investigative controls. As the evaluation proceeds, the data to be collected may differ, the emphasis assigned to given aspects of the data may differ, and what is chosen for interpretation may differ. These all have the potential to lead to alternative ways of framing the diagnosis. In the development of management strategies, alternative diagnostic formulations can be expected to shape the way in which assessment findings are communicated and how the child, the family, and other professionals understand the child's problem.

The fundamental stance of the systemic developmental approach owes much to Piaget's (1936/1952) "clinical interview" techniques, but is essentially that of Vygotsky (1978, 1986). The focus of the assessment is not the Piagetian analysis of the internal workings of the child's mind, but rather the Vygotskian perspective of the child as a "behaver" in his or her environment, which exerts significant influence on the behavior under observation. This formulation is not based on the enrichment of standardized assessment methods by the fruits of clinical interview and/or process analysis. It takes the clinical interview of the child as the fundamental point of departure for intraindividual clinical analysis, seeking to incorporate, with all due rigor, standardized assessment methodology to test the hypotheses generated in the course of the assessment.

The Process Approach

Given the distinction previously discussed between clinical and standardized assessment of children, it is important to note the distinction that should be drawn between the systemic developmental model and the "process approach" as formulated by Kaplan and her colleagues (Goodglass & Kaplan, 1979; Kaplan, 1983, 1988; Kaplan et al., 1999; Milberg, Hebben, & Kaplan, 1986). Kaplan's approach has been to use brain-based knowledge derived from adults with brain lesions to enrich standardized assessment strategies, with the goal of improving diagnostic accuracy by means of detailed analysis of an individual's errors and of his or her behavior en route to solution. This type of strategy is now being applied to perhaps the most widely used standardized measure traditionally used in the assessment of children, the Wechsler Intelligence Scale for Children—Third Edition (WISC-III; Wechsler, 1991), as a Process Instrument (WISC-III-PI; Kaplan et al., 1999).

The systemic developmental approach has sometimes been described as a "process approach with children"; however, this is not an appropriate characterization. Certainly, analyzing the process by which a child tackles a task is part of the individualized stance toward the child that is integral to the clinical assessment in Ginsburg's (1997) view; it is also a necessary component of the developmental clinical analysis, with its emphasis on the role of the task-referenced contextual variables as these are reflected in the child's behavior over time. Nonetheless, the process approach essentially defines a strategy for maximizing the collection of rich, clinically meaningful data. The value of the data collected still depends on the theoretical framework guiding the assessment—a framework that must be reconceptualized to include developmental principles at its core.

The foregoing discussion highlights some of the basic assumptions involved in different models of assessment. The position argued here is that improved assessment models do not depend on the development of better and better-normed tests, but require a "top-down" analysis of the assessment process itself. Such an examination of the assessment process will require an examination of the theoretical framework in which it takes place. The following discussion addresses some of the implications of the BRAIN–CONTEXT–DEVELOPMENT matrix as applied to the clinical setting. As noted earlier, although the three components of the matrix cannot in practice be separated, the discussion focuses on each of them in turn.

BRAIN

Theoretical Assumptions

> *Guiding Principle*:
>
> Brain is the necessary—albeit not sufficient—substrate for behavior.

The basic theoretical assumption associated with BRAIN is the necessity of the construct itself for any clinical analysis that purports to be neuropsychological. A neuropsychological account of behavior must engage with principles of brain–behavior relationships (see Rourke, 1975, 1982), regardless of the well-delineated difficulties in applying adult-derived principles to children (Fletcher & Taylor, 1984). In the systemic developmental approach, integration of BRAIN into the overall assessment strategy has implications for how the problems that neuropsychological assessment is intended to address are framed, what the core unit of analysis is taken to be, how evaluation data are organized, and how the communication of findings is shaped.

This stance has two particular implications. The first reflects the fact that the brain is "owned" by the child. Since (1) a major goal of the assessment process is the portrait of the child, that is, his or her capacities and adaptation, and to be neuropsychological the assessment must incorporate BRAIN, then the assessment must be child-centered.

The second implication follows from the understanding of the brain as the "organ of learning"—necessary, albeit not sufficient, to support the full range of behaviors that the developing child has to learn. This implies that anything that the brain has to learn can conceivably be derailed. In this view, the term *learning disorder* is not restricted to deficits in the acquisition of academic skills (traditionally called *learning disabilities*), but encompasses deficits in communication, language, spatial skills, motor abilities, regulatory capacities, problem-solving skills, social cognition and comportment, and so forth (see also Pennington, 1991). Thus, in this conceptualization, all behavioral capacities are regarded as equivalent in their ability to generate independent deficits and to interact with each other. No one group of capacities is taken to be in any sense primary or more salient, with others acting as moderator variables to influence the interpretation of the primary ones. Some variables may indeed exert moderating influences on others, but this is not assumed to be the case *a priori* as part of the theoretical framework of the assessment process. This definition of *learning disorder* thus permits a more coherent, neuropsychologically based formulation that is responsive to the full range of disorders seen by practicing clinical neuropsychologists in both educational and medical settings.

The concept of *learning disorder*, as defined in terms of the BRAIN–CONTEXT–DEVELOPMENT matrix, is characterized as a "failure to adapt successfully to the learning environment [which] is best understood in the context of a developmental neuropsychological theory" (Holmes-Bernstein & Waber, 1990, p. 329). The problem that brings the child (and family) to the attention of the clinician is one of *adaptation*, not of personal deficit. To illustrate this principle, consider the following question: Can you have dyslexia if you do not live in a society that prizes universal literacy? The answer is no! You can certainly have a biological risk factor for dyslexia, but if nobody ever asks you to read, how would we know that you had it? This means that the definition of dyslexia or any other learning disorder cannot be considered simply a "property" of the child, but rather must be conceptualized as a product of the transactions between that child's brain (i.e., neurobehavioral endowment/current repertoire of skills) and the environment in which the child finds himself or herself. It also follows from this concept of adaptation that documentable biological malfunction is not sufficient in and of itself to define *disorder*; the malfunction must also be experienced as "harmful" by its owner—or, in the case of the child, the members of the child's immediate environment (Wakefield, 1990). As many neuropsychologists working with neurologically involved children can attest, adaptive competence can vary widely, even among individuals whose behavioral functioning might have been expected to be severely constrained by well-documented and severe destruction of brain tissue.

Methodological Considerations

Data Reduction Heuristics

The BRAIN construct plays a major role in the data reduction that is critical to organizing and interpreting the wealth of behavioral observations generated in the course of an assessment. Perhaps the greatest challenge for clinical diagnosis is the limited capacity of the human brain. We clinicians are unable to effectively process and integrate more than a fraction of the data that we can elicit in a clinical interaction (Kerlinger, 1986). This means that all of us, whether we recognize it or not, are forced to use some sort of heuristic strategy to reduce the volume of data to manageable proportions. An important part of the training of future clinicians is explicit recognition of (1) the operation of heuristic strategies and (2) the biases that are associated with them and that influence interpretation. All clinical approaches are subject to bias. Different clinical approaches elicit different biases, however, and require different controls to limit them.

In the approach advocated here, the diagnostic heuristic that helps organize the behavioral data is framed explicitly in BRAIN terms, as represented by a three-axis model consisting of the lateral, anterior–posterior, and cortical–subcortical axes (see also Goldstein, 1986; Rourke, 1982). It is important to note that this is an organizing heuristic and not a localizing statement. Observations are collected and scrutinized within the three-axis framework. The clinician generates and tests hypotheses that are based on the ways in which specific behaviors are believed to cluster together, given current formulations of brain–behavior relationships. In the individual clinical setting, the child's overall behavioral presentation is examined in order to identify clusters of behaviors that can be associated with the integrity (or lack thereof) of one or more specific brain systems. Both the notion of integrity of specific brain systems, and the nature and function of the behavioral clusters that are critical for diagnosis, require further examination.

The Complementary-Contribution Principle

The notion of relative integrity of specific brain systems derives from the complementary-contribution principle formulated by Kaplan (Kaplan, 1976; Goodglass & Kaplan, 1982). It was well known at the time that when adult brain-lesioned patients were asked to draw everyday objects, their products were impaired and the patterns of impairment could be related more or less systematically to the locus of their lesions on the lateral brain axis (Critchley, 1959; McFie & Zangwill, 1960; McFie, Piercy, & Zangwill, 1950). Thus patients with lesions to the right hemisphere made drawings that might be rich in detail and include clearly recognizable attempts to reproduce categorical parts of the stimulus item, but that lacked an appreciation for the gestalt or overall logic of the target. In contrast, patients with left-hemisphere lesions made drawings that represented larger, more global forms, but that lacked detail (often to the extent that they were unrecognizable without knowledge of the stimulus cue). Kaplan's insight, however, was to interpret these different patterns of performance not as reflecting compromised performance of the damaged system, but as representing the intact contribution of the undamaged system doing its best, so to speak, in the absence of its partner. Her insight was formulated as the principle of *complementary contribution*. The implication of these observations from patients with focal brain damage is that what one sees in the drawings of individuals without brain damage—and, by extension, what is going on in normal, on-line information processing by the brain—is the product of both hemispheric systems' working together in complementary fashion.

This principle is an important contribution to the clinical analysis of the child's behavior, and thus potentially to the diagnostic formulation. In the clinical analysis, it cues the clinician to look for relative efficiency versus relative inefficiency of the contributions of different brain systems to a given behavior. Thus, for example, the appreciation of complex visual–spatial material calls on a large number of interacting psychological processes. In the face of such complexity, the description provided by test scores may be too coarse-grained and thus may have limited discriminative power. Test scores in such instances are ideally combined with an examination of the quality of performance and of the process whereby the task was tackled. A child's production can be inspected for evidence that the child has an appreciation of larger gestalt parameters (hypothesized to be dependent on right-hemisphere mechanisms) and for evidence that the child recognizes information about detail (thought to be more dependent on the left hemisphere's contribution to the task). Comparably, on tests involving written language, understanding of discourse parameters or appreciation for the gist of the narrative may provide evidence for input from right-hemisphere mechanisms, while an appreciation for syntax, specific facts, and related material may reflect the left hemisphere's contribution.

Conceptualizing Behavioral Clusters

The identification of diagnostic behavioral clusters is directly dependent on knowledge of brain–behavior relationships as postulated by neuropsychological theory. A *diagnostic behavioral cluster* is a fuzzy set of converging variables whose focus is a neurobehavioral system (Holmes-Bernstein & Waber, 1990). It is thus a group of behavioral variables that are derived from analysis of the historic variables, from direct observations of performance in both clinical and nonclinical settings, and from psychological test performances. All of the members of the diagnostic cluster are postulated to be dependent on the same or closely allied brain systems.

The integration of the three-axis heuristic and the complementary-contribution principle into the clinical analysis strategy has specific implications for the way in which relevant behavioral clusters are identified, conceptualized, and labeled. For example, a diagnostic behavioral cluster labeled by a phrase such as "left-hemisphere-implicating" refers to the co-occurrence in the child's protocol of a group of behaviors that are considered, all other things being equal, to depend on the integrity of left-hemisphere mechanisms. In this example, because the cluster is considered "left-hemisphere-implicating," the workings of left-hemisphere mechanisms are hypothesized to be relatively undermined.

The use of organizing constructs such as "left-hemisphere-implicating" must rest on a clear appreciation for the different levels of organization of data in a clinical analysis. Explicit recognition of the *manifest or index symptom level* versus the *psychological-process level* versus the *neuropsychological level* is important not only for correctly identifying and interpreting the data, but also for formulating the diagnosis. Which level can be invoked in the organization and interpretation of data depends on the nature of the behaviors observed. For instance, the ability to make the judgment that results in the formulation of "left-hemisphere-implicating cluster," which is a statement at the neuropsychological level, must be based on a cross-domain analysis; that is, the behaviors observed are different in kind but are believed to depend on the same brain systems. If the behaviors observed are restricted to only one behavioral domain (such as language), a specific brain system may be involved. However, without independent neurological or neurodiagnostic documentation of that involvement, the conclusion of the neuropsychological analysis can only be framed in psychological or functional terms ("language disorder"), not in terms of possible neural substrates.

The clinical judgment of "left-hemisphere-implicating cluster" also requires identification of behavioral clusters that include both convergent and discriminating variables. That is, the clinical analysis must pay equal attention to behaviors that are intact and behaviors that reflect deficient performance. The phrase "left-hemisphere-implicating" means both that left-hemisphere-mediated functions are relatively insecure and that right-hemisphere-mediated functions are relatively intact. If both left- and right-hemisphere-implicating behavioral clusters are present in the child's protocol, then the clinical hypothesis will need to incorporate the possibility of a global, systemic, or diffuse process in addition to the possibility that more than one discrete behavioral cluster may be present as in the case, for example, of a *contre-coup* head injury.

What the phrase "left-hemisphere-implicating cluster" does *not* mean—at least, not necessarily—is that the left hemisphere in any sense has a lesion in it. At this point in the clinical analysis, the phrase means only that in the presumed balance of functions along the lateral axis, the behaviors associated with left-hemisphere mechanisms appear to be working relatively less efficiently than the behaviors associated with right-hemisphere mechanisms.

The next step, that of characterizing the source of any discrepancy, is a separate and specific clinical judgment. The pattern of discrepant performance need not be a signal of the presence of dysfunction or damage to the brain; it can equally well reflect individual differences between children that are constitutional or developmental in nature. The extent to which the behavioral cluster identified by the clinical analysis can be mapped onto individual difference, dysfunction, or damage in the case of this particular child requires a separate diagnostic decision which must be based on multiple considerations: (1) the child's presenting problem(s), (2) the course of biological and behavioral issues to date, (3) knowledge of potential disorders that can have an impact on a child of this age and sex, (4) familial variables, and (5) socioeconomic and other environmental variables.

As noted, discrepancies in observed behavior can be the result of localized brain damage or neurological dysfunction. However, they can also reflect the impact of atypical development or of a pattern of individual difference that influences how the child deals with complex information. For example, insults to the brain that are nonfocal, inasmuch as they result from systemic exposure to toxic agents, can nonetheless lead to "asymmetrical" neuropsychological profiles as a function of the timing of the exposure in neurobehavioral development (Shaheen, 1984; Waber et al., 1990). Similarly, information-processing deficits that are nonspecific may lead to difficulties or errors in tackling certain types of tasks (but not others) that may be indistinguishable from the impact of specific brain lesions on the same type of materials. Children who process information very slowly, for instance, may have difficulty apprehending the gestalt or configurational aspects of a complex figure as they copy it. In the absence of time constraints and with the target stimulus in full view throughout the task, they may make a reasonably good copy of the figure, representing both larger elements and details. After a delay, however, they all too often recall a set of parts from the original, with little sense of how the parts were logically organized. Their slowed speed of processing appears to limit how the information is coded for later recall, and this results in the loss of gestalt under recall conditions. (See also Geary, Brown, & Samaranayake, 1991, with respect to arithmetic skill development.) Loss of gestalt can be seen in the context of a right-hemisphere lesion; it would be wrong, however, to assume that the converse is true (i.e., that loss of gestalt definitively indicates right-hemisphere damage). The interpretation of any behavior depends on its context, as framed by the task conditions and the child's neurobehavioral repertoire, and the interaction between them.

BRAIN as a Dependent and an Independent Variable

The conceptualization of BRAIN within the overall theoretical framework also influences how data are viewed in the course of the evaluative procedure itself. As clearly stated by Bakker (1984), it is important not to be "neuro-centric" and to limit one's investigation to questions of this type: "What part of the brain is responsible for behavior X?" It is critical to recognize the indivisibility of brain and its context, and to ask, "What is it about the context in which this behavior is happening that is eliciting this response from the brain?" Consider, for example, the following fairly common analysis. A child performs poorly on a block design task; at the same time, the clinician observes behaviors consistent with anxiety. The observation is construed as follows: "The child is anxious, and the anxiety is interfering with performance on the block design task." This might be true, but it is unlikely that anxiety would selectively interfere with one task. In this analysis, "anxiety" is not an observation, but a diagnostic statement. The actual observation can be more precisely stated as follows: "In the face of the block design task, the child is showing a high level of arousal." The critical diagnostic question, then, is this: "What is it about the processing demands of the block design task that is causing this child to be unable to regulate arousal age-appropriately?"

Implications for Management

Clinical management has two major components: (1) education of the child and parents (and other involved professionals), and (2) the development of recommendations to optimize the child's adaptation to the specific demands of his or her unique environment. These are communicated to the parents via the feedback (interpretive, informing) session and the report.

The education component covers general principles that apply to the neurobehavioral development of all children and includes discussion of the various social, adaptive, and academic challenges that must be met over the course of childhood and adolescence. It also includes more specific principles that are derived from the skill profile of this particular child; again, however, these are related to the expectable developmental challenges that all children must try to meet. Examples of the respective roles of BRAIN, CONTEXT, and DEVELOPMENT in children's experience in general and this child's experience in particular are used to illustrate the situations in which the child may be at risk for difficulty and ways in which the risk can be bypassed. An important goal of the discussion is to normalize the child's experience, as well as the parents' experience with the child.

The formulation of recommendations must address the need to manage larger issues—for example, appropriate educational placement and/or peer and family situations and interactions. An alternative school placement, an appropriate classroom setting, and/or a specific type of instructional approach may need to be identified. Family counseling, parent guidance, and/or individual or group therapies may be needed to address psychosocial issues. Recommendations must also provide specific strategies for working with the child. An appropriate strategic plan will include general principles that are likely to apply across domains or activities (managing load, pacing effort, reducing distraction, etc.). It will also provide strategies that focus on specific challenges or tasks (acronym-cued lists of steps for writing assignments, specific instructional approaches for different aspects of mathematics or reading, etc.). The formulation of general principles is typically in response to the BRAIN variable, as manifested in the child's particular neurobehavioral repertoire. For example, the child with regulatory difficulties should be considered at risk in all situations that lack inherent structure. Recommendations should thus include the types of strategies that can help the child to manage load in general across situations (see Bernstein, 1996). Specific recommendations typically respond to the CONTEXT variable; they require a more detailed task and situation analysis, with the child's skills matched as well as possible to the specific demand to be met.

Communicating Findings

The BRAIN construct has at least two valuable roles in the communication of findings to child, family, and other involved professionals. First, it is BRAIN that differentiates the neuropsychologist's role from the roles of the school psychologist and the educational specialist. It is specifically the integrative nature of BRAIN that is most useful in this regard, because it counters what I have dubbed, after frequent encounters with bewildered parents dealing with the educational system, "diagnosis by Swiss cheese." Parents are frequently given a description in terms of psychological test performances. Thus a child may be described as having auditory short-term memory problems, visual–motor integration difficulties, fine motor deficits, and so forth. Parents typically have no way of interpreting all these "holes" in functioning with reference to their child, whom they naturally experience as an integrated individual. The neuropsychological perspective can often provide a framework for explaining the co-occurrence of many behaviors, leaving parents with a much more coherent view of their child and one that is also consistent with their own experience. The brain-referenced explanation offered to parents need not be detailed; broad principles are sufficient to provide the needed framework. The clinician may also wish to offer disclaimers about the limits of present knowledge, whenever it seems appropriate to do so. Nonetheless, the BRAIN construct has important explanatory power with respect to the organization of behaviors that may otherwise seem quite discrepant and thus bewildering to both child and family.

I also use the BRAIN construct as a means of "normalizing" the child's experience. There are two important issues at stake here. One is that of normalizing the child's experience with respect to that of other members of the family. For instance, the parents can be told, "If I were to give you the adult version of the tests I gave to [the child], I could describe your strengths and weaknesses in just the same way." This can be particularly important when the child is being pathologized or treated as intrinsically different from other members of the family because of learning issues, and when the child is not being owned as a true member of the family because the fact of the child's learning disorder is experienced as a narcissistic injury by one or both of the parents. The second issue is that of normalizing the child's experience with respect to the ongoing, expectable developmental challenges of childhood. Just like children developing normally, youngsters with neuro-behavioral conditions must tackle the various tasks associated with development during childhood. Of course, they are likely to need help in so doing if they are to compensate for the impact of their neurobehavioral conditions. Nonetheless, parents need to understand the normality of the expectations that their child must meet, and thus the need to develop ways in which the attendant challenges can be met as successfully as possible.

The Complementary-Contribution Principle

The complementary-contribution principle has an important role to play in the communication of findings and thus the management of the child's well-being. This principle is the basis for identifying strengths, which reflect the contribution of the relatively more intact brain system. This relates to another very important assumption in clinical neuropsychological assessment, which is the requirement to explain the "ups" in performance as well as the "downs." Given that the child has presented with a problem, and the neuropsychologist believes that there are data consistent with, say, "language deficits" or "left-hemisphere dysfunction," it behooves the responsible clinician to find out and explain why a child with this degree of deficit can nonetheless solve many problems as well as or even better than other youngsters of the same age. Why is this important? It is important for a richer understanding of the child, the core of the successful assessment. But it is also the *sine qua non* of successful rehabilitation. One cannot base a coherent rehabilitation strategy on deficits. The utility of planning interventions based on what actually works for the individual child cannot be overstated in the rehabilitation context.

CONTEXT

Theoretical Assumptions

> *Guiding Principle*:
>
> Brain does not operate in isolation.

The lessons of neuroscience are that neither the structure nor the development of the brain is independent of the context in which it operates (Edelman, 1987; Elman et al., 1996; Greenough et al., 1987). The reciprocal relationship between an organism and its environment is also central to theories of behavioral development (Bronfenbrenner, 1993; Bronfenbrenner & Ceci, 1994; Case, 1992; Case & Okamoto, 1996; Ceci, 1996; Fischer & Rose, 1994). An important implication of this principle for the assessment process is that how brain functioning is manifested in behavior at any given moment depends as much on contextual variables as on brain structures. The phrase *contextual variables* must be understood in its widest sense to include the individual's constitutional endowment, previous history, and the full range of environmental influences (demographic, socioeconomic, emotional, situational, etc.) operating at the time the behavior is observed. Observed behavior is the product of transactions between the organism and its environment. Assessment of behavior must therefore be based on close scrutiny of the context in which the brain operates and the behavior is observed.

A second important principle is that of the *construction* involved in the observation of behavior (Globus, 1973). No behavior can be observed independently of an observer and thus of the observer's preconceptions and biases. The observer in the clinical setting is the clinician. Thus the clinician must be understood as a critical element in the context of the assessment, and his or her contribution to what is observed must be scrutinized in detail.

Methodological Considerations

Diagnostic Stance

The inclusion of CONTEXT as a critical theoretical component has implications for the strategic stance the clinician brings to the diagnostic process. Given that brain functioning cannot be defined without reference to context, then a diagnosis in brain terms cannot be based on a simple tally of behaviors that add up to a brain system. In the BRAIN–CON-TEXT–DEVELOPMENT framework, the clinician's primary diagnostic strategy must necessarily be one of ruling out all possible nonbrain (contextual) variables that might give rise to the behavior in question. This strategy not only is responsive to the model currently under discussion, but also has the advantage of requiring that the clinician actively counter the "confirmatory bias" (Tversky & Kahneman, 1974) by seeking potentially falsifying data before offering a hypothesis about BRAIN.

Consider a straightforward, somewhat oversimplified example of this principle in action. The reasoning is as follows: Neuropsychological theory posits a strong relationship between language skills and left-hemisphere brain systems. Formulating an utterance that defines a word (e.g., WISC-III Vocabulary) clearly depends on language ability. Therefore, a Vocabulary scaled score indicates something about the integrity of the left hemisphere. Such reasoning may prove to be correct, in that a low Vocabulary score may be an index of insecure left-hemisphere input to the behavioral profile observed. However, vocabulary knowledge is notoriously subject to educational exposure. This being the case, the low Vocabulary score may only reflect lack of schooling. Conversely, a high Vocabulary score cannot be taken as a guarantee that the left hemisphere is intact. Vocabulary knowledge, because of its overlearned nature, can remain intact when other skills are severely undermined by documentable brain lesions. An individual's educational experience is not intrinsic to BRAIN, but is part of his or her sociocultural context. The clinician must not make the mistake of assuming that the manifest behavior (here, language) leads directly to a brain-referenced diagnosis. The nature of the language stimuli must be analyzed. In this example, the properties of the overlearned verbal knowledge base are determined by contextual variables, which override any simple formulation in terms of a direct brain–behavior relationship. Such CONTEXT variables must be scrutinized explicitly in this model.

The Role of the Clinician

One of the contextual influences that has specific consequences for assessment practice is one that is not addressed frequently enough in clinical practice, in spite of its considerable potential for eliciting error and bias in clinical decision making. This is the behavior of the clinician. A clinician plays at least four roles in assessing an individual: (1) administering and scoring psychological tests; (2) eliciting behavior directly as a member of the child–clinician dyad; (3) analyzing behavioral information; and (4) making diagnostic decisions

(Bernstein & Weiler, in press). The first of these roles is traditionally considered to be the role of the testing psychologist; its rules are prescribed by test manuals and learned in the course of the psychologist's training. The role of diagnostic decision maker is one that has been well studied in a variety of clinical disciplines (e.g., Faust & Nurcombe, 1989; Fisch, Hammond, & Joyce, 1982; Goldberg, 1968; Golden, 1964; Nisbett & Ross, 1980; Oskamp, 1965), although the relevant knowledge base is not always applied consciously in the psychological assessment context. The roles of behavior elicitor and analyzer of behavioral information, however, are not so well defined and depend heavily on the model that drives the assessment. The former reflects the role of the clinician as an integral, and irremovable, component of the context created by the assessment. The latter depends on what the clinician considers relevant data for analysis, as determined by the theoretical framework guiding the assessment process.

Careful observation of experienced clinicians interacting with children in the context of an evaluation reveals that the clinician is a critical part of the context of any assessment. Clinicians' behavior is far from being standardized and responsive in an equal fashion to all children (see Ginsburg, 1997). It is uniquely influenced by a given child, and influences that child's behavior, as is the case in all human interactions. Indeed, it is not possible to eliminate a clinician's influence in his or her interaction with a child. Nor would it be desirable to do so, even if it were possible. If the clinician were to act as a rigid, nonresponsive entity, the very nature of the child's interaction with the environment, of which the clinician is a critical part, would be dramatically changed. But the child's interactions with the environment, which reflect his or her adaptive strengths and weaknesses, are precisely what the assessment is intended to explore. This means that psychological tests, which are administered individually to a child by an adult, cannot be completely objective without changing what it is they are trying to measure—namely, the child's behavior.

It is also important to note that the (necessary) responsiveness of the clinician to the individual child does not mean that the influence of the clinician is subjective and therefore necessarily suspect. It does require that the clinician's behavior in interaction with a child be scrutinized, that the role of specific variables in the child–clinician dyad be operationalized, and that appropriate safeguards for the potential biases that may result from the unique child–adult interaction be built into the investigative design that guides the assessment process (see Bernstein & Weiler, in press, for an extended discussion). In addition, close analysis of individual styles and behaviors with different children must be made part of the training of clinical practitioners.

Interviewing

The CONTEXT construct is invoked most saliently in the examination and understanding of the nature of the child's adaptation to the natural environment. Because the clinician cannot conduct moment-to-moment observations of the ongoing incidents that make up a child's daily life, this has specific implications for the conduct of clinical interviews. Such interviews are major sources of information from the various people who interact with the child under different circumstances; they give the clinician a rich, many-sided view of the child. As a critical source of behavioral data, a clinical interview must be undertaken rigorously, with controls for variability and bias in both interviewer and interviewees. The ability to conduct a skillful interview is a necessary component of the clinician's repertoire. Specific techniques for obtaining information are important. The clinician should beware of soliciting unexamined opinions from interviewees, and should focus instead on eliciting specific anecdotes about a child's performance. These anecdotes allow the clinician to make independent judgments as to the reasons for the child's performance, without editorial input from the other person. What we have called elsewhere the "analytic interviewing" stance (Bernstein & Weiler, in press) is crucial. This requires that the layperson's observations be actively scrutinized for the actual behaviors to which they refer, rather than taken at their diagnostic face value. For example, the description of a child as "anxious" must prompt the clinician to consider what sort of behaviors are likely to lead a layperson to call someone "anxious." These behaviors must then be analyzed from the neuropsychological as well as the psychological perspective. In this case, observed behaviors are likely to include changes in motor and verbal activity or in speech output. The clinician may eventually conclude that these behaviors are correctly interpreted as reflecting anxiety. However, they may be better understood as indicators of heightened arousal, without the fear component of anxiety, or of immature or unstable inhibitory control, or of vulnerability to being overwhelmed secondary to poor self-regulatory capacities. In the analytic interview, the sophisticated clinician will rely on neuropsychological expertise to review the range of possible observed behaviors, to develop hypotheses about these possibilities, and to explore these further by means of carefully framed follow-up queries.

Task Analysis

The analysis of task parameters is the crucial element in incorporating the CONTEXT principle into the overall assessment. The type of analysis to be performed is, in many respects, the place where neuropsychology meets one of its sister psychological disciplines—namely, applied behavior analysis—in the description of neurobehavioral function. The analysis of task parameters is as important for the delineation of risk and the development of a management strategy and interventions as it is for the evaluative process. In this context, *task* needs to be understood in its largest sense: It refers to interactions with persons, developmental challenges, everyday problem solving, and unstructured activities, as well as to formally defined, structured psychological tests.

Task Differences

In the testing setting, contextual demands vary among tasks. This can be relatively straightforward, as in the difference between a visual-perceptual task and one that also involves motor processing, or between comparable tasks that do and do not require memory skills. However, clinicians must also be aware of the potential for other, less immediately noticeable differences between tasks. For example, some tasks engage a child directly in interaction with an adult, such as those requiring listening and speaking. For other tasks, such as constructional or drawing activities, interaction is notably less. This difference may have a significant impact on one child but a negligible influence on another. In all tasks involving verbal interchange, the child and adult form an interactional system. This is not necessarily the case where the child interacts directly with materials. Thus the tasks comprising the Verbal IQ scale of the WISC-III are quite different contextually from those that make up the Performance IQ scale. Some children may be helped enormously by the support inherent in talking with an adult, with all the reciprocal biological regulation and social interaction that this entails. Other children may do much better with the nonverbal materials, because they find the social aspects of verbal interaction too overwhelming to allow for concurrent allocation of resources to the language or knowledge aspects of the tasks. In neither case is it necessarily true that the actual processing demands of linguistic or nonlinguistic stimuli determine the child's behavior.

Again, contextual factors may be influencing, obscuring, or subverting brain–behavior relationships predicted by a too-simple neuropsychological model that does not incorporate developmental and contextual principles.

Scoring Systems

Not only the nature of individual tasks, but also the scoring systems used for even the same task, can create striking differences in the contextual demands of a task as used in the evaluative process. This may reflect the different goals of the developers of the scoring systems, as seen, for example, for the Rey–Osterrieth Complex Figure (Osterrieth, 1944; Rey, 1941). Osterrieth's (1944) scoring system emphasizes the accuracy of specified segments. The Developmental Scoring System (Bernstein & Waber, 1996) highlights not just developmental change, but also the development of an appreciation for the figural logic of the design. In contrast, Kirk's (1985) approach focuses on the sequential logic of the child's approach to the material. A child's preferred information-processing style may interact with the scoring requirements of a given system. The child may produce features that are considered errors or evidence of immaturity by one scoring system but not by another. Similarly, narrative memory performance can differ as a function of the degree to which verbatim versus thematic recall is credited, as can be seen, for example, in a comparison of the scoring criteria for the story memory tasks of the Test of Memory and Learning (Reynolds & Bigler, 1994), the Wide Range Assessment of Memory and Learning (Sheslow & Adams, 1990), and the Children's Memory Scale (Cohen, 1998).

The Child's Individual Style

The potential interaction of the child's individual neurobehavioral profile with task requirements must be borne in mind by the neuropsychologist throughout the evaluation. As the evaluation proceeds and the clinician develops an understanding of the child's overall pattern of abilities, it often becomes evident that the child preferentially deploys one type of problem-solving approach no matter what the task. The child's own neurobehavioral endowment may limit the flexibility of response that is the hallmark of optimal cognitive functioning and may place constraints on how he or she views a given demand. For example, on a figure-copying task, one child may organize the reproduction in terms of the figure's overall gestalt or figural logic, whereas another child may approach it in terms of a sequence of linked elements. Both children may succeed in copying the figure, which permits more than one strategy for solution. However, if a child is limited to only one approach to the material, this processing style may limit how well the material is recalled over time. Similarly, a gestalt style of approach may not be optimal on tasks on which effective problem solving and higher scores depend on the accurate analysis of details (e.g., Story Recall subtest of the TOMAL; Reynolds & Bigler, 1994). Such a child may score at a much improved level, however, on a task on which credit is given for recall in terms of ideas or themes as well as more detailed information (e.g., the WRAML Story Recall task; Sheslow & Adams, 1990). In contrast, a child whose preferred problem-solving style is excessively detail-oriented runs the risk of being overwhelmed by details and failing to see the larger picture that helps organize more complex materials. The contextual demands of a given task can in this way be quite different for two individuals with different ways of dealing with the information. The clinician must be alert to this possibility of interaction between a child's endowment and specific task demands, and should not impose a rigid set of expectations as to what a given task is tapping in every case.

Social/Societal Expectations

Contextual demands must also be evaluated as a function of social class, family values, parental expectations, and school philosophies. Two children with similar cognitive ability profiles may differ markedly in their adaptation. One child with a given family structure or in a particular school may be in serious trouble, while the other may present with much more subtle difficulties. Careful analysis of the specific demands to which each child must respond will be critical to the management plan in both cases.

Implications for Management

The importance of contextual variables in understanding the particulars of a child's adaptation to the different situation cannot be overestimated. Perhaps the most frequent complaint made about a child with learning problems, regardless of its source, is that of inconsistent performance. Parents and teachers demand to know, with varying degrees of resignation, exasperation, or even downright fury, why it is that the child can do something one day that appears completely impossible for him or her the next day. All too frequently the child is perceived as willful: "He can do it, but he won't!" The CONTEXT construct is particularly helpful here. A close analysis of the conditions under which the child is being asked to perform reveals frequently that the demands of the two situations are quite different and that the child's performance is actually responsive to the differences. A very common example of this is the child who has learned to spell given vocabulary words in list form, but who fails to spell the words correctly when he or she must also think about what to say, put the ideas into language, integrate the language with the motor system for writing, and then maintain the correct spelling. Similarly, the child who can recite arithmetic facts fails to compute accurately when struggling with the so-called "long" computations. The difference in performance is not surprising at all when the task differences are clearly highlighted. They may not be so obvious to parents, or even teachers, until they are explained as differences in contextual demand.

Parents and teachers can be taught that the presence or absence of contextual support is important with respect to whether or not a child manifests a problem or is able to cope more or less independently. They can be cued to recognize the conditions under which the child is and is not successful, and then encouraged to identify the various ways in which the context can be shaped to support optimal performance by the youngster.

Perhaps the most important implication of the CONTEXT construct for making recommendations is the principle of *matching*—that is, optimizing the match between the child, with his or her particular neurobehavioral skill profile, and the requirements of academic and social situations. Relevant recommendations encompass environmental engineering (e.g., a different school, a different teacher, smaller classroom settings, minimally distracting situations, blocking of extraneous stimuli); modifications of curriculum expectations (at any grade) or even reordering of curriculum requirements (throughout the high school experience); strategies for reducing the open-endedness of assignments, projects, or activities (e.g., explicit start–stop routines, use of a timer, assignments tailored to independent work ability); tactics for organizing complex stimuli and/or materials (e.g., labeling strategies [Bernstein, 1996, 1998], brainstorming, study and drafting skills); systematic use of technology (e.g., educational and word-processing software, keyboarding, calculators); and specific accommodations to allow the student to demonstrate knowledge in alternative formats or under alternative conditions; as well as particular instructional programs and techniques.

DEVELOPMENT

Theoretical Assumptions

> *Guiding Principle*:
> The child is a developing organism.

The parent discipline of a true neuropsychology of the child cannot be adult neuropsychology (Bernstein & Waber, 1997; Holmes-Bernstein & Waber, 1990; see also Fletcher & Taylor, 1984). The child is not an adult, either in neural status or in behavior. The cardinal feature of the child is that he or she is developing. Thus the parent disciplines of a true neuropsychology of the child must be those that directly address the issue of development—the developmental sciences in neuroscience and psychology (Kolb, 1989; Segalowitz & Hiscock, 1992). Practically, in the clinical context, principles of development must guide the clinical investigative design, the conduct of evaluative procedures, and the interventions proceeding from the assessment. In addition, the influence of a developmental framework for the study of the child on the clinician's whole attitude to the assessment process must be examined (Ginsburg, 1997).

The Developmental Constructionist Stance

The clinician's mandate is to develop an understanding of the individual child, in order to determine the nature of the presenting difficulties and to promote optimal adaptation to the child's own particular environmental demands. The theoretical orientation of the clinician influences the way in which this mandate is carried out. In the systemic developmental approach, the role of DEVELOPMENT cannot be divorced from that of CONTEXT and the ongoing interaction between organism and environment. Thus, the overall stance is one in which the child is understood to be an autonomous constructor of knowledge over time, actively exploring the environment and being directly influenced in its constructions by the experience that the environment provides. This stance will guide both observation and interpretation of behavior, and may be subject to specific bias and error without appropriate controls.

Vertical and Horizontal Analysis

In the clinical context, taking a developmental stance toward clinical analysis means that observed behavior at any point in time is conceptualized as the outcome of the child's developmental course to date. The child's developmental course is the history of the interaction of neural development with the environment and elaboration of the behavior it supports. Taking this history will require close scrutiny of both biological and environmental experiences that shape both behavior and brain. It will also entail careful attention to the possibility of any perturbation in either the building of brain structures or the elaboration of behavioral abilities. When present, the impact of such perturbations will itself become part of the developmental course and will influence the behavioral outcome at every point in the child's subsequent developmental career (Segalowitz & Hiscock, 1992). Developmental perturbations can be the results of neurological damage or dysfunction, of atypical experience, of environmental deprivation, or all of these. Analysis of the child's current presentation in light of a detailed understanding of the developmental course to date is characterized as a *vertical analysis*. This is in contrast to the *horizontal analysis*, which focuses on the current repertoire of behavioral skills and their interactions.

The implications of a vertical, or developmentally referenced, analysis of the child's presentation are not restricted to the clinician's diagnostic strategy and the way in which data are collected and interpreted. The impact of uneven or derailed development secondary to damage or deprivation must be evaluated, as it informs an understanding of the child's ongoing development, subsequent not only to the time of insult but also to the time of evaluation. The child's specific neurobehavioral abilities mean that he or she can be expected to tackle the expectable challenges of ongoing development in his or her own unique fashion. For the clinician, the prediction and mitigation of potential problems to be overcome in meeting these challenges are the primary objectives of a comprehensive management plan.

The consequences of vertical analysis are considerable. First, it puts a high premium on the development of expert interviewing skills. These are not only critical for determining many of the details of the course of development, but also require the capacity for close analysis of contextual variables. Second, it means that the generation of clinical hypotheses is as important in the interview process as it is in the observation of behavior, with or without the use of tests.

Neither horizontal analysis nor vertical analysis of behavior alone is sufficient as the basis for a comprehensive assessment; both types contribute important complementary information to the diagnostic process and to intervention planning. The stance of the clinician in applying them, however, does make a difference to the way in which behavioral observations are collected and interpreted. The methodological concern here is that of the so-called "anchoring and adjustment bias" (Tversky & Kahneman, 1974): A clinician must take explicit note of where he or she starts an analysis, in order to avoid falling into the trap of shaping the analysis to fit the preconceived assumptions of the initial position. The following example highlights the very different initial positions of two different approaches to assessment—the normative developmental and systemic developmental approaches—and illustrates the role of these two types of analysis as they influence hypothesis generation and potential diagnostic classification within these approaches.

Methodological Considerations

Hypothesis Generation

In the normative developmental setting, the first step is to delineate a child's cognitive ability structure on the basis of his or her performance on various psychological tests. This is a horizontal analysis, inasmuch as it focuses on the description of the child's current functioning. Let us say that on the basis of this analysis, the child has quite specific deficits implicating the language domain. For the purposes of generating a diagnosis on which to base an intervention strategy, the clinician may stop at this psychological-process level of analysis and base recommendations on the known risks and outcomes of language disorder in a child of this age. However, an explicitly neuropsychologically framed hypothesis can also be tested: Because linguistic functioning has been strongly associated with left-hemisphere brain mechanisms, such language deficits may imply that left-hemisphere mechanisms are dysfunctional or inefficient in this child. The clinician may seek to test this neuropsychological hypothesis by means of a cross-domain analysis, scrutinizing the child's total protocol for evidence of atypical functioning in other behavioral areas that could also be attributed to left-hemisphere mechanisms. A report of delayed onset of language may be considered a pertinent datum in this search.

In the systemic developmental model, the initial stance is framed in vertical terms. Here the clinician starts by interviewing the child and family, with the goal of determining the progress of this child to this point in time (i.e., the outcome to date). In this case, the interview yields the important datum that generates the hypothesis to be tested, that of delayed onset of language. Relying on the neuropsychological principle that left-hemisphere mechanisms are preferentially mobilized to support linguistic function, the systemic developmental clinician formulates the hypothesis that left-hemisphere mechanisms were unequal to the task of supporting language at the appropriate time, thus requiring the child to find a solution to the challenge of acquiring language in an alternative or less efficient fashion. The clinician then tests the hypothesis that damaged or atypically developed left-hemisphere mechanisms are an important source of this child's presenting complaints. This stance requires both examination of the child's performance on psychological tasks administered during the assessment, and detailed queries about the nature and progress of the child's behavioral adjustment as he or she tackled the expectable developmental challenges of childhood. It also requires that the clinician consider normal developmental processes and progress (Dennis, 1988, 1989) and evaluate the possibility that the delayed acquisition of language itself has contributed to perturbation in the ongoing development of the organism and will remain part of the developmental course thereafter. If this is found to be the case, as is likely, the subsequent trajectory of brain and behavioral development may well be different for this child and may influence the way in which one behavioral domain (language, in this example) is integrated with others in the overall behavioral architecture (Bates, 1997; Locke, 1997; Newport, 1991; Satz, Strauss, & Whitaker, 1990; Teuber & Rudel, 1962). Differences in behavioral architecture, or the ways in which different behavioral domains engage in transactional relationships in ongoing functioning, are as yet poorly understood; however, they can be expected to play a significant role in the elaboration of focused and effective interventions.

Neither a normative developmental nor a systemic developmental approach is inherently better than the other. Nonetheless, the approaches are likely to differ with respect to how the diagnosis is formulated and how the overall management strategy is framed, as well as with respect to the biases to which they are vulnerable and thus the methodological controls that will need to be considered.

Observation and Interpretation

The differences between vertical and horizontal analysis are not restricted to clinical orientation. Different analyses can result in completely different diagnostic formulations that may have significant implications for a patient's well-being. Take the common example of an individual's indulging in verbal commentary during task performance. This is often conceptualized as verbal mediation of behavior. The clinician may then infer that the verbal system is a strength for this individual because it is used for problem solving, and may go further to posit that the left hemisphere is the "better" system and the right hemisphere is the impaired one. In the context of the current discussion, this is a horizontal analysis.

There are at least two things wrong with this type of clinical thinking. First, the behavior has not been adequately observed. The observed behavior does not necessarily represent verbal mediation of behavior; verbal mediation of behavior is a diagnostic inference or interpretation, not an observation. The observation is that the individual is talking during task performance. Whether or not this is mediating the behavior is a separate judgment.

Second, the place of the behavior in the child's current developmental repertoire has not been considered. The distinction between observation and interpretation also applies here. In a child, verbal behavior is subject to developmental forces. Only by about 7 years of age has a child developed sufficient control of inhibitory and executive processes that verbal behavior goes underground, so to speak (cf. Vygotsky's [1986] "inner language" concept). To the extent that a given task challenges the child's problem-solving capacities in a given domain, the child may not be able to allocate cognitive resources efficiently to all other aspects of behavior. One potential result is that inhibitory control cannot be maintained over the verbal system while the problem-solving challenges are being met. This view, which requires consideration of the child's developmental competence with respect to availability of different skills, involves a vertical analysis.

What does this mean for diagnosis? In the developmental context, the clinician must always balance horizontal with vertical analyses. The clinician must consider the possibility that the nature of the observed behavior (here, verbal output) is not the diagnostically important datum. What is important for diagnosis is the fact that the child cannot maintain *age-appropriate inhibitory control* over the behavior—which is elicited by the challenge presented by the information-processing demands of the task in an as-yet-immature organism. The brain mechanisms that support these information-processing demands may be those of the left hemisphere, but they equally well may not be. The observed behavior reflects the fact that the child is unable to maintain age-appropriate inhibitory control of the verbal system, or of the motor system in general. The neuropsychological deficit, however, lies in the specific domain that elicits the loss of inhibitory control. When the clinician presents the child with tasks that call on the deficient skill domain—be it linguistic processing, spatial processing, or emotional processing—additional resources must be allocated to meet the demand. This reallocation of resources makes it harder for a developing child concurrently to maintain appropriate inhibitory control over verbal and motor output. Linguistic processing, spatial processing, and emotional processing involve skills thought to depend on very different neural substrates. In the vertical analysis, the neural substrates associated with the demands of the task, rather than those associated with the observed behavior, point to the neuropsychological diagnosis. To reach a diagnosis, the clinician must analyze task parameters as well as observed behaviors, and must judge them both with reference to the child's developmental status.

Implications for Management

The most important implications of the developmental framework for management come via the concept of *risk*. This is the crucial link between the diagnostic formulation and the management approach. The developmental framework permits a principled analysis of the risks that a given child is likely to face at different points in development, and thus allows the clinician to predict and seek to circumvent the actual manifestations of the risks. Risks must be analyzed in terms of both short- and longer-term goals. They can be identified both horizontally in terms of specific task parameters, and vertically in terms of the natural history of specific disorders or neuropsychological styles (Holmes, 1986).

The implications of the risk construct for management include the following: the ability to provide a principled explanation to the child, parents, and/or teachers of the reason for otherwise puzzling or frustrating "inconsistency" in performance (i.e., different levels of performance in different settings or on different types of tasks); the accurate prediction of specific challenges that the child can be expected to face; the clinician's awareness of a sufficiently comprehensive range of possible challenges to optimal adjustment that may need to be addressed; and the potential for circumventing or mitigating the impact of expectable difficulties. See below for an extended discussion of the concept of risk in relation to all three dimensions—BRAIN, CONTEXT, and DEVELOPMENT.

LINKING EVALUATION TO MANAGEMENT

A major challenge for the assessing clinician is making the link between the evaluative and management components of the assessment. It is important that this link be a principled one. Too often, in the educational setting at least, the relationship between the psychological diagnosis and the recommendations for behavioral and pedagogical interventions is obscure; no rationale is given for *why* this diagnosis leads to that recommendation. In the neurodevelopmental systems model, this link is expressly made via the *systemic circle*.

The Systemic Circle

Figure 18.1 illustrates the evaluation-to-management process in terms of the systemic circle. In this approach, the core unit of analysis is taken to be the child, with the assumption that the child's neurobehavioral functioning cannot be understood without reference to the context in which he or she behaves—that is, the *child–world system* (Holmes-Bernstein & Waber, 1990). The child–world system is evaluated on the basis of the information obtained from the history, from the observations of the child, and from examination of how he or she actually functions in both clinical and nonclinical situations. As illustrated in Figure 18.1, this information yields the diagnostic behavioral cluster, which in turn leads to the diagnostic formulation.

As discussed previously, a diagnostic statement may be formulated at more than one level. Although neuropsychologists may conceptualize their diagnostic formulations in terms of the brain-referenced heuristic as described here, such formulations can be expressed in terms of either neuropsychological or psychological processes, or both. The decision to formulate the diagnosis in neuropsychological terms with a given family should be made

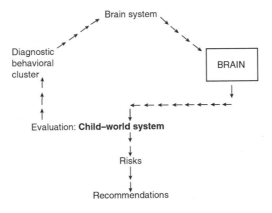

FIGURE 18.1. The systemic circle.

with care, especially when there is no specific neurodiagnostic information available to support the neuropsychological diagnosis. In such situations, a behavioral diagnosis such as "multimodal language disorder" or "nonverbal learning disorder" may be a more appropriate diagnostic characterization. When there is clear clinical or neurodiagnostic evidence for brain abnormality, however, ascribing a child's behavioral or functional difficulties to a "left-hemisphere deficit" or similar neurological referent is appropriate, if not necessary. Conveying that the observed behavior is consistent with what is known about the behavioral effects of a brain lesion is an important element in clinical management. It normalizes the patient's experience as an expected consequence of the brain condition, and thus can help patient and family understand and come to terms with any neuropsychologically based limitations. Depending on the situation, both neuropsychological and psychological diagnoses may need to be specifically referenced to alternative nosological categories (e.g., those of the American Psychiatric Association, 1994) to access different types of services.

In the process of moving from diagnosis to management, the clinician conceptualizes the diagnostic formulation in explicitly brain-referenced terms, rather than in psychological terms. This conceptualization permits access to the box labeled in the figure as BRAIN. In the model, this represents the expertise of the clinician—that is, the clinician's education across a broad range of relevant psychological, educational, and neurological disciplines, in addition to the experience gained from working with children and families. Armed with relevant knowledge about the contribution to behavior of the brain system identified during the evaluative process, the clinician then revisits the child–world system and applies both the CONTEXT and the DEVELOPMENT constructs in a detailed analysis of the expectable challenges that the child will face. These challenges will come from the adaptive, academic, and social spheres and will be both short- and longer-term. The clinician then identifies the risks for this child—that is, the potential limitations on the child's ability to respond effectively to expectable developmental challenges that may accrue as a consequence of his or her neuropsychological profile.

The following example demonstrates the application of the systemic circle model. In the example, a single behavior, constructional apraxia, is isolated. This is done for illustrative purposes only. In a clinical analysis, a brain-referenced diagnostic formulation cannot be made on the basis of a single datum; it requires the identification of a behavioral cluster of converging and discriminating variables that, as a group, identify a specific brain system. For the current example, the diagnostic behavioral cluster includes drawings that illustrate constructional apraxia—in other words, a deficit in the ability to relate elements to each other in a spatial framework. The presence of constructional apraxia in a clinical protocol allows one to say with a relatively high degree of probability that a disturbance of parietal brain systems is present (Critchley, 1959).

The postulation of "a neuropsychological profile referable to parietal systems" is the necessary formulation that serves to access the BRAIN box in this formulation. The clinician can then draw upon his or her knowledge base about the function of the parietal brain systems in general. Armed with this broader-based knowledge, the clinician then explores the implications of this type of deficit for the child's adaptive functioning. Given disrupted development of parietal systems, what is this child at this age, in this family, in this social group, in this type of school setting, and under this academic demand likely to have trouble with? The answer to this query constitutes the child's risk(s) (see below). Note that the same theoretical framework and principles of behavioral analysis govern both evaluation (of behavior in the clinical setting) and management (of behavior in the child's everyday life). The tasks may differ, but the brain that tackles them is taken everywhere the child goes!

The Concept of Risk

As emphasized above, the concept of risk is perhaps the most important and useful contribution of a developmental perspective on behavioral assessment. It is the crucial link between diagnosis and management. Its value is directly related to its potential for prediction and thus for prevention. Specification of risks and the recommendations that follow from them are critical components of the management plan, the primary goal of which is to avert or mitigate the impact of the predicted risks to the greatest extent possible.

In the current formulation, risk is based on CONTEXT, as reflected in the principle of brain–world interaction, and on DEVELOPMENT, as reflected in the changing demands on the child as he or she matures. Risk is not framed only with reference to the presenting complaint. It is defined by examining the child's adaptive strengths and weaknesses in light of what the identified brain systems are postulated to contribute to the normal behavioral repertoire of a child of this age.

The Time-Referenced Symptom

The concept of risk was elegantly captured by the late Rita Rudel in her formulation of the *time-referenced symptom* (Rudel, 1981). This formulation entails that symptoms need not be constant or universal (Pennington, 1991). They not only do, but must, change in response to the differing demands on the child's changing repertoire at different stages in development.

Consider the following example of this principle in action. The child in the office explains that last night he went to the local restaurant, and his sister had pizza but he had "pisgetti." The paraphasic error (i.e., "pisgetti" for "spaghetti") reveals the child's difficulty in sequencing sounds accurately. If the speaker were 3 years old, this utterance would probably not be considered an error, but rather an endearing near-miss in a young child who has not yet mastered the sequencing of complex phonological strings. If the patient is 10 years old, the error is potentially of much greater import, with quite specific diagnostic implications. Developmentally, 10-year-olds are expected to have mastered the ability to produce such sequences very smoothly.

Let us assume that the neuropsychological assessment does indeed proceed with this 10-year-old youngster, and it becomes apparent that this type of sequencing error in ongoing conversation is part of a larger cluster of observations, all of which implicate difficulties in the capacity for sequential processing of elements. The clinician may hypothesize, in neuropsychological terms, that the vulnerability of this particular brain is centered on difficulty in processing elements in sequence. The application to the child's history of the principle "behavior = same brain + different demand," which is derived from the BRAIN–CONTEXT–DEVELOPMENT model, then leads to a finer-grained, more sophisticated understanding of the child's developmental course: Reported behaviors are not simply noted, but are now appreciated as important members of the diagnostic behavioral cluster. Thus a problem in sequencing behavior (a characteristic of this child's BRAIN), which is expressed as speech errors of the "pisgetti" type persisting to age 10, may be manifest during infancy in poor sucking behavior; at the toddler stage, in oral–motor apraxia; in kindergarten or first grade, in a delay in appreciating differences between phonic segments; at age 7, in misreadings such as "girl" for "grill" or vice versa; and, in one child I have worked with, in misuse of time-related concepts such as "before" and "after." In this example, the CONTEXT construct is reflected in the specific tasks that the child must solve at each age (i.e., sustenance, phonology, more elaborated language, reading). DEVELOPMENT is reflected in the change in both expectations and behaviors over time. Note that the tasks that elicit the clinically relevant behavior highlighted here (1) are developmentally referenced and (2) involve adaptive capacities that range from basic human survival skills to those required to cope successfully with socioculturally defined expectations as exemplified in academic skills. Although problems associated with the latter are what typically bring the school-age child to clinical neuropsychological attention, the neuropsychologist must appreciate that the brain was not "designed" to do academic tasks, but was shaped by evolutionary and ecological forces focused on survival and reproductive functions.

The principle illustrated here can, however, be applied quite specifically in the academic context to predict "academic stress points" (Holmes, 1986). For example, a child with language-processing deficits is at risk for various difficulties in the acquisition of written language skills: in first grade, for learning to decode; in fourth grade, for learning to use reading to obtain meaning; in sixth grade and beyond, for learning to express thoughts/ideas in writing (Holmes, 1986; Pardes, 1988). At different times, however, he or she is also at risk for difficulty in listening, which may limit classroom learning; for slow vocabulary development, which depends on reading facility; for regulating emotions, which depends on the ability to use language fluently; and for the development of comfortable social skills, which require fluent conversational skills. A similar analysis of spatial processing, or memory, or motor skills reveals the interdependence of academic learning, social skills development, and emotional well-being for the child's overall adaptation to his or her particular setting.

From Prediction to Prevention

The foregoing discussion highlights the importance of the BRAIN–CONTEXT–DEVELOPMENT principle. Behavior, whether normal or symptomatic, is the product of complexly integrated brain systems responding to and being shaped by specific demands in the environment at a given point in time. The principle applies to the analysis of expectable challenges in the past, demonstrating how careful elicitation of a given child's developmental history contributes directly to diagnosis by adding specific observations to the diagnostic behavioral cluster. It also applies to the analysis of future expectable challenges, and thus to the identification of those that pose risk for this particular child, given his or her neuropsychological abilities and the context in which he or she lives.

The value of the risk concept goes beyond the prediction of risk for the individual, however. As clinicians see more and more children, and identify specific groups of youngsters on the basis of their performance on neuropsychological assessment, they begin to recognize the natural history (Holmes, 1986) of different disorders. Given an understanding of the natural history of disorders associated with different neuropsychological profiles, clinicians have the basic tool of prediction that is crucial to developing prevention strategies/interventions.

Defining Risk

Risk is not defined in terms of a deficit per se. A neuropsychologically defined risk factor in a child need not have functional consequences, as it nearly always does for an adult. In an adult who has developed normally and then sustains a lesion that leads to constructional apraxia, the apraxic deficit may have a severe impact on vocations that involve the manipulation of spatial variables (e.g., plumbing, construction, engineering, architecture). In the pediatric context, however, a direct effect of constructional apraxia on a developmental basis is not likely to be apparent. The real world typically provides so much concrete support that, over the course of development, the child is guided to do what is functionally necessary by dealing with the tools or materials directly. Alternatively, the child may manage to avoid challenging activities; indeed, he or she may well have a history of never being interested in block building or similar activities. This is, however, typically interpreted by caregivers as a reflection of the child's temperament or style, rather than as a strategy to compensate for functional deficits related to neuropsychological impairment. Of course, should the child attempt tasks that place too great a demand on insecure skills, the biological risk factor can be expected to be manifested in dysfunctional or maladaptive behavior. Nonetheless, a great deal of effective adaptation at a basic functional level can be achieved in the presence of significant neuropsychological impairment.

In applying the risk concept, it is important to appreciate that management and intervention are based on analysis of the brain-referenced construct derived from the diagnosis, and not on any given observed behavior. Thus one does not write a report that instructs the reader, in effect, to remediate a behavior such as constructional apraxia. This violates one of the cardinal rules of intervention, that of relevance. The observation of constructional apraxia may be important (as, however, only one element of the overall diagnostic behavioral cluster) to diagnosis. Nonetheless, if such a behavior does not cause a functional problem in the real world, the principle of ecological validity means that it is not addressed in the recommendations.

In contrast, the contribution made to the recommendations by the brain system(s) identified via the diagnostic behavioral cluster cannot be argued. To return to the example of the youngster for whom the diagnostic behavioral cluster identifies parietal brain systems as the relatively weak component of the brain–behavior relationship profile, these brain systems are critical to ongoing behavioral function in the real world. In this case, the identification of parietal brain systems provides the BRAIN component of the model. The clinician's understanding of the role of parietal systems is then brought to bear on the actual CONTEXT of this child at this stage of DEVELOPMENT—that is, to the previously identified child–world system. The question posed by the clinician is as follows: Given insecure parietal system functioning, what risks are faced by this child in this context at this point in development?

In this example, the implicated parietal brain systems constitute a tertiary association area, accepting inputs from multiple different brain regions (Kolb & Whishaw, 1990; Lezak, 1995; Mesulam, 1981). They play an important role in gaze and visual attention, in locating objects in space, and in integrating percepts. A child with this type of difficulty may be at risk for attentional problems or for navigating effectively in space, both of which have the potential for significant functional consequences. Moreover, clinical observation suggests that parietal systems are very important for the understanding of relational concepts in language, such as nuance and metaphor. This being the case, inefficient parietal function can put a child at both social and academic risk. Psychosocial development and emotional well-being may be undermined in the older child or young adolescent if he or she is chronically disadvantaged with peers when jokes and in-group membership require a more sophisticated mastery of subtle linguistic usage. An example is the child with parietal involvement who consistently fails to appreciate verbal (but not physical) humor and laughs because the others are laughing—a subtle behavioral delay that is nonetheless quickly picked up by peers and may be the source of teasing, name calling, or even ostracism. Academic skills that are otherwise relatively advanced, such as reading, may be regularly derailed by an inability to quickly appreciate such notions as "The bird took wing." A student who is explicitly cued to the existence of such curious phrases and directly taught how they work may be able to work out what such a phrase must mean, but this takes time and interferes with both the accuracy and the enjoyment of on-line reading activities.

The foregoing examples highlight the importance of examining the potential for risk in the context of the whole child. Developmental challenges come in both the social and academic realms; they involve behavioral control and social comportment, social cognition and interpersonal skills, communicative competence, motor capacity, and other abilities, as well as the academic skills and attentional and organizational capacities that are so often the focus of complaints in the academic setting.

FINALE

The clinical assessment is not just a tally of skills made in a vacuum; it is a principled undertaking in the context of a theory of the organism. The nature and impact of development have not yet been explored as integral elements at the core of clinical assessment models in pediatric neuropsychology. To incorporate them, however, is not a trivial undertaking. The concept of DEVELOPMENT in the neurobehavioral context cannot be disentangled from the BRAIN that supports behavior and the CONTEXT in which behavior is elaborated.

In the type of neurodevelopmental model advocated here, the guiding theory expressly requires that BRAIN, CONTEXT, and DEVELOPMENT be seen as interacting variables. Their impact is felt at all levels of the assessment and determines how the child–world system at the core of this assessment approach is constructed (Holmes-Bernstein & Waber, 1990). The theoretical framework characterizes the way in which the organism behaves, and thus influences which behaviors are chosen for measurement in order to address the clinical questions. It shapes the assessment methodology (the clinician's diagnostic stance, the types of controls for variability and bias, the way in which actual behaviors are elicited and evaluated, and the types of tools and techniques deemed most effective), and the formulation of the diagnosis (how behaviors are interpreted and conclusions drawn). It determines the way in which management and intervention strategies (the concept of risk, the role of contextual matching, expectable challenges) are framed. BRAIN, CONTEXT, and DEVELOPMENT all make their individual marks on the assessment process and interact complexly therein. Some of the issues have been described here; many more remain to be explored.

NOTE

1. Although it goes beyond the scope of the scope of the present discussion, I would argue that a *theory of pedagogy* is a fourth component of the theoretical framework for the pediatric neuropsychologist who takes his or her responsibilities to the child in the classroom seriously. One important goal of management is an optimal match between the neurobehavioral abilities of the student and the teaching strategies employed in the classroom. Too frequently, neuropsychological clinicians in general practice (as contrasted with rehabilitation specialists) expect this part of the job to be done by educators, but there is no doubt in my mind that an interested neuropsychologist can work very productively as a member of a child's "treatment team," contributing knowledge of how the youngster thinks (shaped by knowledge of the child's neuropsychological strengths and weaknesses) to the teacher's input as to how the child learns (see Bernstein, 1996, 1998).

REFERENCES

American Psychiatric Association. (1994). *Diagnostic and statistical manual of mental disorders* (4th ed.). Washington, DC: American Psychiatric Association.

Bakker, D. J. (1984). The brain as a dependent variable. *Journal of Clinical Neuropsychology, 6,* 1–16.

Bates, E. (1997). Origins of language disorders: A comparative approach. *Developmental Neuropsychology, 13,* 447–476.

Bernstein, J. H. (1996, Fall). Issues in the psycho-educational management of children treated for malignant disease. *P.O.G.O. (Pediatric Oncology Group of Ontario) News,* pp. 9–11.

Bernstein, J. H. (1998). Supporting the "how-to" of learning: Intervention for executive functioning. *Educational Therapist, 19,* 3–5.

Bernstein, J. H., Kammerer, B., Prather, P., & Rey-Casserly, C. (1998). Developmental neuropsychological assessment. In G. P. Koocher, J. C. Norcross, & S. S. Hill, Jr. (Eds.), *Psychologists' desk reference.* New York: Oxford University Press.

Bernstein, J. H., Prather, P. A., & Rey-Casserly, C. (1995). Neuropsychological assessment in pre- and postoperative evaluation. *Neurosurgery Clinics, 6,* 443–454.

Bernstein, J. H., & Waber, D. P. (1996). *Developmental Scoring System for the Rey-Osterrieth Complex Figure.* Odessa, FL: Psychological Assessment Resources, Inc.

Bernstein, J. H., & Waber, D. P. (1997). Pediatric neuropsychological assessment. In T. Feinberg & M. Farah (Eds.), *Behavioral neurology and neuropsychology.* New York: McGraw-Hill.

Bernstein, J. H., & Weiler, M. (in press). Pediatric neuropsychological assessment examined. In G. Goldstein & M. Hersen (Eds.), *Handbook of psychological assessment* (3rd ed.). Amsterdam: Elsevier.

Bornstein, R. (1990). Neuropsychological test batteries in neuropsychological assessment. In A. A. Boulton, G. B. Baker, & M. Hiscock (Eds.), *Neuromethods: Vol. 17. Neuropsychology.* Clifton, NJ: Humana Press.

Bronfenbrenner, U. (1993). The ecology of cognitive development: Research models and fugitive findings. In R. H. Wozniak & K. W. Fischer (Eds.), *Development in context: Acting and thinking in specific environments. The Jean Piaget Symposium series.* Hillsdale, NJ: Erlbaum.

Bronfenbrenner, U., & Ceci, S. (1994). Nature–nurture reconceptualized in developmental perspective: A bioecological model. *Psychological Review, 101,* 568–586.

Case, R. (1992). The role of the frontal lobes in the regulation of cognitive development. *Brain and Cognition, 20,* 51–73.

Case, R., & Okamoto, Y. (1996). The role of central conceptual structures in the development of children's thought. *Monographs of the Society for Research in Child Development, 61*(1–2, Serial No. 246).

Ceci, S. J. (1996). *On intelligence* (2nd ed.). Englewood Cliffs, NJ: Prentice-Hall.

Cohen, M. (1998). *Children's Memory Scale.* San Antonio, TX: Psychological Corporation.

Critchley, M. (1959). *The parietal lobes.* London: Arnold.

Das, J. P., Naglieri, J. A., & Kirby, J. R. (1994). *Assessment of cognitive processes: The PASS theory of intelligence.* Itasca, IL: Riverside.

Deacon, T. W. (1997). *The symbolic species: The co-evolution of language and the brain.* New York: Norton.

Dennis, M. (1988). Language and the young damaged brain. In T. Boll & B. K. Bryant (Eds.), *Clinical neuropsychology and brain function.* Washington, DC: American Psychological Association.

Dennis, M. (1989). Assessing the neuropsychological abilities of children and adolescents for personal injury litigation. *Clinical Neuropsychologist, 3,* 203–229.

Edelman, G. M. (1987). *Neural Darwinism.* New York: Basic Books.

Elman, J., Bates, E., Johnson, M., Karmiloff-Smith, A., Parisi, D., & Plunkett, K. (1996). *Rethinking innateness: A connectionist perspective on development.* Cambridge, MA: MIT Press/Bradford Books.

Faust, D., & Nurcombe, B. (1989). Improving the accuracy of clinical judgment. *Psychiatry, 52,* 197–208.

Fisch, H. U., Hammond, K. R., & Joyce, C. R. B. (1982). On evaluating the severity of depression: An experimental study of psychiatrists. *British Journal of Psychiatry, 140,* 378–383.

Fischer, K. W., & Rose, S. P. (1994). Dynamic development of coordination of components in brain and behavior. In G. Dawson & K. W. Fischer (Eds.), *Human behavior and the developing brain.* New York: Guilford Press.

Fletcher, J. M., & Taylor, H. G. (1984). Neuropsychological approaches to children: Towards a developmental neuropsychology. *Journal of Clinical Neuropsychology, 6,* 39–56.

Fletcher, J. M., Taylor, H. G., Levin, H., & Satz, P. (1995). Neuropsychological and intellectual assessment of children. In H. I. Kaplan & B. Sadock (Eds.), *Comprehensive textbook of psychiatry* (6th ed.). Baltimore: Williams & Wilkins.

Geary, D. C., Brown, S. C., & Samaranayake, V. A. (1991). Cognitive addition: A short longitudinal study of strategy choice and speed-of-processing differences in normal and mathematically disabled children. *Developmental Psychology, 27*, 787–797.

Ginsburg, H. P. (1997). *Entering the child's mind: The clinical interview in psychological research and practice.* New York: Cambridge University Press.

Globus, G. G. (1973). Consciousness and brain: I. The identity thesis. *Archives of General Psychiatry, 29*, 153–160.

Goldberg, L. R. (1968). Simple models or simple processes?: Some research on clinical judgments. *American Psychologist, 23*, 483–496.

Golden, M. (1964). Some effects of combining psychological tests on clinical inferences. *Journal of Consulting Psychology, 28*, 440–446.

Goldstein, G. (1986). The neuropsychology of schizophrenia. In I. Grant & K. M. Adams (Eds.), *Neuropsychological assessment of neuropsychiatric disorders.* New York: Oxford University Press.

Goodglass, H., & Kaplan, E. (1979). Assessment of cognitive deficit in the brain-injured patient. In M. Gazzaniga (Ed.), *Handbook of behavioral neurobiology: Vol. 2. Neuropsychology.* New York: Plenum Press.

Greenough, W. E., Black, J. E., & Wallace, C. S. (1987). Experience and brain development. *Child Development, 58*, 539–559.

Holmes, J. M. (1986). Natural histories in learning disabilities. Neuropsychological difference/environmental demand. In S. J. Ceci (Ed.), *Handbook of cognitive, social and neuropsychological aspects of learning disabilities.* Hillsdale, NJ: Erlbaum.

Holmes-Bernstein, J., & Waber, D. P. (1990). Developmental neuropsychological assessment: The systemic approach. In A. A. Boulton, G. B. Baker, & M. Hiscock (Eds.), *Neuromethods: Vol. 17. Neuropsychology.* Clifton, NJ: Humana Press.

Kaplan, E. (1976). The role of the non-compromised hemisphere in patients with local brain disease. In H.-L. Teuber (Chair), *Alterations in brain functioning and changes in cognition.* Symposium conducted at the annual meeting of the American Psychological Association, Washington, D.C..

Kaplan, E. (1983). Process and achievement revisited. In S. Wapner & B. Kaplan (Eds.), *Toward a holistic developmental psychology.* Hillsdale, NJ: Erlbaum.

Kaplan, E. (1988). A process approach to neuropsychological assessment. In T. Boll & B. K. Bryant (Eds.), *Clinical neuropsychology and brain function.* Washington, DC: American Psychological Association.

Kaplan, E., Fein, D., Delis, D., & Morris, R. (1999). *The WISC-III-PI (Wechsler Intelligence Scale for Children, Third Edition, Process Instrument): Manual.* San Antonio, TX: Psychological Corporation.

Kerlinger, F. N. (1986). *Foundations of behavioral research* (3rd ed.). Fort Worth, TX: Holt, Rinehart & Winston.

Kirk, U. (1985). Hemispheric contributions to the development of graphic skill. In C. T. Best (Ed.), *Hemispheric function and collaboration in the child.* New York: Academic Press.

Kolb, B. (1989). Brain development, plasticity and behavior. *American Psychologist, 44*, 1203–1212.

Kolb, B., & Whishaw, I. Q. (1990). *Fundamentals of human neuropsychology* (3rd ed.). New York: Freeman.

Korkman, M., Kemp, S., & Kirk, U. (1998). *NEPSY: A developmental neuropsychological assessment.* San Antonio, TX: Psychological Corporation.

Lezak, M. (1995). *Neuropsychological assessment* (3rd ed.). New York: Oxford University Press.

Locke, J. L. (1997). A theory of neurolinguistic development. *Brain and Language, 58*, 265–326.

Lowman, R. L. (1996). Introduction to the special section on what every psychologist should know about assessment. *Psychological Assessment, 8*, 339–340.

Matarazzo, J. D. (1990). Psychological assessment versus psychological testing. *American Psychologist, 45*, 999–1017.

McFie, J., Piercy, M. F., & Zangwill, O. C. (1950). Visual spatial agnosia associated with lesions of the right cerebral hemisphere. *Brain, 73*, 167–190.

McFie, J., & Zangwill, O. C. (1960). Visual-constructive disabilities associated with lesions of the left cerebral hemisphere. *Brain, 83*, 243–260.

McKenna, P., & Warrington, E. K. (1986). The analytical approach to neuropsychological assessment. In I. Grant & K. M. Adams (Eds.), *Neuropsychological assessment of neuropsychiatric disorders.* New York: Oxford University Press.

Mesulam, M.-M. (1981). A cortical network for directed attention and unilateral neglect. *Annals of Neurology, 10*, 309–325.

Milberg, W. P., Hebben, N., & Kaplan, E. (1986). The Boston process approach to neuropsychological assessment. In I. Grant & K. M. Adams (Eds.), *Neuropsychological assessment of neuropsychiatric disorders.* New York: Oxford University Press.

Newport, E. (1991). Contrasting conceptions of the critical period for language. In S. Carey & R. Gelman (Eds.), *The epigenesis of mind: Essays in biology and cognition.* Hillsdale, NJ: Erlbaum.

Nisbett, R. E., & Ross, L. (1980). *Human inference: Strategies and shortcomings of social judgment.* Englewood Cliffs, NJ: Prentice-Hall.

Oskamp, S. (1965). Overconfidence in case-study judgments. *Journal of Consulting Psychology, 29,* 261–265.

Osterrieth, P. A. (1944). Le test de copie d'une figure complexe. *Archives de Psychologie, 30,* 206–356.

Pardes, J. R. (1988). Beyond the diagnosis. In R. G. Rudel, J. M. Holmes, & J. R. Pardes (Eds.), *Assessment of developmental learning disorders: A neuropsychological approach.* New York: Basic Books.

Pennington, B. F. (1991). *Diagnosing learning disorders.* New York: Guilford Press.

Piaget, J. (1952). *The origins of intelligence in children* (M. Cook, Trans.). New York: International Universities Press. (Original work published 1936)

Rapp, P. E. (1997). Foreword. In F. Masterpasqua & P. A. Perna (Eds.), *The psychological meaning of chaos.* Washington, DC: American Psychological Association.

Rey, A. (1941). L'examen psychologique dans le cas d'encephalopathie traumatique. *Archives de Psychologie, 28,* 286–340.

Reynolds, C. R., & Bigler, E. D. (1944). *Test of Memory and Learning (TOMAL).* Austin, TX: PRO-ED.

Rourke, B. P. (1975). Brain–behavior relationships in children with learning disabilities: A research program. *American Psychologist, 30,* 911–920.

Rourke, B. P. (1982). Central processing deficiencies in children: Toward a developmental neuropsychological model. *Journal of Clinical Neuropsychology, 4,* 1–18.

Rourke, B. P. (1989). *Nonverbal learning disabilities: The syndrome and the model.* New York: Guilford Press.

Rourke, B. P., Bakker, D. J., Fisk, J. L., & Strang, J. D. (1983). *Child neuropsychology: An introduction to theory, research, and clinical practice.* New York: Guilford Press.

Rourke, B. P., Fisk, J. L., & Strang, J. D. (1986). *Neuropsychological assessment of children.* New York: Guilford Press.

Rudel, R. G. (1981). Residual effects of childhood reading disabilities. *Bulletin of the Orton Society, 31,* 89–102.

Satz, P., Strauss, E., & Whitaker, H. (1990). The ontogeny of hemispheric specialization: Some old hypotheses revisited. *Brain and Language, 38,* 596–614.

Segalowitz, S. J., & Hisclock, M. (1992). The emergence of a neuropsychology of normal development: Rapprochement between neuroscience and developmental neuropsychology. In I. Rapin & S. J. Segalowitz (Eds.), *Handbook of neuropsychology: Vol. 6. Child neuropsychology.* Amsterdam: Elsevier.

Shaheen, S. J. (1984). Neuromaturation and behavioral development: The case of childhood lead poisoning. *Developmental Psychology, 20,* 542–550.

Sheslow, D., & Adams, W. (1990). *The Wide Range Assessment of Memory and Learning (WRAML).* Wilmington, DE: Wide Range.

Taylor, H. G. (1988). Neuropsychological testing: Relevance for assessing children's learning disabilities. *Journal of Consulting and Clinical Psychology, 56,* 795–800.

Taylor, H. G., & Fletcher, J. M. (1990). Neuropsychological assessment of children. In G. Goldstein & M. Hersen (Eds.), *Handbook of psychological assessment* (2nd ed.). New York: Pergamon Press.

Taylor, H. G., & Fletcher, J. M. (1995). Progress in pediatric neuropsychology [Editorial]. *Journal of Pediatric Psychology, 20,* 695–701.

Teuber, H.-L., & Rudel, R. G. (1962). Behavior after cerebral lesions in children and adults. *Developmental Medicine and Child Neurology, 4,* 3–20.

Thatcher, R. W. (1992). Cyclic cortical reorganization during early childhood development. *Brain and Cognition, 20,* 24–50.

Tramontana, M. G., & Hooper, S. R. (1988). Child neuropsychological assessment: Overview of current status. In M. G. Tramontana & S. R. Hooper (Eds.), *Assessment issues in child neuropsychology.* New York: Plenum Press.

Tversky, A., & Kahneman, D. (1974). Judgment under uncertainty: Heuristics and biases. *Science, 183,* 1124–1131.

Vanderploeg, R. D. (1994). Interview and testing: The data collection phase of neuropsychological evaluations. In R. D. Vanderploeg (Ed.), *Clinician's guide to neuropsychological assessment.* Hillsdale, NJ: Erlbaum.

Vygotsky, L. S. (1978). *Mind in society: The development of higher psychological functions.* Cambridge, MA: Harvard University Press.

Vygotsky, L. S. (1986). *Thought and language.* Cambridge, MA: MIT Press.

Waber, D. P., Urion, D. K., Tarbell, N. J., Niemeyer, C., Gelber, R., & Sallan, S. E. (1990). Late effects of central nervous system treatment of acute lymphoblastic leukemia are sex-dependent. *Developmental Medicine and Child Neurology, 32*, 238–248.

Wakefield, J. C. (1990). The concept of mental disorder. *American Psychologist, 47*, 373–388.

Wechsler, D. (1991). *Wechsler Intelligence Scale for Children—Third Edition (WISC-III)*. San Antonio, TX: Psychological Corporation.

Willis, W. G. (1986). Actuarial and clinical approaches to neuropsychological diagnosis: Applied considerations. In J. E. Obrzut & G. W. Hynd (Eds.), *Child neuropsychology: Vol. 2. Clinical practice*. Orlando, FL: Academic Press.

19

CLINICAL IMPLICATIONS AND PRACTICAL APPLICATIONS OF CHILD NEUROPSYCHOLOGICAL EVALUATIONS

IDA SUE BARON

The chapters of this volume demonstrate that the practice of child neuropsychology has changed considerably in recent years. As evidence of the field's increasing sophistication, child neuropsychologists frequently play integral roles within pediatric medical and child rehabilitative settings, and they contribute actively to a variety of research protocols. Courses on child neuropsychology are beginning to appear as core parts of the curriculum in graduate programs, and postdoctoral training is now offered in this area (Hammeke, 1993).

Critics may argue that the many technological advances in neurodiagnosis over the last two decades have detracted from the value of child neuropsychological assessment. Cases in point include the precise enhancement of brain regions made possible by sophisticated neuroimaging techniques, and the increasing identification of genetic/molecular bases of developmental disorders. Advances such as these, however, have only further stimulated the growth of the field and the recognition of the many different effects of underlying neurological dysfunction or disorder on the developing child.

The increasing sophistication of neuropsychological assessment has been central to the evolution of child neuropsychology as a field of study. A primary goal of a clinical child neuropsychologist is to generate conditions that allow for the observation of a range of neurobehavioral functioning. True to the tradition of adult neuropsychology, assessment data are commonly obtained within the structure of a formal psychometric evaluation (i.e., by the accumulation of quantitative information about a child's abilities). Comprehensive child evaluations, however, also require careful attention to qualitative aspects of functioning, through observation, history taking, and interview with selected individuals in the child's milieu. Another of the clinical child neuropsychologist's primary goals is to describe neurobehavioral strengths and weaknesses as a means of achieving an ecologically valid understanding of the child (Taylor & Schatschneider, 1992a). Relevant aims are to anticipate the child's responses in a variety of real-life situations and to provide a framework for implementing techniques to assist the child in making an optimal adaptation to academic, familial, and other environmental circumstances.

It is inevitable that children will question authority and assert their independence as they mature into adolescents. Child neuropsychology, too, is finding its adolescent voice. Individuals within the field are reevaluating the principles and models that guided the earlier practice of child neuropsychology, rejecting claims that are based strictly on adult data, and striving for new approaches to treatment and better understanding of the ecological validity of their findings (Baron, Fennell, & Voeller, 1995; Fletcher & Taylor, 1984). Markers of this progress in child neuropsychology include the greater attention given to the importance of theory-driven research, the articulation of child neuropsychological models (Cooley & Morris, 1990; Denckla, 1996b; Rourke, 1989; Wilson, 1992; Wilson & Risucci, 1986), and a movement away from a reliance on models developed to account for adult brain–behavior relationships (Fennell & Bauer, 1989; Bernstein & Waber, 1990). Other signs of the field's evolution include an increase in the variety of assessment instruments applicable to the young ages (Baron & Gioia, 1998; Butterbaugh, 1988), a wider range of child populations referred clinically (Yeates, Ris, & Taylor, 1995) and studied experimentally, an increasing literature devoted specifically to child neuropsychology, and the application of treatment approaches that are theoretically based and that can be evaluated for clinical effectiveness (Bakker, Licht, & Kappers, 1995; Denckla & Reader, 1992; Franzen, Roberts, Schmits, Verduyn, & Manshadi, 1996; Rourke, Fisk, & Strang, 1986; Ylvisaker, Szakeres, Hartwick, & Tworek, 1994). These changes have taken place in a relatively short period of time. Along with these changes, long-held beliefs about the limitations of young children have been called into question by findings from allied fields, such as developmental and cognitive psychology. These findings have suggested that young children may be more cognitively capable than was originally assumed (Klahr & Robinson, 1981).

Despite these advances, many practical aspects of a child neuropsychological evaluation have rarely been formally addressed in the literature. Although my colleagues and I have addressed practical issues in assessing children in a recent book (Baron et al., 1995, pp. 151–217), it is principally through externship and internship experiences, or through supervised on-the-job experience, that individuals obtain the competence to translate raw data into meaningful practical recommendations. It is unfortunate that so little information is available on methods for linking the didactic, formal aspects of an evaluation with a family's real-life concerns. The primary aim of this chapter is to demonstrate how to apply the clinical knowledge obtained about a child in a formal assessment to the real-world setting. To meet this objective, I first consider recent changes that have occurred in the conduct of child neuropsychological assessment. I then review some general points to keep in mind in carrying out the parent interpretive session. Third, I provide some examples of how to link the knowledge obtained about a child with practical recommendations that have general applicability at home and at school. These recommendations are presented as illustrations of potential parent-supervised interventions, and are appropriate in working with children with specific cognitive deficits. They are not presented as prescriptions, but as models that I hope will spur the reader to consider a wide range of possibilities and to generate other recommendations according to the specifics of the individual case. These recommendations also exemplify the types of communication that educate and encourage parents on ways to become more active participants in the intervention process. A central purpose in providing feedback and recommendations is to enlighten parents about their child's strengths and weaknesses, and thus to help them become more informed and effective advocates for their child's needs.

CHANGES IN THE ASSESSMENT OF CHILDREN

Prior to recent developments, a child neuropsychological evaluation was often considered complete if it included a measure of general intelligence (IQ), a test of academic achievement, a drawing test, and a brief language screening. Occasionally, motor screening, sensory-perceptual assessment, and/or a reasoning test might be included. The narrow scope of the evaluation was due in part to (1) limited theoretical knowledge about brain–behavior relationships in the maturing child, (2) limited test instrumentation, (3) restricted normative data, (4) limited clinical experience about the effects of brain injury and disease on the developing brain, and (5) an overreliance on models of adult functioning without empirical data on children to support such assumptions.

One problem with many of these earlier evaluations was their reliance on a single, global measure of cognitive functioning. A further shortcoming related to the fact that when supplemental measures of specific functions were administered they were not validated with respect to brain functions (Fletcher & Taylor, 1984). It quickly became apparent to clinicians that such tests were inadequate. Test results failed to enhance understanding of presenting problems or to identify problems associated with earlier brain insults. The search for better ways to evaluate brain–behavior relationships in children began and is still continuing. With recent improvements in test construction, measurement (Francis, Shaywitz, Stuebing, Shaywitz, & Fletcher, 1994; Spreen & Strauss, 1991), and statistical analysis (Sawrie, Chelune, Naugle, & Luders, 1996; Francis, Fletcher, Stuebing, Davison, & Thompson, 1991; Francis, Fletcher, Rourke, & York, 1992), tools for more reliable and valid test administration and interpretation are increasingly available (Brown, Rourke, & Cicchetti, 1989).

As highlighted in the other chapters of this book, numerous cognitive domains are now routinely assessed by child neuropsychologists, with functions frequently fractionated within domains. The domains of a child neuropsychological evaluation are often considered to be independent of one another, but these domains probably make interactive and overlapping contributions to children's day-to-day functioning. Even performance on relatively specific cognitive tasks is multiply determined. Domains now considered basic in any thorough evaluation include the earlier emphasized areas of general intelligence, academic achievement, and visual–motor functioning, as noted above. However, an evaluation will also include an assessment of subcomponents of attention (e.g., sustained attention, divided attention, vigilance); executive functioning; receptive and expressive language; visual–perceptual and visual–analytic ability; motor and sensory-perceptual functioning (i.e., auditory, tactile, visual) of the two sides of the body; learning and retrieval of verbal and nonverbal material; and psychological/social-emotional status (Baron et al., 1995; Fletcher & Taylor, 1997; Yeates & Taylor, 1998).

Procedures commonly used to assess each of these domains are listed in Table 19.1. The tests listed are merely examples, and the choice of these is not intended to exclude the use of other appropriate tests. Selection of tests from within each domain should be based on the need for (1) sampling each domain to evaluate integrity of function, and (2) further investigating aspects or subcomponents that will clarify the nature of the child's detected

TABLE 19.1. Common Procedures Used to Assess Neuropsychological Domains

Executive functioning
  Category Test
  Wisconsin Card Sorting Test
  Tower of Hanoi
  Verbal Fluency
  Raven's Progressive Matrices
  Trail Making Test
  WISC-III Mazes
  Reciprocal motor movements
  WISC-III Similarities

Attention/concentration/orientation/vigilance
  Continuous-performance test
  Cancellation tests
  Stroop Color–Word Test
  Paced Auditory Serial Addition Task
  WISC-III Freedom from Distractibility Index
  Symbol Digit Modalities Test
  WISC-III Symbol Search, Coding

Receptive and expressive language
  Aphasia Screening Test
  WISC-III Vocabulary
  Peabody Picture Vocabulary Test—III
  Gardner Expressive One Word Picture
    Vocabulary Test—Revised
  Gardner Receptive One Word Picture
    Vocabulary Test—Revised
  Auditory Analysis Test
  Token Test
  Boston Naming Test
  Comprehensive Evaluation of Language
    Functions—Revised
  Test of Language Development—2
  Automatic language sequences
  Paragraph production

Sensory-perceptual functioning
  Reitan–Kløve Sensory-Perceptual Examination
    Double Simultaneous Tactile, Auditory,
      Visual Stimulation
    Finger Recognition
    Fingertip Symbol/Number Writing
    Visual Fields

Motor functioning
  Lateral Dominance Examination
  Right–Left Orientation Test
  Apraxia Examination
  Finger Tapping Test
  Grip Strength (Dynamometer) Test

  Grooved Pegboard Test
  Purdue Pegboard Test
  Luria Motor Sequences
  Rapid alternating movements

Visual–spatial analysis and constructional skills
  Beery-Buktenica Developmental Test of
    Visual–Motor Integration
  Benton Judgment of Line Orientation Test
  Benton Facial Recognition Test
  WISC-III Block Design, Object Assembly,
    Picture Arrangement
  Hooper Visual Organization Test
  Money Road Map Test
  Draw-A-Clock
  Free drawings

Learning and retrieval
  Selective Reminding Test
  California Verbal Learning Test—Children's
    Version
  Rey–Osterrieth Complex Figure
  Benton Visual Recognition Test
  Continuous Recognition Memory Test
  WISC-III Information
  Story recall
  Paired associates
  Sentence memory
  Composite memory batteries
    Wide Range Assessment of Memory and
      Language
    Test of Memory and Learning
    Children's Memory Scale

Academic achievement
  Wechsler Individual Achievement Test
  Wide Range Achievement Test—Third Edition
  Woodcock Johnson Psycho-Educational
    Battery—Revised
  Peabody Individual Achievement Test—
    Revised

Personality/social-emotional/adaptive functioning
  Vineland Adaptive Behavior Scales
  Child Behavior Checklist
  Personality Inventory for Children—Revised
  Children's Depression Inventory
  Reynolds Depression Scale
  State–Trait Anxiety Inventory for Children
  Conners Rating Scales

weakness within a specific domain. For example, assessment of more basic language components may not be necessary if higher-order language skills appear intact on a screening. However, if the child makes dysphonetic spelling errors, a more complete evaluation of language components will be helpful, along with tests from other domains that will provide data about the integrity of specific brain regions or of neuropsychological functional systems important for language processing in general and spelling ability in particular. Thus auditory-perceptual tests that have direct implications for the integrity of temporal lobe processing, or fine and gross motor tests that highlight lateralized cerebral dysfunction and involve intraindividual comparison, can be selected to define a cognitive profile. Other language domain tests and academic achievement tests will help determine whether the deficit extends to more broadly affected language functions, and will provide data about how the child's performance compares to that of other children of the same age and grade. Recommendations will depend on the eventual profile of intact and dysfunctional abilities, and, importantly, on a clinical interpretation that incorporates the data obtained in a detailed individual developmental, medical, academic, psychological, and family history.

Kaufman (1994), among others, has described methods for interpreting results from intelligence testing, and Taylor and Schatschneider (1992b) have noted some of the limitations of using summary IQ scores to describe the sequelae of early brain insults. Therefore, I do not elaborate on IQ testing here, except to emphasize that such testing has a usefulness to child neuropsychologists that goes beyond the calculation of summary IQ scores. The clinical utility of IQ testing stems more from the pattern of individual subtest scores, qualitative features of a child's performance, and resulting cognitive profiles and their correlation with neurological disease or insult.

INTERPRETATION: TRANSLATION OF DATA INTO REAL-LIFE RECOMMENDATIONS

General Considerations

As noted above, a subject rarely covered in textbooks, and one mastered through clinical experience rather than didactics, is the *interpretation* of assessment results and the translation of these data into practical recommendations. The interpretation of the child's history, clinical evaluation findings, the parent interview, and supplemental social, educational, and medical data is what best distinguishes child neuropsychological assessment from other modes of evaluation and leads most directly to meaningful outcomes for the child and family.

Interpretation is often forbidding to the novice. An unfamiliarity with the profiles and patterns of test results, and with the behavioral sequelae of brain insult, makes it difficult to translate "test numbers" into meaningful explanations of a child's behavior. Furthermore, if one has focused primarily on a specific child population (such as children with learning disabilities), it may be difficult to interpret results from assessment of children with other conditions (such as those with chronic neurological illness). Exposure to a diversity of cases, together with a grounding in normal and abnormal child development, is thus needed for facility in interpretation and formulation of appropriate recommendations.

At the interpretive session, the clinical child neuropsychologist condenses all historical and assessment data to highlight neurocognitive issues, and then proposes a plan of action based on the full evaluation. A successful interpretive session will enable parents to become active advocates for their child. It is therefore crucial to enlist the parents' support by comparing behaviors in the test session to behaviors in the real world, and by having parents participate in developing the recommendations.

How is one's interpretation made meaningful to nonprofessionals, and how can one be sure that this interpretation has heightened parents' understanding? These are questions that all child neuropsychologists face, and some answer these questions more easily than others. Some examples of attempts to relate information to parents and to highlight the importance of selected aspects of the evaluation are provided below. My reason for choosing these examples is to demonstrate the connection between objective raw data and practical recommendations that parents can use to help change a child's behavior. The examples include children with specific deficits in the domains of executive functioning, motor and sensory-perceptual functioning, visual–motor/visual-perceptual functioning, and memory and attention. The emphasis in these case illustrations is not on academic remediation, but on practical and "doable" interventions that a parent can easily employ to supplement what teachers and specialists offer in the structured academic or therapeutic setting. These recommendations are not offered as substitutes for formal therapies by appropriately trained professionals, but as examples of how to translate evaluation data into recommendations for dealing with real-life situations.

Before I present these examples, however, it is important to outline general guidelines for communicating technical information to parents. The following guidelines have applicability, regardless of the profile of function documented in testing:

• Be aware of the reasons for which parents are seeking an evaluation. Ask them why they have brought their child for evaluation, what they expect to learn, and what questions they wish answered.

• Because only a limited amount of factual data is likely to be retained, present the results in a way that directly answers parents' concerns and makes the test data meaningful. The written report will allow for more detailed presentation of findings and will serve to remind parents of the discussion content.

• When conveying impressions about the child's general intellectual level, ask the parents to estimate the range in which they would expect their child's score to fall, and to indicate how the measured intelligence of the child compares to intelligence estimates for other family members. For example, one must consider whether a child's IQ is inconsistent with the family norm but falls within acceptable levels compared to normative data, or whether a child's IQ is consistent with the family norm but nevertheless places the child at a disadvantage relative to higher-functioning classmates.

• Encourage descriptive statements about the child's behavior in different settings, to facilitate an understanding of the implications of findings for the child's practical abilities and limitations in these varying settings.

• Consider the child's chronological age before making recommendations. For example, although writing or spelling tutoring is often appropriate for a young child, the benefits of such help might be questioned in the case of a teenager who has never improved despite early intervention. In the latter instance, it might be better to provide academic challenges geared to the individual's strengths, explore vocational opportunities that do not rely on the deficit area, as well as to encourage the use of assistive devices.

• Explore further any weaknesses discovered in testing that have not already been reported in real-life settings. The significance of these weaknesses will depend on parent-reported examples of the child's adaptive functioning. The identification of a weakness on testing does not automatically translate into a neuropsychological deficit. Although what appears to be a weakness may be an early manifestation of a deficit that will emerge more clearly as the child matures, it may also be normal variation in ability structure for the child and therefore not a cause for undue concern.

• Consider the possibility that mild or subtle difficulties may explain poor academic performance in the classroom (e.g., lowered grades, frustration related to specific academic subject matter) and poor behavior at home (e.g., expressed dislike for school, acting-out behavior).

• Present a balanced appraisal of the child's capabilities. Parents may need help "letting go" of a problem that has been intractable but is not likely to impede the child seriously in adult life. For example, a learning-disabled teenager may benefit from the use of a calculator in completing arithmetic problems, but the use of the assistive device may have resulted in parent–child arguments and parental insistence that this tool not be used.

• Remind parents to pay close attention to their child's social-emotional functioning, as well as cognitive state, as the child progresses through school. In this way, parents can intervene in a timely manner should a problem emerge (e.g., as the complexity of school-work increases or as peer pressure builds).

• Consider the recency of medical diagnoses or central nervous system (CNS) treatments in interpreting findings. Neuropsychological test results obtained prior to recovery from an acute insult or during an active phase of CNS treatment may underestimate or overestimate functioning. In these instances, parents need to know that the current profile may not reflect future capabilities.

• Determine whether other family members have problems similar to the child's, since this may make it easier for a parent and child to accept the child's difficulties and to offer emotional support.

Case Example: Deficits in Executive Functioning

Measures of executive functioning have received much recent attention in the child neuropsychological literature (Lyon & Krasnegor, 1995). Assessment of this domain requires the administration of tasks that enable the prediction of an individual child's behavior in novel circumstances, and in situations demanding organization, mental shifting, decision making, planning, reasoning, response inhibition, and the creative generation of ideas and concepts (Denckla, 1989, 1996a, 1996b; Levin et al., 1996; Welsh & Pennington, 1988; Welsh, Pennington, & Grossier, 1991; Weyandt and Willis, 1994). Tests of executive functioning offer critical insights into children's' adaptive abilities and tap processes substantially different from those assessed by intelligence tests or measures from other neuropsychological domains. For example, sometimes individuals with a high IQ will be rigid, incapable of making good choices, unable to make mental shifts adaptively, unable to develop effective problem-solving strategies, and generally ineffective in using their high intelligence to best advantage in specific circumstances. On the other hand, persons with lower IQ may be flexible, creative, generative, and able to adapt efficiently to a wide variety of circumstances. If IQ results were the sole criterion for success, these latter persons would be regarded as "overachievers." Therefore, the qualities that are measured within the domain of executive functions provide unique clues to the child's style, adaptability, motivation, and resourcefulness.

The importance of measuring executive functioning is evident to anyone who has had to explain to a parent why an intellectually gifted child fails to remember homework assignments, leaves textbooks at school, or shares qualities associated with the "absent-minded professor." An appraisal of executive functions has direct implication for the interpretive session with parents. Explanations of executive abilities can help the child neuropsychologist to communicate to the parents an accurate picture of their child's typical way of responding (i.e., likely reaction to daily occurrences or circumstances within the home or school setting). Being able to communicate these impressions to the parents, even after what they may perceive as a relatively brief evaluation, may convince them of the accuracy of the child neuropsychologist's clinical judgments about their child, and thus may make them more open to other test interpretations. The ability to translate test scores into recognizable behavior patterns is especially valuable when there is resistance to the idea that a single assessment procedure can offer much insight, or when assessment is perceived to be of limited utility due to the artificial nature of the testing environment.

A case example involving a 7-year-old girl helps to underscore this point. Review of background information revealed that a recent educational evaluation had been conducted and had yielded evidence of average intelligence and average academic achievement. The results of a screening for attention-deficit/hyperactivity disorder (ADHD) were negative. An explanation for her poor school performances (i.e., low grades) was not provided; hence her parents sought additional evaluation. A thorough neuropsychological examination was completed, and results revealed markedly poor performances on several tests of reasoning and conceptual flexibility. Despite these difficulties, she performed well in all other test domains. There was no evidence of learning disability or of psychiatric disorder.

Although this child's poor performances on tests of executive functioning were inconsistent with expectations, her specific weaknesses in this area suggested that she was more rule-based than other children her age and less able to adapt to changing circumstances or rules. Such a child may find novelty, varying environmental conditions, and new academic lessons initially overwhelming, and may cling to previously established behavior patterns, even if these are no longer appropriate for the circumstances. A child with this pattern of strengths and weaknesses may find it more comfortable to "back off" from tasks perceived as difficult rather than to attempt them and fail. As a result, the child may withdraw from active academic involvement, exhibit little motivation to succeed, and/or drift off or become inattentive in class, despite having the cognitive potential to be a successful student.

After a discussion of their daughter's strengths, these possibilities were broached with the parents during the interpretive session. They confirmed that such behaviors were characteristic of their daughter. The discussion then focused on specific ways in which her executive weaknesses interfered with school performance, and on ways to assist her to overcome these problems. Accommodations suggested for her included the following:

- Providing a preparatory list of expected topics and assignments in consultation with her teacher.
- Offering a concrete description of appropriate behavior in a specific situation and rehearsing this behavior.
- Explaining in a step-by-step fashion the differences between new situations or demands and old ones.
- Rehearsing alternative responses for each specific situation.
- Increasing organization/planning skill through list making and use of visual cues and graphic organizers (e.g., a daily or weekly calendar).
- Monitoring assignments and reviewing poor performances by emphasizing differences between what was expected and what was produced.

- Providing liberal positive feedback for efforts to improve.
- Opening a dialogue between parents and child that fosters discussion of the school day in a nonjudgmental, informative, and supportive way.

Case Example: Deficits in Motor and Sensory-Perceptual Functions

Child neuropsychologists commonly assess motor and sensory-perceptual functioning. Lateralized performance in these domains may highlight major inconsistencies in functioning between the two sides of the body, and thus between the two cerebral hemispheres. Inferences about an individual child's functioning are generally based either on the pathognomonic signs or on differential scores (Francis, Fletcher, & Rourke, 1988). Deficits in the sensory-perceptual domain may be less obvious and are more likely to go unnoticed in real-life situations than are motor impairments. The assessment and identification of motor or sensory-perceptual disturbance has a useful role in documenting the severity of an underlying neurological condition and in monitoring of cognitive decline or recovery. These assessments are especially useful in following children with vascular problems, hydrocephalus, and traumatic brain injury, but are also applicable to children with other neurological conditions (Denckla, 1985; Dewey & Kaplan, 1992; Williams & Dykman, 1994).

A discrepancy between expected and actual motor or sensory-perceptual performances may reveal subtle abnormalities in these functions that have not been identified in natural settings. These abnormalities may nevertheless be recognized as clumsiness on the sports field or awkwardness in the classroom. Similarly, a hearing deficit may escape notice despite the child's tendency to turn up the volume on the television set, or a visual impairment may be overlooked even though the child has begun to hold the pages of a book too close or to lower his or her head to the printed page. A lateralized motor and/or sensory-perceptual deficit noted during testing may also correlate with academic problems, as when a right-handed child with left-hemisphere dysfunction develops difficulties in written language skills. In such cases, neuropsychological findings provide concrete illustrations of how the child's behavior is affected by a specific underlying neurological problem.

The results of motor and sensory-perceptual testing can also serve as a basis for practical recommendations. For example, as a result of graphomotor impairment, a child may elect to produce a minimal amount of written work. Because of discrepancies between the child's verbal expressive skills and written expressive output, the child may be perceived as not trying hard enough (a common teacher misperception). Evidence of graphomotor weakness in testing will clarify the child's true capabilities, and will justify a number of adaptations to make learning easier and to enable more reliable assessment of what the child has learned (Baron & Goldberger, 1993). Examples of classroom adaptations are listed below:

- Extending time limits for written examinations and written productions.
- Encouraging one-word responses, and making use of true–false or multiple-choice formats rather than lengthy essay questions.
- Encouraging examination and essay production through dictation on an audiocassette recorder or to another individual.
- Recording the teacher's oral presentations for later replay, to minimize the need for rapid or extensive written transcription during class time.
- Decreasing demands for copying from the chalkboard.

- Providing written handouts whenever possible.
- Decreasing emphasis on written production (e.g., by grading content separately from neatness or form of the written production).
- Extending time limits or eliminating these constraints.
- Decreasing repetitive writing.
- Increasing the use of computer word processing, to avoid the need for laborious written formulation.

Adaptations for the home setting vary with the child's age, but may usefully incorporate some of the following:

- Providing a variety of writing materials that are comfortable and that have intrinsic interest (e.g., that vary in size, writing color, and artistic possibilities).
- Having the child accompany the parent to the store to purchase interesting writing instruments and paper materials.
- Reinforcing the child's efforts to write and offering opportunities to do so in non-academic contexts. Examples include a phone book for the child to list friends, their addresses, and their telephone numbers; a list of grocery store items the child would like the parent to purchase; a list of friends to invite to a party, or a list of party activities; a diary about a school or family trip; an essay about the family pet; and a letter to extended family members.
- Encouraging the development of computer keyboard skills; these skills become increasingly important as the child progresses through the grades.
- Encouraging familiarity with computer word-processing programs, especially with programs that provide internal spelling and grammatical checks.
- Encouraging parents to recognize that writing may always be a challenge for their child, despite intervention, and that many successful people learn to compensate (e.g., by using a computer or dictating).

Case Example: Deficits in Visual-Perceptual and Visual–Motor Skills

Children's performances on measures of visual-perceptual and visual–motor functions may help to account for weaknesses in spatial abilities, social judgment, or other nonverbal functions. Weaknesses in this area are often observed in the context of relatively intact elementary verbal skills. Routine vision screening generally confirms that impairments in acuity or other primary sensory capacities are not present.

An illustration of visual-perceptual/visual–motor impairments is provided by a 7-year-old boy with a history of an encapsulated low-grade astrocytoma located in the middle and posterior right temporal lobe. The tumor had been successfully resected at age 2, and 5 years later his parents were requesting an evaluation to determine whether any residual impairment had resulted from the tumor or its treatment. Their son had not received chemotherapy or radiation therapy.

Administration of the Wechsler Intelligence Scale for Children—Third Edition (WISC-III; Wechsler, 1991) revealed superior Verbal and Full Scale IQs, but only high-average Performance IQ (the difference was not statistically significant). His academic progress had been excellent, with no obvious signs of impairment in this area. His parents had requested the evaluation for their own edification, and not in response to any specific con-

- Utilizing rehearsal and repetition strategies (e.g., flash cards, audiocassette replay of verbal information).
- Building on strengths by using multimodality cueing strategies.
- Teaching crossed-modality cueing (e.g. use of color, shape, or visual associations to stimulate retention of verbal material).
- Reducing demands for retention of multistep commands while increasing single-step requests.
- Encouraging the use of daily planners, event calendars, and homework-due charts.
- Having teachers provide written handouts for their verbal homework assignments and written outlines for lecture material.
- Encouraging cross-checking with a "study buddy."

Behavioral factors and individual learning styles also bear consideration in evaluating memory complaints. For example, shy children may be reluctant to speak out in class even if they know the answer, or boastful children may be so eager to give an answer that they omit important information. Other potential bases of memory complaints are attention deficits (Schmitter-Edgecombe, 1996) and executive dysfunction (Gnys & Willis, 1991). If children do not pay attention and information is not encoded, it will not be available for later retrieval. Similarly, if children cannot inhibit actions that interfere with successful learning, they will not show evidence of learning in subsequent testing of their knowledge. Thus, children with ADHD, or even those with attentional weaknesses that do not meet strict criteria for this disorder, may appear to have memory problems. More generally, memory problems may be due to inappropriate, inaccurate, or incomplete learning. Alternative accounts of memory difficulties, therefore, must be distinguished from true amnestic impairments. Only by doing so will it be possible to target interventions appropriately.

The case of a 6-year-old female identical twin illustrates the practical implications of these distinctions. The girl was referred for evaluation because she did not follow directions at home and seemed unable to remember what was said to her, despite repetition. A careful history revealed some extraordinary circumstances and relevant family medical history. Although she was the biological child of American parents and lived with her family in the United States at the time of the assessment, her nursery school and kindergarten years had been spent in an impoverished country because of her father's overseas assignment. The country was at war, and conditions were not conducive to consistent school attendance. One day she was kidnapped on her way to school, but was released unharmed shortly afterwards. A long separation from her father, who traveled for business, further complicated adjustment to this stressful setting. Her development was reported to be normal, but her parents felt that she lagged behind her twin sister by about "4 to 6 weeks." An older brother had delayed speech and delayed fine and gross motor abilities, and was diagnosed with ADHD and anxiety problems. The family history was also significant for learning difficulties, "mild Tourette syndrome," and ADHD in her father. Her current first-grade teacher did not report behavioral or academic problems. The child comprehended and followed all instructions well during the testing session. Some attentional variability was clinically evident, and test results revealed that attention/concentration was her weakest area of measured ability. Her level of general intelligence fell between low-average and average levels. She initiated and inhibited actions well, and she performed age-appropriately on tests requiring organization, planning, and mental flexibility. Language skills were appropriate for her chronological age. She also performed well on a verbal selective reminding test (Morgan, 1982), demonstrating efficient learning of the word list, age-appropriate skill on a measure of consistent long-term retrieval, and excellent delayed free retrieval (my own administration procedure). Her performance on this list-learning task attested to her capacities for verbal encoding, storage, and delayed recall.

Several alternative explanations of the "memory" problem were considered in the interpretive session. The girl's parents were first informed that her general intellectual level placed her at a relative disadvantage compared to her classmates, who in her community functioned primarily at the average to high-average intellectual level. Her abilities also appeared to fall below those of her identical twin, which might contribute to feelings of frustration or diminished self-esteem. Second, she had not had the same opportunities to acquire basic academic skills as had her classmates, since she had only recently begun her education in the United States. This lack of opportunity was likely to be reflected in her schoolwork. Her errors on simple math computations, inability to "recall" how to write some letters, and poor grasp of readiness concepts suggested that intensive tutoring or resource help was needed to bring her up to grade level. Third, she had experienced considerable emotional trauma overseas, and her parents' marital relationship was also strained. It was important to consider adjustment issues and family dynamics as potential influences on school-related performance. Fourth, she had selective impairment on attentional tasks, and clinical observations were of greater attentional variability than is typical for a young child in a structured testing environment. The possibility of an attentional deficit thus deserved strong consideration as one basis for her "memory" difficulties. Her family history of ADHD was consistent with this possibility and reinforced the need for careful monitoring of her progress.

Although treatment of attention deficits is beyond the scope of this chapter, there is a considerable literature on various therapeutic approaches (e.g., Barkley, 1998). Several strategies that may prove particularly useful for parents and teachers are listed below:

- Confirming the child's understanding of verbal directions (e.g., by asking for repetition of what was stated).
- Having the child rehearse learning tasks or assignments.
- Helping the child work more efficiently by reinforcing short, concentrated periods of activity and by progressively increasing the length of these periods.
- Using multimodal presentations that combine auditory/verbal, visual, tactile, and/ or kinesthetic cues.
- Giving directions and instructions in a step-by-step fashion, with clearly articulated verbal presentations and sufficient time for processing.
- Supplementing lectures with written outlines, handouts, or text containing essential details of the curriculum.
- Seating the child within the classroom in a position that permits easy face-to-face interaction with the teacher and that limits distractions (e.g., a seat away from a window or a distracting child, a study carrel).
- Referring parents to local organizations and support groups serving families of children with attentional problems.
- Assigning a "study buddy" to work with the child in a supportive and nonobtrusive manner, and to provide opportunities for developing social skills.

CONCLUSION

One of the child neuropsychologist's major clinical roles is to integrate information from a wide variety of sources, in an effort to assist parents in understanding the bases of presenting complaints. This role requires the neuropsychologist to identify children's strengths as well as weaknesses. Too often an emphasis is placed on what is wrong with a child, rather than on the balance of the child's assets and liabilities. When a parent states, "But my child is talented in . . . , gifted in . . . , has a strength in . . . ," it is important to note these characteristics. The conclusions reached about a child are incomplete if these talents are not considered. This search for a balance in the overall picture of how a child functions is also critical in maintaining a child's self-esteem, highlighting positive aspects of parents' and teachers' efforts to help the child, and recommending treatment modalities and techniques that can utilize areas of strength. Awareness of the child's strengths may also be useful in providing vocational guidance and in suggesting extracurricular activities that would be likely to enhance socialization and self-esteem.

As noted above, the number and range of test instruments and procedures that enable determination of neuropsychological functioning have increased considerably in recent years. It is expected that neuropsychologists will maintain current awareness of the statistical measurement properties of preferred instruments, normative data appropriate for the clinical populations they evaluate, recent research on studies of different clinical disorders that present in childhood, comorbidities that are complicating factors in the differential considerations about the bases for a child's behavior, and the emergence of subtypes within diagnostic groups as these occur. A focus on ecological validity has emerged and is expected to be an even more prominent consideration—increasingly so as research is conducted on the effectiveness of individual, family, and school interventions based on neuropsychological principles and data.

The practical benefits of child neuropsychological assessment thus depend on an appreciation of the full spectrum of the child's adaptive functioning, as well as on an understanding of the specific intervention options that will support the child's continued optimal developmental maturation. Among the future directions in the field that hold exciting prospects is the application of neuropsychological principles and methods to the very youngest children. Such investigation may result in the stimulation of novel strategies that build on a child's inherent maturational steps, but that enable the child to maximize neurodevelopmental outcome (e.g., despite environmental impedences). The correlation of the neurobehavioral manifestations of congenital and early acquired neurological disease or injury and of formal neuropsychological data with the results of advanced neuroimaging techniques also holds promise for extending our knowledge of brain development and the important influences that maintain or disrupt development at different stages of maturation. This effort is important if child neuropsychologists are to continue to apply neuropsychological principles in an ecologically meaningful way for children, families, and society.

REFERENCES

Bakker, D., Licht, R., & Kappers, J. (1995). Hemispheric stimulation techniques in children with dyslexia. In M. G. Tramontana & S. R. Hooper (Eds.), *Advances in child neuropsychology* (Vol. 3, pp. 144–177). New York: Springer-Verlag.

Barkley, R. A. (1998). *Attention deficit hyperactivity disorder: A handbook for diagnosis and treatment*. New York: Guilford Press.

Baron, I. S., & Gioia, G. A. (1998). Neuropsychology of infants and young children. In G. Goldstein, P. D. Nussbaum, & S. Beers (Eds.), *Neuropsychology* (pp. 9–34). New York: Plenum Press.

Baron, I. S., & Goldberger, E. (1993). Neuropsychological disturbances of hydrocephalic children with implications for special education and rehabilitation. *Neuropsychological Rehabilitation, 3,* 389–410.

Baron, I. S., Fennell, E. B., & Voeller, K. K. S. (1995). *Pediatric neuropsychology in the medical setting*. New York: Oxford University Press.

Bauer, P. J. (1996). What do infants recall of their lives?: Memory for specific events by one- to two-year olds. *American Psychologist*, *51*, 29–41.

Bernstein, J. H., & Waber, D. P. (1990). Developmental neuropsychological assessment: The systemic approach. In A. A. Boulton, G. B. Baker, & M. Hiscock (Eds.), *Neuromethods: Vol. 17. Neuropsychology* (pp. 311–371). Clifton, NJ: Humana Press.

Boyd, T. A. (1988). Clinical assessment of memory in children: A developmental framework for practice. In M. G. Tramontana & S. R. Hooper (Eds.), *Assessment issues in child neuropsychology*. New York: Plenum Press.

Brown, S. J., Rourke, B. P., & Cicchetti, D. (1989). Reliability of tests and measures used in the neuropsychological assessment of children. *Clinical Neuropsychologist*, *3*, 353–368.

Butterbaugh, G. J. (1988). Selected psychometric and clinical review of neurodevelopmental infant tests. *Clinical Neuropsychologist*, *2*, 350–364.

Clodfelter, C. J., Dickson, A. L., Newton Wilkes, C., & Johnson, R. B. (1987). Alternate forms of selective reminding for children. *Clinical Neuropsychologist*, *1*, 243–249.

Cooley, E. L., & Morris, R. D. (1990). Attention in children: A neuropsychologically based model for assessment. *Developmental Neuropsychology*, *6*, 239–274.

Delis, D. C., Kramer, J. H., Kaplan, E., & Ober, B. A. (1994). *California Verbal Learning Test: Children's Version*. San Antonio, TX: Psychological Corporation.

Denckla, M. B. (1985). Motor coordination in dyslexic children. Theoretical and clinical implications. In F. H. Duffy & N. Geschwind (Eds.), *Dyslexia: A neuroscientific approach to clinical evaluation* (pp. 187–195). Boston: Little, Brown.

Denckla, M. B. (1989). Executive function, the overlap zone between attention deficit hyperactivity disorder and learning disabilities. *International Pediatrics*, *4*, 155–160.

Denckla, M. B. (1996a). Research on executive function in a neurodevelopmental context: Application of clinical measures. *Developmental Neuropsychology*, *12*, 5–15.

Denckla, M. B. (1996b). A theory and model of executive dysfunction: A neuropsychological perspective. In G. R. Lyon & N. A. Krasnegor (Eds.), *Attention, memory, and executive function* (pp. 263–278). Baltimore: Paul H. Brookes.

Denckla, M. B., & Reader, M. (1992). Education and psychosocial interventions: Executive dysfunction and its consequences. In R. Kurlan (Ed.), *Handbook of Tourette syndrome and related tic and behavioral disorders* (pp. 431–451). New York: Marcel Dekker.

Dennis, M., Spiegler, B. J., Fitz, C. R., Hoffman, H. J., Hendrick, E. B., Humphreys, R. P., & Chuang, S. (1991). Brain tumors in children and adolescents: II. The neuroanatomy of deficits in working, associative and serial-order memory. *Neuropsychologia*, *29*, 829–847.

Dennis, M., Spiegler, B. J., Hoffman, H. J., Hendrick, E. B., Humphreys, R. P., & Becker, L. E. (1991). Brain tumors in children and adolescents: I. Effects on working, associative, and serial-order memory of IQ, age at tumor onset and age of tumor. *Neuropsychologia*, *29*, 813–827.

Dewey, D., & Kaplan, B. J. (1992). Analysis of praxis task demands in the assessment of children with developmental motor deficits. *Developmental Neuropsychology*, *8*, 367–379.

Fennell, E. B., & Bauer, R. M. (1989). Models of inference in evaluating brain–behavior relationships in children. In C. R. Reynolds (Ed.), *Handbook of child clinical neuropsychology* (pp. 167–180). New York: Plenum Press.

Fletcher, J. M., & Taylor, H. G. (1984). Neuropsychological approaches to children: Towards a developmental neuropsychology. *Journal of Clinical Neuropsychology*, *6*, 39–56.

Fletcher, J. M., & Taylor, H. G. (1997). Children with brain injury. In E. J. Mash & L. G. Terdal (Eds.), *Assessment of childhood disorders* (3rd ed., pp. 453–480). New York: Guilford Press.

Francis, D. J., Fletcher, J. M., & Rourke, B. P. (1988). Discriminant validity of lateral sensorimotor tests in children. *Journal of Clinical and Experimental Neuropsychology*, *10*, 779–799.

Francis, D. J., Fletcher, J. M., Rourke, B. P., & York, M. J. (1992). A five-factor model for motor, psychomotor, and visual–spatial tests used in the neuropsychological assessment of children. *Journal of Clinical and Experimental Neuropsychology*, *14*, 625–637.

Francis, D. J., Fletcher, J. M., Stuebing, K. K., Davison, K. C., & Thompson, N. R. (1991). Analysis of change: Modeling individual growth. *Journal of Consulting and Clinical Psychology*, *59*, 27–37.

Francis, D. J., Shaywitz, S. E., Stuebing, K. K., Shaywitz, B. A., & Fletcher, J. M. (1994). The measurement of change: Assessing behavior over time and within a developmental context. In G. R. Lyon (Ed.), *Frames of reference for the assessment of learning disabilities* (pp. 29–58). Baltimore: Paul H. Brookes.

Franzen, K. M., Roberts, M. A., Schmits, D., Verduyn, W., & Manshadi, F. (1996). Cognitive remediation in pediatric traumatic brain injury. *Child Neuropsychology*, *2*, 176–184.

Gathercole, S. (1998). The development of memory. *Journal of Child Psychology and Psychiatry, 39,* 3–27.

Gnys, J. A., & Willis, W. G. (1991). Validation of executive function tasks with young children. *Developmental Neuropsychology, 7,* 487–501.

Hammeke, T. A. (1993). The association of postdoctoral programs in clinical neuropsychology (APPCN). *Clinical Neuropsychologist, 7,* 197–204.

Hitch, G. J., & Halliday, M. S. (1983). Working memory in children. *Journal of the Royal Society of London B, 302,* 325–340.

Kail, R. V., Jr., & Hagen, H. W. (1977). *Perspective on the development of memory and cognition.* New York: Wiley.

Kaufman, A. S. (1994). *Intelligent testing with the WISC-III.* New York: Wiley.

Klahr, D., & Robinson, M. (1981). Formal assessment of problem-solving and planning processes in preschool children. *Cognitive Psychology, 13,* 113–148.

Levin, H. (1989). *Buschke–Levin Selective Reminding Test.* Galveston: University of Texas Medical Branch.

Levin, H., Fletcher, J. M., Kufera, J. A., Harward, H., Lilly, M. A., Mendelsohn, D., Bruce, D., & Eisenberg, H. M. (1996). Dimensions of cognition measured by the Tower of London and other cognitive tasks in head-injured children and adolescents. *Developmental Neuropsychology, 12,* 17–34.

Lyon, G. R., & Krasnegor, N. A. (Eds.). (1995). *Attention, memory, and executive function.* Baltimore: Paul H. Brookes.

Morgan, S. F. (1982). Measuring long-term storage and retrieval in children. *Journal of Clinical Neuropsychology, 4,* 77–85.

Pennington, B. F. (1991). *Diagnosing learning disorders: A neuropsychological framework.* New York: Guilford Press.

Rourke, B. P. (1989). *Nonverbal learning disabilities: The syndrome and the model.* New York: Guilford Press.

Rourke, B. P., Fisk, J. L., & Strang, J. D. (1986). *Neuropsychological assessment of children: A treatment-oriented approach.* New York: Guilford Press.

Rybash, J. M., & Colilla, J. L. (1994). Source memory deficits and frontal lobe functioning in children. *Developmental Neuropsychology, 10,* 67–73.

Sawrie, S. M., Chelune, G. J., Naugle, R. I., & Luders, H. O. (1996). Empirical methods for assessing meaningful neuropsychological change following epilepsy surgery. *Journal of the International Neuropsychological Society, 2,* 556–564.

Schmitter-Edgecombe, M. (1996). The effects of divided attention on implicit and explicit memory performance. *Journal of the International Neuropsychological Society, 2,* 111–125.

Sheslow, D., & Adams, W. (1990). *Wide Range Assessment of Memory and Learning administration manual.* Wilmington, DE: Jastak.

Spreen, O., & Strauss, E. (1991). *A compendium of neuropsychological tests: Administration, norms, and commentary.* New York: Oxford University Press.

Taylor, H. G., & Schatschneider, C. (1992a). Child neuropsychological assessment: A test of basic assumptions. *Clinical Neuropsychologist, 6,* 259–275.

Taylor, H. G., & Schatschneider, C. (1992b). Academic achievement following childhood brain disease: Implications for the concept of learning disabilities. *Journal of Learning Disabilities, 25,* 630–638.

Waber, D., & Holmes, J. (1986). Assessing children's memory productions of the Rey–Osterrieth Complex Figure. *Journal of Clinical and Experimental Neuropsychology, 8,* 563–580.

Wechsler, D. (1991). *Wechsler Intelligence Scale for Children—Third Edition: Manual.* San Antonio, TX: Psychological Corporation.

Welsh, M. C., & Pennington, B. F. (1988). Assessing frontal lobe functioning in children: Views from developmental psychology. *Developmental Neuropsychology, 4,* 119–230.

Welsh, M. C., Pennington, B. F., & Grossier, D. B. (1991). A normative-developmental study of executive function: A window on prefrontal function in children. *Developmental Neuropsychology, 7,* 131–149.

Weyandt, L. L., & Willis, W. G. (1994). Executive functions in school-aged children: Potential efficacy of tasks in discriminating clinical groups. *Developmental Neuropsychology, 10,* 27–38.

Williams, J., & Dykman, R. A. (1994). Nonverbal factors derived from children's performances on neuropsychological test instruments. *Developmental Neuropsychology, 10,* 19–26.

Wilson, B. C. (1992). The neuropsychological assessment of the preschool child: A branching model. In F. Boller & J. Grafman (Series Eds.) and I. Rapin & S. J. Segalowitz (Vol. Eds.), *Handbook of Neuropsychology: Vol. 6. Child neuropsychology* (pp. 377–394). Amsterdam: Elsevier.

Wilson, B. C., & Risucci, D. A. (1986). A model for clinical–quantitative classification: Generation 1. Application to language-disordered preschool children. *Brain and Language, 27,* 281–309.

Yeates, K. O., Blumenstein, E., Patterson, C. M., & Delis, D. C. (1995). Verbal learning and memory follow-ing pediatric closed-head injury. *Journal of the International Neuropsychological Society, 1,* 78–87.

Yeates, K. O., Enrile, B. E., Loss, N., Blumenstein, E., & Delis, D. C. (1995). Verbal learning and memory in children with myelomeningocele. *Journal of Pediatric Psychology, 20,* 801–815.

Yeates, K. O., Ris, M. D., & Taylor, H. G. (1995). Hospital referral patterns in pediatric neuropsychology. *Child Neuropsychology, 1,* 56–62.

Yeates, K. O., & Taylor, H. G. (1998). Neuropsychological assessment of older children. In G. Goldstein, P. D. Nussbaum, & S. Beers (Eds.), *Neuropsychology* (pp. 35–61). New York: Plenum Press.

Ylvisaker, M., Szekeres, S. F., Hartwick, P., & Tworek, P. (1994). Cognitive intervention. In R. C. Savage & G. F. Wolcott (Eds.), *Educational dimensions of acquired brain injury* (pp. 121–184). Austin, TX: PRO-ED.

PART V

Commentary

20

REVIEW AND FUTURE DIRECTIONS

BYRON P. ROURKE

The primary purpose of this chapter is to provide a review of the contributions to this book that pertain to specific neurological and possibly related medical conditions (Chapters 2–17). For each chapter, I have highlighted some of the dimensions that I feel are of particular importance to the scientist–practitioner in pediatric neuropsychology. Where I thought it relevant to do so, I have provided other references that were not mentioned by the particular author(s) of each chapter, but that interested readers may wish to consult. I conclude the chapter with some general observations.

COMMENTS ON SPECIFIC CHAPTERS

The groups headed by Fletcher in Houston and Dennis in Toronto (see Fletcher, Dennis, & Northrup, Chapter 2) have substantially advanced our understanding of early hydrocephalus. Exhaustive studies of a wide range of neurobehavioral and linguistic domains have contributed a unique and valuable perspective to the knowledge base about this set of disorders. Furthermore, the testing of theoretically important dimensions of neuropsychological development has characterized these efforts, and it should stand as a model for our field.

The authors of Chapter 2 summarize what is known about the effects of early hydrocephalus of varying etiologies on important dimensions of significant developmental epochs. Their suggestions for future research in this very interesting area are sound, and I hope that these will be followed.

Investigators interested in an associated condition, collosal agenesis of the corpus callosum viewed within the context of the syndrome of nonverbal learning disabilities (NLD), may find Smith and Rourke (1995) of interest. Also, the characterization of the intact and deficient linguistic dimensions investigated by Dennis and colleagues is reflected in the characterization of the preserved and deficient linguistic dimensions evident in NLD that arises from a variety of causes, including early hydrocephalus (Rourke & Tsatsanis, 1996).

Seizure disorders have been studied extensively, and reports of this research are found almost everywhere in journals with a neuroscience emphasis. What may not be obvious to the pediatric neuropsychologist is the extensive knowledge base that has been elucidated through this exercise. Much of this is nicely summarized in Chapter 3 by Williams and Sharp. Furthermore, their contribution serves as a primer on seizure types and on treatments for childhood epilepsies.

A critical view of the incidence of learning disabilities, attentional deficits, and psychosocial functioning is especially noteworthy in this chapter. The interactions of seizure types and pharmacotherapies with respect to disorders in these areas is of special interest for the practicing pediatric neuropsychologist. Indeed, the combination of basic science, clinical pharmacology, and clinical neuropsychology that runs through this presentation is a format with which the informed pediatric neuropsychologist should feel particularly comfortable.

In Chapter 4, Morris, Krawiecki, Kullgren, Ingram, and Kurczynski provide a very useful summary of the epidemiology and major types of brain tumors in children. Their overview of the various etiologies and risk factors sets the stage for a discussion that deals with a variety of clinical presentations, natural history, and treatment modalities. Developmental outcomes, especially relating to the potential perils of radiation treatment, are well described within the limitations posed by the relative paucity of reliable data that have been generated in this area.

The inadequacy of IQ tests for the full description of the long-term outcome for children with brain tumors is a position that virtually all pediatric neuropsychologists salute. The necessity for comprehensive neuropsychological evaluation within the context of long-term follow-up is also a point of convergence for all of us who are involved in such studies (Rourke, 1976, 1995c). The attempt to "drive" this type of investigation in terms of a neurodevelopmental model (e.g., Buono et al., 1998) is especially welcome in a field that is becoming richer in terms of data, but is still relatively poor in terms of model and theory development and testing. It is clear that the studies this group has carried out should be a major paradigm for the foreseeable future.

Finally, the points raised in this chapter underscore the necessity for a thorough understanding of the natural history of brain disorders in children. The wide variability in personal, academic, and psychosocial outcomes noted by many clinical investigators points to the need to identify the characteristics leading to these different developmental paths. The identification of reliable subtypes of neuropsychological and psychosocial functioning advocated herein can be expected to shed considerable light on what is probably a specific set of neurodevelopmental histories. Indeed, attempts to search for the homogeneous set of sequelae for which less sophisticated researchers yearn seem doomed to failure.

For some pediatric neuropsychologists, questions regarding the effects of traumatic brain injury (TBI) are their most common referral challenges. Other professionals and caregivers are particularly interested in the short- and long-term outcomes for children so afflicted. Will the child's abilities decline over time? Will there be some psychosocial problems? Will the child be capable of benefiting from education, now and in the foreseeable future? Are there some treatments that might prove helpful?

There is a sense in which these questions are asked in a more or less similar manner for virtually all of the childhood diseases and disorders discussed in this book. But in the case of TBI, we are now in a position to address these questions in an informed manner. This does not mean that the answers to these questions can be framed with great confidence in every instance. What is meant is this: An abundance of information in the literature now suggests that there are indeed fairly predictable outcomes. The bases for these predictions are reviewed in a thorough manner by Yeates in Chapter 5.

Of special importance is the finding that outcomes are variably dependent upon age of injury, neurological status (including length of coma and posttraumatic amnesia), types of neuropsychological problems manifested when a child is able to undergo a comprehensive evaluation, and social/family/environmental conditions that both pre- and postdate the injury. The inclusion of academic and psychosocial outcomes as objects of systematic inquiry is especially welcome, given the importance of these developmental demands.

Yeates's call for careful developmental analysis of the sequelae of TBI parallels such advocacy in most other chapters of this book. It may also be useful to note that a start has been made in the development of a typology of psychosocial outcomes following TBI (Butler, Rourke, Fuerst, & Fisk, 1997). Such efforts, together with those outlined in this chapter, should put to rest the widely held notion that there is a common psychosocial outcome following significant TBI and that this outcome is uniformly negative. Indeed, it appears to be the case that TBI classified as "severe" from several perspectives is very often associated with no or very few psychosocial deficits (Butler et al., 1997).

Reflection on the implications of the multidimensional nature of the outcome measurements reviewed in this chapter, perhaps especially relating to the psychosocial functioning of the child's family, should enhance the design of investigations aimed at providing the data we need to answer the very important questions posed to us. These beguilingly simple questions will be amenable to efficacious, although somewhat complex, answers once these ramifications are seriously considered and thoroughly investigated.

In Chapter 6, Anderson and Taylor describe the various types of meningitis and continue with a thorough coverage of their pathophysiologies. This discussion provides the backdrop against which to consider their medical and neuropsychological sequelae. Findings relating to the differential impact of one type of the disease (e.g., the finding that nonverbal skills and executive functions are more clearly compromised than other abilities) in the North American studies are of particular interest. Such differences were not as apparent in the Australian studies reported. The authors go to great pains to point out why these sets of results are different. A study of their reasoning yields much of import for the pediatric neuropsychologist as a "consumer" of research in this and other areas covered in this book.

Among the many laudable features of this very informative chapter, the reader may be especially impressed by the authors' emphasis upon the interactions of sociocultural, and especially family, factors with short- and long-term outcomes. That these factors, in conjunction with access to remedial resources, may be more important determinants of outcome than are illness-related variables is a point that should be considered in most, if not all, of the chapters in this volume.

Moore and Denckla begin Chapter 7 with a succinct but thorough overview of the salient medical features of neurofibromatosis (NF). This is a necessary prolegomenon to the sections that follow it.

The inadequacies of many early neuropsychological investigations of NF are highlighted, and the incidence and (sub)types of learning disabilities (LD) found are emphasized. In their research on LD in NF, the authors appear to have found that individual children with NF may exhibit more than one type of LD. This reminds me of a neuropsychological colleague's assertion that we need to remember that children may have "measles and a broken leg." Of course, the intriguing research question arising from such an observation is that it may be very fruitful to attempt to determine the etiology of the "measles" and the "broken leg," and to learn how these can coexist in the same individual. Of relevance within this context, it should also be borne in mind that persons who exhibit NLD are thought to have very pervasive linguistic deficits (Rourke, 1989; Rourke & Tsatsanis, 1996), and that distinct types of "disabilities" in arithmetic can arise from very different patterns of neuropsychological assets and deficits (Rourke, 1982, 1993; Rourke & Conway, 1997; Rourke & Strang, 1983).

Comparisons with other reasonably well-researched single-gene abnormalities constitute a singularly important feature of this chapter. Such comparisons are likely to shed considerable light upon the neurological bases for differing phenotypic patterns of neuropsychological assets and deficits, as well as what appears to be the "final common pathway" for several neurodevelopmental disorders—for example, Williams syndrome (Anderson & Rourke, 1995) and velocardiofacial syndrome (Fuerst, Dool, & Rourke, 1995). As regards the possible relationship of the syndrome of NLD to such disorders, the interested reader may wish to consult Crowe and Hay (1990) and Bawden et al. (1996).

The neuroimaging results presented in this chapter are fascinating, and it would appear that systematic use of this technology in conjunction with comprehensive neuropsychological evaluations of children is becoming a particularly fruitful path to follow. The authors' suggestions for future directions for research involving such technologies would appear to be particularly relevant, especially if carried out within the developmental/longitudinal framework that they envision. Finally, it might be helpful to know whether and to what extent children and adolescents with these genetic disorders exhibit the subtypes of psychosocial functioning that have been documented in several studies of children and adolescents who exhibit LDs but have no known genetic abnormality (Rourke & Fuerst, 1991; Tsatsanis, Fuerst, & Rourke, 1997).

Chapter 8, by Shapiro and Balthazor, contains a useful summary of much that is known about metabolic and degenerative disorders in children. Its emphasis on the usefulness of neuropsychological study of such youngsters as a method of assessing the efficacy of treatments aimed at the central nervous system (CNS) is especially welcome.

The outline of the neurological and other medical dimensions of these comparatively rare diseases is useful, as are the neuropsychological characteristics that have been found to characterize the stages of disease progression. Standard batteries of tests employed in multicenter trials would certainly seem to be required if the full extent of the neuropsychological dimensions at each stage of progression (and treatment, such as bone marrow transplant) are to be understood.

As for the reference to the syndrome of NLD, the interested reader may wish to peruse more recent references that include modifications of the original model in light of subsequent tests of deductions from it (e.g., Rourke, 1988, 1989, 1995b). It should be noted that adrenoleukodystrophy appears to result in virtually all of the neuropsychological assets and deficits proposed in the neurodevelopmental model of NLD (Rourke, 1995a). Also, the relationship between NLD and the leukodystrophies is covered in Dool, Fuerst, and Rourke (1995).

An area that has been marked by controversy and indeed by acrimony—that is, the neuropsychological impact of environmental neurotoxicants—is now enjoying the fruits of a reasonably firm scientific basis. Few pediatric neuropsychologists would dismiss the findings of the negative developmental impact of lead and high concentrations of organic mercury. And virtually none would suggest that children, from conception onward, should not be protected from these and other known environmental neurotoxicants.

The studies reviewed by Dietrich in Chapter 9 range from early ones (which were, for the most part, afflicted with inadequate methodology and narrow outcome measures) to those of more recent vintage (which utilize sophisticated methodology and a range of outcome measures that do justice to the complexity of brain–behavior relationships). Large-scale studies spanning significant developmental epochs are now underway.

From a scientist–practitioner standpoint, the author's closing words regarding the importance of keeping abreast of new developments in this emerging field should be taken very much to heart:

> A working knowledge of this area not only will enhance the clinical and scientific acumen of the pediatric neuropsychologist, but may eventually help to identify as yet undiscovered environmental risks to normal CNS development. Clinicians after all, were the first to identify some of the best-known environmental and pharmaceutical chemical risks to CNS development. (p. 228)

As in so many other areas of neuropsychological endeavor, good science and good practice go hand in hand (Rourke, 1995c).

The advances in perinatal medicine over the past two to three decades have decreased mortality among low-birthweight (LBW) and very-low-birthweight infants. Indeed, very large numbers of children who until the 1950s–1960s would have expired soon after birth are now surviving. The neuropsychological characteristics of these children are of considerable interest to those who seek to understand the implications of this condition, and to those who are responsible for the care and nurturance of children so designated.

In Chapter 10, Picard, Del Dotto, and Breslau do an admirable job of describing the medical complications of LBW. A focus on the neuropathologies associated with this condition is, of course, necessary in the current context.

Their description of the results of their own studies of the developmental outcomes of children with LBW is brief and to the point. Their conclusions relating to the gradient of LBW sequelae, their comparisons between children with LBW and those with normal birthweight, and especially their generation of subtypes of children with LBW have broad implications for pediatric neuropsychology.

The arbitrariness of cutoffs established some time ago for children with varying degrees of LBW comes as no surprise. Indeed, in studies using cutoffs to designate sectors of a continuum (in this case, birthweight), the null hypothesis to be tested should be that there is no gradient in neuropsychological sequelae.

Although the neuropsychological measures used in their studies were somewhat limited, these investigators were able to generate subtypes of children with LBW. It would be of considerable interest to investigate the reliability of this typology and then to explore its external validity. Doing this within a developmental context, and especially following a cohort of such children over a considerable length of time, would add immeasurably to our understanding of the emergent subtypes and their relationship to neurological and neuropsychological dimensions. The probability of so doing would be considerably enhanced by including more measures of the principal neuropsychological variables. Also, it would seem very heuristic to include reliable and valid measures of personality and psychosocial functioning in these investigations, so that these important dimensions could be evaluated within the context of subtyping investigations (see Butler et al., 1997, and Rourke & Fuerst, 1991, for examples of such approaches).

One of the very few disorders that has occupied center stage in pediatric neuropsychological analysis for some time is Turner syndrome. The pioneering efforts of Money and colleagues, referred to by Berch and Bender in Chapter 11, alerted us to the potentially heuristic investigations of this genetic anomaly. And, to put it mildly, this investigative effort has been quite successful.

Berch and Bender present a very clear and concise summary of what is known about the disorder. They emphasize its complexity, and they point to the wide individual variation in its neuropsychological/adaptive presentations. They also highlight the problems with the use of small samples, limited dimensions of measurement, and other oversights that plagued much of the early research on this syndrome.

Their suggestions for future investigative efforts mirror those that are enunciated throughout this book: larger data sets, comprehensive neuropsychological batteries, and emphasis upon dimensions of psychosocial functioning. The interested reader may wish to refer to Rovet (1995) for a description of a research program that embodies these dimensions.

In Chapter 12, Welsh and Pennington examine a wide range of evidence bearing on the question of whether phenylketonuria (PKU), particularly early-treated PKU, results in a relatively specific neuropsychological phenotype. The authors assert that "PKU is a disorder in which the links among gene, enzyme, biochemistry/neurochemistry, brain functioning, and behavior are clearer than in most other neurodevelopmental disorders" (p. 276), and they provide a careful analysis of these relationships.

These authors also promote the "executive function" hypothesis as an explanation of the set of neuropsychological assets and deficits associated with PKU, treated or untreated. However, the notion that there are "prefrontal skills," and presumably some specific prefrontal dysfunction that may account for deficiencies in such skills, has yet to be demonstrated. For example, the Wisconsin Card Sorting Test is not associated specifically with prefrontal functioning in adults (Mountain & Snow, 1993).

The authors may wish to consider the white matter model of NLD (e.g., Rourke, 1989, 1995a) as an alternative model for this neuropsychological phenotype. Indeed, as the authors state, the "one consistent result across different research paradigms (autopsy, MRI, animal models) in the existence of defective myelination" (p. 281). Given the clear evidence of white matter perturbations in PKU (especially within subcortical and posterior regions of the brain), as well as the evidence of visual–spatial–organizational, psychomotor, psychosocial, and related deficits within the context of relatively intact linguistic skills, it may be valuable to consider this model in future research.

The series of interrelated studies presented by Waber and Mullenix in Chapter 13 constitutes an excellent model for investigative efforts in our field. The implications of acute lymphoblastic leukemia (ALL) are addressed within a context of experimental (animal and human), pharmacological, and neuroradiological dimensions. And a model developed to capture the long-term effects of treatment is presented.

Issues regarding the relevance of sex differences, research questions for enhancing practice, and formulation of batteries of neuropsychological tests may be of particular interest for more general applications in pediatric neuropsychology. As a highly relevant practical outcome, the role and impact of neuropsychological research in the mitigation of late effects without compromising efficacy is nicely described and explained.

The authors point out that the most important negative outcomes for the child who is treated and survives ALL are LD. For an extensive analysis of some dimensions of this issue, the interested reader may wish to consult Picard and Rourke (1995), which focuses on the relationship of the syndrome of NLD and the long-term sequelae of treatment for ALL.

The concluding sentences of this chapter bear repeating:

> The overriding goal of neuropsychological research is not to determine whether a particular agent is toxic, but to clarify the factors to be considered in specifying the costs and benefits of treatment. Decisions regarding treatment should be based on a set of complex considerations having to do with the age and sex of the child, as well as the effects of particular combinations (and even timing of combinations) of treatment agents. (p. 317)

Applications of these suggestions to other fields of research and practice in pediatric neuropsychology should be promulgated. For example, such considerations *mutatis mutandis* can be seen to apply to the pure and applied aspects of environmental neurotoxin research outlined in Chapter 9 by Dietrich.

The importance of the study of sickle cell disease (SCD) is quite adequately summarized in Chapter 14 by Ris and Grueneich:

> Research into SCD is challenging in multiple respects (biological, psychosocial, and methodological). It serves as an exemplar of how medical and behavioral research must proceed hand in hand—each informing the other—in order to capture the full range of morbidity and its complex interactions, and to gauge treatment effects. There are few genetic diseases producing such devastating effects with such a high incidence, and therefore with such a high payoff for significant advances in treatment. (p. 333)

I would add two points here: First, the study mounted by these investigators and described in this chapter is a model for achieving the explicit and implicit aims captured within the quotation above. Second, the search for subtypes of neuropsychological manifestations within SCD that these investigators have launched is laudable; continued efforts along these lines could be quite contributory to demonstrating linkages between SCD variables and phenotypic outcome, including the possibility of the interaction of multiple neuropsychological bases for the subtypes isolated.

As for the reference to the syndrome of NLD, the interested reader may again wish to consult more recent references that include modifications of the original model in light of subsequent tests of deductions from it (e.g., Rourke, 1988, 1989, 1995a).

Most of the available data regarding the possible relationships between diabetes and neuropsychological deficits have been gathered from adults. As Rovet describes in Chapter 15, she and her colleagues have attempted to rectify this by mounting several interrelated, longitudinal investigations of these relationships in children and adolescents. This research and other well-controlled studies have suggested very strongly that the impact of diabetes and related side effects (e.g., hypoglycemic episodes, seizures) have far different effects upon developing children than upon persons with adult-onset diabetes.

As is true of many other investigations covered in this volume, the systematic investigation of brain–behavior relationships in children with diabetes has led to quite different conclusions than would be anticipated on the basis of the results of studies of adults with the same disorder. Also, the author's contention that the study of this disease may elucidate many dimensions of the developing brain is well taken and, in a heuristic sense, invaluable.

In Chapter 16, Fennell provides an excellent example of attempts to determine interrelationships among a particular systemic illness, its various treatment modalities, and neuropsychological outcomes. The systematic analysis of pediatric end-stage renal disease provides a suitable context for a discussion of various forms of treatment, including kidney transplantation. The data gathered on patients who are otherwise quite similar, but have been subjected to various forms of therapy, are compelling. Additional studies in this area, carried out in the systematic manner advocated by Fennell and her group of investigators, should provide data that will allow for more informed decision making about various forms of intervention. It is quite probable that the information generated in such studies will be somewhat different from that available for adults similarly afficted (e.g., Ratner, Adams, Levin, & Rourke, 1983).

Also, the call for long-term developmental follow-up is well taken. The paucity of data regarding the psychosocial dimensions of this illness in its various forms is an area of concern that can be rectified by systematic studies of end-stage renal disease. Including children with other, comparable forms of chronic illness in such investigations may very well provide evidence concerning what is common among children with these illnesses, as well as what might be unique neuropsychological and psychosocial outcomes in the case of end-stage renal disease.

Pulsifer and Aylward present a succinct account in Chapter 17 of the changing nature of neuropsychological assets and deficits associated with pediatric human immunodeficiency virus (HIV). This presentation highlights the differences between early and later studies, the probable influence of medical treatments, and the very different—and more hopeful—picture that has emerged in the long-term follow-up of children whose initial prognosis appeared to be particularly bleak.

Suggestions for future research in this area are reasonable. They also echo themes from other chapters of this book: namely, the need for long-term follow-up, methodological rigor, and consideration of differences that may arise from different etiologies and (especially) differing patterns of family function and dysfunction.

The interested reader may also wish to consult findings relating to the presence or absence of white matter lesions in children with HIV (Brouwers, van der Vlugt, Moss, Wolters, & Pizzo, 1995). These are of particular interest to those of us who wish to test the white matter model of NLD (Rourke, 1995a).

GENERAL OBSERVATIONS

1. It is reassuring to note that virtually all of the contributors to this work see the merit of comprehensive neuropsychological assessment of children if the aim is to understand and deal with the developmental trajectories of the diseases and disorders considered. Although this approach has been advocated for some time (e.g., Rourke, 1976; Rourke, Bakker, Fisk, & Strang, 1983; Rourke, Fisk, & Strang, 1986), it does no harm to iterate it.

2. The elucidation of white matter neuropathologies in many of the chapters is also of some note, especially because such pathologies have been seen as causative in various developmental disorders (Fuerst & Rourke, 1995). That authors address issues relating to somatosensory perception in conjunction with this focus is consistent with the findings of other investigations in this area (e.g., Casey & Rourke, 1992).

3. It is abundantly apparent that the consideration of subtypes of neuropsychological functioning in children who have various forms of neuromedical impairment is no less important than are such considerations for adults with well-studied neurological diseases such as Alzheimer's disease (e.g., Fisher et al., 1996; Fisher, Rourke, et al., 1997). Failure to appreciate the necessity to search for homogeneous subtypes within such disorders is tantamount to scientific malpractice, with consequent negative impact on clinical practice. Failure to appreciate that it is possible to identify subtypes constitutes a failure to appreciate the existing literature (e.g., Rourke, 1985; Harnadek & Rourke, 1994).

4. The advocacy of sophisticated, systematic biostatistical methodology, and the explication of the scientific benefits to be reaped thereby, are welcome within a variety of contexts. Some of us have been advocating such methodology for a very long time (e.g., Rourke, 1975) and have made some effort to summarize it (e.g., Rourke, Costa, Cicchetti, Adams, & Plasterk, 1992).

5. Viewing childhood disorders within a developmental context is a common theme that is advocated by virtually all of the contributors to this book. Such considerations are as important in the elucidation of specific syndromes (e.g., Casey, Rourke, & Picard, 1991) as they are for broader issues within our field (e.g., Rourke & Fuerst, 1995).

6. The sophisticated use of neuroimaging techniques is a particularly welcome dimension of research on many of the disorders addressed in this work. There is no doubt that the systematic use of these technologies, especially in conjunction with the monitoring of concurrent "mental" activity, will yield an abundance of important heuristic data.

7. The relative paucity of sophisticated utilization of event-related potentials (e.g., Dool, Stelmack, & Rourke, 1993; Stelmack, Rourke, & van der Vlugt, 1995) for the understanding of developmental disabilities should be of concern to the editors when it is time for a second edition of this volume.

8. The interactions between attention-deficit/hyperactivity disorder and LD (e.g., Casey, Rourke, & Del Dotto, 1996) are very frequent referral concerns for the pediatric neuropsychologist and should be covered in a text that deals with our field. Furthermore, much less frequently occurring disorders (and hence concerns), such as neuropsychological differences between persons with high-functioning autism and Asperger syndrome (e.g., Klin, Sparrow, Volkmar, Cicchetti, & Rourke, 1995; Klin, Volkmar, Sparrow, Cicchetti, & Rourke, 1995), are important areas of pediatric neuropsychological research that merit attention because of their theoretical and clinical relevance. In the editors' defense, it should be pointed out that they made a conscious decision not to include considerations of these issues in this work. Perhaps they may change their minds in the second edition!

9. Treatment considerations are replete within the work, as they should be. For the most part, however, these are referred to in rather general terms. The interested reader may wish to consult presentations that deal with specific programs for subtypes of children who exhibit deficits thought to obtain in many of these disorders (Rourke, 1995d; Rourke & Tsatsanis, 1996).

Finally, it is apparent that this volume contains an abundance of valuable information and insights regarding the types of diseases, disorders, and dysfunctions that occupy center stage for the practicing pediatric neuropsychologist. Almost without exception, any shortcomings, including those mentioned in this chapter, are more a function of economy of presentation and space than of any inherent limitations in the work of the very accomplished investigators who have contributed their work to this landmark volume.

REFERENCES

Anderson, P., & Rourke, B. P. (1995). Williams syndrome. In B. P. Rourke (Ed.), *Syndrome of nonverbal learning disabilities: Neurodevelopmental manifestations* (pp. 138–170). New York: Guilford Press.

Bawden, H., Dooley, J., Buckley, D., Camfield, P., Gordon, K., Riding, M., & Llewellyn, G. (1996). MRI and nonverbal cognitive deficits in children with neurofibromatosis 1. *Journal of Clinical and Experimental Neuropsychology, 18*, 784–792.

Brouwers, P., van der Vlugt, H, Moss, H., Wolters, P., & Pizzo, P. (1995). White matter changes on CT brain scan are associated with neurobehavioral dysfunction in children with symptomatic HIV disease. *Child Neuropsychology, 1*, 93–105.

Buono, L. A., Morris, M. K., Morris, R. D., Krawiecki, N., Norris, F. H., Foster, M. A., & Copeland, D. R. (1998). Evidence for the syndrome of Nonverbal Learning Disabilities in children with brain tumors. *Child Neuropsychology, 4*, 144–157.

Butler, K., Rourke, B. P., Fuerst, D. R., & Fisk, J. L. (1997). A typology of psychosocial functioning in pediatric closed-head injury. *Child Neuropsychology, 3*, 98–133.

Casey, J. E., & Rourke, B. P. (1992). Disorders of somatosensory perception in children. In I. Rapin & S. J. Segalowitz (Eds.), *Handbook of neuropsychology: Vol. 6. Child neuropsychology* (pp. 477–494). Amsterdam: Elsevier.

Casey, J. E., Rourke, B. P., & Del Dotto, J. E. (1996). Learning disabilities in children with attention deficit disorder with and without hyperactivity. *Child Neuropsychology, 2*, 83–98.

Casey, J. E., Rourke, B. P., & Picard, E. M. (1991). Syndrome of nonverbal learning disabilities: Age differences in neuropsychological, academic, and socioemotional functioning. *Development and Psychopathology, 3*, 331–347.

Crowe, S. F., & Hay, D. A. (1990). Neuropsychological dimensions of the fragile X syndrome: Support for a non-dominant hemisphere dysfunction hypothesis. *Neuropsychologia, 28*, 9–16.

Dool, C. B., Fuerst, K. B., & Rourke, B. P. (1995). Metachromatic leukodystrophy. In B. P. Rourke (Ed.), *Syndrome of nonverbal learning disabilities: Neurodevelopmental manifestations* (pp. 331–350). New York: Guilford Press.

Dool, C. B., Stelmack, R. M., & Rourke, B. P. (1993). Event-related potentials in children with learning disabilities. *Journal of Clinical Child Psychology, 22*, 387–398.

Fisher, N. J., Rourke, B. P., Bieliauskas, L., Giordani, B., Berent, S., & Foster, N. L. (1996). Neuropsychological subgroups of patients with Alzheimer's disease. *Journal of Clinical and Experimental Neuropsychology, 18*, 349–370.

Fisher, N. J., Rourke, B. P., Bieliauskas, L. A., Giordani, B., Berent, S., & Foster, N. L. (1997). Unmasking the heterogeneity of Alzheimer's disease: Case studies of individuals from distinct neuropsychological subgroups. *Journal of Clinical and Experimental Neuropsychology, 19*, 713–754.

Fuerst, D. R., & Rourke, B. P. (1993). Psychosocial functioning of children: Relations between personality subtypes and academic achievement. *Journal of Abnormal Child Psychology, 21*, 597–607.

Fuerst, D. R., & Rourke, B. P. (1995). Psychosocial functioning of children with learning disabilities at three age levels. *Child Neuropsychology, 1*, 38–55.

Fuerst, K. B., Dool, C. B., & Rourke, B. P. (1995). Velocardiofacial syndrome. In B. P. Rourke (Ed.), *Syndrome of nonverbal learning disabilities: Neurodevelopmental manifestations* (pp. 119–137). New York: Guilford Press.

Fuerst, K. B., & Rourke, B. P. (1995). White matter physiology and pathology. In B. P. Rourke (Ed.), *Syndrome of nonverbal learning disabilities: Neurodevelopmental manifestations* (pp. 27–44). New York: Guilford Press.

Harnadek, M. C. S., & Rourke, B. P. (1994). Principal identifying features of the syndrome of nonverbal learning disabilities in children. *Journal of Learning Disabilities, 27*, 144–154.

Klin, A., Sparrow, S. S., Volkmar, F., Cicchetti, D. V., & Rourke, B. P. (1995). Asperger syndrome. In B. P. Rourke (Ed.), *Syndrome of nonverbal learning disabilities: Neurodevelopmental manifestations* (pp. 93–118). New York: Guilford Press.

Klin, A., Volkmar, F. R., Sparrow, S. S., Cicchetti, D. V., & Rourke, B. P. (1995). Validity and neuropsychological characterization of Asperger syndrome: Convergence with nonverbal learning disabilities syndrome. *Journal of Child Psychology and Psychiatry, 36*, 1127–1140.

Mountain, M., & Snow, W. G. (1993). Wisconsin Card Sorting Test as a measure of frontal pathology: A review. *Clinical Neuropsychologist, 7*, 108–118.

Picard, E. M., & Rourke, B. P. (1995). Neuropsychological consequences of prophylactic treatment for acute lymphocytic leukemia. In B. P. Rourke (Ed.), *Syndrome of nonverbal learning disabilities: Neurodevelopmental manifestations* (pp. 282–330). New York: Guilford Press.

Ratner, D., Adams, K. M., Levin, N. W., & Rourke, B. P. (1983). Effects of hemodialysis of the cognitive and sensory–motor functioning on the adult chronic hemodialysis patient. *Journal of Behavioral Medicine, 6,* 291–331.

Rourke, B. P. (1975). Brain–behavior relationships in children with learning disabilities: A research program. *American Psychologist, 30,* 911–920.

Rourke, B. P. (1976). Issues in the neuropsychological assessment of children with learning disabilities. *Canadian Psychological Review, 17,* 89–102.

Rourke, B. P. (1982). Central processing deficiencies in children: Toward a developmental neuropsychological model. *Journal of Clinical Neuropsychology, 4,* 1–18.

Rourke, B. P. (Ed.). (1985). *Neuropsychology of learning disabilities: Essentials of subtype analysis.* New York: Guilford Press.

Rourke, B. P. (1988). The syndrome of nonverbal learning disabilities: Developmental manifestations in neurological disease, disorder, and dysfunction. *Clinical Neuropsychologist, 2,* 293–330.

Rourke, B. P. (1989). *Nonverbal learning disabilities: The syndrome and the model.* New York: Guilford Press.

Rourke, B. P. (Ed.). (1991). *Neuropsychological validation of learning disability subtypes.* New York: Guilford Press.

Rourke, B. P. (1993). Arithmetic disabilities, specific and otherwise: A neuropsychological perspective. *Journal of Learning Disabilities, 26,* 214–226.

Rourke, B. P. (1995a). Introduction and overview: The NLD/white matter model. In B. P. Rourke (Ed.), *Syndrome of nonverbal learning disabilities: Neurodevelopmental manifestations* (pp. 1–26). New York: Guilford Press.

Rourke, B. P. (Ed.). (1995b). *Syndrome of nonverbal learning disabilities: Neurodevelopmental manifestations.* New York: Guilford Press.

Rourke, B. P. (1995c). The science of practice and the practice of science: The scientist–practitioner model in clinical neuropsychology. *Canadian Psychology, 36,* 259–287.

Rourke, B. P. (1995d). Treatment program for children with NLD. In B. P. Rourke (Ed.), *Syndrome of nonverbal learning disabilities: Neurodevelopmental manifestations* (pp. 497–508). New York: Guilford Press.

Rourke, B. P., Bakker, D. J., Fisk, J. L., & Strang, J. D. (1983). *Child neuropsychology: An introduction to theory, research, and clinical practice.* New York: Guilford Press.

Rourke, B. P., & Conway, J. A. (1997). Disabilities of arithmetic and mathematical reasoning: Perspectives from neurology and neuropsychology. *Journal of Learning Disabilities, 30,* 34–46.

Rourke, B. P., Costa, L., Cicchetti, D. V., Adams, K. M., & Plasterk, K. J. (Eds.). (1992). *Methodological and biostatistical foundations of clinical neuropsychology.* Lisse, The Netherlands: Swets & Zeitlinger.

Rourke, B. P., Fisk, J. L., & Strang, J. D. (1986). *Neuropsychological assessment of children: A treatment-oriented approach.* New York: Guilford Press.

Rourke, B. P., & Fuerst, D. R. (1991). *Learning disabilities and psychosocial functioning: A neuropsychological perspective.* New York: Guilford Press.

Rourke, B. P., & Fuerst, D. R. (1995). Cognitive processing, academic achievement, and psychosocial functioning: A neuropsychological perspective. In D. Cicchetti & D. Cohen (Eds.), *Developmental psychopathology* (Vol. 1, pp. 391–423). New York: Wiley.

Rourke, B. P., & Strang, J. D. (1983). Subtypes of reading and arithmetical disabilities: A neuropsychological analysis. In M. Rutter (Ed.), *Developmental neuropsychiatry* (pp. 473–488). New York: Guilford Press.

Rourke, B. P., & Tsatsanis, K. D. (1996). Syndrome of nonverbal learning disabilities: Psycholinguistic assets and deficits. *Topics in Language Disorders, 16,* 30–44.

Rovet, J. (1995). Turner syndrome. In B. P. Rourke (Ed.), *Syndrome of nonverbal learning disabilities: Neurodevelopmental manifestations.* New York: Guilford Press.

Ryan, T. V., Crews, Jr., W. D., Cowan, L., Goering, A. M., & Barth, J. T. (1998). A case of triple X syndrome manifesting with the syndrome of nonverbal learning disabilities. *Child Neuropsychology, 4,* 225–232.

Smith, L. A., & Rourke, B. P. (1995). Callosal agenesis. In B. P. Rourke (Ed.), *Syndrome of nonverbal learning disabilities: Neurodevelopmental manifestations* (pp. 45–92). New York: Guilford Press.

Stelmack, R. M., Rourke, B. P., & van der Vlugt, H. (1995). Intelligence, learning disabilities, and event-related potentials. *Developmental Neuropsychology, 11,* 445–465.

Tsatsanis, K. D., Fuerst, D. R., & Rourke, B. P. (1997). Psychosocial dimensions of learning disabilities: External validation and relationship with age and academic functioning. *Journal of Learning Disabilities, 30,* 490–502.

INDEX